Illustrated Manual of

Laboratory Diagnosis

Indications and Interpretations

Illustrated Manual of

Laboratory Diagnosis

Indications and Interpretations

SECOND EDITION

R. Douglas Collins, M.D.

Associate Professor of Medicine, Medical University of South Carolina, and Director of Education for the Department of Internal Medicine, Spartanburg General Hospital, Spartanburg, South Carolina; Diplomate of the American Board of Internal Medicine

Color Illustrations by Joseph Alemany, B.A.

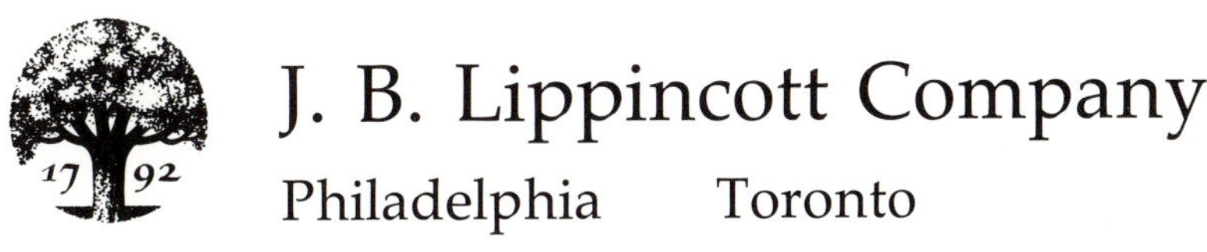

J. B. Lippincott Company

Philadelphia Toronto

Second Edition

ISBN 0-397-50340-7

Library of Congress Catalog Card Number 74-23530

Printed in the United States of America

1 3 5 6 4 2

Library of Congress Cataloging in Publication Data

Collins, R Douglas.
Illustrated manual of laboratory diagnosis.

Includes bibliographical references.
1. Medicine, clinical—Laboratory manuals. I. Title.
[DNLM: 1. Diagnosis, Laboratory. QY4 C712i]
RB36.C65 1975 616.07'5 74-23530
ISBN 0-397-50340-7

Dedicated to
THE GREATEST TEACHER OF THEM ALL

Preface

The purpose of this edition, as of the first, is to aid medical students and practicing physicians in the clinical evaluation and interpretation of laboratory data. The modern laboratory is now able to perform scores of tests that give a solid scientific foundation to clinical judgment, and able to facilitate a diagnosis that would not have been suspected upon initial examination. For effective use, however, the physician must understand the rationale behind each test, and know how to use the information received appropriately and efficiently.

The textbook approach to the problems raised by this necessity remain too detailed and time-consuming for the practicing physician, and textbook emphasis too often has been placed upon techniques rather than interpretation and clinical application. Furthermore, the orientation is likely to be toward the pathologist or technician rather than the physician, and there is often insufficient correlation with other diagnostic modalities.

To reach this goal in the second edition we have retained the following principles:

1. Only laboratory tests with widespread clinical application have been discussed.
2. Discussions are oriented toward the clinician. For the most part, laboratory technique has been omitted, since most laboratory tests are now performed by trained technicians under the direction of a qualified pathologist.
3. The material is presented in an organized fashion: first the normal physiology underlying a laboratory test, and then the alterations of the normal physiology as they occur in each disease. When possible, the cause of each alteration is also discussed.
4. The alterations of the normal physiology in each disease are illustrated by full-color diagrams to simplify the learning and recall process.
5. In discussing each condition, those tests most helpful in diagnosis are repeatedly emphasized.
6. Diseases are indexed with those laboratory tests most useful in their diagnosis.
7. Symptoms are also indexed with those laboratory tests most useful in determining their cause.
8. Discussions are succinct and to the point. The material is generally acceptable information, and so references have been held to a minimum.

The continuing progress in clinical diagnosis since 1968 has required the inclusion of new chapters—on the interpretation of autoanalyzer results, on the office laboratory, and on sequential tests appropriate to follow the course of a disease during treatment. There is a new chapter on multiphasic screening of asymptomatic patients; the chapter on hormones has been completely revised, as have discussions of enzyme disorders, radioisotopes, toxic substances and the hyperlipoproteinemias. All chapters have been rigorously reviewed for accuracy.

It is not possible to name all those associated with this new edition, but the assistance of Joyce Betenbaugh with the chapter on the autoanalyzer and the expert typing of Annette Little cannot go unnoticed, nor can the able assistance of Stuart Freeman, Editor, Medical Books, and the rest of the staff of the J. B. Lippincott Company.

R. Douglas Collins, M.D.

Introduction

Use of the laboratory in clinical medicine has undoubtedly increased the proportion of accurate diagnoses. Moreover, it has refined clinical diagnosis by providing confirmation of clinical impressions, and diagnosis is made earlier, at a time when therapy is more likely to result in a cure. Along with these assets reliance on laboratory tests presents certain hazards. For example, the patient may become physically and even psychologically ill from some of these procedures. An erroneous result may set the physician off on a wild goose chase or commit him to radical or expensive therapy. For the busy physician, laboratory tests may become a substitute for a good physical examination. Thus the clinician must know what tests to order in each case and how to interpret them.

WHAT TESTS TO ORDER

Routine Tests. The laboratory has not eliminated the need for a good history and physical examination. On the other hand, certain laboratory tests are as essential in the initial work-up of a patient as a rectal or a vaginal examination. These tests are listed on page 307. They need not be indicated by the clinical impression and present a minimum hazard to the patient. Clinicians who object to routine tests are reminded of the many patients with anemia and leukemia who have been saved from surgery by the routine CBC, and the many diabetics who would have been overlooked without routine blood sugars.

Indicated Tests. Following the history and physical, the clinician may find himself in one of four situations:

1. He may be still bewildered by the patient's complaints and have no concrete evidence to support a diagnosis. In this case he may elect to put the patient on a tranquilizer or a placebo and see him again for follow-up. However, when the patient presents with a serious complaint such as weight loss or fever, it may be unwise to follow such a course. These patients are usually admitted to the hospital for a work-up. Of what should such a work-up consist? The tests most useful to the author in working up these symptoms are listed in Appendix II.

2. The clinician may not have a clear-cut clinical diagnosis but may have a good idea of what organ or organs are involved. In this case he may confirm his impression by ordering function tests of the organ or organs in question. These are found in Appendix IV.

3. Most frequently the clinician has established a strong clinical impression from the history and physical and needs the laboratory tests merely for confirmation. Those tests most useful in diagnosing a specific disease are listed in Appendix III.

4. Finally, the clinician may be so certain of his diagnosis that he can institute therapy without laboratory confirmation. This is often the case in common respiratory diseases and gastroenteritis.

These tests are not to be transferred verbatim to the order sheet. Rather, the clinician should use his judgment in selecting, "*à la carte,*" the most appropriate tests in each case. In the hospital, laboratory tests may be ordered in either of two ways. One method is to order a whole battery of tests on the first hospital day. This may save the patient time and money by cutting down on the number of hospital days. Therapy may be initiated earlier. However, the patient may become ill from the numerous procedures, and the cost of such a battery of tests may be prohibitive unless an autoanalyzer is available. The other method is to order one or two tests at a time and await their results. This may cut the laboratory expense, but frequently it increases the length and cost of the hospital stay. The author has found judicious application of the first method less costly, less time-consuming, and rarely a hazard to the patient. Furthermore, by this method diagnoses have been uncovered that might otherwise have been missed.

There are other important subtleties in effective ordering of laboratory tests. In general, it is wise to begin the work-up with the simple and innocuous procedures and to reserve hazardous procedures for later. This does not always apply. When clinical suspicion is high, it is often senseless to waste time and money on simple but less accurate procedures when more definitive tests will be required in any case. For example, an EEG is often superfluous in a case of papilledema with focal neurological signs when a radiocontrast study or brain scan is indicated anyway. Or, as another example, it is redundant to order a sedimentation rate and C-reactive protein in cases of acute myocardial infarction already proven by an electrocardiogram or enzyme studies.

One must be as practical as possible in the laboratory work-up. Laboratory tests that exclude the treatable diseases in the differential diagnosis should be requested if there is the slightest possibility of their existence. For example, although there is no specific therapy for most causes of chronic transverse myelitis, a gastric analysis should be performed to exclude pernicious anemia, and a Wassermann to exclude syphilis.

When the clinical picture is almost pathognomonic, one or two tests may suffice. When it is vague, more tests may be required. The clinician in ordering should carefully distinguish the less accurate or screening tests and the more specific tests. Frequently, he must use a battery of tests to substantiate a diagnosis owing to the inaccuracy of the available tests. An outstanding example of this is hyperthyroidism, in which the T_4, RAI, and T_3 uptake are not reliable enough when used alone, and therefore all tests must be ordered at once.

HOW TO INTERPRET LABORATORY TESTS

No laboratory result can be taken at face value. There are many possibilities of error both in the performance of the test and in its interpretation.

1. **Improper collection and handling of the specimen** is a common source of laboratory error. How often are urine specimens for culture collected under unsterile techniques? How often are throat cultures a swab of saliva? Blood collected from the finger may be diluted with tissue fluid, distorting hematologic values. Specimens for culture frequently sit overnight before being plated. Stools for ovum and parasites may sit around the laboratory for hours before being examined. There are many other examples of this type of error. The only way to be certain of this part of the technique is to collect the specimen personally, a procedure frequently practiced by the author.

2. **An unreliable laboratory** is worse than no laboratory at all. Of course, a laboratory is only as good as its technicians. The physician should check the qualifications and experience of both the director and the technicians of any laboratory before using it. If these are top-notch, there are still other factors that must be considered before a laboratory can be considered to be reliable.

A good laboratory uses standard reference solutions. A good laboratory keeps a continuous record of all tests done over a 3- or 4-month period. In this way a series of abnormal results may be readily detected and signal the need for checking the standard or the other parts of the laboratory procedure. A good laboratory periodically checks the accuracy of its results with a larger reference laboratory. This is the reason that most good laboratories participate in the evaluation program sponsored by the American College of Pathologists.

The clinician should periodically check the laboratory by duplicating specimens on the same patient and on patients with diseases that would be expected to give abnormal results. It is not unusual to get abnormal urine reports such as pus cells on tap water.

One of the best ways the clinician can check the laboratory is to perform the test personally. Of course, the clinician is not expected to run PBI's or blood sugars himself, but a look at a blood smear or urinary sediment should never be below a physician's dignity and can often clarify suspicions of the laboratory.

3. **Inadequate Knowledge of Normal Values.** Table I lists the normal values for the procedures that are standard in most laboratories. However, normal values vary from laboratory to laboratory, the variability depending on the test method applied. This is the reason that most laboratories report their normal values along with each test result. When they do not, the clinician should ask for a copy.

4. **Unreliable Laboratory Procedures.** The clinician must know the reliability of the test procedure applied. Platelet counts and erythrocyte counts are unreliable even in the best hands. The determination of the PBI, to get a correct result, requires meticulous handling of the glassware. Bioassay methods such as those applied in determining certain hormone concentrations are notoriously inaccurate. Methods of determining the urinary aldosterone, blood ammonia, or serum iron are also often inaccurate even in the best laboratories. Rather than base a diagnosis on one of these tests, the clinician initially should utilize less diagnostic but more accurate laboratory tests.

5. **Insufficient Understanding of the Physiology Behind the Chemical or Cellular Element Tested.** The clinician must know what

other metabolic alterations will cause an abnormal test result in addition to the one suspected. For example, a high BSP is not pathognomonic of liver disease. Congestive heart failure and shock will give the same result because of inadequate circulation of the substance through the liver. The hemoglobin may be normal in the presence of anemia if there is associated dehydration. Countless other examples could be cited. It is hoped that the chapters in this book will give the reader a better understanding of this aspect of interpretation.

6. **False Negative Results.** Laboratory tests do not "rule out" disease. A test giving a negative result in the face of strong clinical suspicion to the contrary should be repeated several times, and even then the clinical diagnosis often should prevail. It may be worth having an outside laboratory repeat the test.

7. **False Positive Results.** A positive test result does not establish a diagnosis beyond a shadow of doubt. False positive results are common. The high PBI in a person who has ingested iodide cough medicine, the high triglyceride levels obtained after a meal, the high red cell counts in dehydrated patients are all good examples of this pitfall. Others are cited throughout the pages of this book.

In summary, listening to the patient, examining him with all the equipment that may be carried in the doctor's bag, and utilizing the best laboratory procedures available are all indispensable in clinical diagnosis. The importance of each must be determined separately in each case. The clinician must never underestimate the value of the laboratory in clinical diagnosis, but a healthy degree of skepticism is essential in interpreting laboratory results.

Contents

1 Disorders of Serum Acid and Alkaline Phosphatases 3

Normal Metabolism 3
Value of the Tests 3
Interpreting the Color Plates 3
Disorders of Production 5
Metastatic Bone Tumors 5
Metastatic Prostatic Carcinoma 6
Osteitis Deformans (Paget's Disease) 7
Osteogenic Sarcoma 8
Rickets and Osteomalacia 9
Disorders of Excretion 10
Carcinoma of the Head of the Pancreas 10
Chlorpromazine Hepatitis 11
Miscellaneous 12
Metastatic Carcinoma of the Liver 12

2 Disorders of Serum Bilirubin 13

Normal Metabolism 13
Disorder of Production 15
Hereditary Spherocytosis 15
Disorders of Metabolism 16
Viral Hepatitis 16
Laennec's Cirrhosis 17
Disorders of Excretion 18
Carcinoma of the Head of the Pancreas 18
Chlorpromazine Hepatitis 19
Choledocholithiasis 20

3 Disorders of Serum Calcium 21

Normal Metabolism 21
The Approach to the Diagnosis 22
Disorder of Intake 23
Malnutrition 23
Disorders of Absorption 24
Boeck's Sarcoid 24
Hypovitaminosis D 25
Malabsorption Syndrome 26
Disorder of Transport 27
Nephrotic Syndrome 27
Disorders of Storage 28
Cushing's Syndrome 28
Metastatic Carcinoma of the Bone 29
Disorders of Excretion 30
Chronic Nephritis 30
Renal Tubular Acidosis 31
Disorders of Regulation 32
Hyperparathyroidism 32
Hypoparathyroidism 33
Miscellaneous 34
Pseudopseudohypoparathyroidism 34

4 Disorders of Blood Electrolytes 35

Normal Metabolism 35
The Diagnostic Approach 37
Disorders of Intake 39
Dehydration 39
Starvation 40
Disorder of Absorption 41
Malabsorption Syndrome 41
Disorder of Transport 42
Congestive Heart Failure 42
Disorders of Secretion 43
Pyloric Obstruction 43
Diarrhea 44

4 Disorders of Blood Electrolytes—*Continued*

Pathological Diaphoresis ... 45
Disorders of Excretion ... 46
Acute Renal Failure ... 46
Pulmonary Emphysema ... 47
Salicylate Toxicity ... 48
Disorders of Regulation ... 49
Adrenal Cortical Insufficiency ... 49
Diabetes Insipidus ... 50
Primary Aldosteronism ... 51
Mercurial Diuretics ... 52
Chlorothiazide Diuretics ... 53
Renal Tubular Acidosis ... 54
Chronic Renal Failure ... 55
Miscellaneous ... 56
Diabetic Acidosis ... 56

5 Disorders of Blood Glucose ... 58

Normal Metabolism ... 58
The Approach to the Diagnosis ... 59
Disorder of Intake ... 60
Malnutrition ... 60
Disorders of Absorption ... 61
Idiopathic Steatorrhea ... 61
Tachyalimentation Hypoglycemia ... 62
Disorder of Production ... 63
Galactosemia ... 63
Disorders of Storage ... 64
Advanced Cirrhosis of the Liver ... 64
Glycogen-Storage Disease (von Gierke's Disease) ... 65
Disorder of Excretion ... 66
Renal Glycosuria ... 66
Disorders of Regulation ... 67
Addison's Disease ... 67
Cushing's Syndrome ... 68
Anterior Pituitary Insufficiency ... 69
Acromegaly ... 70
Hyperthyroidism ... 71
Pheochromocytoma ... 72
Chronic Pancreatitis ... 73
Islet Cell Adenoma ... 74
Miscellaneous ... 75
Diabetes Mellitus ... 75
Other Causes of Hyperglycemia ... 75

6 Disorders of the Hormones ... 76

Functions of Certain Hormones ... 76
Normal Metabolism ... 76
The Approach to the Diagnosis ... 79
Disorders of Pituitary Hormones ... 83
Acromegaly ... 83
Basophilic Adenoma of the Pituitary ... 84
Panhypopituitarism ... 85
Pituitary Hypogonadism ... 86
Disorders of Thyroid Hormone ... 87
Hyperthyroidism ... 87
Subacute Thyroiditis ... 88
Myxedema ... 89
Disorders of Adrenal Hormones ... 90
Addison's Disease ... 90
Primary Aldosteronism ... 91
Cushing's Syndrome ... 92
Adrenogenital Syndrome ... 93
Disorders of Ovarian Hormones ... 94
Turner's Syndrome ... 94
Polycystic Ovaries (Stein-Leventhal Syndrome) ... 95
Menopausal Syndrome ... 96
Miscellaneous ... 97
Pregnancy ... 97
Chorionepithelioma ... 98
Seminoma ... 99
Klinefelter's Syndrome ... 100

7 Disorders of Serum Lipids ... 101

Nature of Body Lipids ... 101
Normal Metabolism ... 101
The Approach to the Diagnosis ... 103
Disorder of Intake ... 105
Early Starvation ... 105
Disorder of Absorption ... 106
Idiopathic Steatorrhea ... 106

7 **Disorders of Serum Lipids**—*Continued*
- Disorders of Transport ... 107
  - Malnutrition ... 107
  - Nephrotic Syndrome ... 108
- Disorder of Production ... 109
  - Portal Cirrhosis ... 109
- Disorder of Storage ... 110
  - Xanthoma Disseminatum ... 110
- Disorder of Utilization ... 111
  - Diabetes Mellitus ... 111
- Disorder of Excretion ... 112
  - Obstructive Jaundice ... 112
- Disorder of Regulation ... 113
  - Hypothyroidism ... 113
- Miscellaneous ... 114
  - Acanthocytosis ... 114
  - Type I Hyperlipoproteinemia ... 115
  - Type II Hyperlipoproteinemia ... 116
  - Type III Hyperlipoproteinemia ... 117
  - Type IV Hyperlipoproteinemia ... 117
  - Type V Hyperlipoproteinemia ... 118

8 **Disorders of Blood Nonprotein Nitrogen Substances** ... 119
- Normal Metabolism ... 119
- Disorder of Intake ... 121
  - Starvation ... 121
- Disorders of Production ... 122
  - Bleeding Gastric Ulcer ... 122
  - Cirrhosis of the Liver ... 123
- Disorders of Transport ... 124
  - Congestive Heart Failure ... 124
  - Hypovolemic Shock ... 125
- Disorder of Storage ... 126
  - Muscular Dystrophies ... 126
- Disorders of Excretion ... 127
  - Obstructive Uropathy ... 127
  - Chronic Glomerulonephritis ... 128
- Disorder of Regulation ... 129
  - Hyperthyroidism ... 129

9 **Disorders of Blood Oxygen Content** ... 130
- Normal Metabolism ... 130
- The Approach to the Diagnosis ... 131
- Disorders of Intake and Excretion ... 135
  - Asthmatic Bronchitis ... 135
  - Pulmonary Emphysema ... 136
  - Ankylosing Spondylitis ... 137
- Disorders of Absorption ... 138
  - Sarcoidosis ... 138
  - Pulmonary Hemangioma ... 139
  - Pulmonary Embolism ... 140
- Disorder of Transport ... 141
  - Congestive Heart Failure ... 141
- Disorder of Regulation ... 142
  - Barbiturate Intoxication ... 142

10 **Disorders of Plasma Proteins** ... 143
- Normal Metabolism ... 143
- Methods of Study ... 144
- Disorder of Intake ... 145
  - Starvation ... 145
- Disorder of Absorption ... 146
  - Idiopathic Steatorrhea ... 146
- Disorders of Production ... 147
  - Portal Cirrhosis ... 147
  - Acute and Chronic Bacterial Infections ... 148
  - Familial Idiopathic Dysproteinemia ... 149
  - Hypogammaglobulinemia ... 150
  - Alpha-1 Antitrypsin Deficiency ... 151
  - Viral Hepatitis ... 152
  - Multiple Myeloma ... 153
- Disorder of Excretion ... 154
  - Nephrotic Syndrome ... 154

11 **Disorders of Serum Creatine Phosphokinase, Transaminases, and Lactic Dehydrogenases** ... 155
- Normal Metabolism ... 155
- Disorders of Production ... 157

11 Disorders of Serum Creatine Phosphokinase, Transaminases, and Lactic Dehydrogenases—*Continued*
Myocardial Infarction ... 157
Cardiac Failure ... 158
Viral Hepatitis ... 159
Dermatomyositis ... 160
Disorder of Excretion ... 161
Extrahepatic Biliary Obstructions ... 161
Miscellaneous ... 162
Pulmonary Infarction ... 162

12 Disorders of Serum Uric Acid ... 163

Normal Metabolism ... 163
Disorders of Production ... 165
Gout ... 165
Leukemia ... 166
Disorders of Excretion ... 167
Chronic Glomerulonephritis ... 167
Toxemia of Pregnancy ... 168
Fanconi Syndrome ... 169

13 Miscellaneous Blood Chemistries ... 171

Disorders of Serum Amylase and Lipase ... 171
Disorders of Urinary Catecholamines ... 172
Disorders of Copper Metabolism ... 173
Disorders of Urine 5-Hydroxyindoleacetic Acid ... 173
Disorders of Serum Iron ... 174
Disorders of Serum Magnesium ... 175
Disorders of Melanin Metabolism ... 175
Disorders of Porphyrin Metabolism ... 176
The Detection of Toxic Substances in the Blood and Urine 178

14 Renal Function Tests ... 180

Urine Formation ... 180
Laboratory Tests ... 180
Primary Purpose ... 182

15 Radioactive Isotopes in Diagnosis ... 183
Gastrointestinal Tract ... 183
Hemopoietic System ... 183
Endocrine System ... 186
Nervous System ... 188
Liver ... 188
Respiratory System ... 189
Pancreas ... 189
Bone ... 189

16 Comparative Analysis of Body Fluids ... 190

Obtaining the Specimen ... 190
Volume ... 191
pH ... 192
Specific Gravity ... 192
Examination for Clotting ... 193
Appearance ... 193
Blood ... 194
Casts ... 196
Crystals ... 196
Biochemical Alterations ... 197
Cytology ... 199

17 The Autoanalyzer ... 200

Apparatus and Test Method ... 200

18 Disorders of the Erythrocytes ... 210

Normal Metabolism ... 210
The Approach to the Diagnosis ... 212
Disorders of Red Cell Production ... 213
Hypochromic Anemia of Infancy ... 213
Idiopathic Steatorrhea ... 214
Pernicious Anemia ... 215
Myelophthisic Anemia ... 216
Idiopathic Aplastic Anemia ... 217
Polycythemia Vera ... 218
Disorders of Transport ... 219
Bleeding Peptic Ulcer, Acute Stage ... 219
Bleeding Peptic Ulcer, Subacute Stage ... 220
Chronic Menorrhagia ... 221
Disorders of Red Cell Destruction ... 222

18 **Disorders of the Erythrocytes**—*Continued*
Hereditary Spherocytosis ... 222
Sickle Cell Anemia ... 223
Thalassemia Major ... 224
Acquired Hemolytic Anemia ... 225
Hemolytic Transfusion Reactions ... 226
Erythroblastosis Fetalis ... 230
Miscellaneous ... 231
Acute Myeloblastic Leukemia ... 231
Cirrhosis of the Liver ... 232
Chronic Congestive Splenomegaly (Banti's Syndrome) ... 233
Hypothyroidism ... 234
Simple Chronic Anemia ... 235

19 **Disorders of the Leukocytes** ... 236
Normal Metabolism ... 236
The Primary Approach to the Diagnosis ... 238
The White Count of Infants and Children ... 239
Disorders of Production ... 240
Acute Leukemia ... 240
Chronic Myelogenous Leukemia ... 241
Chronic Lymphocytic Leukemia ... 242
Multiple Myeloma ... 243
Gaucher's Disease ... 244
Hodgkin's Disease ... 245
Waldenström's Macroglobulinemia ... 246
Disorders of Regulation ... 247
Addison's Disease ... 247
Cushing's Syndrome ... 248
Disorder of Destruction ... 249
Lupus Erythematosus ... 249
Miscellaneous ... 250
Acute Viral Infections ... 250
Acute Bacterial Infections ... 251
Chronic Bacterial Infections ... 252
Infectious Mononucleosis ... 253
Agranulocytosis ... 254
Trichinosis ... 255
Agnogenic Myeloid Metaplasia ... 256

20 **Disorders of Hemostasis** ... 257
Normal Mechanisms of Hemostasis ... 257
The Approach to the Diagnosis ... 259
Disorders of Platelets ... 262
Idiopathic Thrombocytopenic Purpura ... 262
Hereditary Hemorrhagic Thrombasthenia (Glanzmann's Disease) ... 263
Stage I Disorder ... 264
Hemophilia A (Classical Hemophilia) ... 264
Stage II Disorders ... 265
Dicumarol Therapy ... 265
Hemorrhagic Disease of the Newborn ... 266
Obstructive Jaundice ... 267
Stage III Disorder ... 268
Abruptio Placentae ... 268
Disorders of Vascular Resistance ... 269
Vascular Hemophilia (von Willebrand's Disease) ... 269
Anaphylactoid Purpura (Henoch-Schönlein Purpura) ... 270
Hereditary Hemorrhagic Telangiectasia ... 271
Scurvy ... 272
Miscellaneous ... 273
Heparin Therapy ... 273
Acute Leukemia ... 274
Cirrhosis of the Liver ... 275
Ehlers-Danlos Syndrome ... 276
Polycythemia Vera ... 277

21 **The Laboratory Diagnosis of Infectious Diseases** ... 278
Smears and Cultures ... 278
Animal Inoculation ... 289
Serologic Tests ... 290
Skin Tests ... 291

22 **The Office Laboratory** ... 293
Hematology ... 293
Blood Chemistries ... 295
Urinalysis ... 295
Stool ... 296
Bacteriology ... 296
Cytology ... 297
Immunological Tests ... 297

22 The Office Laboratory—*Continued*
Semen Analysis 297
Special Procedures 297
Skin Tests 298
Miscellaneous 298

23 Following Diseases With Laboratory Tests 299

24 Multiphasic Screening of Asymptomatic Patients 303

Conclusion 304

Appendix I Normal Values 305

Appendix II Laboratory Work-up of Symptoms 307

Appendix III Laboratory Work-up of Diseases 319

Appendix IV Relatively Innocuous Nonspecific Tests of Organ Involvement 330

Index 333

Illustrated Manual of

Laboratory Diagnosis

Indications and Interpretations

1 Disorders of Serum Acid and Alkaline Phosphatases

The phosphatases are one group of the many groups of enzymes found in the body. Aside from their specificity and location, they have no special characteristics to distinguish them from the other enzyme groups. They are of clinical significance because of the measurable changes that occur in their serum concentrations in diseases of the prostate, hepatobiliary, and skeletal systems. Skillful interpretation of these changes has become helpful not only in the diagnosis but also in the prognosis of disease states in these systems. Diagnoses cannot be made in most cases by simply matching phosphatase levels with signs and symptoms. Rather, serial determinations and correlation with other laboratory data are essential for the logical and accurate utilization of their values.

NORMAL METABOLISM

Production. The body contains many phosphatases. These have been categorized on the basis of the pH at which they exhibit maximum activity. Of clinical significance are the low specificity alkaline and acid phosphatases. The alkaline phosphatases are maximally active at pH's of 9 to 10 and have a rather widespread tissue distribution, the intestinal mucosa showing the greatest activity, followed by kidney, bone, thyroid, liver, etc. Physiologically, they are necessary for the hydrolysis of organic phosphates, and in this role they become important in digestion and mucosal absorption. A second role is found in the body's osteoblastic tissue. Metabolic activity of the osteoblasts is associated with varying degrees of increased alkaline phosphatase activity. Regenerating and proliferating liver tissue is rich in this enzyme.

Transportation. In the normal state, both alkaline and acid phosphatase are found circulating in the blood, although in somewhat different concentrations. Acid phosphatase levels of 0.2 to 0.8 Bodansky units (1 to 4 King-Armstrong units) per 100 ml. are normal. The alkaline phosphatase ranges between 1 and 4 Bodansky units (8 to 14 King-Armstrong units) per 100 ml. in normal adults. Slightly higher concentrations (5 to 15 Bodansky units) are found in the growth phase of development, this being due to increased osteoblastic activity during these years. General debility and anemia have been associated with somewhat lower values.

Excretion. Alkaline phosphatase until recently was believed to be excreted in much the same way as bilirubin by way of the hepatobiliary system. The exact pathway remains unknown, but the mechanism is now believed to be different from that of the bile pigments. Acid phosphatase excretion pathways have not yet been elucidated.

VALUE OF THE TESTS

Alkaline Phosphatase. This test is very useful in distinguishing obstructive and hepatocellular jaundice. In hepatocellular jaundice it is infrequently elevated, whereas in obstructive jaundice elevation is the rule. Elevation in hepatomegaly without jaundice suggests metastatic liver disease. The test is very useful in differentiating various bone diseases and hyperparathyroidism (p. 32) when combined with determinations of serum calcium and phosphorus and roentgenograms.

Acid Phosphatase. This test is most useful in diagnosing carcinoma of the prostate that has spread beyond the capsule.

INTERPRETING THE COLOR PLATES

A minimum of explanation has been included on each plate. The basic color plate, the first plate of each series, demonstrates the nor-

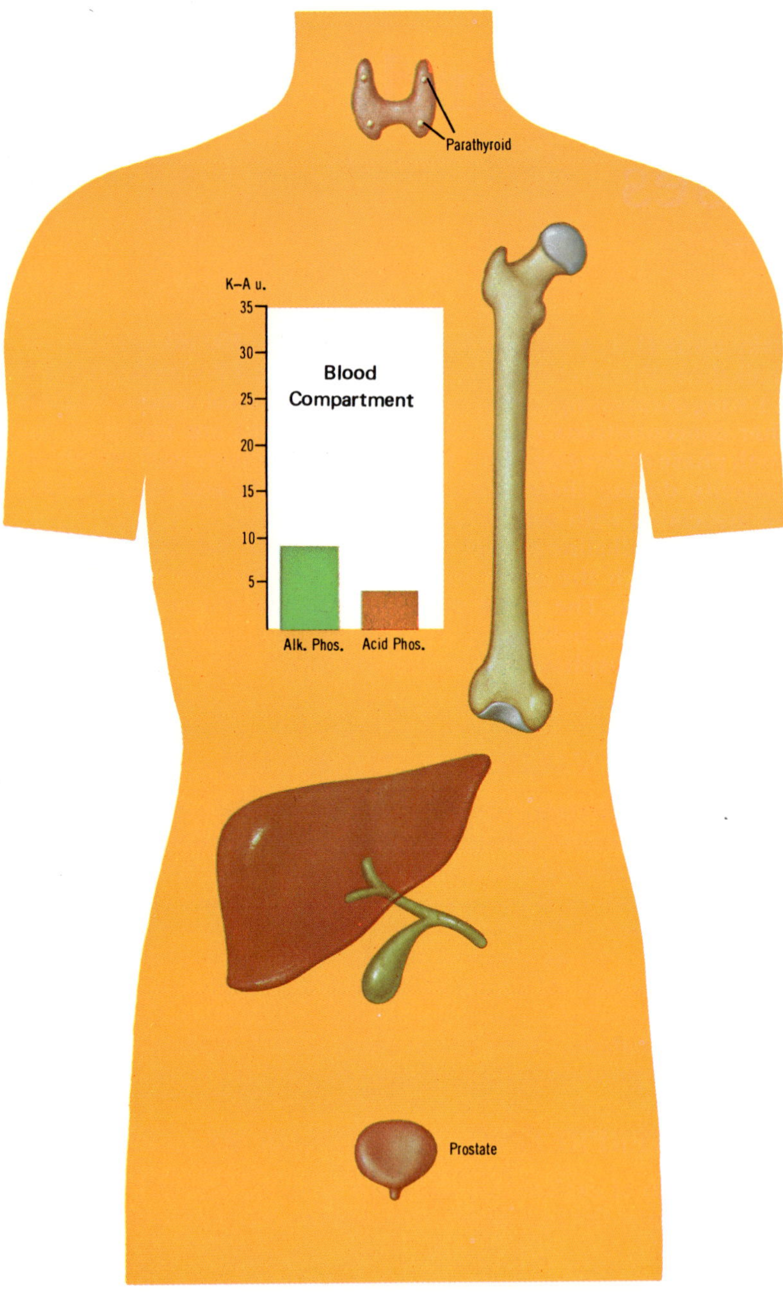

mal values and the normal metabolism. The results of laboratory tests dealing with constituents of blood or serum are shown in the white rectangle labeled Blood Compartment.

The changes in each disease are indicated in black. If there is no change, the plate is left unaltered. Hypertrophy or increase in tissue elements is shown by circles superimposed on each other. Atrophy, damage, or decrease in tissue function is indicated by stippling or solid black. Total absence of a chemical substance or tissue is indicated by an X. A block of a physiological function is also indicated by an X.

METASTATIC BONE TUMORS

Metastatic neoplasms of the bone may stimulate osteoblastic activity leading to an *elevated alkaline phosphatase.* When these metastases are from the prostate, there is usually an *elevated acid phosphatase also* (p. 6). Roentgenograms of the bones and bone biopsy confirm the diagnosis. Bone alkaline phosphatase can be differentiated from liver alkaline phosphatase because it is heat-stable.

Other osteoblastic metastases are carcinoma of the breast, Hodgkin's disease, and carcinoma of the thyroid and kidney.

Metastatic carcinomas from the lung, rectum, kidney, and breasts may produce osteolytic lesions with no significant rise in alkaline phosphatase activity.

Summary of Laboratory Findings:

Alkaline phosphatase: Increased

Acid phosphatase: Normal or increased

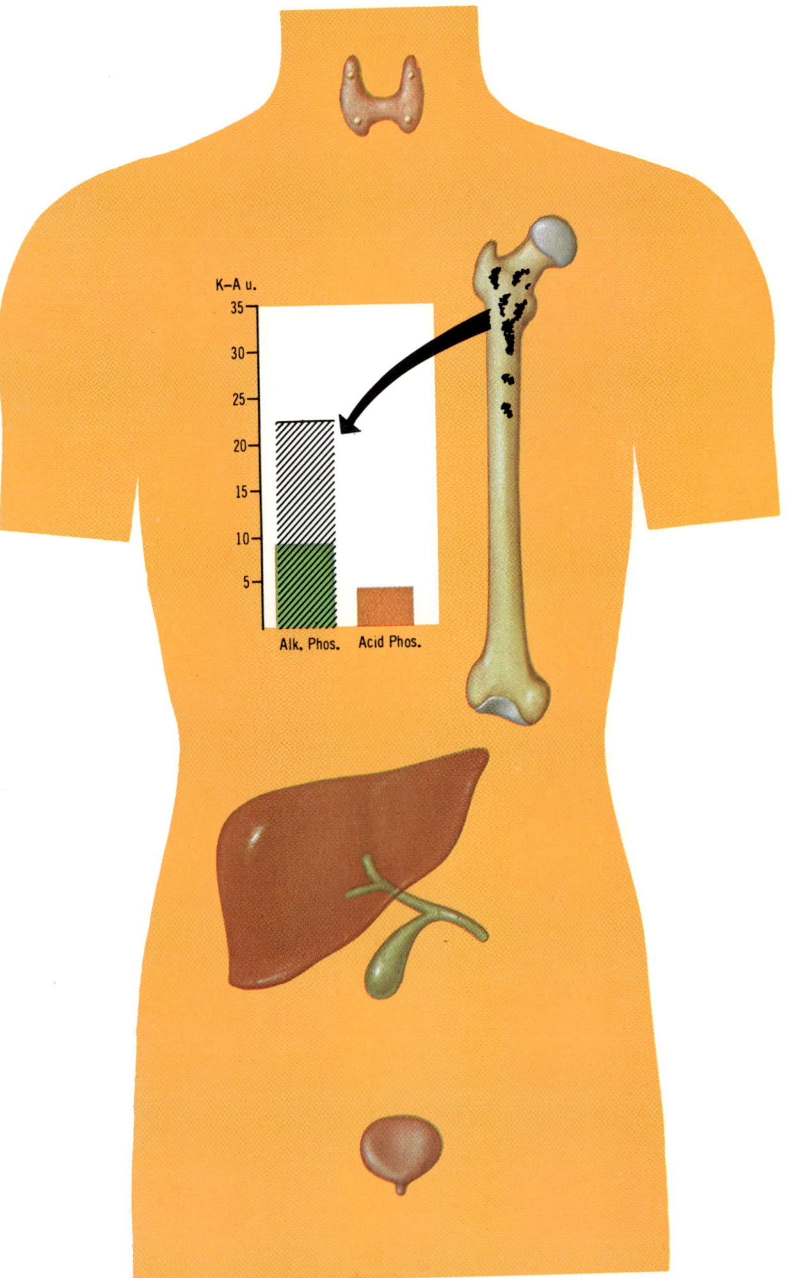

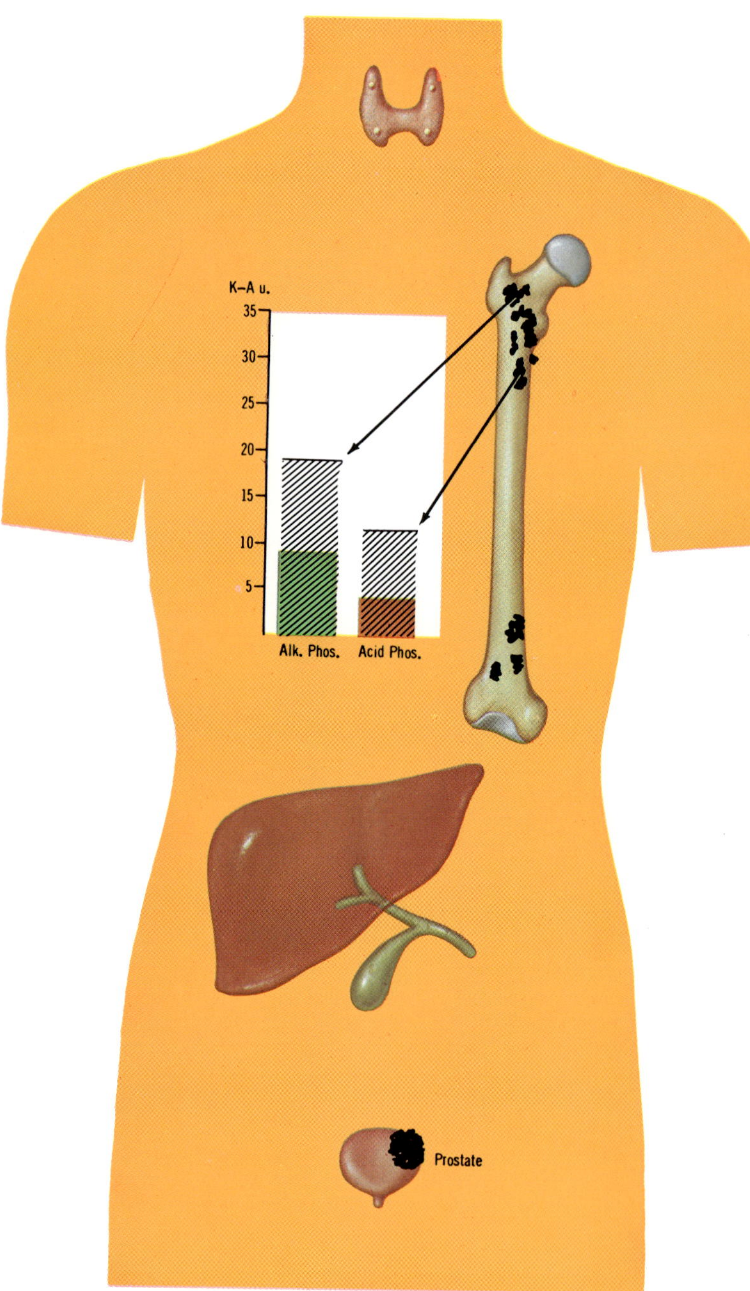

METASTATIC PROSTATIC CARCINOMA

Because prostatic epithelium characteristically produces large amounts of acid phosphatase, it is not surprising that metastatic prostatic carcinoma is often associated with a *high serum acid phosphatase.* The alkaline phosphatase is also increased. Only in the highly anaplastic types of metastatic prostatic cancer is the serum acid phosphatase normal. Serial determinations are useful in following the course of the disease after treatment. Acid phosphatase is not usually elevated in localized prostatic carcinoma unless it extends through the capsule. Without bone metastasis the alkaline phosphatase would be normal. The diagnosis is confirmed by roentgenograms of the bone and bone or prostatic biopsy.

The acid phosphatase is also elevated in the reticuloendothelioses, such as Gaucher's disease, and in hemopoietic disturbances.

Summary of Laboratory Findings:

Alkaline phosphatase: Increased

Acid Phosphatase: Increased

OSTEITIS DEFORMANS (PAGET'S DISEASE)

In Paget's disease of the bone, the *serum alkaline phosphatase* concentration may *reach* its *highest known levels* (100 Bodansky units or greater), thus reflecting tremendous osteoblastic activity in the involved areas of the skeleton as depicted in x-ray films of the skull and long bones. The high levels are sometimes reflected in an increased acid phosphatase also. The basic process underlying this condition is idiopathic localized bone destruction and reabsorption, followed by compensatory abnormal new bone formation. Serial determinations of the alkaline phosphatase are useful in following this disease. A dramatic rise in the serum alkaline phosphatase may indicate the development of an osteogenic sarcoma, a common complication in this disease.

Summary of Laboratory Findings:

Alkaline phosphatase: Markedly increased

Acid phosphatase: Normal or increased

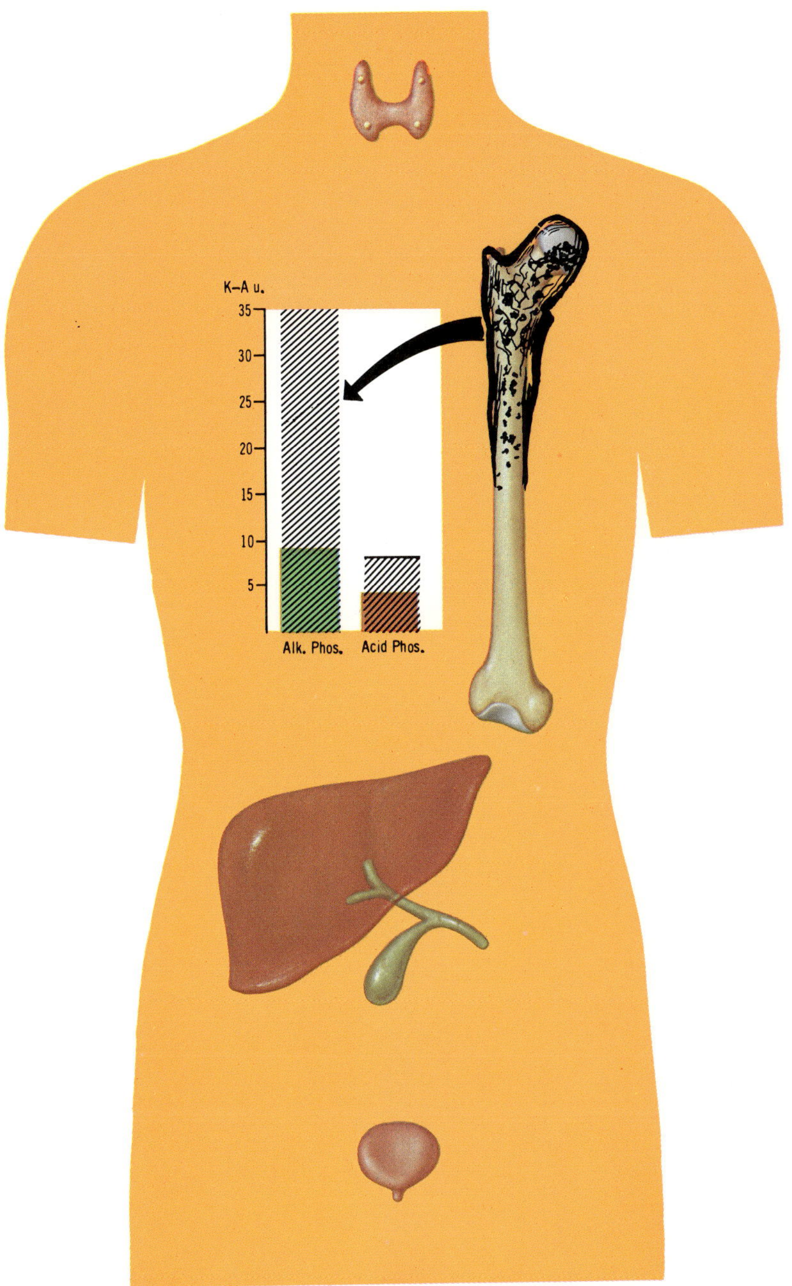

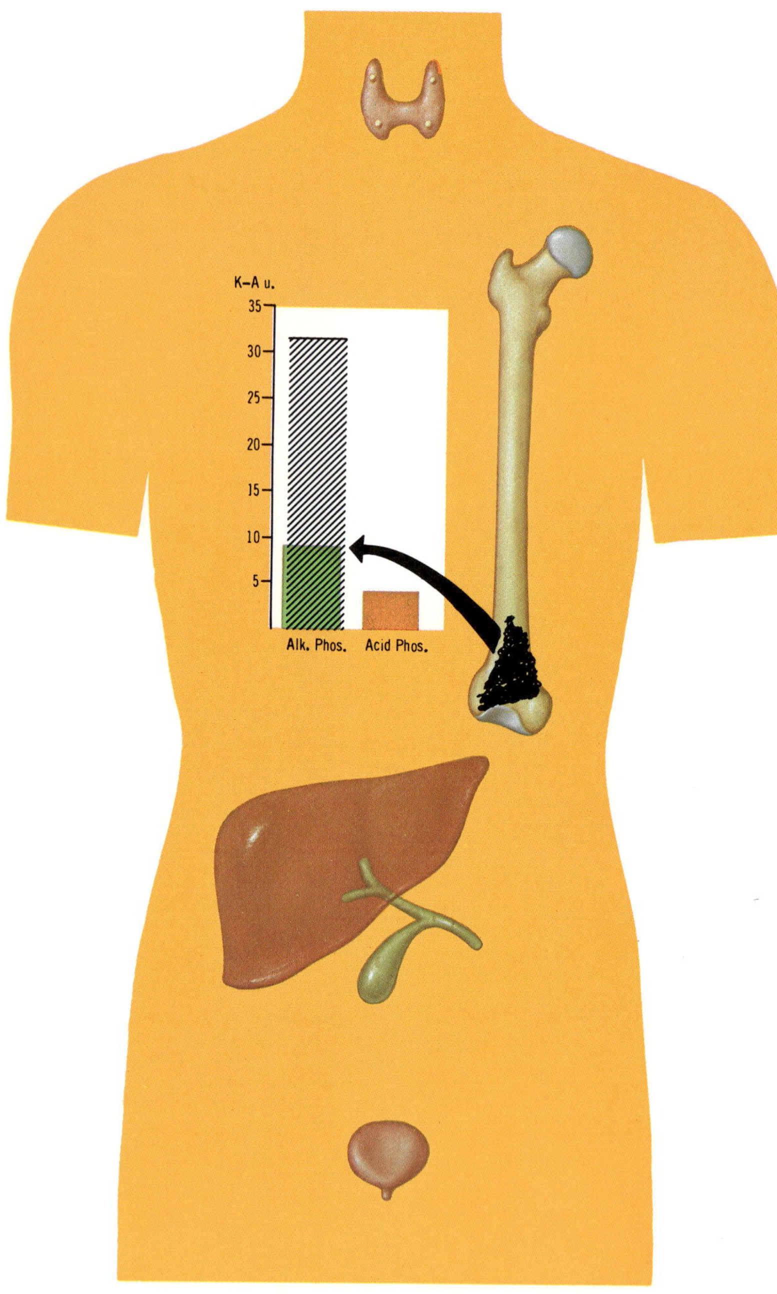

OSTEOGENIC SARCOMA

There are two types of osteogenic sarcoma, an osteoblastic and an osteolytic. The osteoblastic type, as might be expected, is associated with a marked *increase* of *alkaline phosphatase* (20 to 40 times normal). Serum calcium and phosphorus levels are normal. The diagnosis is established by roentgenograms of the bone and bone biopsy.

Several other primary bone tumors (chondrosarcomas, malignant giant-cell tumors) are accompanied by an elevated alkaline phosphatase.

Summary of Laboratory Findings:

Alkaline phosphatase: Increased

Acid phosphatase: Normal

RICKETS AND OSTEOMALACIA

In these disorders the low blood calcium stimulates parathyroid activity (A), which in turn induces reabsorption of bone to compensate for the low blood calcium. The bone reacts with increased osteoblastic activity, and thus the *serum alkaline phosphatase rises.* (See also p. 25). Roentgenograms of the bones and response to vitamin D help to confirm the diagnosis. Primary hyperparathyroidism produces a similar picture.

Whenever a low blood calcium results from inadequate intake or absorption or increased urinary excretion, a similar rise in alkaline phosphatase occurs.

Summary of Laboratory Findings:

Alkaline phosphatase: Increased

Acid phosphatase: Normal

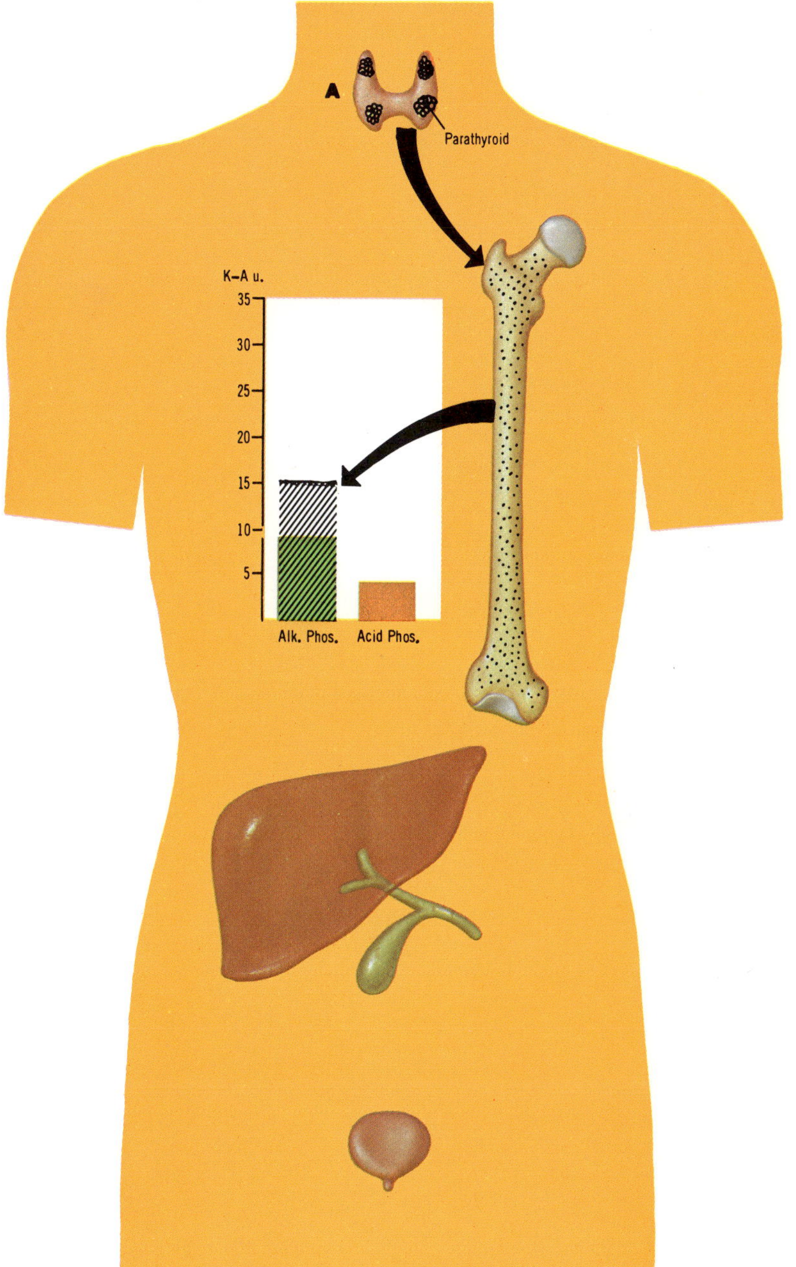

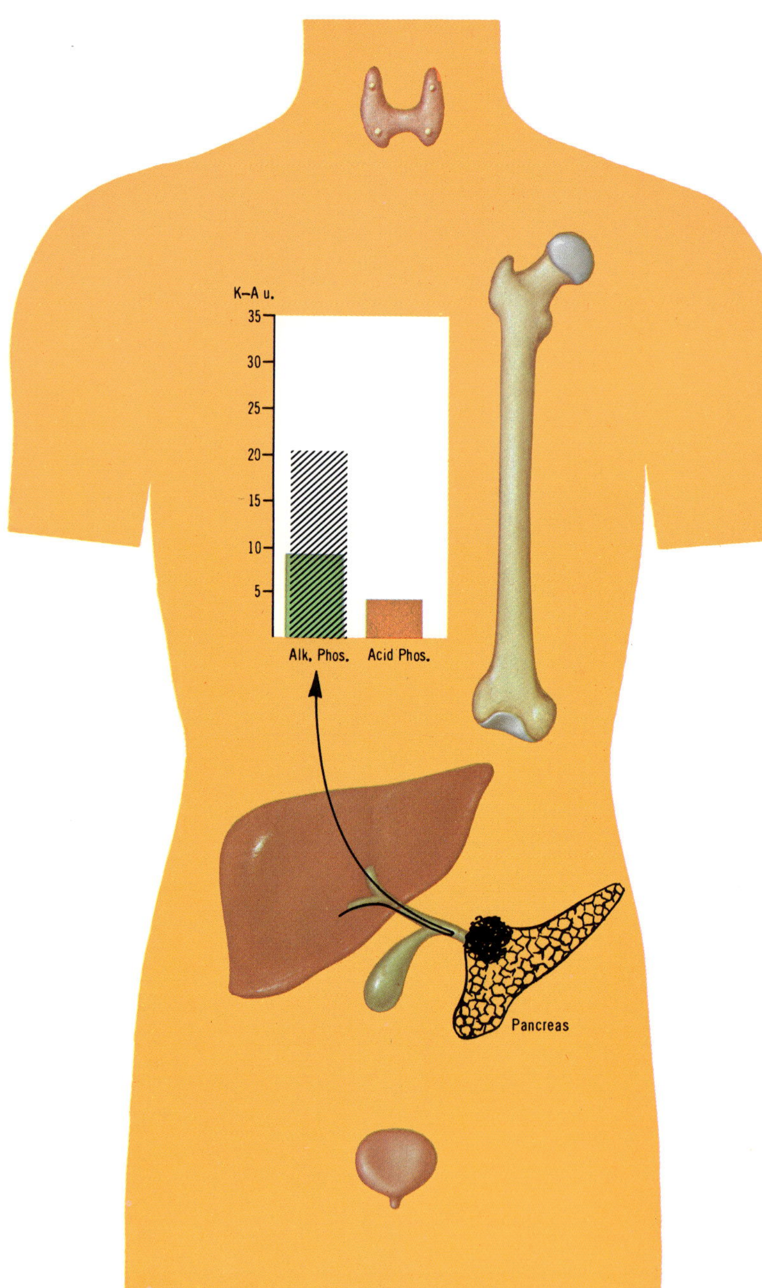

CARCINOMA OF THE HEAD OF THE PANCREAS

When this neoplasm compresses and obstructs the common bile duct, an *elevation* of the serum *alkaline phosphatase* occurs and is accompanied by a parallel rise in the serum concentrations of bilirubin, cholesterol, and phospholipids. Whether the rise in alkaline phosphatase is due to increased hepatic synthesis of alkaline phosphatase or the backflow of hepatobiliary-produced enzyme is still debated. The diagnosis is usually established by exploratory laparotomy.

Any disorder that may produce obstruction of the common duct (carcinoma of the ampulla of Vater, stone) may produce a similar picture. A simultaneous elevation of the leucine amino peptidase (LAP) enzyme serves to confirm the presence of biliary obstruction.

Summary of Laboratory Findings:

Alkaline phosphatase: Increased

Acid phosphatase: Normal

CHLORPROMAZINE HEPATITIS

In this disorder a hypersensitivity reaction induces intrahepatic cholestasis, resulting in an *elevated alkaline phosphatase* along with a high serum bilirubin and cholesterol. In contrast, viral hepatitis is not usually associated with a marked increase in alkaline phosphatase unless it involves the cholangioles. The diagnosis is best established by history, a therapeutic trial of cortisone, and liver biopsy, but other useful tests are discussed on page 19.

Summary of Laboratory Findings:

Alkaline phosphatase: Increased

Acid phosphatase: Normal

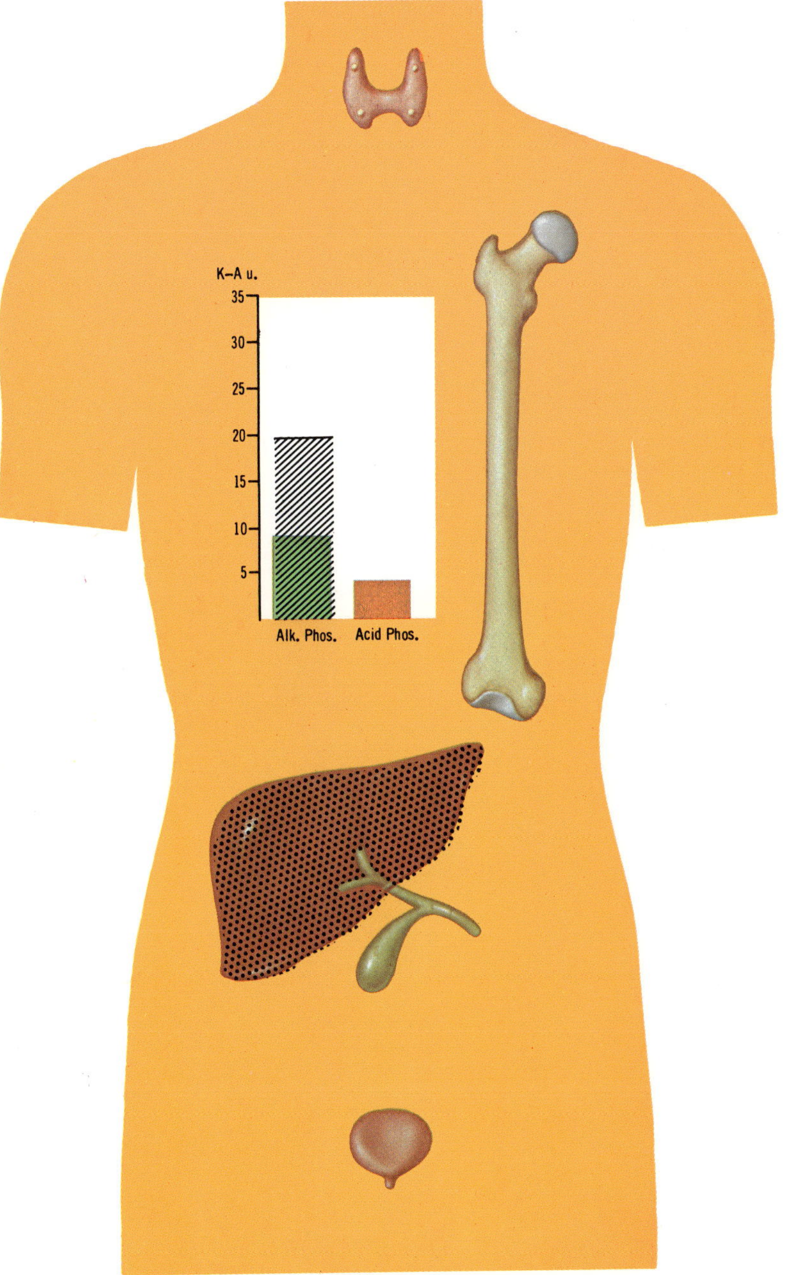

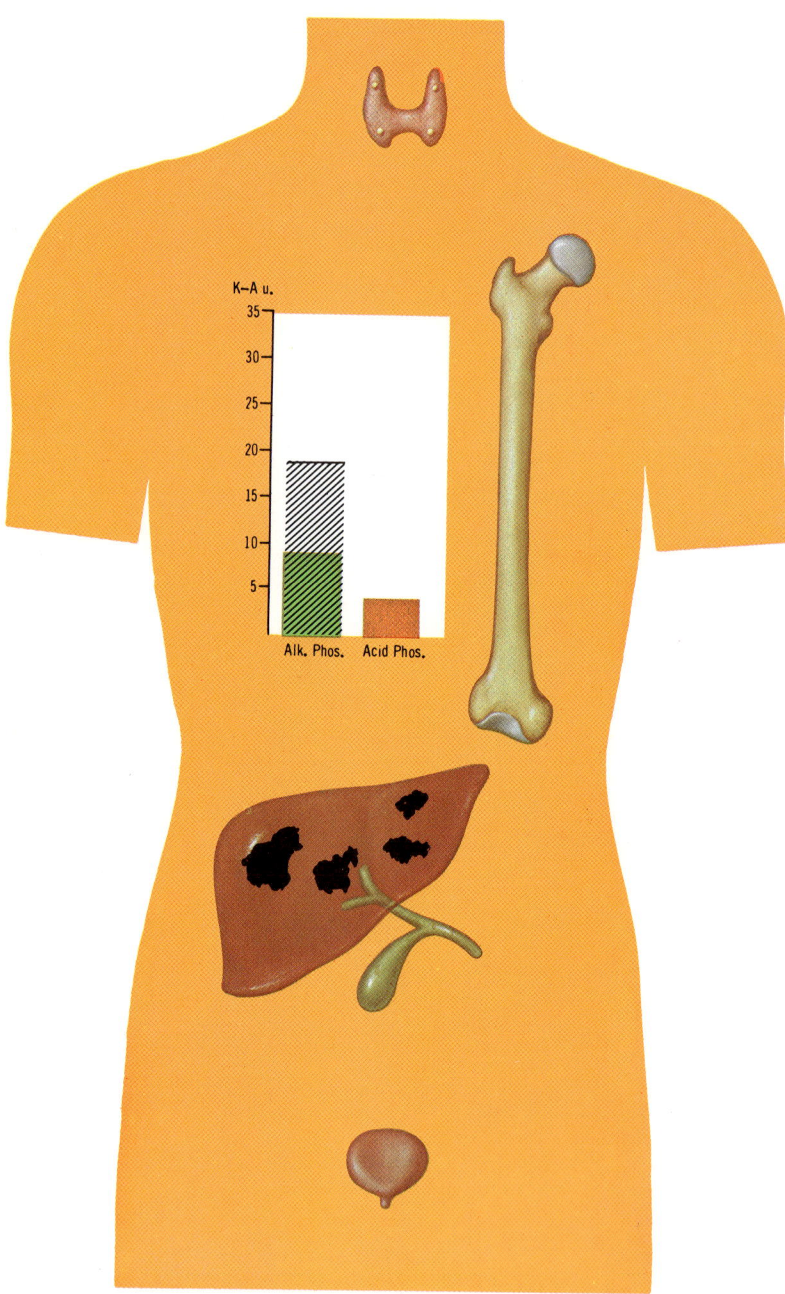

METASTATIC CARCINOMA OF THE LIVER

Barring osseous metastasis, a marked *increase* in the *serum alkaline phosphatase* without an accompanying increase in the serum bilirubin is highly suggestive of hepatic metastasis when there is a known primary tumor elsewhere in the body. In contrast, primary hepatomas are not associated with any consistent change in the serum alkaline phosphatase levels. Again, definitive diagnosis is made by liver biopsy, liver scan, or exploratory laparotomy. Selective arteriography is also useful.

Summary of Laboratory Findings:

Alkaline phosphatase: Increased

Acid phosphatase: Normal

2 Disorders of Serum Bilirubin

The functional status of the liver and its biliary drainage system can be evaluated by a series of laboratory studies collectively known as the "liver profile." Although these tests are not specific for any one disease state, they are helpful, when correlated with the history and physical examination, in making diagnoses in pathological conditions involving the liver and biliary tract. Of the many tests that comprise this profile, none perhaps is as informative as the serum bilirubin concentration. It has been not only the foundation of the laboratory diagnosis of liver disease but also an instrument in furthering understanding of liver physiology.

NORMAL METABOLISM

Production. Bilirubin is a by-product of hemaglobin metabolism and is derived mainly from this substance. A certain amount (25–30%), however, is derived from other substances, such as myoglobin, catalases, and cytochromes. Each day because of physiological red cell destruction, 7 to 8 gm. of hemoglobin becomes available for disintegration. The site of this disintegration lies within the cells of the reticuloendothelial system (liver, spleen, bone marrow, etc.). Within these cells the protein moiety or globin portion of the hemoglobin molecule leaves the molecular proper and returns to the body's protein pool for subsequent reutilization. The remaining protein-deficient substance, called heme, then loses its iron and is referred to as protoporphyrin. This ring-shaped structure is then opened to form a linear tetrapyrrole that is, in fact, bilirubin, the golden-hued pigment that accumulates in abnormal quantities in the jaundiced patient. Bilirubin tetrapyrrole is then released from the reticuloendothelial cells and enters the blood stream. Because it is highly insoluble in aqueous media under physiological conditions, it depends on protein binding, mainly to albumin, to remain in solution in the plasma.

Metabolism. In 1916, van den Bergh, a German investigator, discovered that serum bilirubin could be quantitated by reacting it with a diazo compound if alcohol were first added to the mixture. This bore clinical significance even at that time. He further noticed that bilirubin of bile was different from bilirubin of the serum in that bile bilirubin would react with the diazo compounds even without the previous addition of alcohol (direct van den Bergh reaction). Many years of investigation into identifying the changes that take place were necessary before it was possible to account for these differences in the two bilirubins. Today it is known that the water-insoluble serum bilirubin is transported in the plasma to the liver parenchymal cells, where it is conjugated with glucuronic acid in the presence of glycuronyl transferase and uridine triphosphate to form bilirubin diglucuronide. Conjugation with sulfates also occurs, but to a lesser degree than with glucuronic acid. Both these substances are water-soluble. The glycuronide conjugation system is not unique to bilirubin but rather is an ubiquitous system used to render water-insoluble compounds water-soluble, often for the purpose of excretion.

Excretion. Bilirubin is a waste product and thus must be excreted. In its conjugated water-soluble form it can be readily eliminated into the bile, where, indeed, it accounts for the pigmentation of that substance. The excretory process of conjugated bilirubin has been shown to be distinct from the conjugation process in the hepatic cells. In fact, clinical jaundice can result from a defective excretory mechanism in the presence of normal conjugation (chronic idiopathic jaundice: Dubin-Johnson syndrome). It should be noted also that water-soluble bilirubin can be cleared and excreted by the kidneys in cases of its accumulation in the blood (e.g., obstructive jaundice).

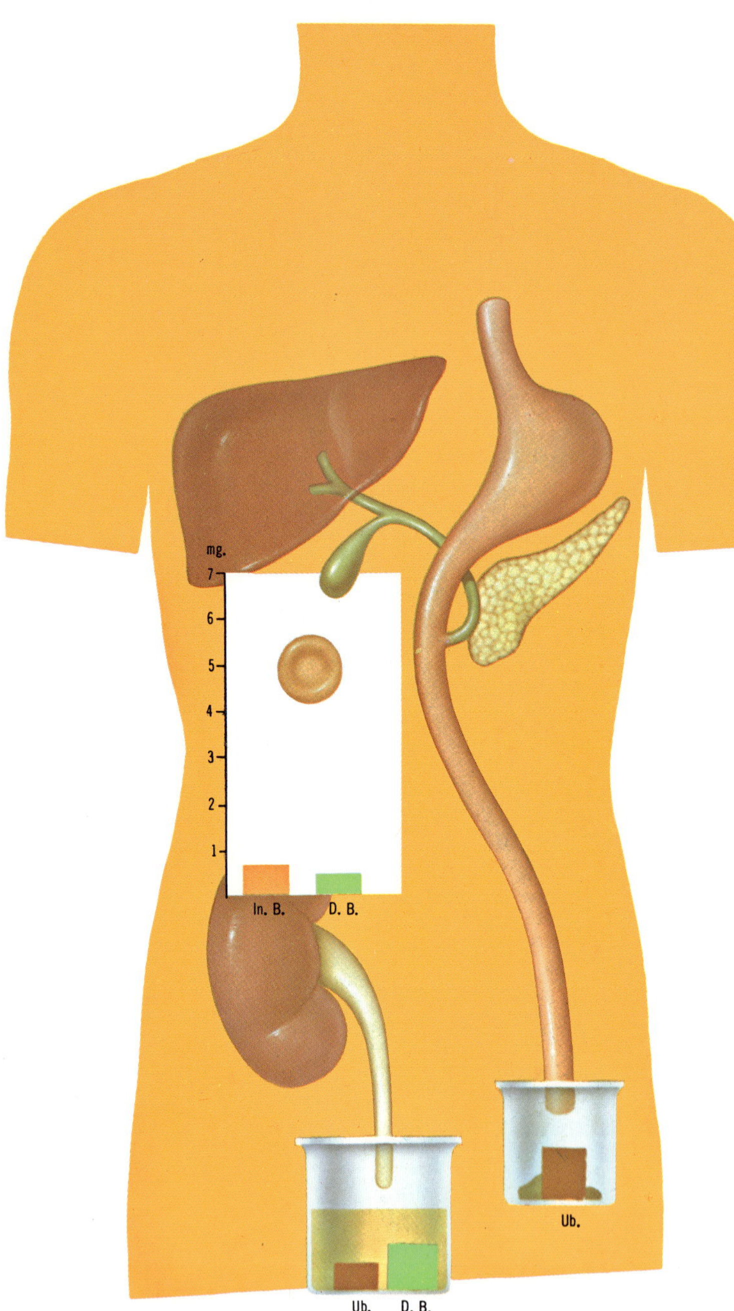

After being transferred into the bile, bilirubin passes successively through the bile canaliculi, cholangioles, the hepatic ducts, the common bile duct, and into the duodenum. Once in the gastrointestinal tract, bilirubin is changed by the colon bacteria to other compounds, i.e., the uro and the sterco bilinogens and bilins. It is the stercobilins that give the characteristic colors to feces. Absence of bilirubin products makes feces light, gray, or colorless, as in obstructive jaundice. In a 24-hour period approximately 50 to 300 mg. of bilirubin are excreted as stercobilinogen in a normal adult. This, again, is derived from 7 to 8 gm. of hemoglobin plus that derived from myoglobins, catalases, and cytochromes.

A small amount of the fecal urobilinogen is reabsorbed from the intestine into the portal circulation. This amount is then almost totally cleared from the blood by the liver cells (enterohepatic circulation) and is then re-excreted as bilirubin. Tiny amounts, however, escape hepatic clearance and are excreted in the urine as urobilinogens (0-4 mg./24 hours). This becomes important as a diagnostic instrument in cases of hepatic parenchymal disease. In such disease states there will be decreased clearing through the diseased liver, and thus increased amounts of urobilinogen will be present in the urine. In complete obstruction of the bile ducts, with one exception (p. 20), there will be no urobilinogen in the urine.

In summary, then, it can be stated that the cellular mechanisms involved in the various stages of bilirubin formation, conjugation, and excretion are incompletely understood. What is known, however, suggests that these mechanisms are complex. In disease these mechanisms can be impaired at various points, the result of which is clinical jaundice.

Bromsulphalein Dye Excretion. The liver handles the excretion of this dye somewhat analogous to the way it handles bilirubin. When the bilirubin is normal, this is a very sensitive test of hepatic function. Thus it is an excellent screening test. Its only drawback is the occasional allergic reaction. Normally less than 5% remains in the serum 45 minutes after intravenous injection. In jaundice due to hemolytic anemias the BSP is usually normal, another helpful differential point.

Abbreviations Used in Plates:

In. B. = Indirect bilirubin in mg. per 100 ml.

D. B. = Direct bilirubin in mg. per 100 ml.

Ub. = Urobilinogen in mg. per 24 hr.

HEREDITARY SPHEROCYTOSIS

In this disorder the intrinsically defective red cells hemolyze (A) at a rapid rate, leading to an increased formation of bilirubin. The liver can compensate for this to some degree by excreting more bilirubin, with the result that the *stool* and *urinary urobilinogen increase*. When the hemolysis is severe, hepatic reserve is exceeded, and the *serum indirect bilirubin rises*. Since there is little or no parenchymal liver disease in this condition, tissue enzymes (SGOT, etc.), thymol turbidity, and the cephalin flocculation do not rise. The diagnosis is confirmed by the red–cell fragility test, reticulocyte count, blood smear, radioactive chromium red-cell survival time, and BSP.

Hemolytic disorders such as this one may, however, be associated with bilirubin stones, which can cause obstructive jaundice. Constitutional hepatic dysfunction (Gilbert's syndrome) also may produce a high serum indirect bilirubin and is occasionally associated with a hemolytic anemia. Sickle cell anemia, Cooley's anemia, and other hemolytic diseases may cause the same picture.

Summary of Laboratory Findings:

Serum bilirubin, indirect: Increased

Serum bilirubin, direct: Normal

Urine bilirubin: Normal

Urine urobilinogen: Increased

Stool urobilinogen: Increased

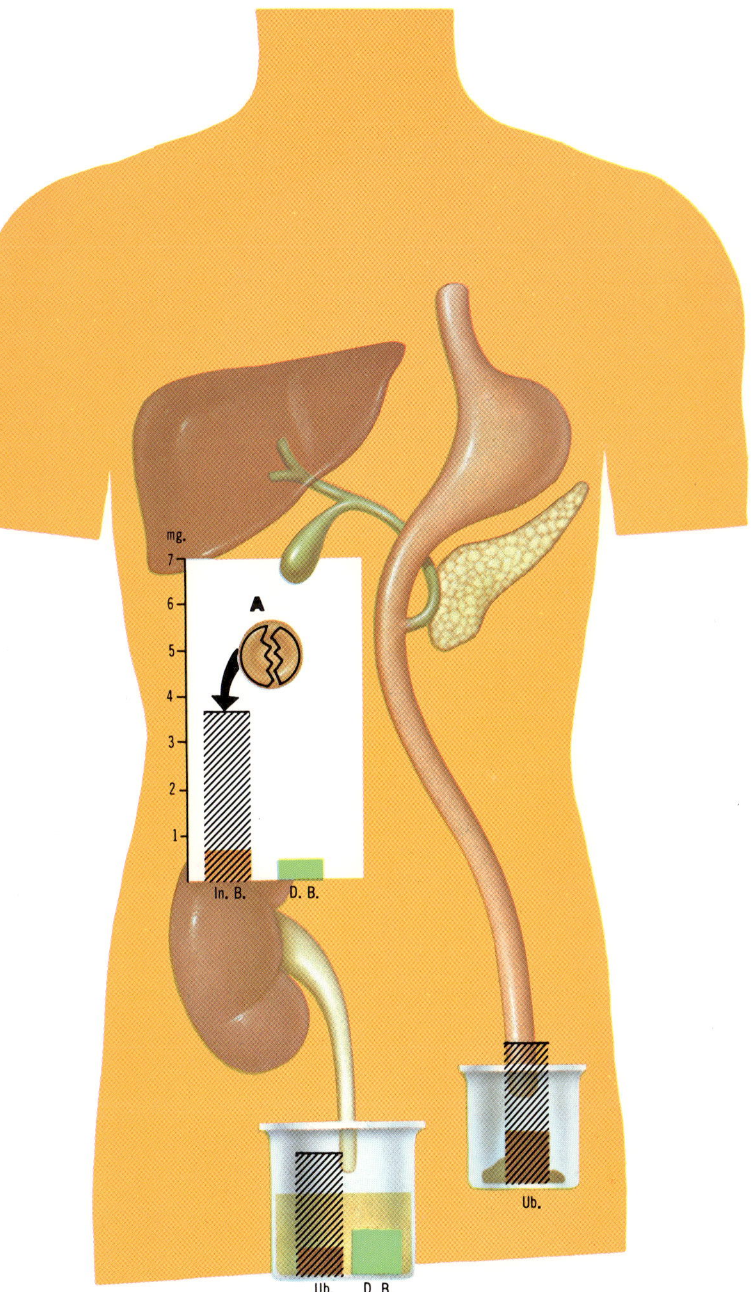

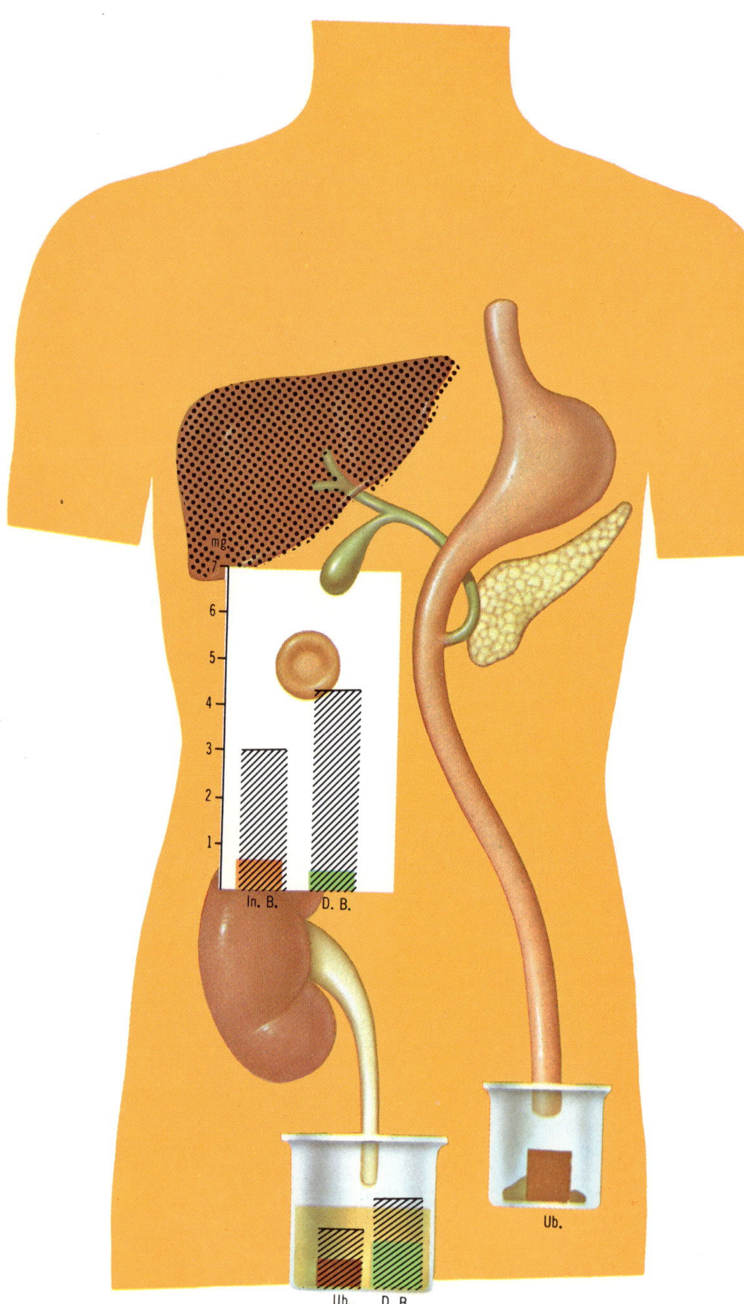

VIRAL HEPATITIS

In this disorder the combination of hepatocellular damage and intrahepatic cholestasis leads to a *rise* in both the *indirect* and the *direct bilirubin*. The latter increases the most and is found in the *urine* even before it rises in the serum. These alterations progress in intensity for several weeks and then slowly subside. The *urine urobilinogen* is *increased* during the preicteric stage.

The cephalin-cholesterol flocculation and thymol turbidity are usually strongly positive, and the serum transaminases rise considerably, as further indications of hepatocellular damage. The gamma glutamyl transpeptidase (GGT) is a sensitive indicator of hepatic function and is often elevated in biliary obstruction when the transaminase is normal. Alkaline phosphatase levels are only mildly elevated unless intrahepatic cholestasis is severe. The BSP is usually elevated in the numerous anicteric cases of this disease. Liver biopsy often confirms the diagnosis. The HAA (Australia antigen) is positive in type B (serum hepatitis) but becomes negative if the disease subsides.

Summary of Laboratory Findings:

Serum bilirubin, indirect: Increased
Serum bilirubin, direct: Increased
Urine bilirubin: Increased
Urine urobilinogen: Normal or increased
Stool urobilinogen: Normal or decreased

LAENNEC'S CIRRHOSIS

The degeneration, necrosis, and fibrosis of hepatic tissue in the *advanced* stages of this disorder lead to an inability to convert indirect bilirubin to the soluble glucuronide. As a result, the *indirect bilirubin* may *rise*. Perhaps because the fibrosis induces intrahepatic biliary obstruction, the *direct bilirubin* also *rises*. Occasionally direct bilirubins of 20 mg. or more are reached, and sequential liver scans may be necessary to rule out obstruction.

The associated biliary obstruction may result also in a rise of the alkaline phosphatase and serum cholesterol unless hepatocellular damage is severe. Concurrently with episodic hepatocellular necrosis, the thymol turbidity and cephalin-cholesterol flocculation become positive and the transaminases rise. As the disease becomes advanced, albumin production and cholesterol esterification by the liver are impaired. Finally, as the liver loses its ability to store glucose, there is intermittent hypoglycemia. Early in the course of the disease an impairment of bromsulphalein excretion may be the only abnormality. The diagnosis is established by liver biopsy.

Summary of Laboratory Findings:

Serum bilirubin, indirect: Increased

Serum bilirubin, direct: Increased

Urine bilirubin: Increased

Urine urobilinogen: Normal or increased

Stool urobilinogen: Normal

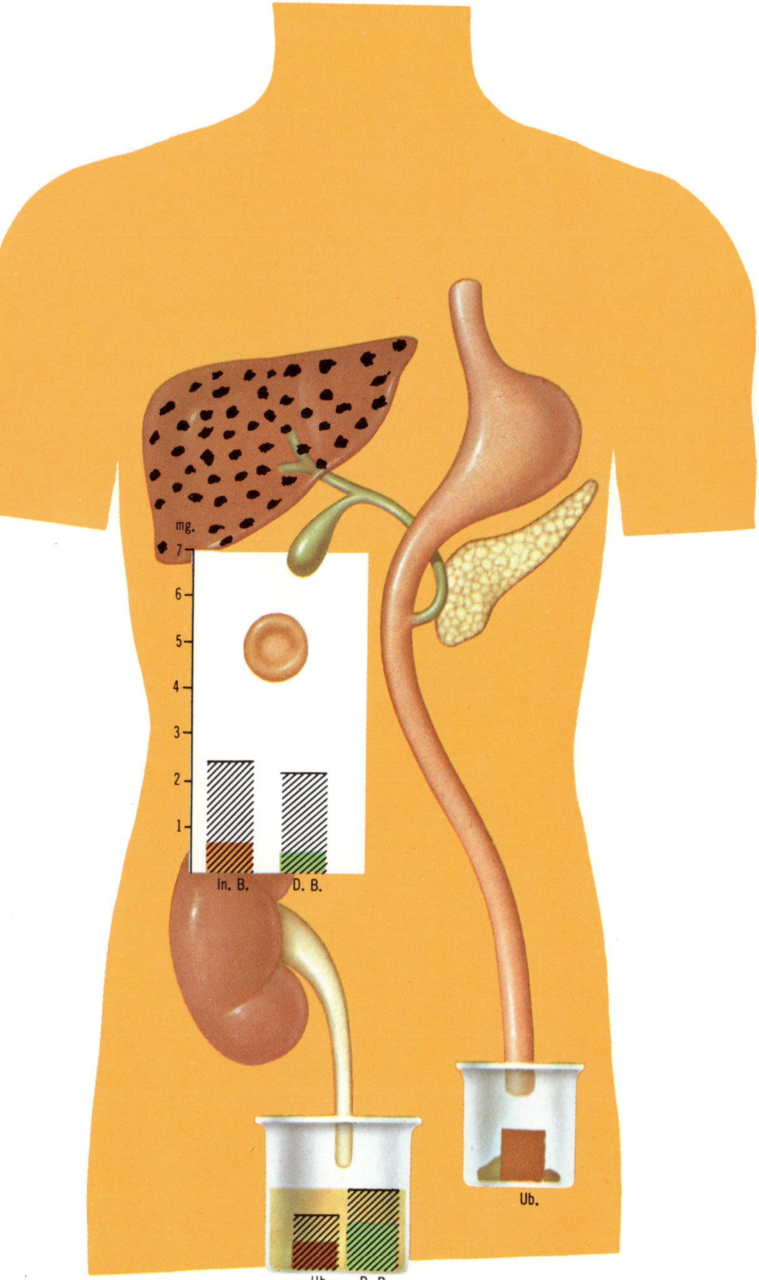

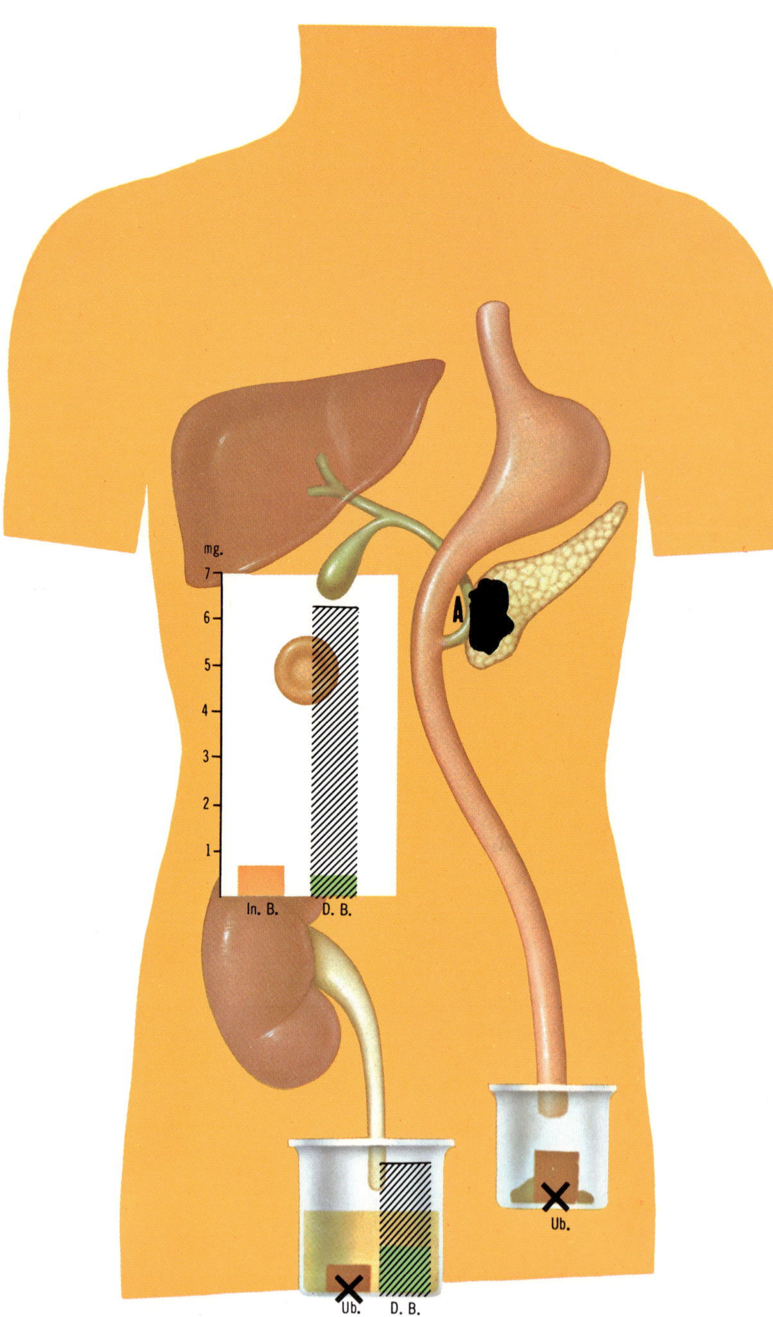

CARCINOMA OF THE HEAD OF THE PANCREAS

This neoplasm compresses the bile ducts (A), resulting in extrahepatic biliary obstruction. The direct reacting *serum bilirubin rises* and *appears* in the *urine*. When biliary obstruction is complete, no bilirubin enters the duodenum, and as a result *no urobilinogen appears* in the *stool* or *urine*.

Excretion of alkaline phosphatase and cholesterol is blocked, and the blood levels of both also rise. All indices of hepatocellular damage, such as the thymol turbidity and serum transaminase, are normal or only slightly altered unless there is associated liver disease. The lack of bile in the intestines prevents the absorption of vitamin K and other fat-soluble vitamins. Consequently, plasma prothrombin may be reduced. However, parenteral administration of vitamin K returns the prothrombin to normal.

Carcinoma of the bile duct, the gallbladder, and ampulla of Vater may give a similar picture. The last condition is often distinguished by a variation in the bilirubin from day to day and occult blood in the stool. Definitive diagnosis depends on an exploratory laparotomy, since a liver biopsy is contraindicated in these disorders.

Summary of Laboratory Findings:

Serum bilirubin, indirect: Normal

Serum bilirubin, direct: Increased

Urine bilirubin: Increased

Urine urobilinogen: Decreased

Stool urobilinogen: Decreased

CHLORPROMAZINE HEPATITIS

Intrahepatic cholestasis in this disorder leads to a *rise* in the *direct reacting serum bilirubin* and *overflow into the urine. Fecal* and *urinary urobilinogen* are *decreased or absent.* Flocculation and turbidity tests, serum transaminase activity, and serum proteins are usually normal, since hepatocellular damage is minimal. Eosinophilia and positive skin tests for the drug help to substantiate the diagnosis. Differentiation from common bile duct obstruction may be made by giving a cortisone derivative for 5 days. This will usually cause a 50 per cent drop in the serum bilirubin for toxic hepatitis but not for extrahepatic bile duct obstruction, except in the occasional case due to a stone. Androgens, sulfonylureas, cinchophen, and other drugs may give a similar picture. Some drugs (iproniazid, etc) may cause, in addition, scattered areas of hepatocellular necrosis, in which case the thymol turbidity and the serum transaminase may be elevated. Primary biliary cirrhosis may be differentiated by a high titer of mitochondrial antibodies.

Summary of Laboratory Findings:

Serum bilirubin, indirect: Normal or slightly increased

Serum bilirubin, direct: Markedly increased

Urine bilirubin: Increased

Urine urobilinogen: Decreased

Stool urobilinogen: Decreased

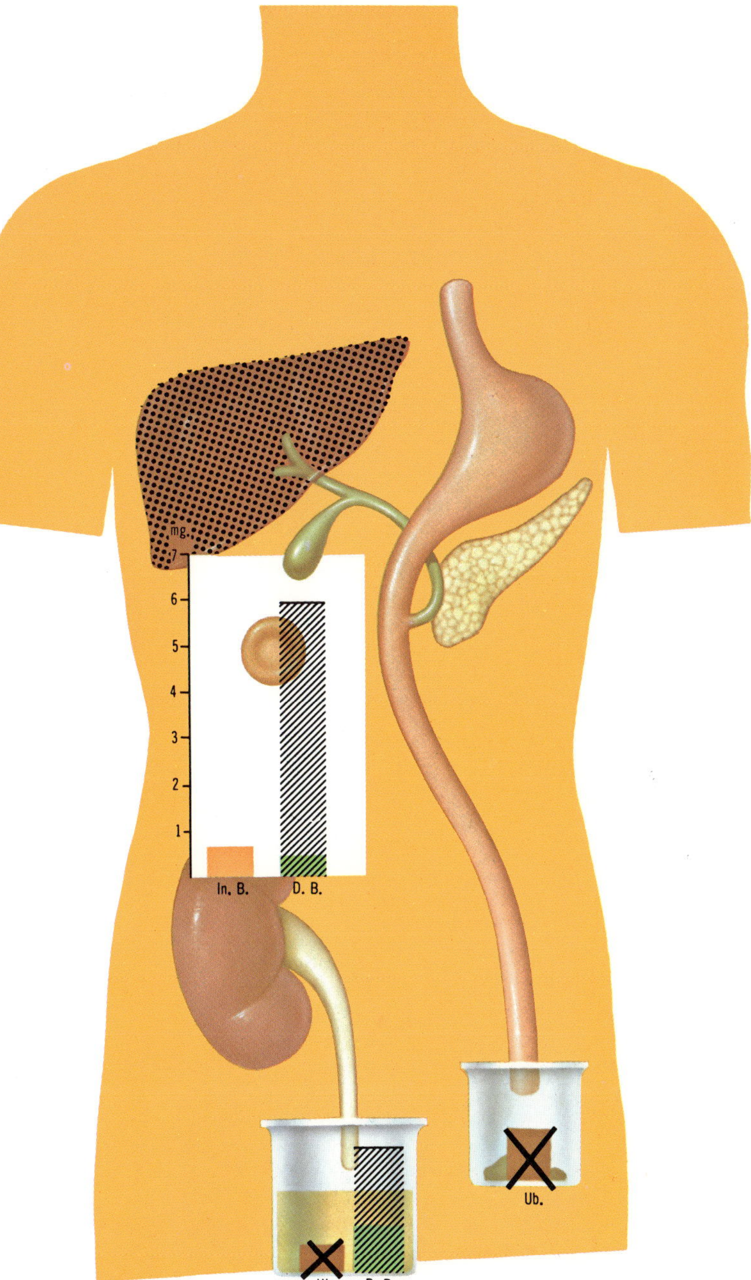

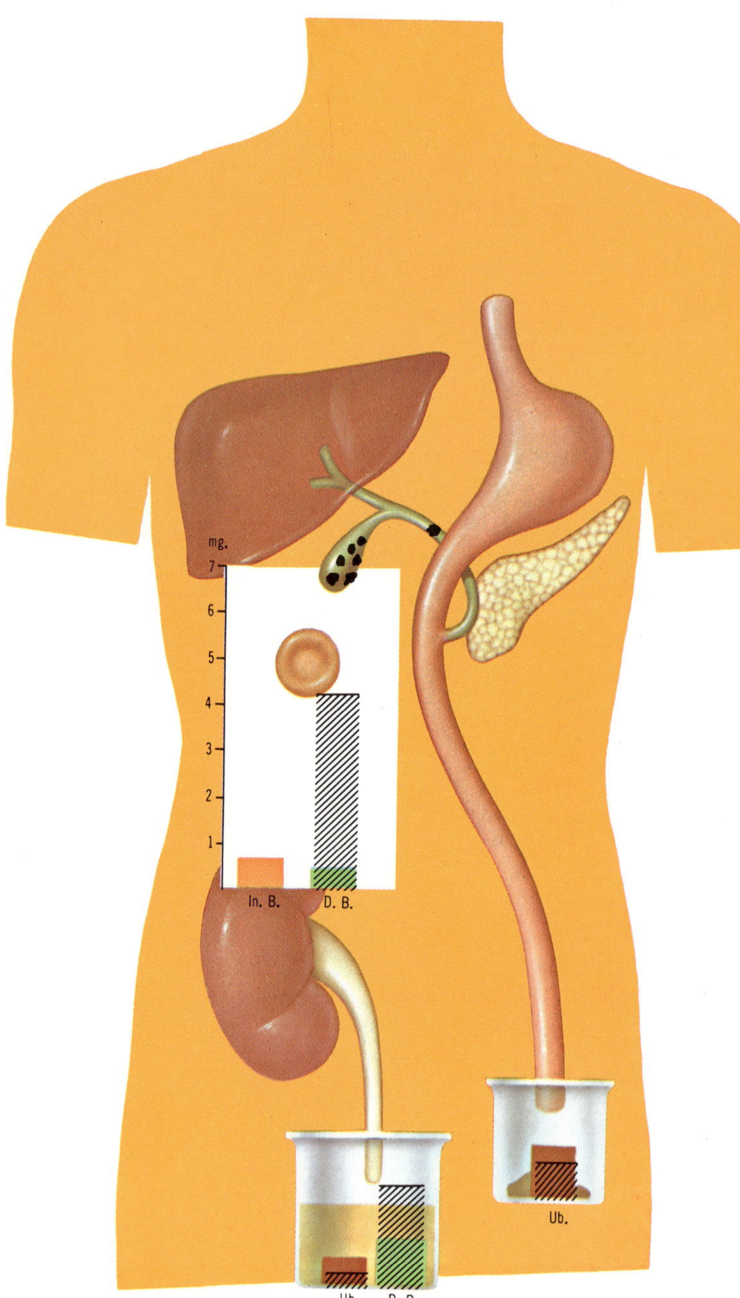

CHOLEDOCHOLITHIASIS

When gallstones pass into the common bile duct, they cause extrahepatic cholestasis. The *direct reacting serum bilirubin rises* in the *blood* and *urine*. *Fecal* and *urine urobilinogen* are *diminished* but rarely disappear, for the obstruction is seldom complete. Urine urobilinogen may be high if there is an associated cholangitis. The obstruction frequently is variable, because stones may pass, or inflammation and edema of the bile duct may occur intermittently. Consequently, the serum bilirubin often changes from day to day. This helps to differentiate this condition from neoplasms obstructing the bile ducts, in which a stable or progressive rise of the bilirubin is the rule. Thymol turbidity, flocculation tests, and serum transaminase are normal in most cases.

The diagnosis is usually confirmed by a cholecystogram or cholangiogram after the jaundice subsides. Sometimes exploratory laparotomy or percutaneous transhepatic cholangiography are necessary to establish the diagnosis. Recently, retrograde cholangiography has been performed by catheterizing the ampulla of Vater through the duodenoscope.

Summary of Laboratory Findings:

Serum bilirubin, indirect: Normal

Serum bilirubin, direct: Increased intermittently

Urine bilirubin: Increased

Urine urobilinogen: Decreased

Stool urobilinogen: Decreased

3 Disorders of Serum Calcium

Since disorders of calcium metabolism are associated with alterations in serum phosphates and alkaline phosphatase as well as calcium, the metabolism of these elements will be considered together.

NORMAL METABOLISM

Intake. *Calcium* and *phosphorus* enter the body through the alimentary canal. The daily requirements are 500 to 800 mg. of calcium and 1.0 to 1.5 gm. of phosphorus.

Absorption. *Calcium* and *phosphorus* are absorbed by the small intestine with the help of vitamin D and the parathyroid hormone. Absorption is assisted by an acid pH in the intestine. Large amounts of phosphorus, fats, or phytic acid in the diet inhibit calcium absorption. Less than 50 per cent of the dietary calcium is absorbed, the rest being excreted in the feces.

Transport. *Calcium* is transported in the blood in two forms. Half of it is in an un-ionized protein-bound form, and the other half is ionized with phosphate. The total concentration is normally 9 to 11 mg. per 100 ml. (4.5 to 5.5 mEq. per liter), and the ionized fraction is 4.5 to 5.0 mg. per cent. The ionizable fraction is distributed throughout the extracellular fluid, but neither the protein-bound nor the ionizable fraction is present in significant quantities in the intracellular fluid. The inorganic *phosphate* of the plasma ranges from 3 to 4 mg. per cent in adults and 4.5 to 6.5 mg. per cent in children. Unlike calcium, it is present in large quantities in the cell. There is a reciprocal relationship between the concentrations of calcium and of phosphate in the blood.

Storage. Approximately 1,100 gm. of *calcium* are stored in the bones of a 70-kg. adult (2 to 3% of body weight). About 80 to 90 cent of the total body *phosphate* is "stored" in bone; the remainder is widely distributed in both the intracellular and extracellular fluid. Both the calcium and phosphate of bone are in a constant state of exchange with that in the blood and the extracellular fluid, but equal amounts are being released and precipitated at all times, provided that there is sufficient ingestion. Vitamin D probably exerts a calcemic effect on bone, and parathyroid hormone stimulates resorption of bone.

Excretion. *Calcium* and *phosphate* are excreted in the urine and feces. Most of the calcium in the feces is that which has escaped absorption. The rest is from digestive secretions. In 24 hours 100 to 150 mg. of calcium is excreted in the urine. Of the calcium filtered through the glomerulus, about 99 per cent is reabsorbed. The amount of reabsorption is apparently influenced by vitamin D and parathyroid hormone (see below). Urinary phosphate accounts for about 60 per cent of the total excretion under normal conditions. The rest is excreted in the feces. Phosphate is filtered through the glomerulus, and about four fifths is reabsorbed by the tubules, the remainder passing into the urine. The amount of urinary phosphate excretion is influenced by parathyroid hormone and vitamin D, as well as the glomerular filtration rate.

Regulations. Numerous factors govern the concentration of serum *calcium* and *phosphorus,* the most important being the parathyroid hormone. A fall in serum calcium stimulates the secretion of this hormone; as a consequence, calcium is mobilized from bone by resorption, calcium absorption from the intestine and the renal tubules is enhanced, and phosphate secretion by the renal tubules is increased, or its reabsorption by the renal tubules is inhibited. A rise in serum calcium stimulates the secretion of calcitonin from either the thyroid or parathyroid gland, returning the serum calcium to normal. Vitamin D influences serum calcium by raising intestinal absorption of calcium. In its absence the serum calcium may fall, with consequent stimulation of parathyroid activity and the series of in-

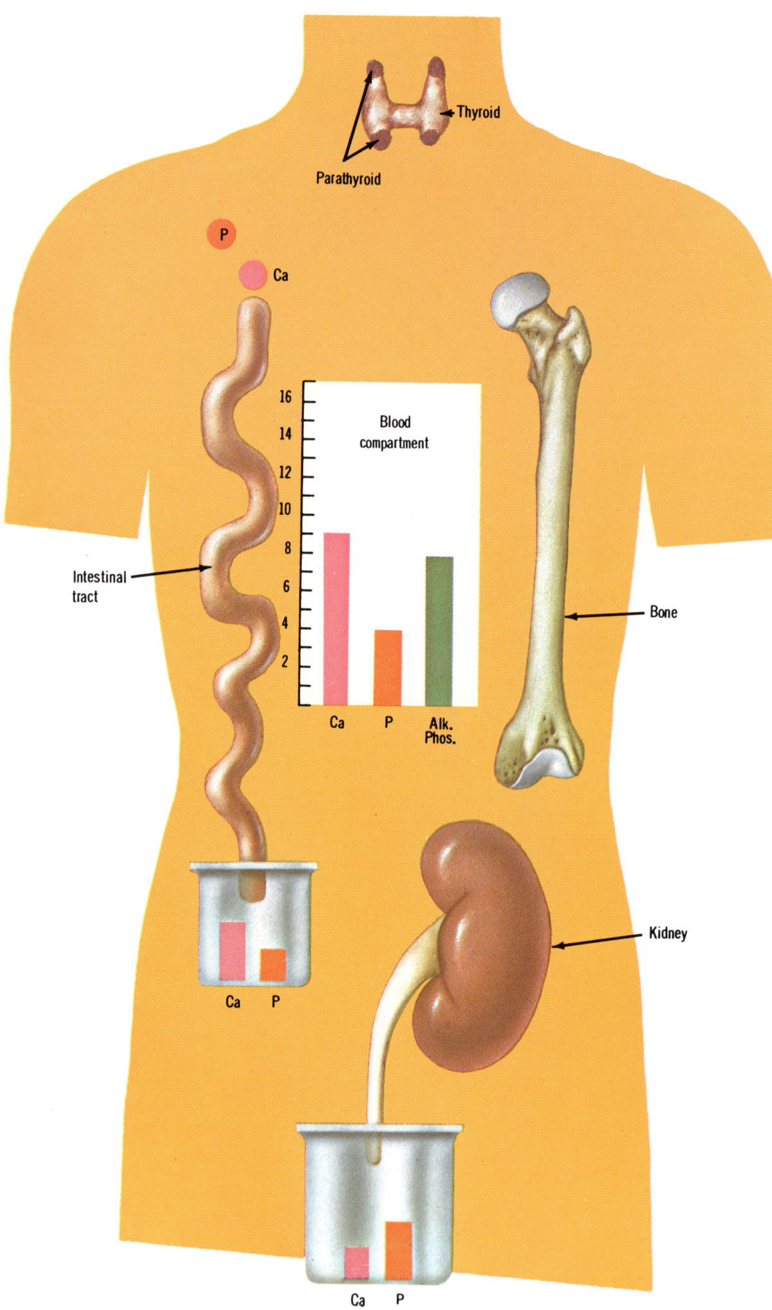

teractions previously outlined. The total serum concentration of calcium varies directly with the concentration of the serum protein. The ionizable fraction varies indirectly with the pH. A high pH (alkalosis) decreases the ionizable fraction, and a low pH (acidosis) increases it.

Alkaline Phosphatase. The metabolism of alkaline phosphatase is discussed elsewhere (p. 3). Because this enzyme is produced by osteoblasts, its serum concentration will rise whenever there is an increase in osteoblastic activity, as in the period following bone resorption.

THE APPROACH TO THE DIAGNOSIS

A disorder of calcium metabolism might be suspected whenever a patient presents with renal calculi, bone disease, convulsions, or tetany. Vague complaints such as malaise, fatigue, polyuria, or polydipsia might also suggest this disorder. Under these circumstances calcium, phosphate, and alkaline phosphatase determinations are routinely ordered. They should be repeated. In addition, a 24-hour urine calcium test is invariably indicated, preferably after a calcium-free diet for 3 days. An increased 24-hour urine calcium suggests hyperparathyroidism or renal tubular acidosis. A decreased 24-hour urine calcium suggests hypoparathyroidism, hypovitaminosis D, or malabsorption syndrome. Definitive diagnosis may be established by performing the various tests listed under each of these disorders. Radioimmunoassay of parathyroid hormone can now be done, but hopefully a more accurate method will be developed.

Body deficits of calcium, whether due to decreased intake or excessive output, induce the compensatory mechanism of secondary hyperparathyroidism. This confuses the blood picture by returning the calcium toward normal and often increasing the alkaline phosphatase. Conditions associated with this are thus made difficult to distinguish from primary hyperparathyroidism.

Abbreviations Used in Plates:

Ca = Calcium in mg. per 100 ml.

P = Phosphates in mg. per 100 ml.

Alk. Phos. = Alkaline phosphatase in King-Armstrong units

MALNUTRITION

In this disorder there is lack of dietary ingestion of calcium. Consequently, the serum *calcium tends to fall,* but this stimulates parathyroid activity (A) and, in turn, resorption of bone and renal tubular secretion of phosphate. Thus, *serum calcium* may be normal, but *serum phosphates drop,* and *alkaline phosphatase* often *rises.*

Summary of Laboratory Findings:

Serum calcium: Normal or decreased
Serum phosphates: Decreased
Serum alkaline phosphatase: Increased
Urine calcium: Decreased

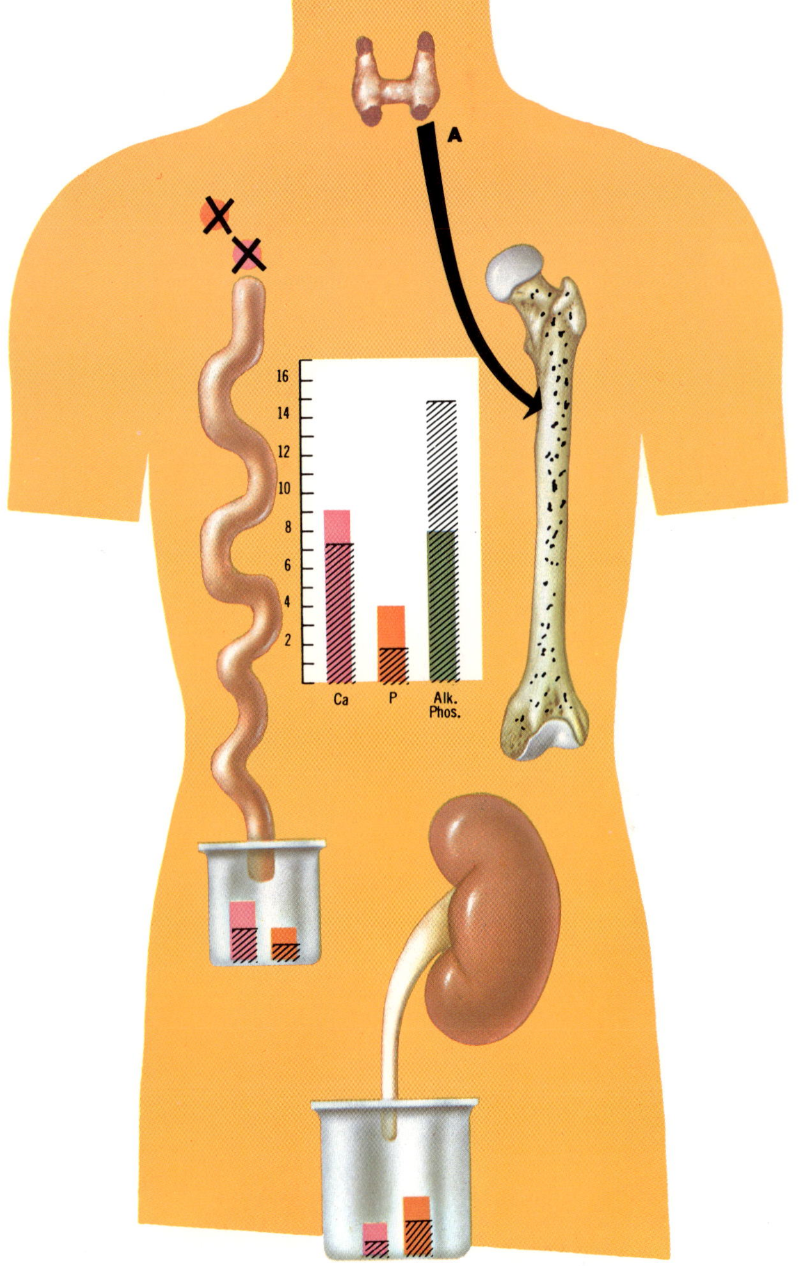

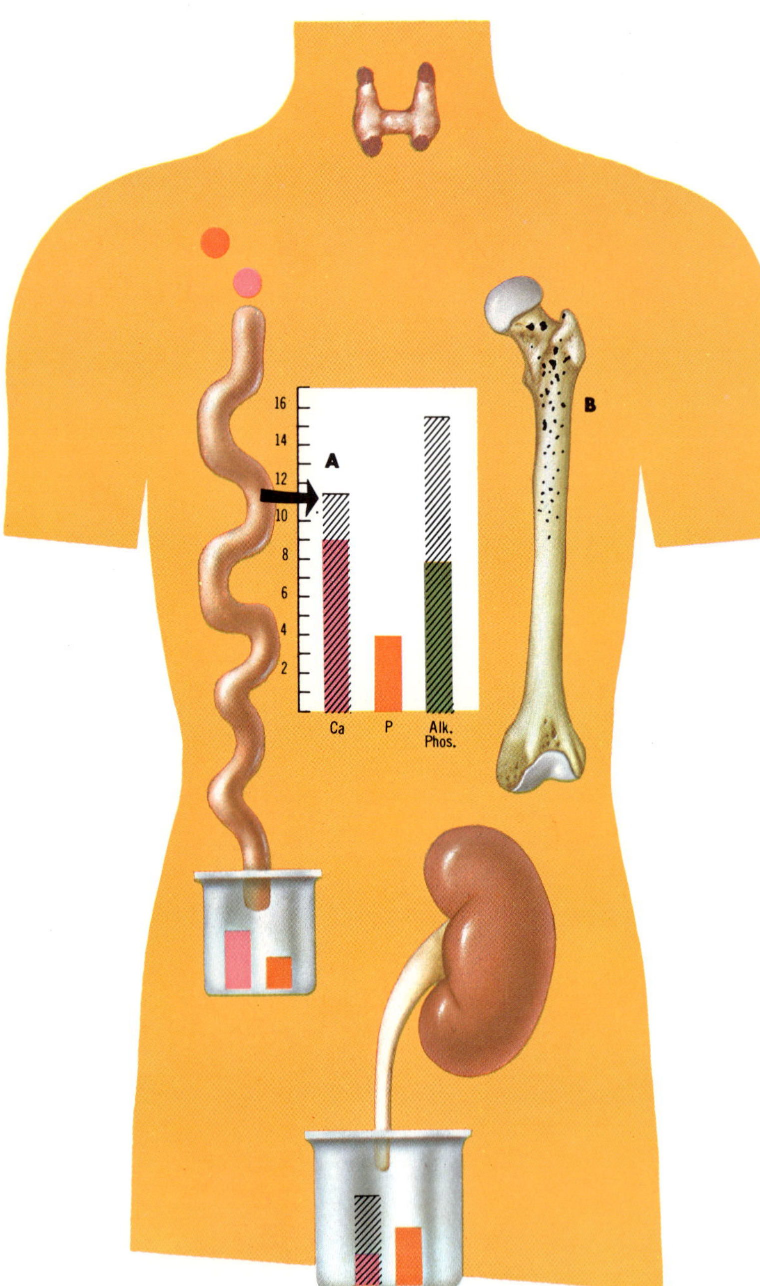

BOECK'S SARCOID

Increased sensitivity to vitamin D in this disorder promotes intestinal absorption of calcium (A) and *elevates* the *serum calcium*. Osteolytic lesions (B) may contribute to this change and also induce a *high alkaline phosphatase*. The diagnosis is confirmed by roentgenograms of the hands and chest, skin tests, and lymph node biopsy.

Summary of Laboratory Findings:

Serum calcium: Increased

Serum phosphates: Normal

Serum alkaline phosphatase: Increased

Urine calcium: Increased

HYPOVITAMINOSIS D

In this condition the daily intake of calcium may be normal, but the lack of sufficient vitamin D prevents adequate absorption of calcium, and it is excreted in the stool. Thus the *serum calcium* is characteristically *low* but may be normal. The low serum calcium stimulates the same series of events discussed under malnutrition (secondary hyperparathyroidism) (see p. 23). Thus the *blood phosphates* are often *lowered,* and the *alkaline phosphatase* is *elevated.* X-ray films of the long bones and a good response to vitamin D support the diagnosis.

Summary of Laboratory Findings:

Serum calcium: Normal or decreased
Serum Phosphates: Decreased
Serum Alkaline phosphatase: Increased
Urine calcium: Decreased

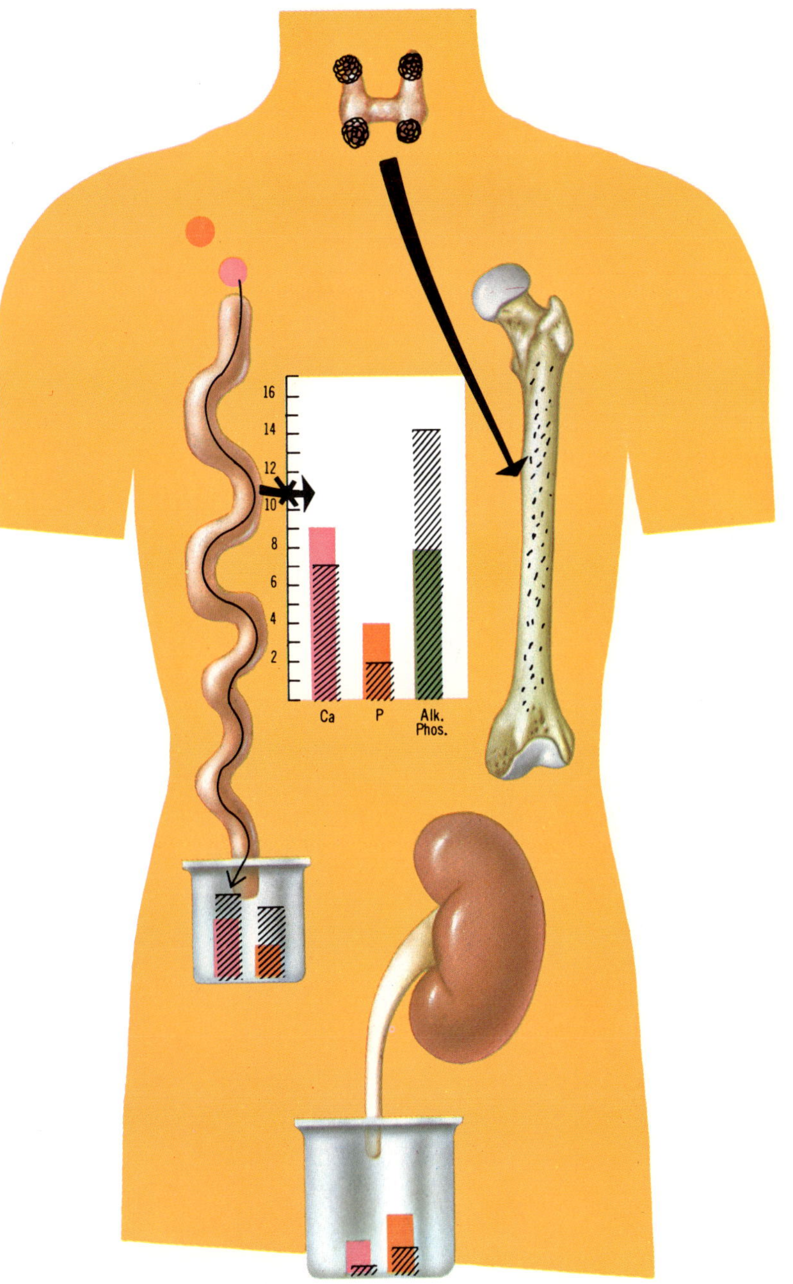

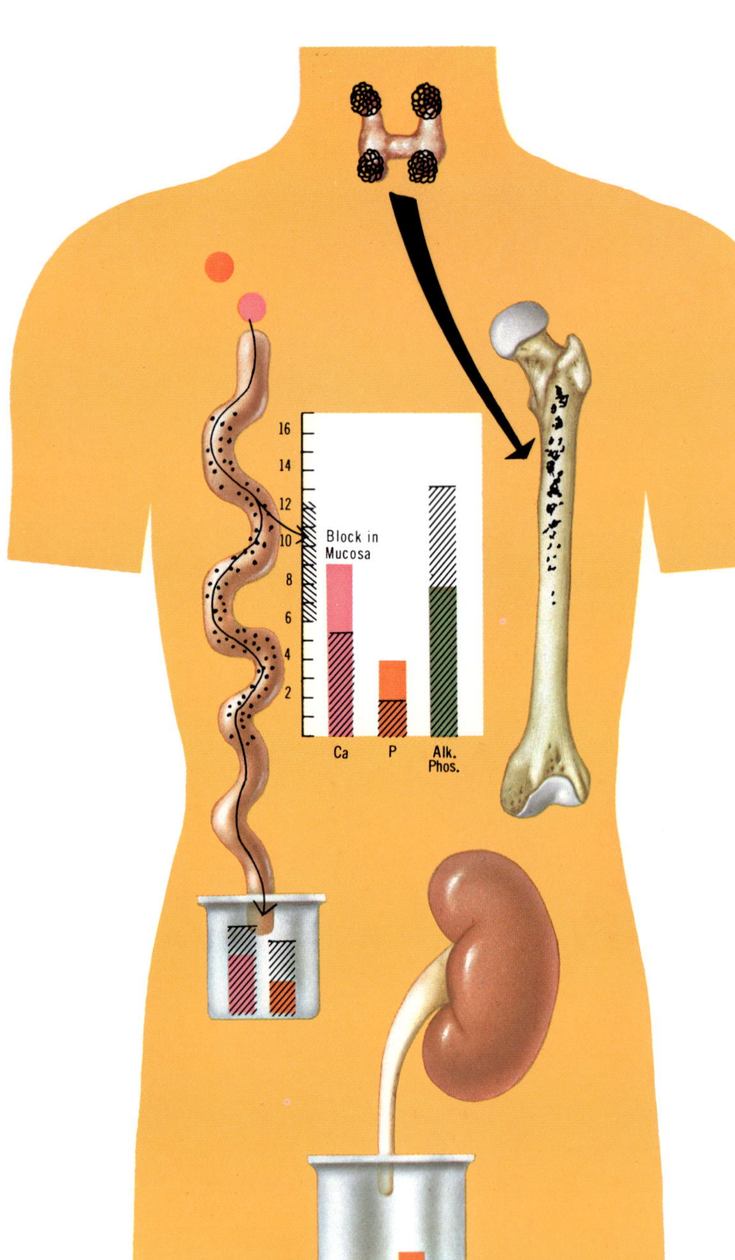

MALABSORPTION SYNDROME

Whether the result of inadequate breakdown of fat (as in pancreatic disease) or of inability to absorb broken down fat, the net effect is the retention of abnormal amounts of fat in the alimentary canal. The fat combines with calcium to form an insoluble nonabsorbable soap. The *serum calcium* is *reduced,* and secondary hyperparathyroidism ensues, with the resulting *changes* in *serum phosphates* and *alkaline phosphatase.* Fat-soluble vitamins (vitamin D, etc.) are poorly absorbed in this condition, further limiting calcium absorption. The diagnosis is confirmed by analysis of stool fat content, D-xylose absorption, and other tests (p. 41).

Summary of Laboratory Findings:

Serum calcium: Decreased

Serum phosphates: Decreased

Serum alkaline phosphatase: Increased

Urine calcium: Decreased

NEPHROTIC SYNDROME

The *serum calcium* is *lowered* in this disorder because of the associated reduction in serum proteins, which are lost in the urine (A). Because the ionizable fraction is not appreciably reduced in concentration, a secondary hyperparathyroidism does not result unless uremia develops. Urinalysis, renal function tests, serum cholesterol and protein electrophoresis, and renal biopsy help to establish the diagnosis.

Other causes of hypoproteinemia (cirrhosis of the liver, malnutrition, and malabsorption syndrome, etc.) may produce hypocalcemia on the same basis.

Summary of Laboratory Findings:

Serum calcium: Decreased

Serum phosphates: Normal

Serum alkaline phosphatase: Normal

Urine calcium: Normal

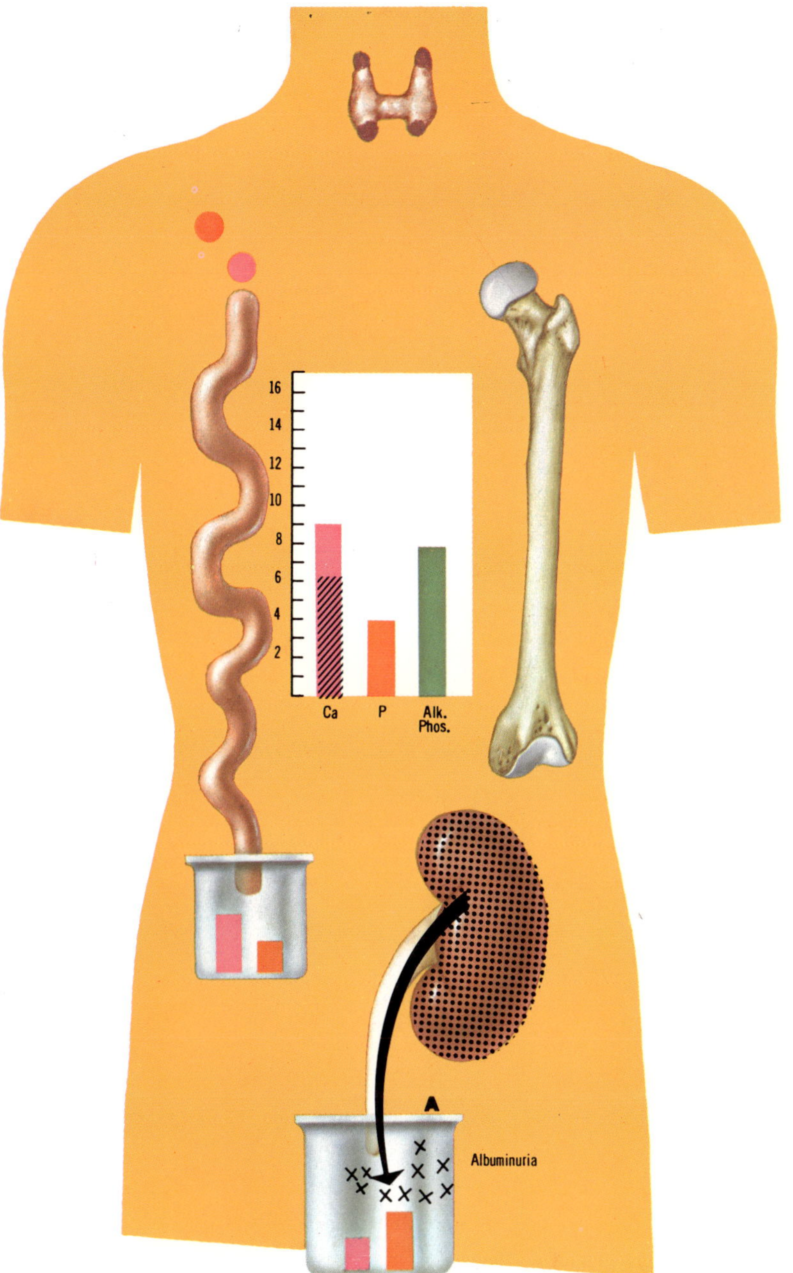

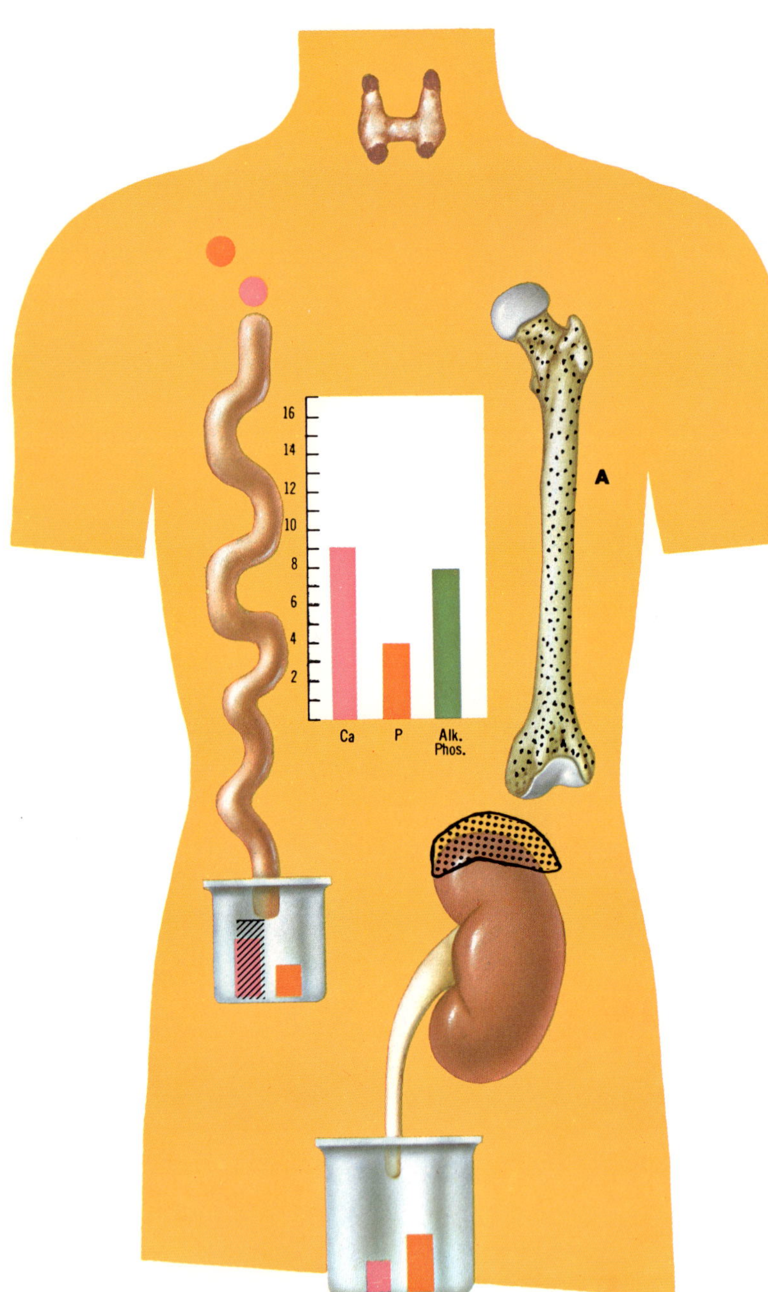

CUSHING'S SYNDROME

Excessive production of cortisol in this disorder impedes the formation of new bone, and consequently less calcium is deposited in the bone, resulting in osteoporosis (A). More of the dietary calcium is excreted in the urine and feces. The *blood level does not usually rise.* In addition, cortisol antagonizes the action of vitamin D on the intestinal mucosa, preventing calcium absorption. Definitive diagnosis is made by determination of plasma and urinary steroids (p. 92).

Other endocrine disorders may also be associated with osteoporosis.

Summary of Laboratory Findings:

Serum calcium: Normal

Serum phosphates: Normal

Serum alkaline phosphatase: Normal

Urine calcium: Normal

METASTATIC CARCINOMA OF THE BONE

The primary feature of this disorder is invasion and breakdown of bone with associated release of calcium into the blood. Calcium is readily excreted, and thus the *serum calcium* usually *does not rise.* However, on occasion the invasion is so massive that the serum calcium rises, and steroids are needed to bring the level of calcium down. The osteoblasts attempt to keep up with the breakdown, and thus there is an *elevated serum alkaline phosphatase.* The diagnosis is confirmed by roentgenograms and scans of the long bones and by bone biopsy.

Summary of Laboratory Findings:

Serum calcium: Increased or normal

Serum phosphates: Normal

Serum alkaline phosphatase: Increased

Urine calcium: Increased

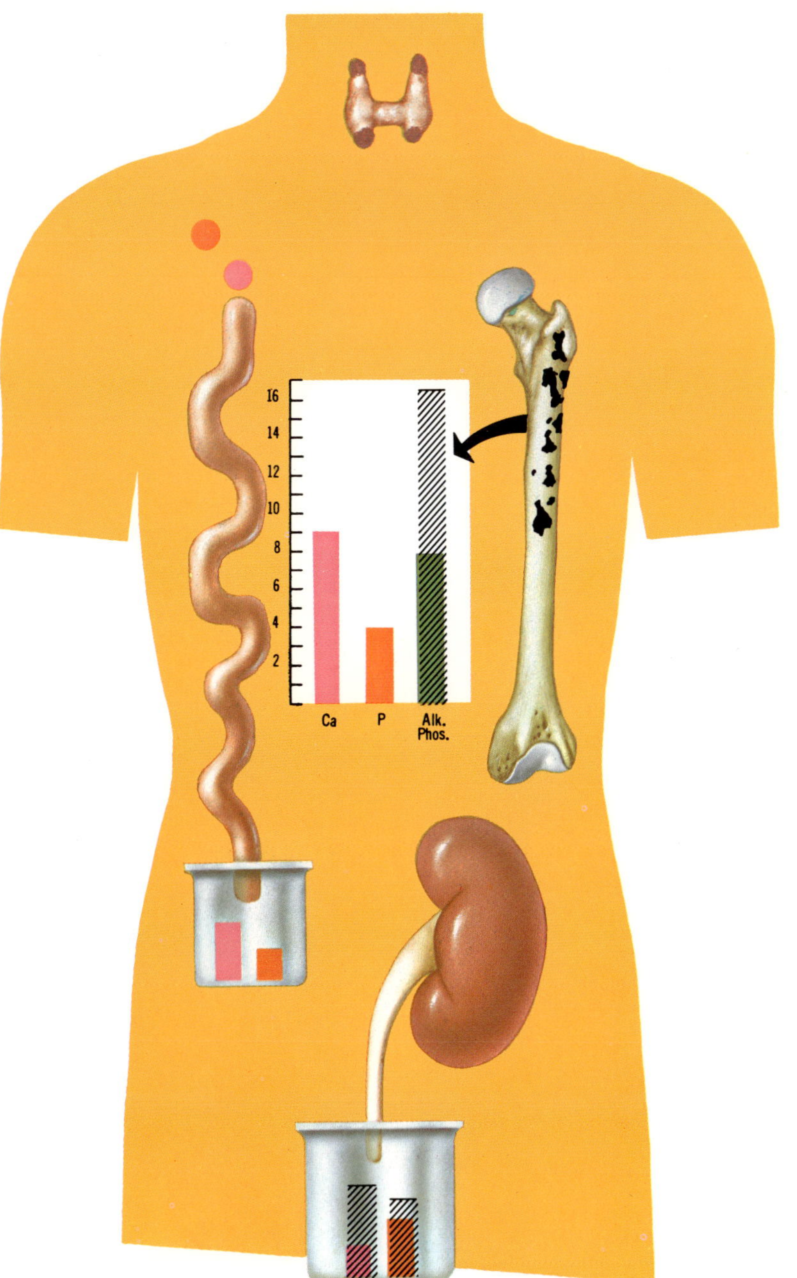

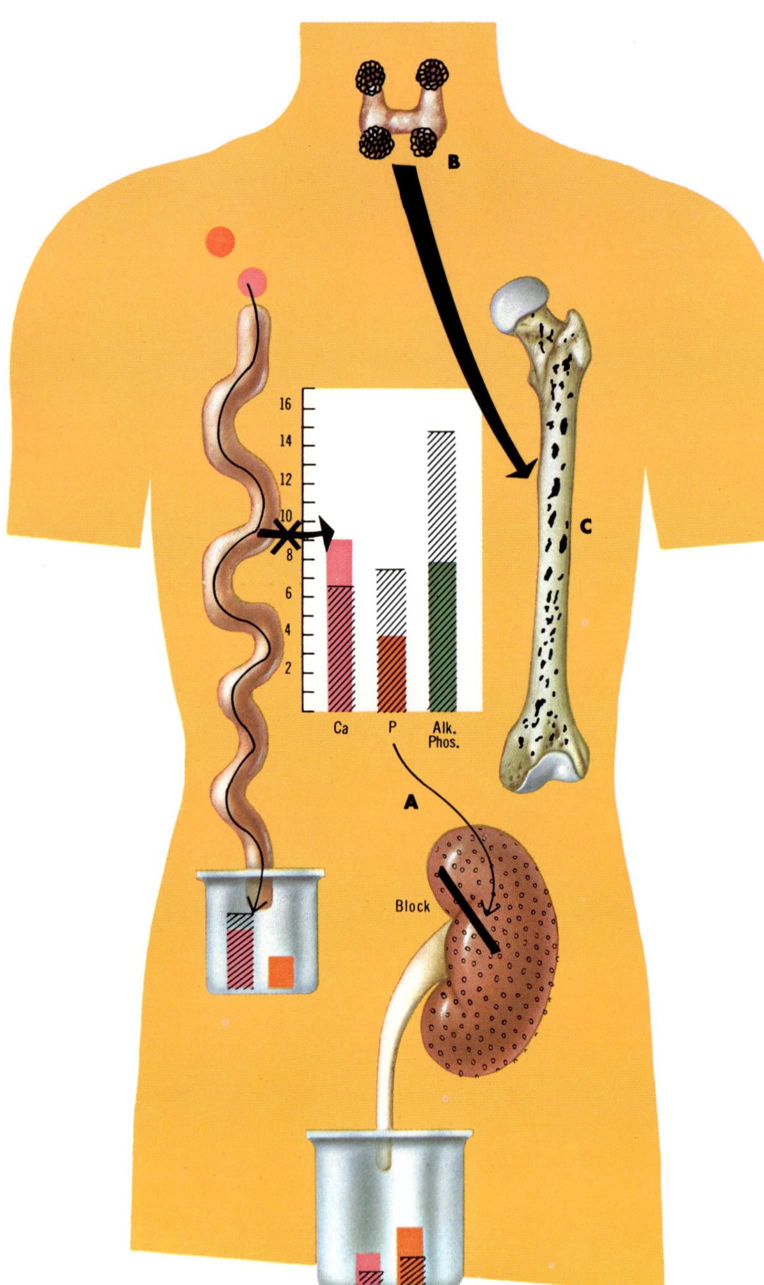

CHRONIC NEPHRITIS

In this disorder a decrease in renal clearance of phosphorus (A) results in a *high blood phosphate*. More of the phosphorus is excreted in the feces. In addition, intestinal absorption of calcium is impaired, and more dietary calcium passes into the feces. This is because the diseased kidneys cannot form the active metabolite of vitamin D, 1, 25-dihydroxycholecalciferol, from 25-OHCC (formed from vitamin D_3 in the liver). There is a *drop* in *blood calcium*, which activates the parathyroids (B), inducing bone resorption (C). A secondary osteoblastic reaction may occur, resulting in an elevated *alkaline phosphatase*. Radiographically, there may be a mixture of osteoporosis, osteomalacia, and osteitis fibrosa. Bone biopsy, response to vitamin D, and renal function tests are all useful in distinguishing this condition from primary hyperparathyroidism, but exploration of the neck may still be necessary because of the question, "Which came first, the chicken or the egg?" In other words, is the renal disease secondary to the hyperparathyroidism or is the hyperparathyroidism secondary to primary renal disease?

Summary of Laboratory Findings:

Serum calcium: Decreased

Serum phosphates: Increased

Serum alkaline phosphatase: Increased

Urine calcium: Decreased

RENAL TUBULAR ACIDOSIS

In this condition the renal tubular reabsorption of calcium and phosphates is defective (A), and these are lost in the urine. As a result, the *serum calcium* and *phosphate* may *drop*, and a secondary hyperparathyroidism can develop with the associated *increase* in *serum alkaline phosphatase* and attempt to return the serum calcium to normal. Diagnosis is established by the finding of acidosis, alkaline urine, and persistently high urine calcium and phosphates. With a limited calcium intake, rickets or osteomalacia may be found radiographically.

The Fanconi syndrome, hyperglobulinemia, amphotericin B toxicity, and acetazolamide therapy may produce a similar picture.

Summary of Laboratory Findings:

Serum calcium: Normal or decreased

Serum phosphates: Decreased

Serum alkaline phosphatase: Increased

Urine calcium: Increased

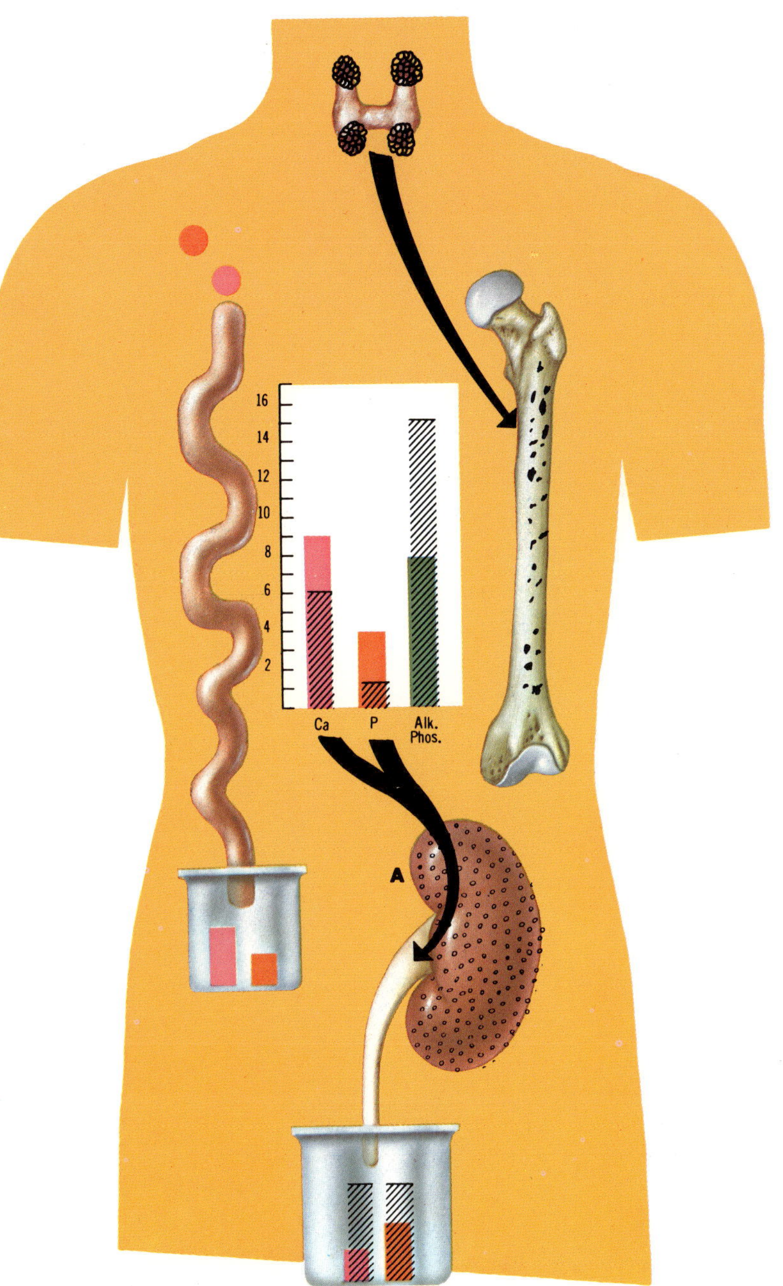

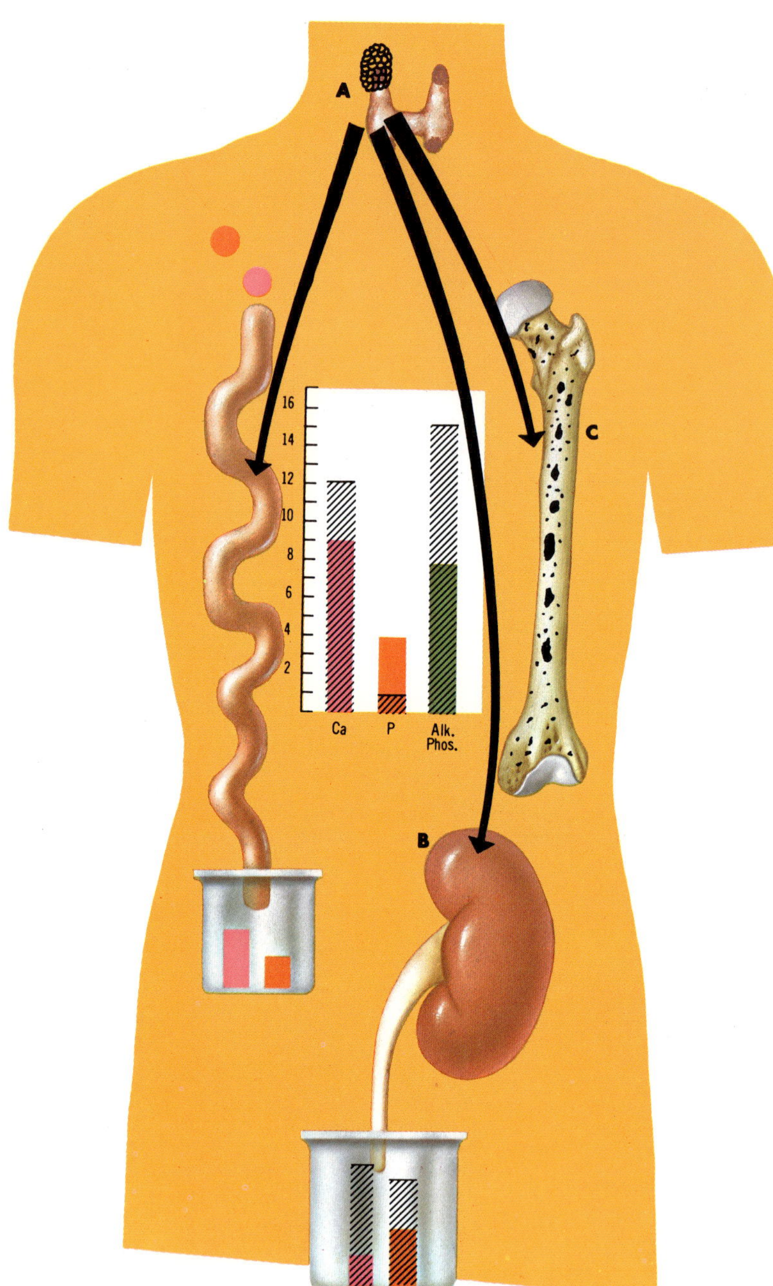

HYPERPARATHYROIDISM

Whether due to an adenoma (A) (90% of the cases), hyperplasia, or carcinoma (rare), this disorder is associated with increased secretion of parathyroid hormone. The parathyroid hormone elevates the serum calcium by accelerating bone resorption and increasing renal tubular and intestinal absorption of calcium.* It *lowers* the *serum phosphates* by accelerating renal tubular secretion (B) of phosphates or inhibiting their reabsorption. The *alkaline phosphatase* may be *elevated* from the secondary osteoblastic reaction to bony resorption (C). The *24-hour urine calcium* is *elevated,* a reflection of the bony resorption and the increased intestinal absorption of calcium.

The diagnosis is substantiated by radiological findings of osteitis fibrosa cystica and/or nephrocalcinosis, as well as absence of the lamina dura of the teeth. In doubtful cases a cortisone suppression test or estimation of the bone turnover rate with radioactive calcium should be done. Cortisone will not lower the serum calcium in patients with hyperparathyroidism. Another excellent test to help confirm the diagnosis is the phosphate reabsorption test. An index value of less than 80% indicates diminished tubular reabsorption of phosphate and suggests the diagnosis. Radioimmunoassay of parthormone can be done but is not reliable, and therefore it should not be used routinely.

Summary of Laboratory Findings:

Serum calcium: Increased

Serum phosphates: Decreased

Serum alkaline phosphatase: Increased

Urine calcium: Increased

* Duncan, G. G.: Diseases of Metabolism. ed. 5, p. 250. Philadelphia, W. B. Saunders, 1964.

HYPOPARATHYROIDISM

In the absence of parathyroid hormone there is a decrease in renal tubular secretion of phosphate, causing a *high serum phosphate.* Moreover, the decrease in intestinal absorption, renal tubular reabsorption, and bony resorption of calcium causes a *low serum calcium.* The *alkaline phosphatase* is, quite logically, *normal.* These tests establish the diagnosis in the majority of cases. In doubtful cases the response to intravenous loading with calcium may be determined. Normally, *plasma phosphate rises,* whereas urine phosphate drops, but in hypoparathyroidism there is a brisk phosphate diuresis. Another excellent test for doubtful cases is to measure the 24-hour urine calcium after the patient consumes sodium phytate orally for 3 days. This will depress absorption of calcium, and the hypoparathyroid individual cannot compensate for this and so will excrete very little calcium in the urine.

Pseudohypoparathyroidism produces a similar picture. It may be differentiated by the Ellsworth-Howard test, in which parathyroid hormone is injected intravenously. The renal tubular cells of these subjects do not respond to parathyroid hormone, and so they do not demonstrate a phosphate diuresis. However, hypoparathyroid subjects will. Increased secretion of thyrocalcitonin, as occurs in medullary carcinoma of the thyroid, may also lower the serum calcium, but the phosphorus will be low also.

Summary of Laboratory Findings:

Serum calcium: Decreased
Serum phosphates: Increased
Serum alkaline phosphatase: Normal
Urine calcium: Decreased

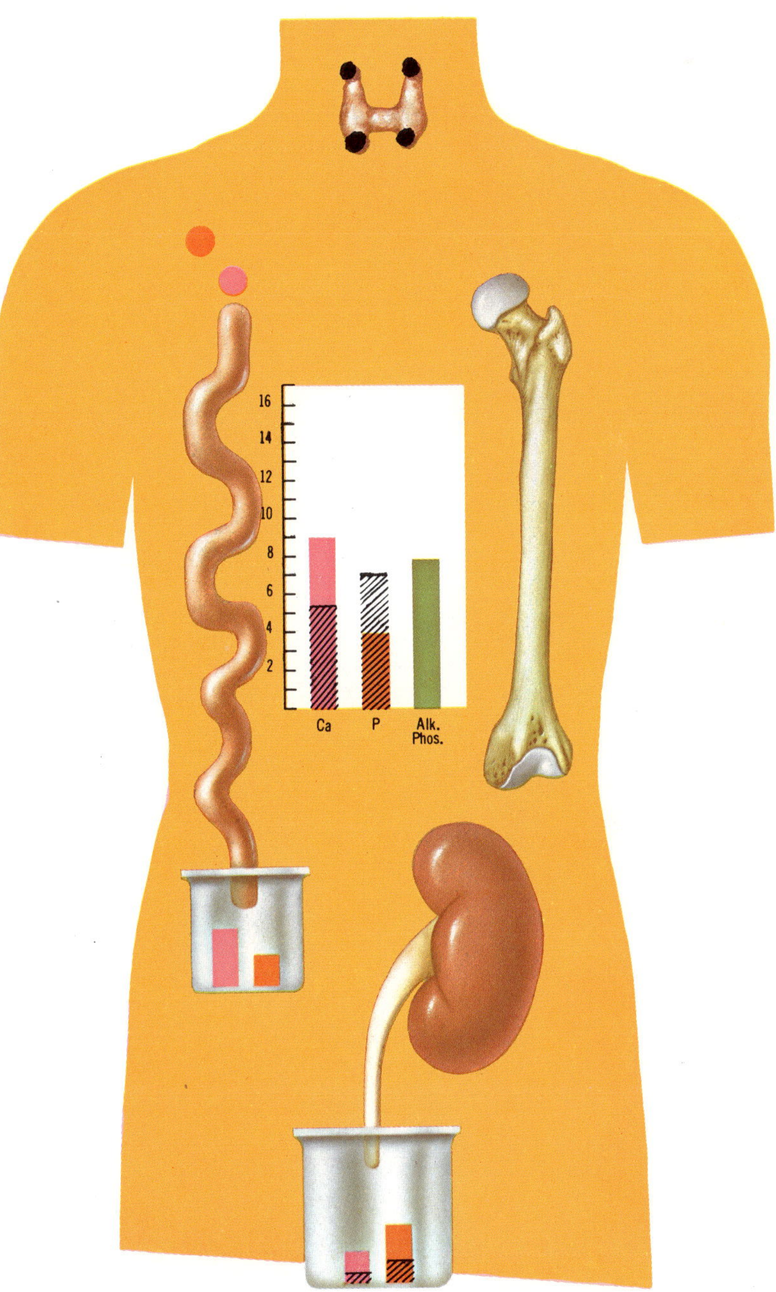

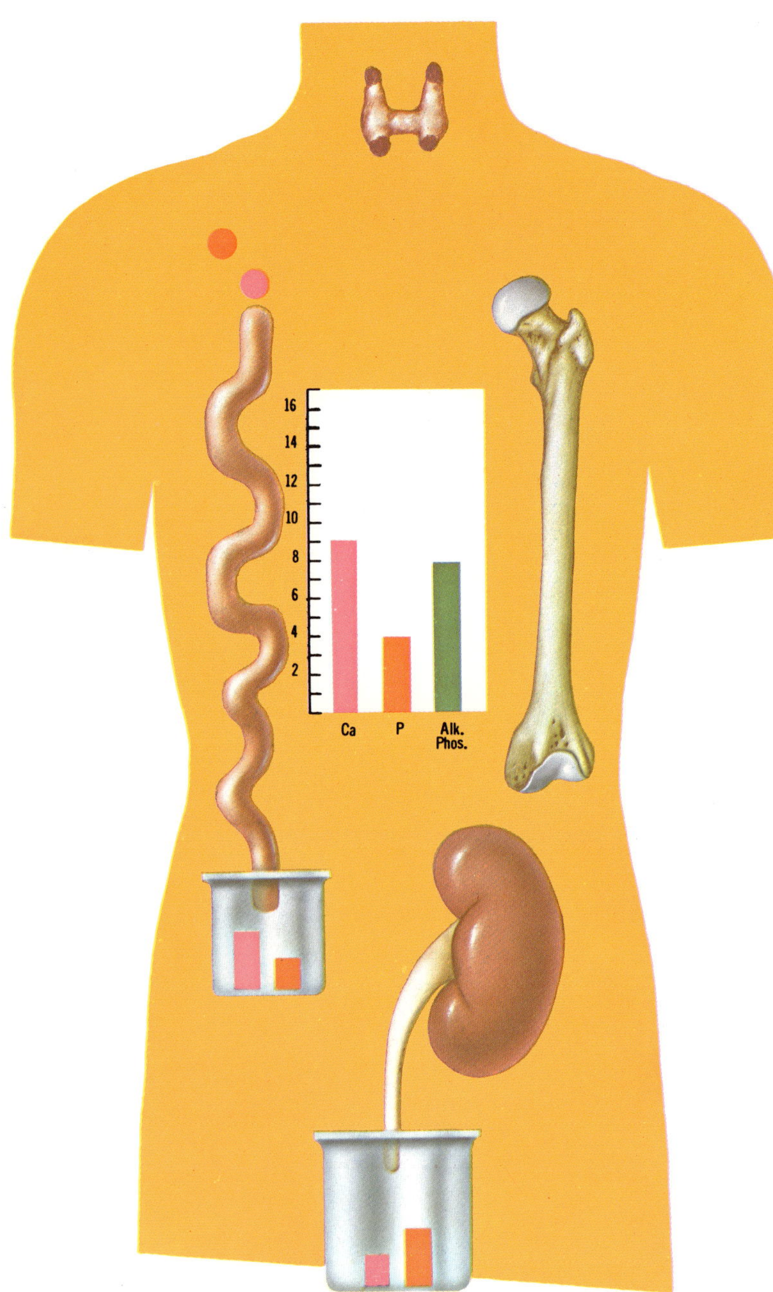

PSEUDOPSEUDOHYPOPARATHYROIDISM

This reader will note that the *calcium* and *phosphate* are *normal* in this disorder, but that the alkaline phosphatase may be reduced. These subjects have the physical appearance of those with pseudo-hypoparathyroidism (short statue, short fingers, etc.) without the disturbed calcium metabolism.

Summary of Laboratory Findings:

Serum calcium: Normal

Serum phosphates: Normal

Serum alkaline phosphatase: Normal or decreased

4 Disorders of Blood Electrolytes

Since the blood electrolytes, sodium, potassium, chloride, and bicarbonate, as well as water, so frequently alter reciprocally in disease processes, they will be considered together. An extra block is left vacant in the drawing to display either foreign anions or those anions that play a significant role only in isolated disease states. Aside from bicarbonate, intake of each of these ions should be equivalent to output under healthy circumstances.

NORMAL METABOLISM*

Intake. Sodium, potassium, water, and chloride enter the body by ingestion with foodstuffs. In this manner the average normal adult ingests 70 to 100 mEq. of potassium, 69 to 208 mEq. of sodium and chloride, and 1,500 to 3,000 ml. of water daily. Carbon dioxide is, of course, not ingested.

Absorption. Potassium, sodium, chloride, and water are all probably absorbed by an as yet unknown active diffusion process. The absorption of water may be influenced by adrenocortical hormone.

Transport. All the major electrolytes and water are transported in the blood and lymphatics. The power for their transport is supplied primarily by the heart and the skeletal muscle. The normal concentrations are: sodium, 135 to 147 mEq./liter; potassium, 3.5 to 5.0 mEq./liter; chloride, 100 to 106 mEq./liter; bicarbonate, 24 to 30 mEq./liter. A large amount of carbon dioxide is transported inside the red cells.

Production. Carbon dioxide and water are products of body metabolism of carbohydrate, fat, and protein. Approximately 300 ml. of water is produced in this manner each day. Sodium, chloride, and potassium, on the other hand, are fully exogenous in origin, but potassium and water are released from storage by cellular catabolism.

Storage. *Sodium* and *chloride* exist primarily in the extracellular and intravascular space in practically equivalent concentrations, but there are 35 mEq./liter of sodium and 25 mEq./liter of chloride in the cells. In addition, a sizable amount of sodium is deposited in the bone and can be released as a safety device in acidosis.

Potassium, on the other hand, is mainly an intracellular cation. Its concentration here is approximately 160 mEq./liter. Potassium may be released into the extracellular space by catabolism. Its concentration extracellularly is essentially the same as that in the blood. Potassium moves into the cell with the absorption of glucose.

Bicarbonate is an extracellular ion, in concentration similar to that of the blood, but a ready supply is constantly pouring in from the catabolism of carbohydrate, protein, and fat. Of course, this is at first carbon dioxide, then carbonic acid, and thereafter much of it is transformed to sodium bicarbonate by the buffers of the plasma and red cell.

Water in the amount equivalent to 40 per cent of body weight is stored intracellularly, and an amount equivalent to 15 to 20 per cent of body weight is stored extracellularly.

Secretion. Over 8 L. of fluid are secreted and reabsorbed in the gastrointestinal tract each day. Ordinarily, this is of little clinical significance. However, this allows for a sizable exodus of water and electrolytes in pathological conditions associated with vomiting and diarrhea. The four types of secretions, gastric, biliary, pancreatic, and small intestinal, all contain sodium, potassium, chloride, and bicarbonate, but in different concentrations. The values of each of these appear in Table 4-1.

It is not necessary to know the exact concentrations of these ions in the various secretions for practical purposes. However, one should keep in mind that the gastric juice contains little or no bicarbonate

* See plate on p. 38.

Table 4-1. Concentration of Electrolytes in Four Types of Body Secretions*

Fluid	Na+ *mEq./L.*	K+ *mEq./L.*	$-HCO_3$ *mEq./L.*	Cl− *mEq./L.*
Stomach	20-100	5-25		90-155
Pancreas	110-150	3-10	70-110	40-80
Bile	120-150	3-12	30-50	80-120
Small Intestine	80-150	2-10	20-40	90-131

* Duncan, G. G. (ed.): Diseases of Metabolism. ed. 5. Philadelphia, W. B. Saunders, 1964.

but large amounts of hydrogen and chloride ion, whereas the pancreatic, biliary, and intestinal fluids contain substantial amounts of bicarbonate but little hydrogen ion. All of these secretions contain sizable amounts of potassium, but gastric secretions contain significantly more than the others.

Excretion. The excretion of sodium, potassium, chloride, and water ordinarily is equivalent to intake, so that an equilibrium is maintained. The kidney, the major excretory organ, excretes in the urine 80 to 90 per cent of the sodium, potassium, and chloride that is ingested. This amounts to about 111 mEq. of sodium, 119 mEq. of chloride, and 25 to 100 mEq. of potassium in 24 hours. Although the kidney can reduce sodium chloride excretion to a bare minimum in deficiency states, significant potassium excretion continues.

The remainder of these electrolytes is lost in the sweat and stools. The sweat contains these electrolytes at hypotonic concentrations. There are approximately 10 to 80 mEq./liter of sodium and chloride and 1 to 15 mEq./liter of potassium in sweat.

Bicarbonate is excreted by the kidney in varying amounts according to body needs. Carbon dioxide, on the other hand, is excreted by the lungs (see below).

Unlike the electrolytes, the greater part of the water ingested daily may not be excreted by the kidney in the normal adult. Approximately 800 ml. is lost by way of the lungs and the skin by vaporization (insensible perspiration). Varying with the body and environmental temperature and humidity, the sensible water loss through sweating can be negligible or up to 8 L. a day. Nevertheless, the average adult excretes between 600 and 1,600 ml. of water in the urine each day, the amount depending on ingestion and the quantity of waste solutes to be excreted.

In disease states in which the body needs to conserve water, insensible water loss through the lungs and skin, as well as the obligatory water loss through the kidney in the excretion of wastes, continues. Thus the body compensatory mechanisms for water loss are limited.

Regulation

Several regulatory mechanisms have been hinted at in the above discussion. Two organs, the *kidney* and the *lung,* are primarily responsible for the control of body fluid, electrolyte and acid-base balance. Although variable amounts of fluid and electrolytes may be lost by way of the sweat glands and the gastrointestinal tract, these organs do not adjust their rate of secretion to meet body fluid and electrolyte requirements. Ingestion of fluid in response to thirst is important in maintaining water balance but of little effect on electrolyte equilibrium.

The Kidney

The kidney, under the influence of aldosterone hormone from the zona glomerulosa of the adrenal cortex and the antidiuretic hormone (ADH) from the posterior pituitary, plays a major role in the regulation of the tonicity, volume, and acidity of body fluids. The mechanism of this control is fascinating.

Tonicity. If the plasma, and hence the glomerular filtrate (a protein-free plasma filtrate with the same electrolyte composition as plasma), is hypertonic, the osmoreceptors in the supraoptic nucleus are stimulated to release antidiuretic hormone (ADH). This activates the distal tubule to reabsorb more water from the filtrate, diluting the blood and concentrating the urine. If the plasma is hypotonic, then the secretion of ADH is inhibited, and the distal tubule reabsorbs less water from the filtrate, concentrating the blood and diluting the urine.

Volume. If the blood and the extracellular fluid are low in volume, volume receptors, probably located in the juxta-glomerular apparatus, secrete renin which activates angiotensin to stimulate the adrenal cortex to secrete aldosterone, and more sodium is reabsorbed from the filtrate in exchange for potassium and hydrogen ions. The resulting hypertonicity of the plasma will lead to ADH secretion and water retention, as described above. Thus the volume is returned to normal. A large plasma volume will lead to suppression of aldosterone secretion in like manner, with a consequent decrease in tubular reabsorption of sodium. Intravascular and extracellular volume is adjusted by the intracellular volume in many disease states. When there is water loss with resulting hypertonicity of extracellular fluid, water moves out of the cell. When there is excess extracellular water and hypotonicity, the reverse occurs.

Acidity. Were it not for the remarkable homeostatic mechanisms in the kidney, the blood would quickly become acid. In the first place, the average diet contains substances with acid end-products (ammonium salts, sulfur containing amino acids, phosphoric acid compound). Furthermore, carbon dioxide is constantly being poured into the blood as an end-product of cellular metabolism. To a lesser degree, keto-acids are being produced in fat metabolism. These substances are buffered by the bicarbonate, phosphate, and other buffer systems so that the blood pH does not change radically from the normal range of 7.30 to 7.45. These buffers must be maintained, particularly the sodium bicarbonate. The kidney and lung are primarily responsible for this.

The kidney's part of the job is to recover bicarbonate and sodium from the glomerular filtrate. The kidney accomplishes this by three mechanisms: (1) by reabsorbing all the sodium bicarbonate from the glomerular filtrate, (2) by acidifying urinary buffer salts such as disodium phosphate, and (3) by excreting hydrogen ion as the ammonium salt of strong acids.

All three mechanisms are based on one fundamental process. This is the tubular secretion of hydrogen ion in exchange for sodium in the tubular urine. A readily available source of hydrogen ion is provided by the conversion of water and carbon dioxide to carbonic acid under the influence of carbonic anhydrase in the tubular cell. The hydrogen ion of the carbonic acid is then exchanged for the sodium of sodium bicarbonate, sodium disphosphate, and strong acid salts (e.g., sodium chloride) of the glomerular filtrate in the following manner:

$$NaHCO_3 \xrightarrow{H^+} H_2CO_3 + Na^+$$
$$Na_2HPO_4 \xrightarrow{H^+} NaH_2PO_4 + Na^+$$
$$NaCl \xrightarrow[NH_3]{H^+} NH_4Cl + Na^+$$

(Ammonium is added by the tubular cells in the last equation.)

The sodium released by these mechanisms combines with the bicarbonate of the tubular cell and enters the blood as sodium bicarbonate. In alkalotic states all of the above mechanisms may be depressed to a varying degree, with consequent excretion of sodium and bicarbonate, etc., and an alkaline urine.

The Lung

Extra carbon dioxide produced by the metabolism of carbohydrate, fat, and protein or the buffering of acids stimulates the respiratory center to increase respirations, so that the extra carbon dioxide is excreted through the lung, and the pH is maintained. The rate and depth of respiration may be doubled, with an increase of pCO_2 of as little as 0.3 per cent. In disorders of acid-base balance the respiration rate can be increased or decreased in this way to bring the pH back to normal.

Other Mechanisms

Water excretion may be influenced by thyroid hormone, which increases urine solute by increasing both catabolism and the oral intake of food stuffs.

The electrolyte composition of the extracellular fluid may be altered by the pH of the blood through other than renal mechanisms. For example, in acidosis hydrogen ion moves into the cell in exchange for potassium. In alkalosis sodium ion moves into the cell in exchange for potassium, which is then excreted. Thus the cell itself becomes an effective buffer.

THE DIAGNOSTIC APPROACH

The laboratory study of an electrolyte disorder is of value only when correlated with a clinical appraisal of the state of hydration, body weight, intake and output, past and present, and acid-base equilibrium. Ocular tension, periocular wrinkling, skin turgor, and the appearance of the tongue and urine will establish the state of hydration. Inquiry regarding diet and fluid intake, previous vomiting, diarrhea, hyperventilation, polyuria or oliguria will assist in estimating past losses or gains of fluid and electrolytes. Observing the rate and depth of respiration will often give a clue to the blood pH. These clinical data give meaning to the *laboratory determinations* of *serum sodium, chloride, carbon dioxide combining power, potassium,* and *protein.* These tests, along with urinary specific gravity and pH, establish the diagnosis in most cases. In doubtful cases arterial blood

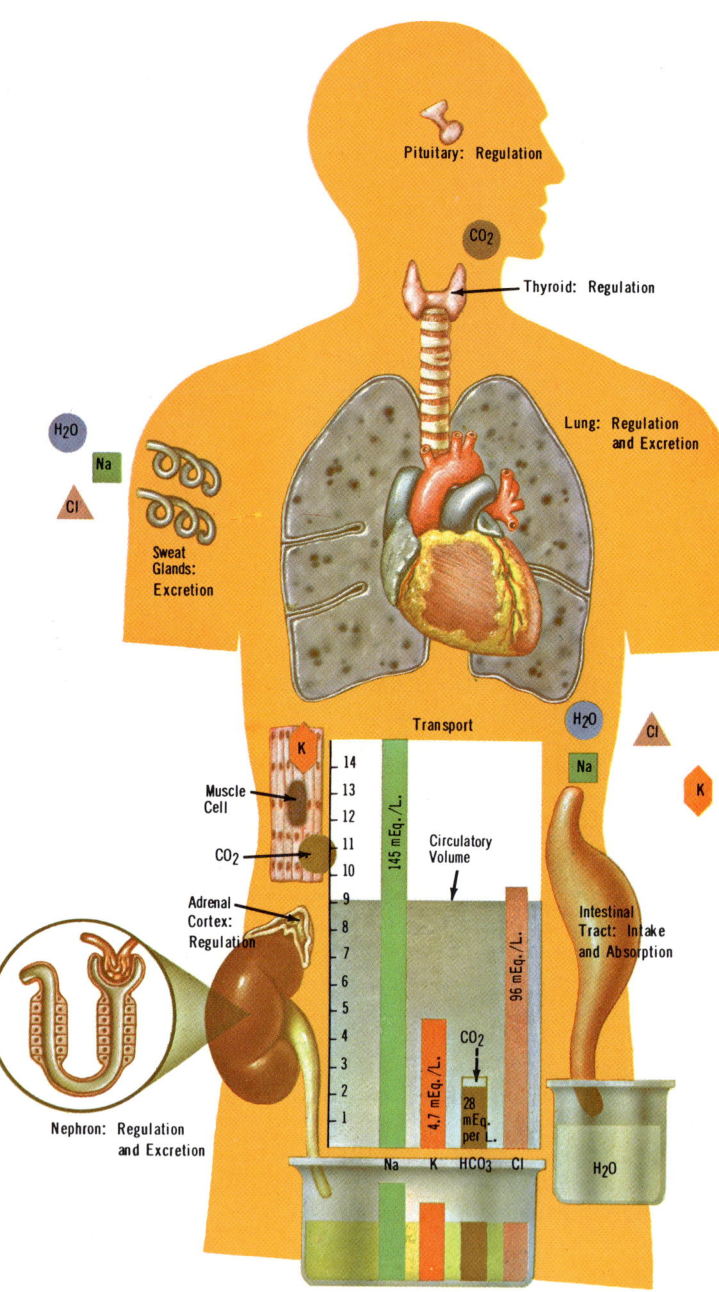

gases and pH and 24-hour urine sodium, chloride, and potassium are invaluable.

Repeated determinations of blood electrolytes and recording of the intake and output will be rewarding. The change in these values may often be more significant than single determinations. An ECG will be of assistance in evaluating changes in body potassium. Blood volume and venous pressure will give a clue to dehydration or circulatory overload.

A word of caution is indicated. It should be remembered that these tests are determinations of electrolyte concentrations, and therefore they are not absolute values but vary with the circulatory volume and other factors. Accordingly, they give no direct knowledge of the total amount of the electrolyte in question. In addition, these values are a reflection of only a small quantity of the total body fluid, and intracellular electrolyte concentrations are almost impossible to determine.

Abbreviations Used in Plates:

Na = Sodium in mEq. per liter × 10
K = Potassium in mEq. per liter
HCO_3 = Bicarbonate ion in mEq. per liter × 10
Cl = Chloride in mEq. per liter × 10

DEHYDRATION

Decreased oral intake of water leads to depletion of intracellular and extracellular body water stores because the obligatory loss of water through the skin, lung, and kidney continues. Blood levels of *electrolytes*, particularly *sodium* and *chloride, increase* markedly. This is quite conceivable in view of the resulting hemoconcentration, but in addition tubular reabsorption of sodium and chloride is enhanced by the stimulus of a contracted circulatory volume on the "osmoreceptor-aldosterone" system. Urine volume drops, whereas the concentration of urine solutes rises.

Summary of Laboratory Findings:

Serum sodium: Increased
Serum potassium: Normal
Serum bicarbonate: Normal or decreased
Serum chlorides: Increased
Blood volume: Decreased
Urine sodium: Increased
Urine potassium: Increased
Urine pH: Decreased
Urine volume: Decreased

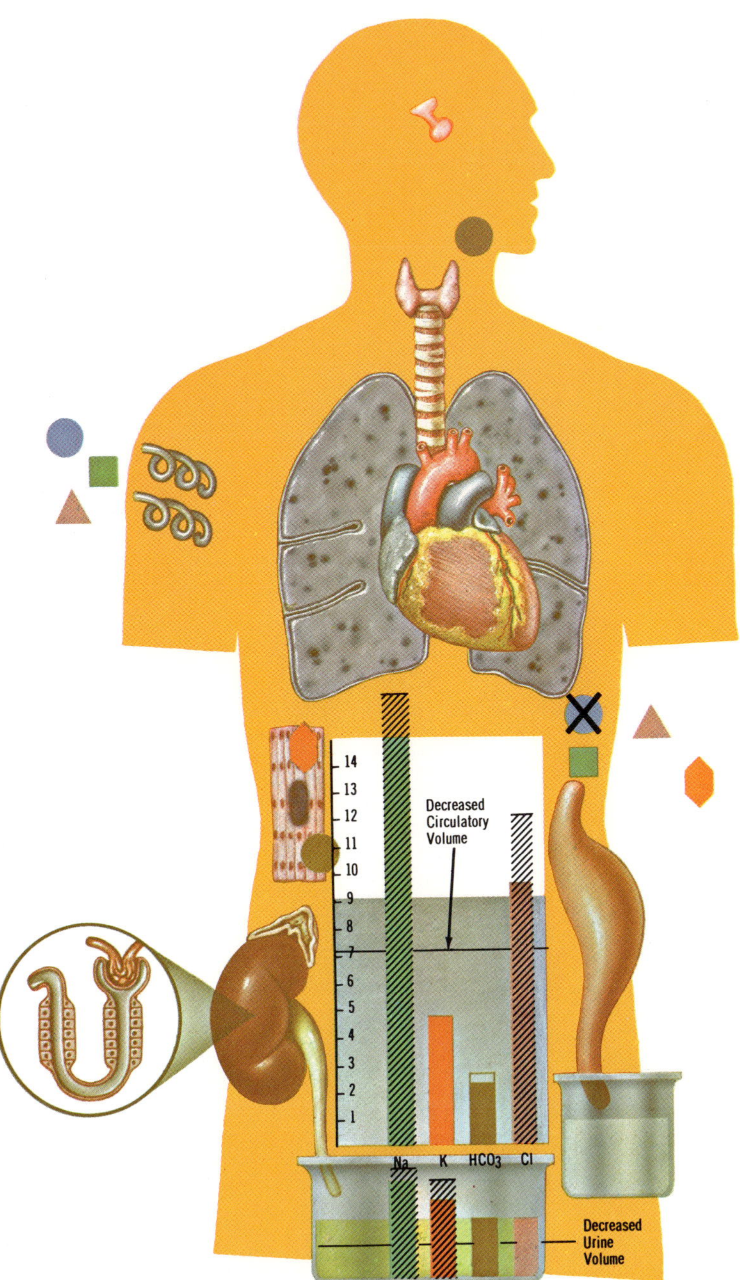

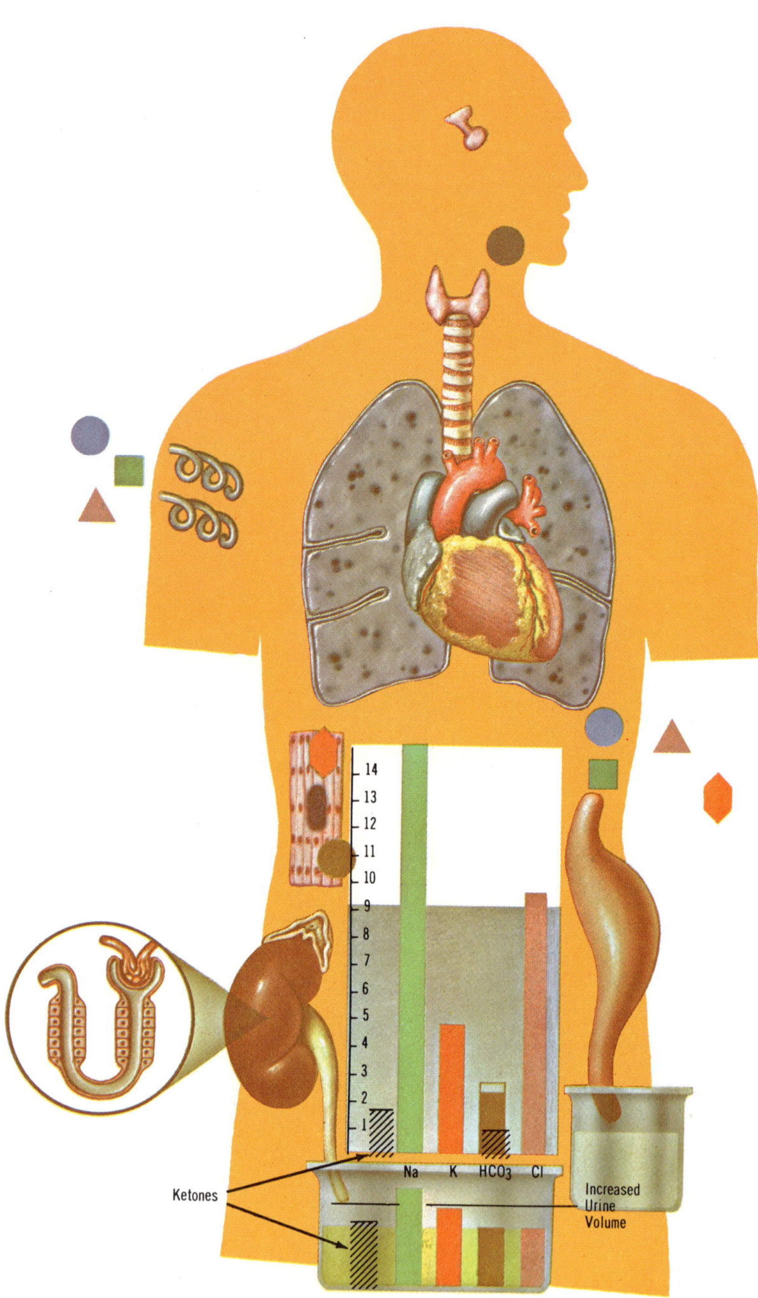

STARVATION

The major alteration in starvation is the addition of *organic acids* to the *blood electrolytes,* as in diabetic acidosis. With the lack of carbohydrate intake and the depletion of glycogen stores, the cells are forced to rely on fats, proteins, and their breakdown products, the ketones, for energy. As in diabetic acidosis, the supply of keto-acids exceeds the demands of the cells, and the *plasma levels* of these *organic acids rise.* Plasma *bicarbonate decreases,* since it is utilized in neutralizing these acids. However, the by-product, carbon dioxide, is blown off by the lungs, so that the resulting metabolic acidosis is well compensated.

Summary of Laboratory Findings:

Serum sodium: Normal
Serum potassium: Normal
Serum bicarbonate: Decreased
Serum chlorides: Normal
Blood volume: Normal or decreased
Urine sodium: Normal or increased
Urine potassium: Increased or normal
Urine pH: Decreased
Urine volume: Increased and urine contains ketones

MALABSORPTION SYNDROME

The poor absorption of water and salts in this disorder (A) leads to *hyponatremia, hypokalemia,* and a drop in circulatory volume. Obviously not all cases of the malabsorption syndrome are severe enough to present this picture. Serum carotene affords a good screening test for this disease, but D-xylose absorption, urine 5-HIAA (5-hydroxyindoleacetic acid), and mucosal biopsy are best for establishing the diagnosis.

Summary of Laboratory Findings:

Serum sodium: Decreased
Serum potassium: Decreased
Serum bicarbonate: Normal or decreased
Serum chlorides: Normal
Blood volume: Decreased
Urine sodium: Decreased
Urine potassium: Decreased
Urine pH: Normal or decreased
Urine volume: Normal

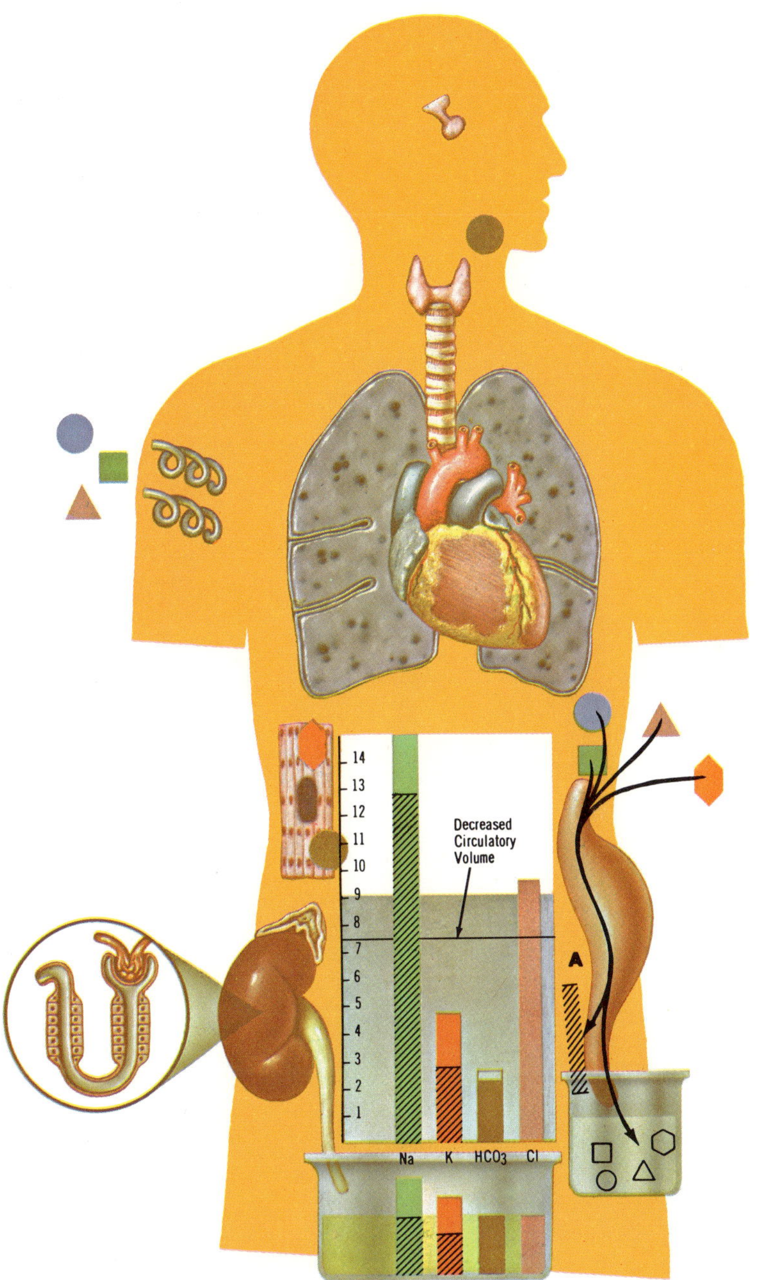

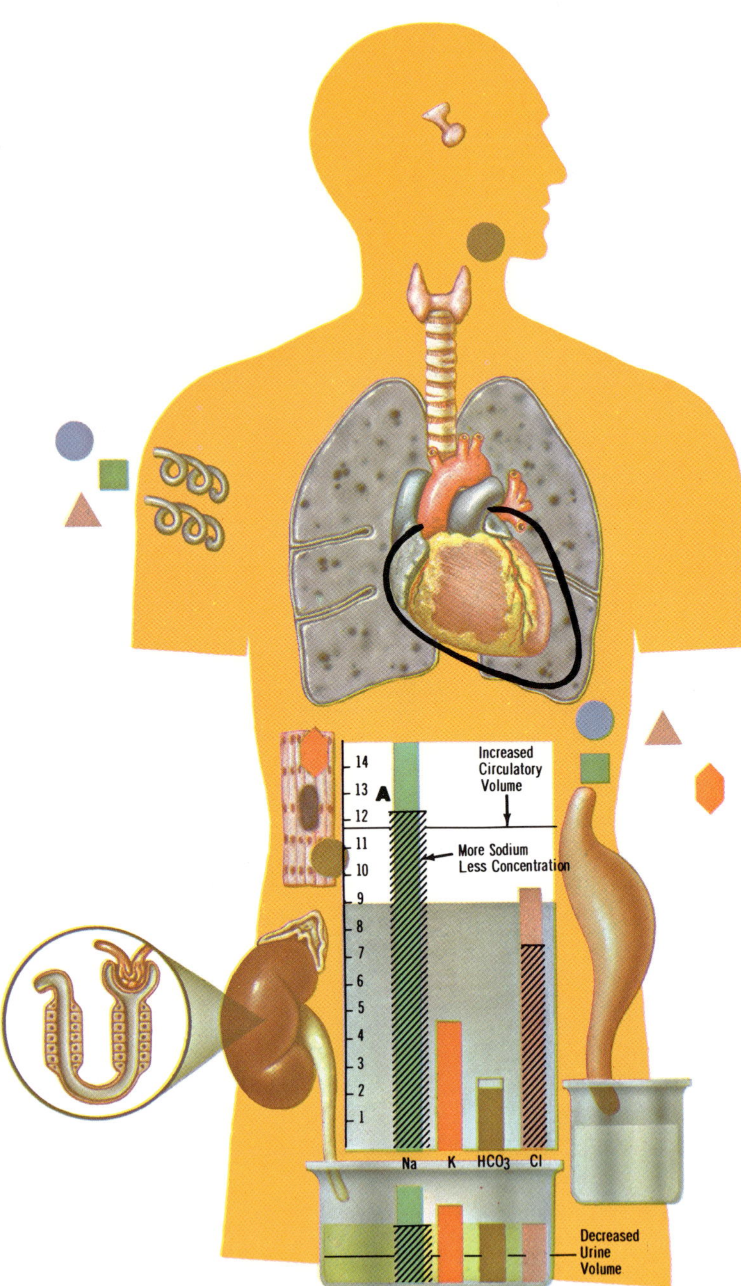

CONGESTIVE HEART FAILURE

Circulatory insufficiency in this disorder leads to retention of sodium and water by the kidney and an increase in total body water and sodium (A). The *serum* concentration of *sodium will vary* in proportion to the amounts of water retained with the sodium, but it is *usually normal*. In the late stages of failure more water may be retained, and dilutional hyponatremia may develop. Although there is dispute regarding the exact mechanism of the retention of sodium in this disorder, it is agreed that decreased output of sodium by the kidney is responsible. Decreased glomerular filtration rate, increased tubular reabsorption of sodium under aldosterone influence, and other mechanisms have been proposed. Perhaps all of them are responsible in individual cases. Retention of water may be secondary to the retention of sodium, but an increased secretion of ADH is also known to occur. This would account for the dilutional hyponatremia in the late stages of this disorder. Blood volume studies, venous pressure and circulation time, and chest roentgenograms help to confirm the diagnosis.

The syndrome of inappropriate secretion of antidiuretic hormone (SIADH) may resemble the dilutional hyponatremia of congestive heart failure, but the urine sodium will be high (> 30 mEq/liter). This is found with many neoplasms (e.g., oat-cell carcinoma of the lung), myxedema, drugs (chlorpropamide, vincristine, etc.) and all types of traumatic, vascular, inflammatory, and degenerative diseases of the brain.

Summary of Laboratory Findings:

Serum sodium: Normal or decreased
Serum potassium: Normal
Serum bicarbonate: Normal
Serum chlorides: Decreased
Blood volume: Increased
Urine sodium: Decreased
Urine potassium: Normal
Urine pH: Normal
Urine volume: Decreased

PYLORIC OBSTRUCTION

In this condition fluid and all the major blood electrolytes except bicarbonate are lost by "excretion" through an abnormal pathway. The constricted pylorus (A) prevents the passage of gastric juice into the intestine, where under normal conditions it is absorbed. Instead, it accumulates in the stomach and is vomited (B). Large amounts of *water, potassium, hydrogen ion,* and *chloride* in excess of *sodium* are lost, with a corresponding *drop in their blood levels.* Loss of hydrogen ion leads to a metabolic alkalosis, and thus the respiratory rate is depressed, so that carbon dioxide is retained in the form of carbonic acid. This compensates somewhat for the alkalosis. In addition, reabsorption and production of bicarbonate by the kidney come almost to a halt, a decline that allows for loss of fixed base. Later, because the alkalosis blocks carbohydrate metabolism, and the cells demand fat breakdown for energy, the *blood ketones rise,* a result that leads the pH back to the acid side.

The situation is further aggravated by the fact that insensible water losses through the lung and skin and obligatory water loss by way of the kidney cannot be prevented by the intake of water. The diagnosis is established by an upper G.I. series.

Such alterations in the blood electrolytes may also occur in prolonged gastric suction, potassium deficits from whatever cause, and administration of alkaline salts such as antacids.

Summary of Laboratory Findings:

Serum sodium: Decreased
Serum potassium: Decreased
Serum bicarbonate: Increased
Serum chlorides: Decreased
Blood volume: Decreased
Urine sodium: Decreased
Urine potassium: Normal
Urine pH: Increased
Urine volume: Decreased

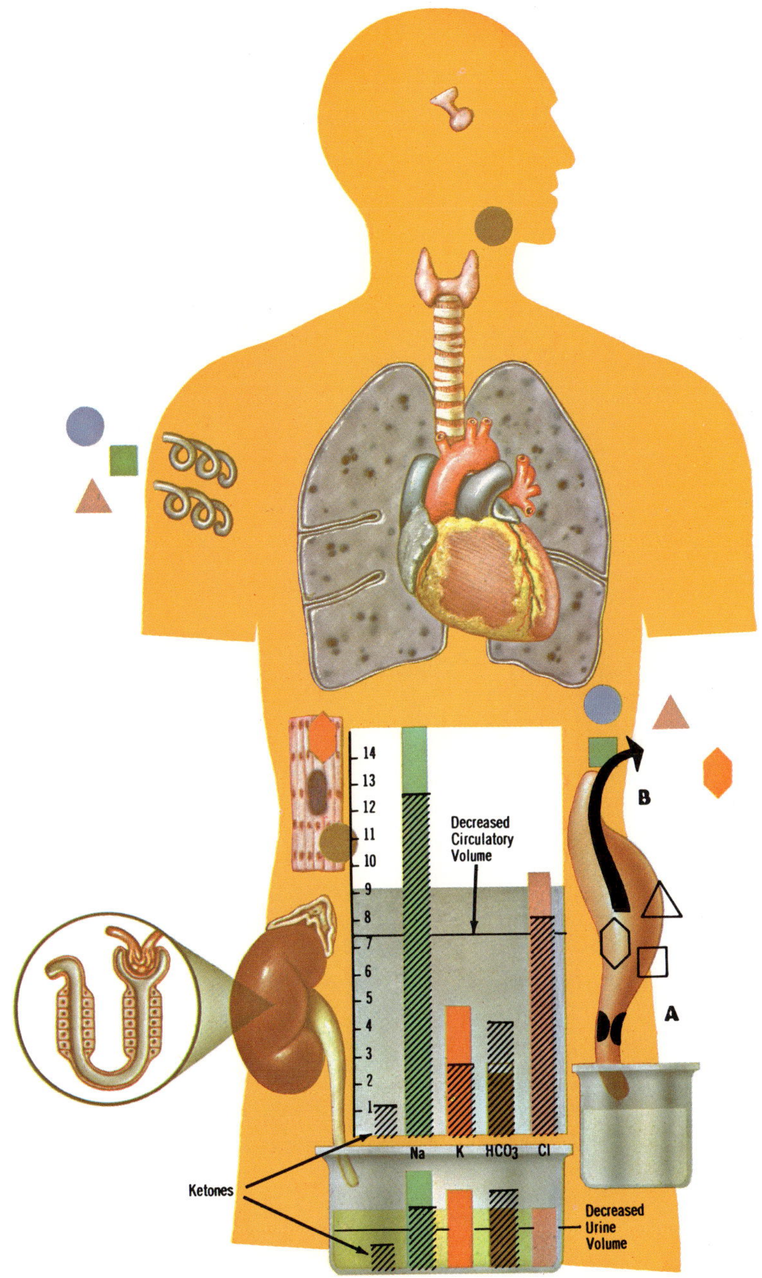

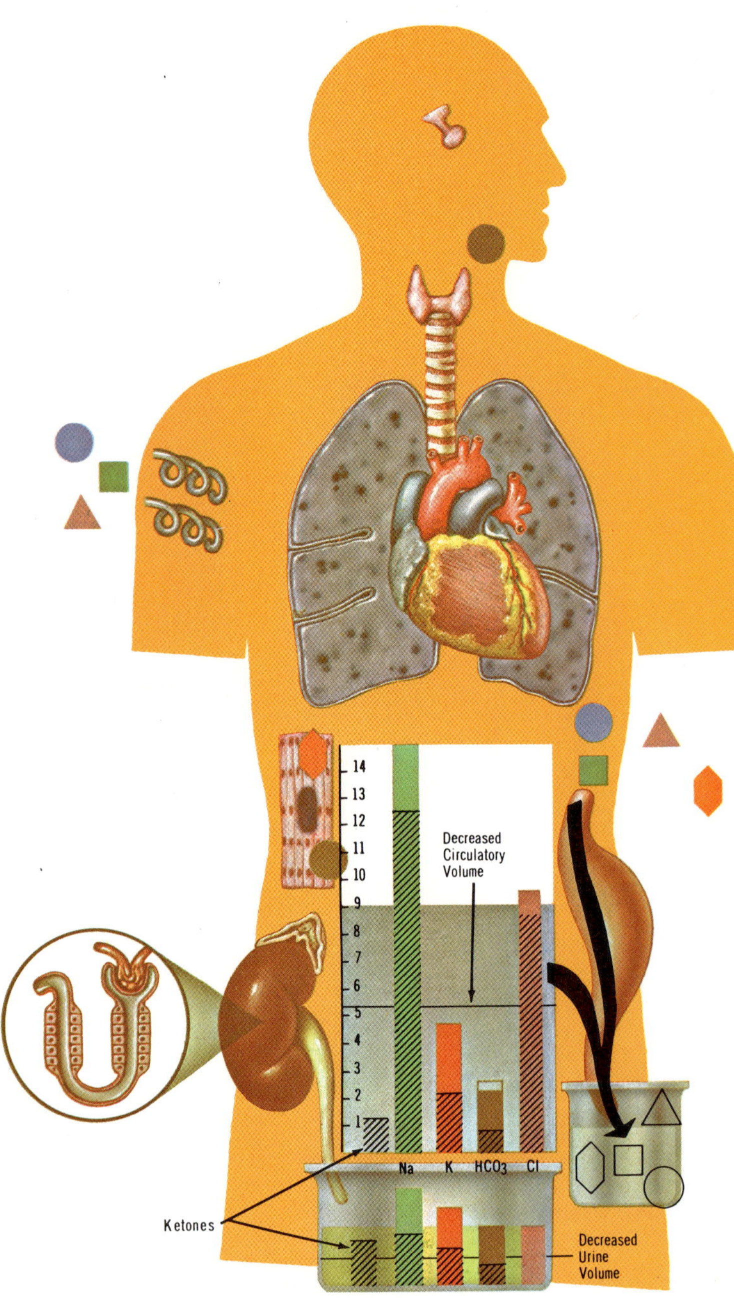

DIARRHEA

Here the prime mover is "excretion" of water and all the electrolytes by an abnormal route. With increased peristalsis of the bowel, there is insufficient time for adequate reabsorption of the bile, pancreatic, and intestinal secretions.

This could amount to a loss of as much as 5 L. of water and electrolytes daily. The *blood* levels of *sodium, potassium, bicarbonate,* and *chloride* all *decrease,* but since the intestinal juices contain more bicarbonate than chloride, this anion diminishes to a greater extent, with resulting metabolic acidosis. However in the secretory diarrhea of cholera larger amounts of chloride are lost. *Ketonemia,* produced by the lack of carbohydrate intake, which necessitates the metabolism of fat for energy, aggravates the acidosis. In severe cases shock may develop, reducing the compensatory action of the kidney and enchancing the acidosis.

Summary of Laboratory Findings:

Serum sodium: Decreased
Serum potassium: Decreased
Serum bicarbonate: Decreased
Serum chlorides: Decreased
Blood volume: Decreased
Urine sodium: Decreased
Urine potassium: Normal or decreased
Urine pH: Decreased
Urine volume: Decreased

PATHOLOGICAL DIAPHORESIS

Excessive sweating, such as that which occurs in people working in environments with high temperatures, leads to marked loss of water and moderate losses of sodium and chloride (A). One would expect a rise in serum concentrations of *sodium* and *chloride*, because water loss is in excess of salt loss. In actuality there is a *drop* in these values, since these patients replace the water by ingestion (B) but not the salt.

Summary of Laboratory Findings:

Serum sodium: Decreased
Serum potassium: Normal
Serum bicarbonate: Normal
Serum chlorides: Decreased
Blood volume: Normal
Urine sodium: Decreased
Urine potassium: Normal
Urine pH: Normal
Urine volume: Normal

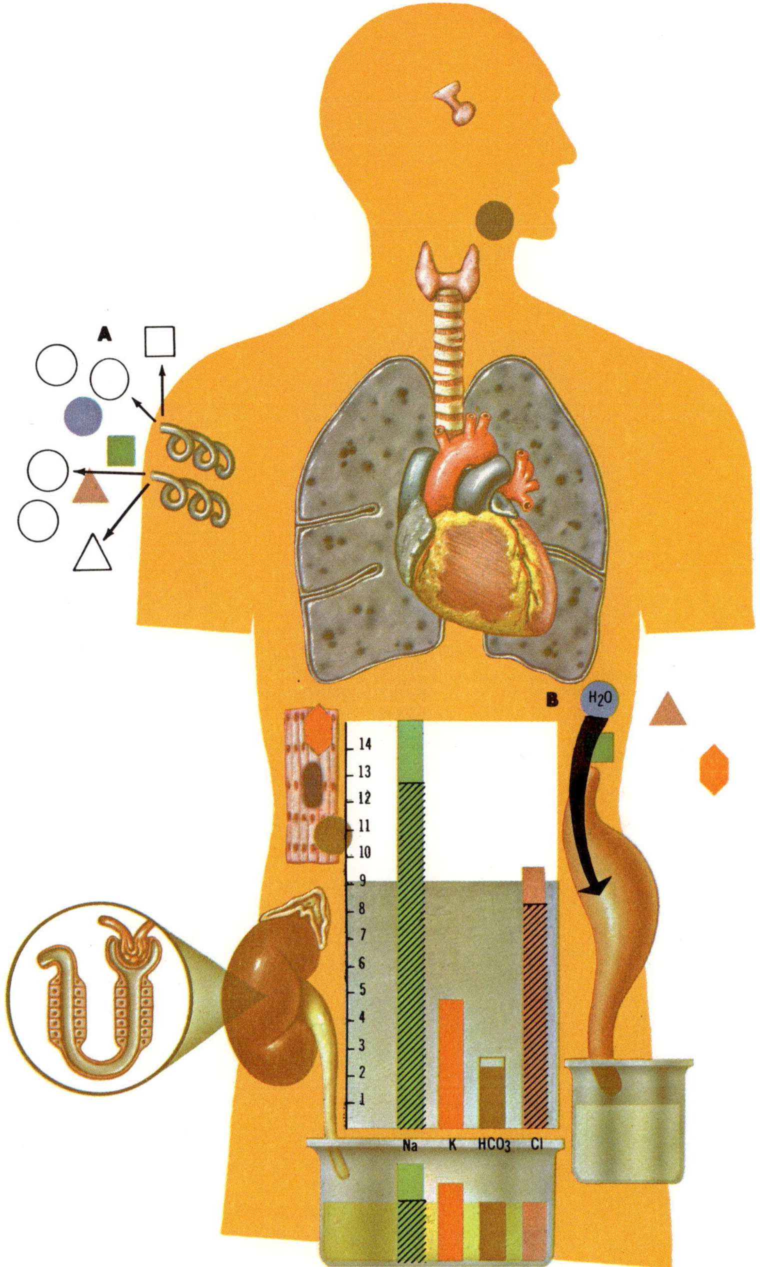

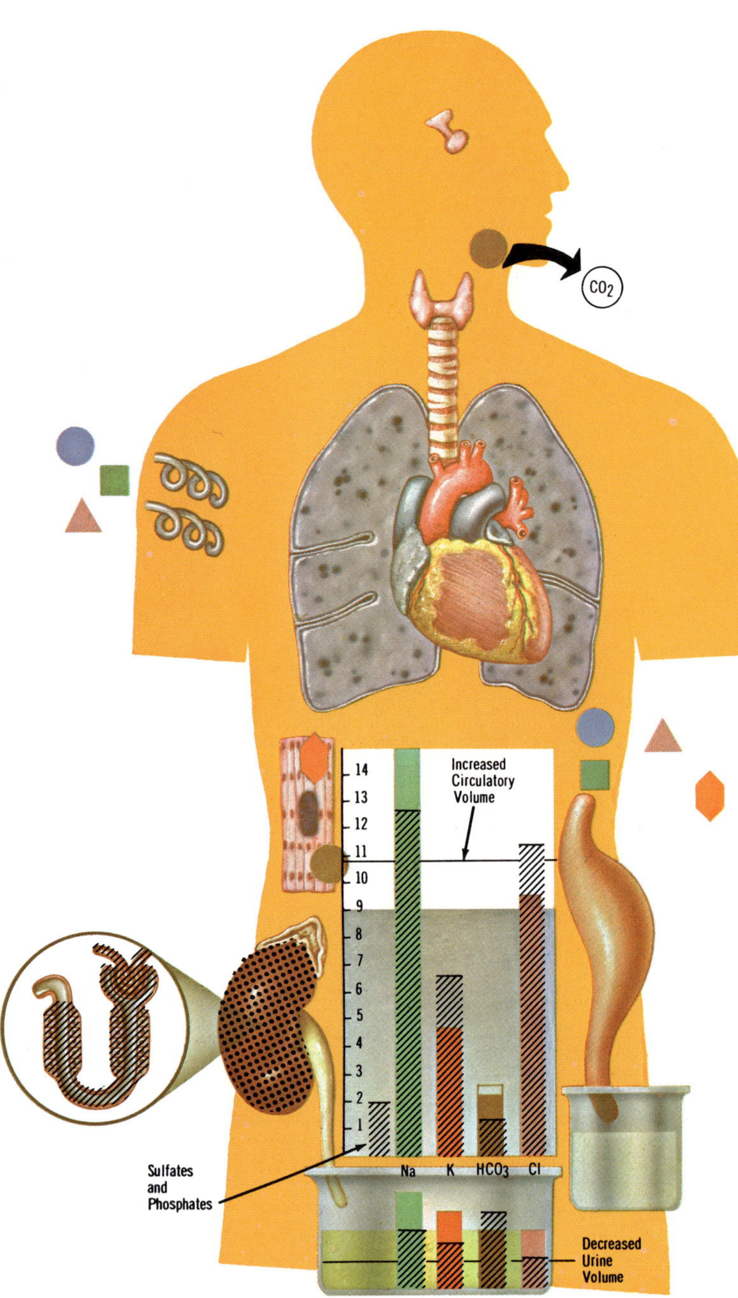

ACUTE RENAL FAILURE

In acute renal failure the excretion of water and all the major electrolytes is blocked, and these accumulate in the body. Although the concentration of *potassium* and *chloride increase,* the concentration of *sodium usually decreases.* The reason is that the associated retention of water is proportionately greater than the retention of sodium. Unless oral intake of fluids is restricted, congestive heart failure may develop.

An important additional factor is the retention of inorganic acids, such as *sulfates, phosphates,* and other products of protein catabolism that are insignificant under normal circumstances. These are at first neutralized by bicarbonate and other buffers, with consequent *reduction* in plasma *bicarbonate.* The damaged tubular cells are unable to replace the bicarbonate or to excrete the hydrogen ion, and a metabolic acidosis ensues. The lung can compensate to a certain extent by hyperventilation and increased excretion of carbon dioxide.

Acute renal failure may result from a variety of drugs, poisons, heavy metals, transfusions or other hemolytic reactions, shock, dehydration, severe glomerulonephritis, or obstructive uropathy.

Summary of Laboratory Findings:

Serum sodium: Decreased
Serum potassium: Increased
Serum bicarbonate: Decreased
Serum chlorides: Increased
Blood volume: Increased
Urine sodium: Decreased
Urine potassium: Decreased
Urine pH: Normal or alkaline
Urine volume: Decreased

PULMONARY EMPHYSEMA

Carbon dioxide excretion is impaired in this condition (A). This results from poor respiratory exchange in the distended bullous portions of the lung and poor capillary perfusion, preventing the escape of carbon dioxide from the blood. The rise of the blood *carbon dioxide* in the form of carbonic acid leads to a lowering of the pH. The kidney acts to compensate for the respiratory acidosis by retaining bicarbonate and producing more through the carbonic anhydrase system. *Chloride drops,* since it is excreted to compensate for the increased anions. The urine is usually acid.

Respiratory acidosis occurs in other pulmonary diseases, such as pneumonia, pneumothorax, and pulmonary edema, as well as in states leading to hypoventilation, such as poliomyelitis and anesthesia. In cases of alveolar-capillary block, such as sarcoidosis and silicosis, carbon dioxide as a rule is not retained.

Frequent daily blood gas and electrolyte determinations are of value in following this disorder. Arterial oxygen saturation (p. 136) before and after pure oxygen will often help to distinguish pulmonary emphysema from cyanotic congenital heart disease and pulmonary arteriovenous fistulas. Chest roentgenograms, fluoroscopy, and pulmonary function studies also assist in establishing the diagnosis.

Summary of Laboratory Findings:

Serum sodium: Normal
Serum potassium: Normal
Serum bicarbonate: Increased
Serum chlorides: Decreased
Blood volume: Normal or increased
Urine sodium: Decreased
Urine potassium: Normal
Urine pH: Decreased
Urine volume: Normal

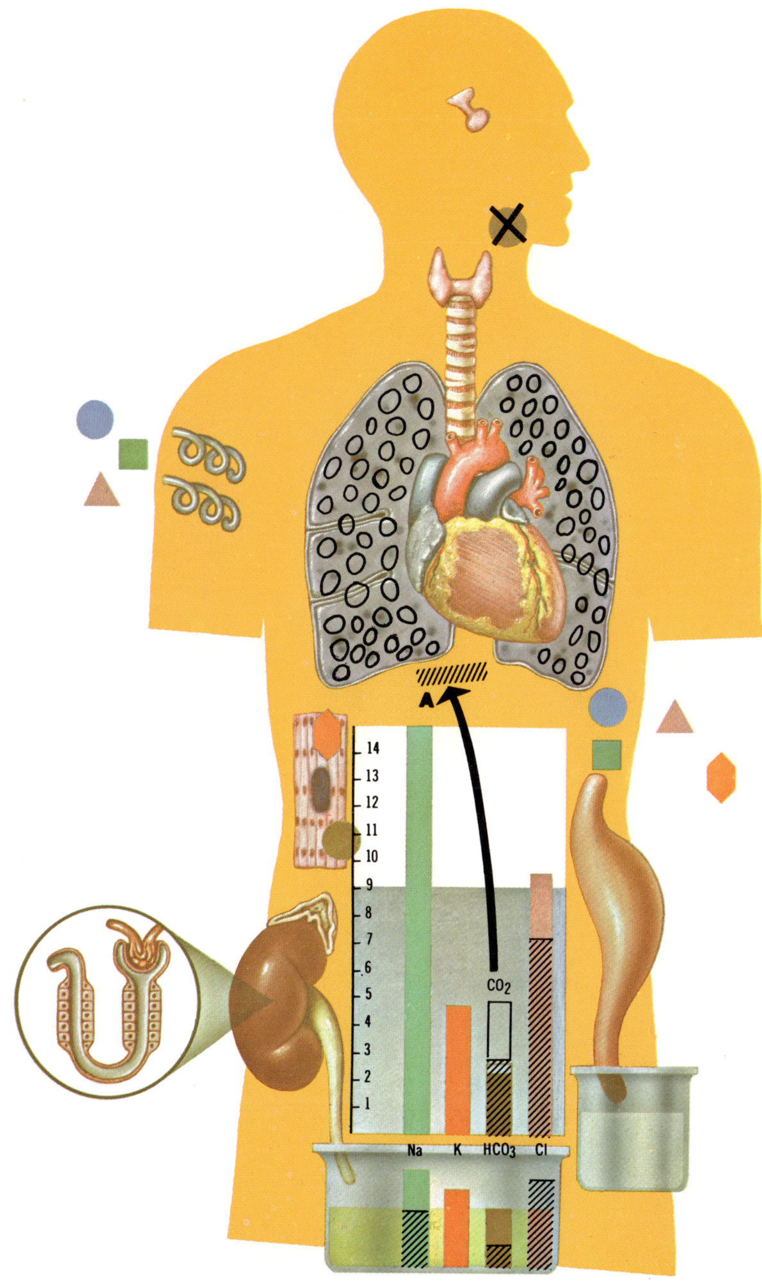

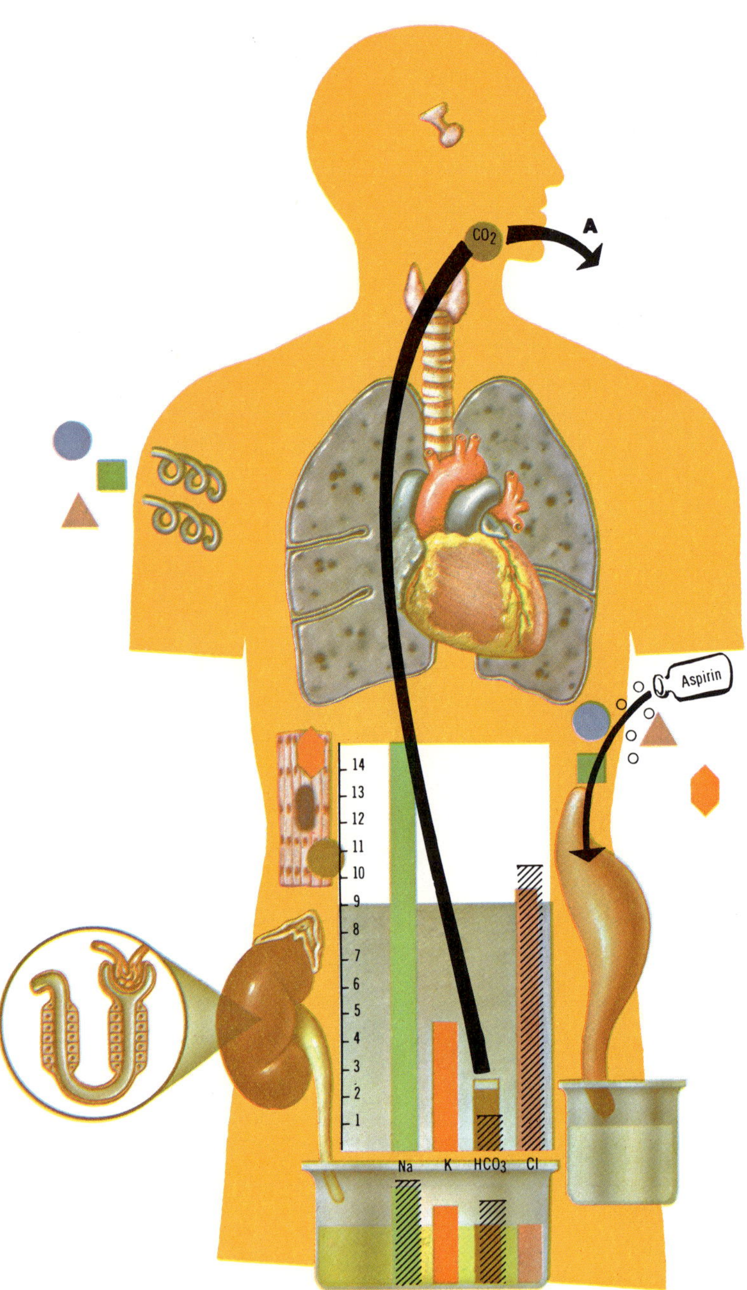

SALICYLATE TOXICITY

In this condition the primary change is an increased excretion of *carbon dioxide* (A). Stimulation of the respiratory center by the high concentration of blood salicylates results in hyperventilation and blowing off of carbon dioxide. The blood pH increases. To compensate for the loss of carbonic acid and to bring the pH back to normal, the kidney excretes bicarbonate. Thus blood bicarbonate decreases. To make up for the deficit in anions, the blood chloride shows a relative *increase*. In later stages ketones may accumulate and thus cause a metabolic acidosis. Apparently, alkalosis inhibits the metabolism of glucose, and the cells must rely on the mobilization and oxidation of fatty acids for energy. The diagnosis is established by examining the urine for salicylates.

Fever, high altitude, hyperventilation syndrome, and head trauma will produce the same picture.

Summary of Laboratory Findings:

Serum sodium: Normal
Serum potassium: Normal or decreased
Serum bicarbonate: Decreased
Serum chloride: Increased
Blood volume: Normal
Urine sodium: Increased
Urine potassium: Normal or increased
Urine pH: Increased
Urine volume: Normal

ADRENAL CORTICAL INSUFFICIENCY

In this condition there is insufficient aldosterone (and possibly hydrocortisone) secretion to induce the renal tubules to conserve salt. Large amounts of *sodium chloride* and some fixed base (*bicarbonate*) are *excreted* in the urine, and the *blood levels* of these electrolytes *diminish*. The salt takes with it substantial quantities of *water*, and consequently the *circulatory volume decreases*.

If this were not hindered by the greater tubular reabsorption of water, possibly based on the lack of aldosterone antagonism of ADH, blood volume would be severely reduced. The *increased* plasma *potassium* is less well understood. At least one tubular influence of adrenal cortical secretions is postulated to be that of the secretion of potassium in exchange for sodium. This would, of course, cease in adrenal insufficiency, with retention of potassium. Spironolactone, a potent antagonist of aldosterone, produces a similar picture.

The poor retention of chloride and the increased reabsorptive powers of water in this disorder have been made the basis of two tests. The Cutler-Power-Wilder test shows a continued substantial excretion of sodium plus chloride in the urine despite a low salt diet. The Robinson-Power-Kepler test demonstrates a poor output of urine in response to a measurable intake of water (p. 81). Diagnosis is established by direct measurement of urinary corticosteroids (p. 90).

Summary of Laboratory Findings:

Serum sodium: Decreased
Serum potassium: Increased
Serum bicarbonate: Normal or decreased
Serum chlorides: Decreased
Blood volume: Decreased
Urine sodium: Increased
Urine potassium: Normal or decreased
Urine pH: Normal or alkaline
Urine volume: Normal or decreased

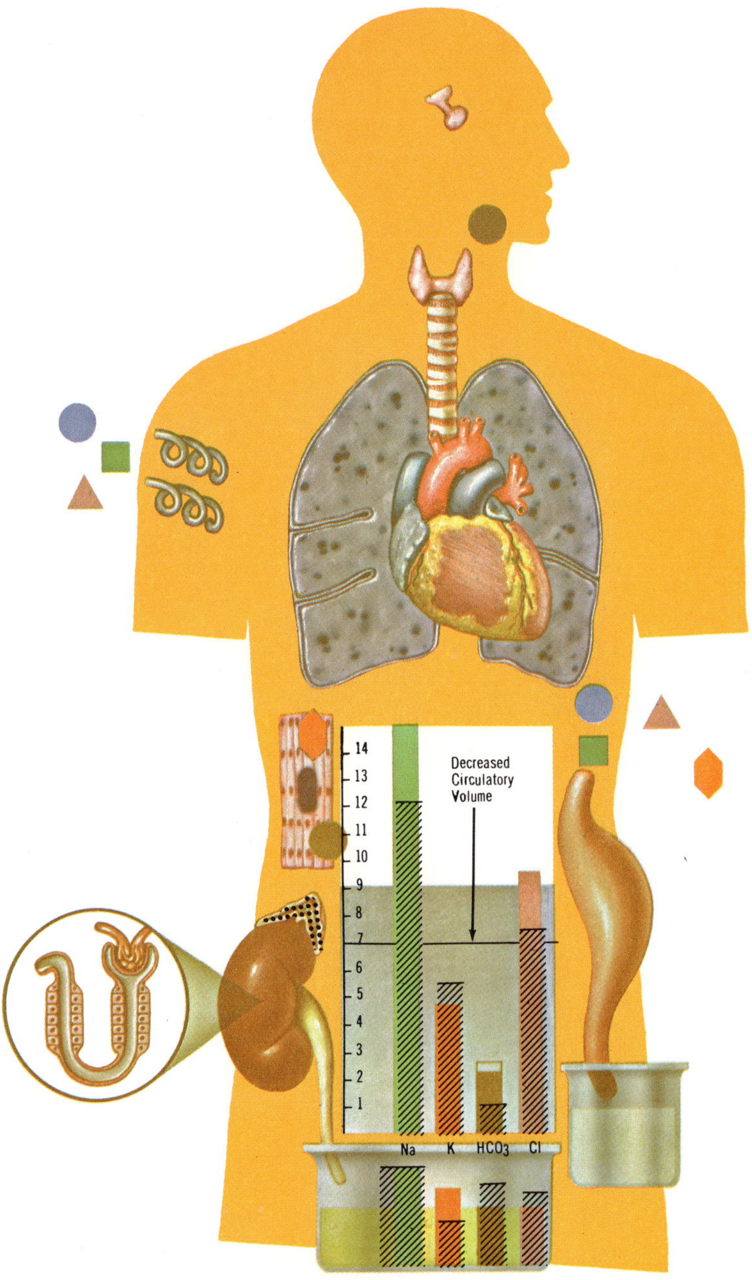

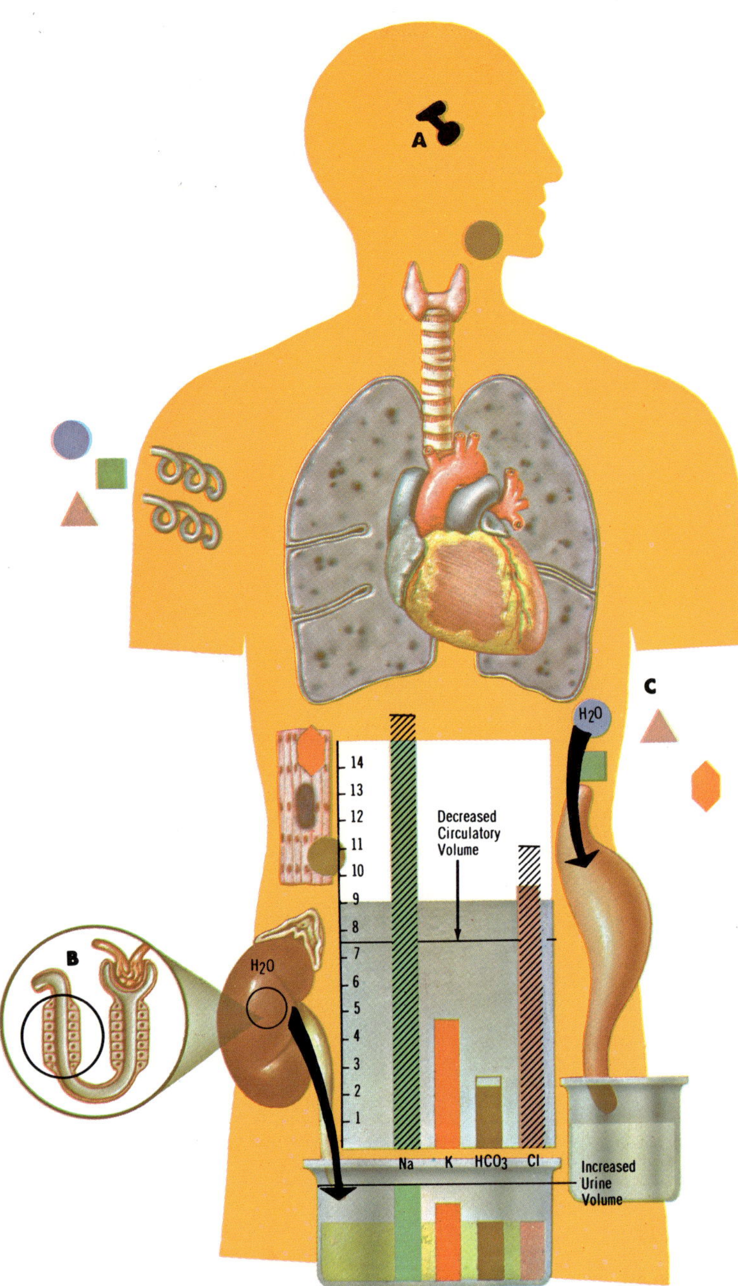

DIABETES INSIPIDUS

This condition is characterized by excessive excretion of water. In the face of decreased antidiuretic hormone (ADH) secretion (A) by the posterior pituitary, distal tubules and collecting tubules of the kidney (B) lose their ability to reabsorb water. As much as 10 L. of water may be lost each day. The body attempts to make up this deficit by increasing oral intake of water (C). Apparently, this compensation is incomplete, since the serum *sodium* and *chloride* are usually elevated, a reflection of the hemoconcentration. Common causes of this disorder are pituitary tumor, syphilis, encephalitis, and trauma. Many cases are, however, idiopathic.

Nephrogenic diabetes insipidus, a hereditary disorder, may produce the same alteration in blood electrolytes. In this condition the renal tubule fails to respond to an adequate secretion of antidiuretic hormone (ADH). Acquired nephrogenic diabetes insipidus may result from lithium carbonate, demeclocycline, and methoxyflurane anesthesia. Hypercalcemia and hypokalemia may cause a partial nephrogenic diabetes insipidus.

When nephrogenic diabetes insipidus is secondary to chronic glomerular nephritis, the other alterations of electrolytes regularly occurring in this disorder are apparent. The administration of Pitressin will be of help in differentiating nephrogenic diabetes insipidus from the pituitary type. In true diabetes insipidus there is an abrupt reduction in the urine output in response to Pitressin. Also in patients with diabetes insipidus, unlike normal subjects, an intravenous infusion of hypertonic saline (Hickey-Hare test) fails to suppress diuresis.

Summary of Laboratory Findings:

Serum sodium: Normal or increased
Serum potassium: Normal
Serum bicarbonate: Normal
Serum chlorides: Increased
Blood volume: Decreased
Urine sodium: Normal
Urine potassium: Normal
Urine pH: Normal
Urine volume: Increased

PRIMARY ALDOSTERONISM

A benign adenoma (A), hyperplasia, or carcinoma of the glomerulosa layer of the adrenal cortex is usually the cause for this disorder. In these cases there is secretion of excessive amounts of aldosterone hormone, which activates the distal tubule to reabsorb large amounts of sodium (B) in exchange for potassium and hydrogen ion. As a result, the total body and serum concentration of *sodium increases*, and the serum *bicarbonate increases*, whereas the serum *potassium decreases*. The development of metabolic alkalosis induces further loss of potassium. In addition, there is inhibition of tubular reabsorption of water. The reabsorption of sodium counterbalances this by stimulating thirst and increased water intake, as well as by stimulating ADH secretion with consequent increased tubular reabsorption of water, so that there is often an increase in body water and circulatory volume. Diagnosis is established by 24-hour urine potassium and aldosterone levels and plasma renin.

Summary of Laboratory Findings:

Serum sodium: Increased
Serum potassium: Decreased
Serum bicarbonate: Increased
Serum chlorides: Decreased
Blood volume: Normal or increased
Urine sodium: Decreased
Urine potassium: Increased
Urine pH: Normal or decreased
Urine volume: Increased

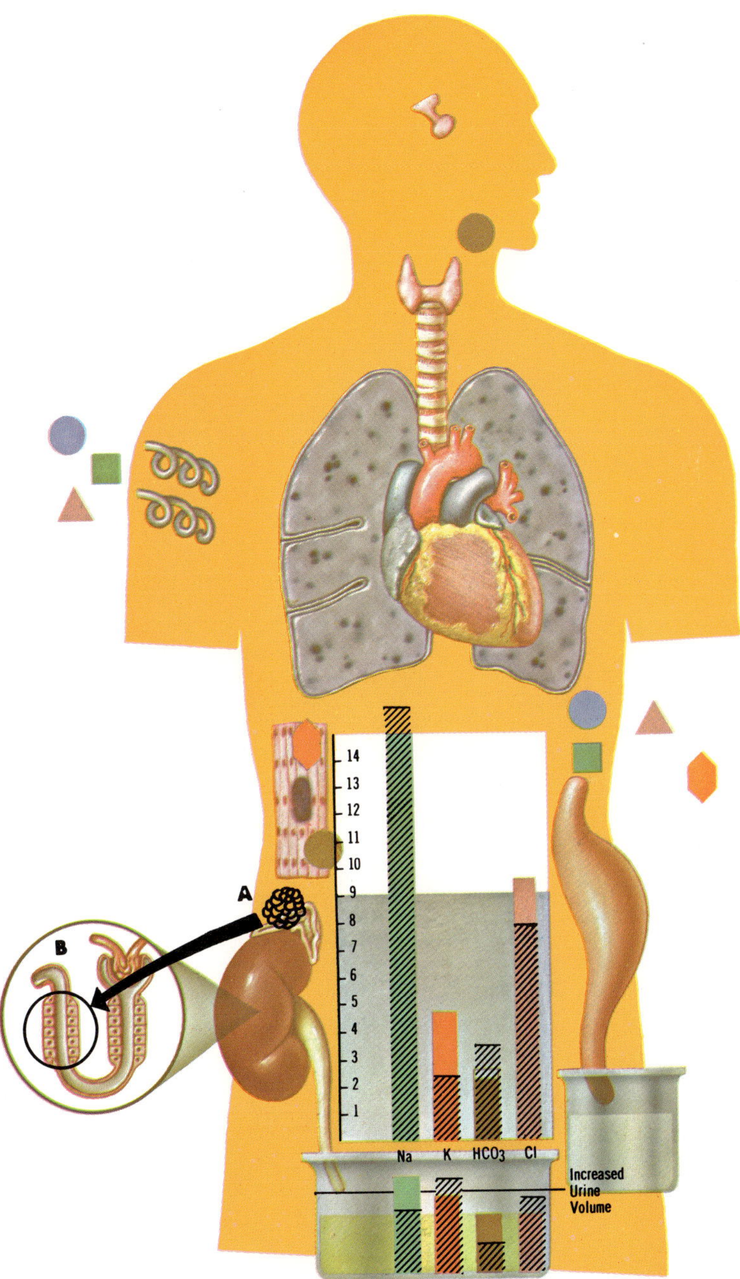

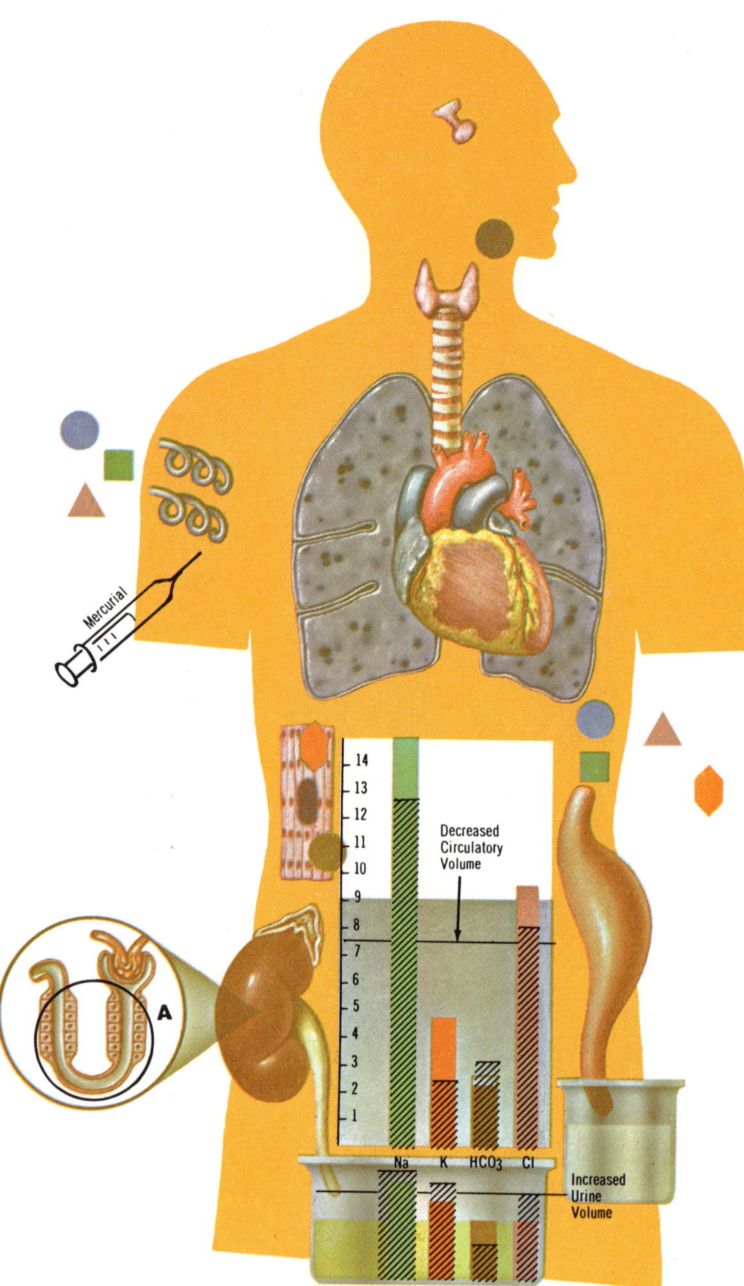

MERCURIAL DIURETICS

Although the mechanism of action is unclear, mercurial diuretics cause the excretion of large amounts of sodium and chloride via the urine (A). The blood levels of *sodium* and *chloride decrease,* whereas the urine levels increase. Reabsorption of sodium with bicarbonate in the proximal tubule is uninhibited, so that the serum bicarbonate increases to make up the deficit in anions (chloride loss), and the result is a metabolic alkalosis. The metabolic alkalosis hinders hydrogen ion excretion, and, instead, potassium ion is excreted in exchange for sodium. The level of serum *potassium* is therefore *reduced.*

Summary of Laboratory Findings:

Serum sodium: Decreased
Serum potassium: Decreased
Serum bicarbonate: Increased
Serum chlorides: Decreased
Blood volume: Decreased
Urine sodium: Increased
Urine potassium: Increased
Urine pH: Decreased
Urine volume: Increased

CHLOROTHIAZIDE DIURETICS

This drug is a potent carbonic anhydrase inhibitor, and thus it inhibits reabsorption of bicarbonate and the excretion of hydrogen ion through the tubules (A). This would result in a picture similar to that of renal tubular acidosis (page 54) if it were not for an additional direct action on the renal tubule to depress salt reabsorption. This action is analogous to that of mercurial diuretics but apparently acts on a different transport system. The result is the expected *drop* in serum *sodium* and *potassium;* but since both serum *bicarbonate* and *chloride* are also *decreased,* neither acidosis nor alkalosis developes to a significant degree. Ethacrynic acid and furosemide produce a similar picture, but because they act both on the ascending loop of Henle and the proximal tubule as well they may produce severe volume, sodium, and potassium depletion.

Summary of Laboratory Findings:

Serum sodium: Decreased
Serum potassium: Decreased
Serum bicarbonate: Decreased
Serum chlorides: Decreased
Blood volume: Decreased
Urine sodium: Increased
Urine potassium: Increased
Urine pH: Normal or increased
Urine volume: Increased

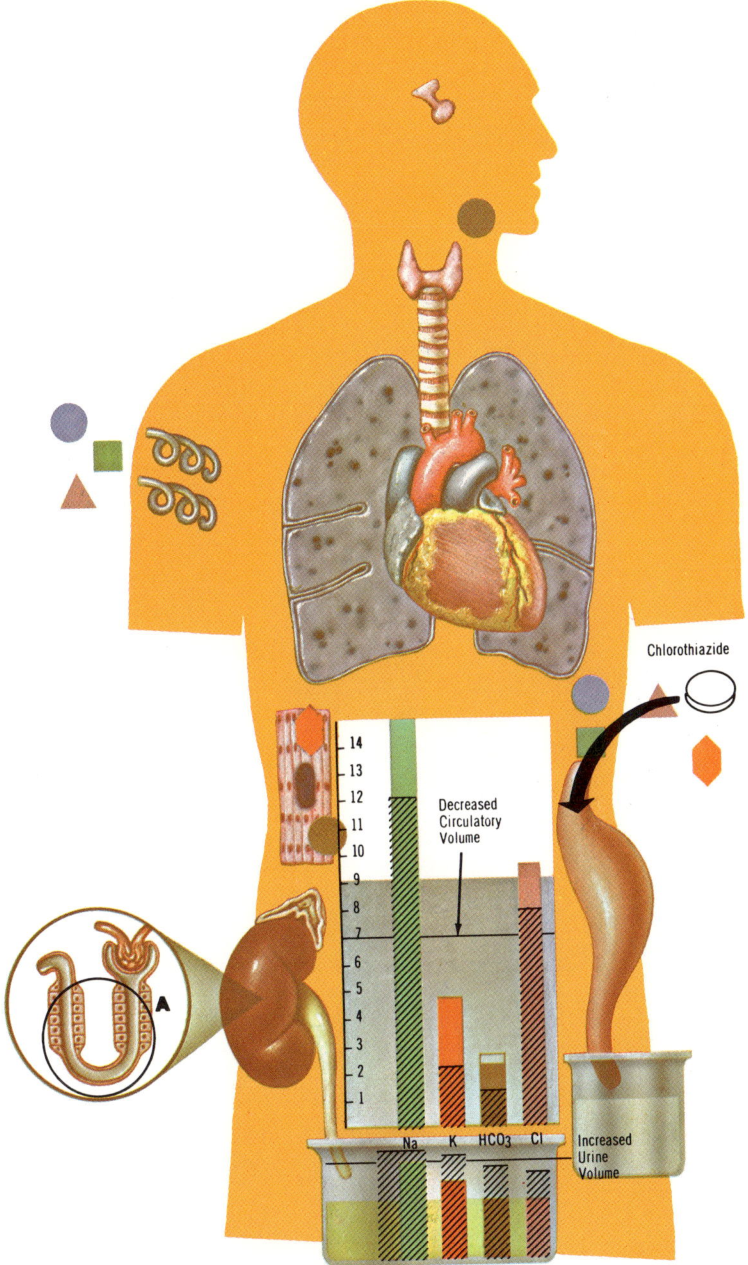

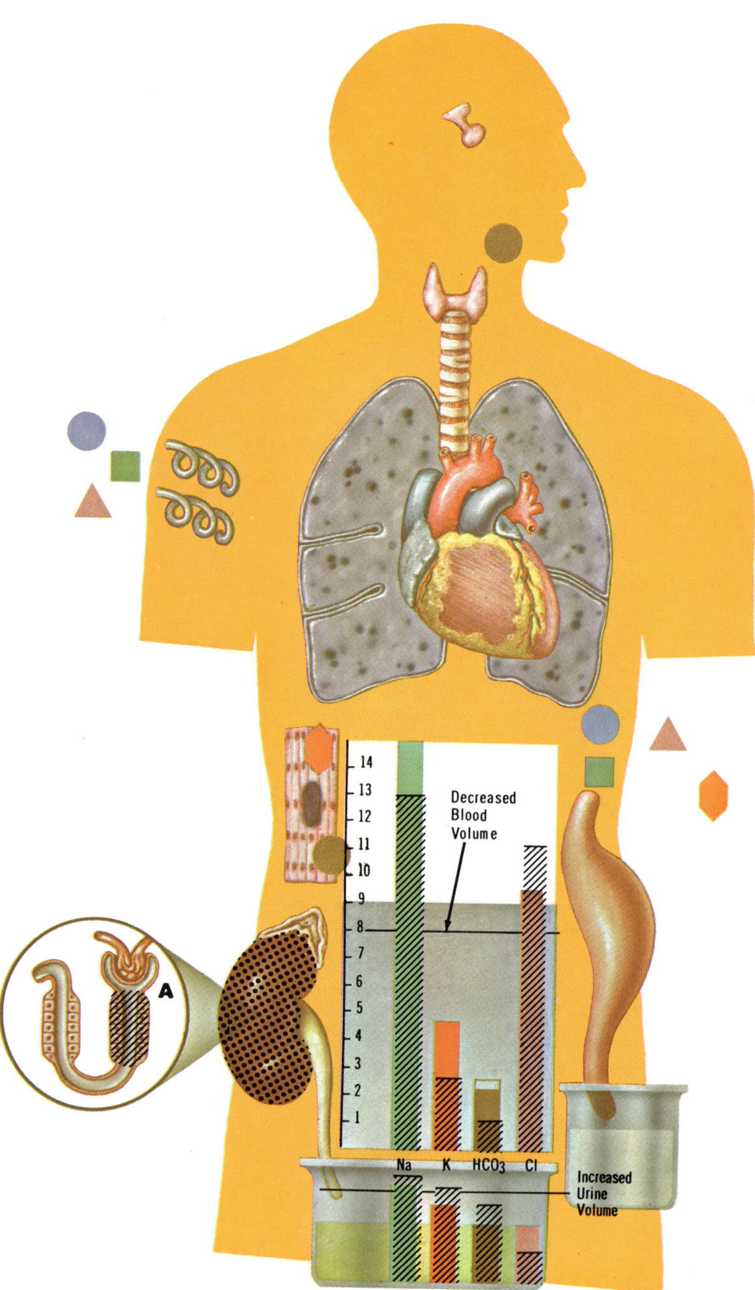

RENAL TUBULAR ACIDOSIS

In this hereditary disorder there is a tubular defect (A) in the excretion of hydrogen ion and the reabsorption of bicarbonate from the glomerular filtrate. Serum *bicarbonate falls,* whereas serum *chloride increases* to make up the deficit of anions. The tubules, unable to secrete hydrogen ion in exchange for sodium, secrete potassium ion instead. Thus serum *potassium* also *diminishes.* Blood pH drops, an indication of metabolic acidosis.

A similar alteration in electrolytes occurs in acetazolamide (Diamox) administration for the same reasons, and in ammonium chloride ingestion.

Summary of Laboratory Findings:

Serum sodium: Decreased
Serum potassium: Decreased
Serum bicarbonate: Decreased
Serum chlorides: Increased
Blood volume: Decreased
Urine sodium: Increased
Urine potassium: Increased
Urine pH: Increased
Urine volume: Increased

CHRONIC RENAL FAILURE

The electrolyte derangement of chronic renal insufficiency can best be explained by a loss of the kidney's regulatory powers in electrolyte and acid-base equilibrium. Indeed, although there is often destruction of a large percentage of the glomeruli, glomerular filtration necessary for average needs is maintained. Thus water, sodium, potassium, and chloride are not usually retained.

On the other hand, tubular damage (A) impairs the unique regulatory capacity of the kidney to reabsorb water and electrolytes selectively and to retain fixed base. The tubules fail to respond to the salt-retaining stimulus of aldosterone or the water-retaining stimulus of ADH. Thus *sodium, potassium,* or *water* may not be conserved, and their plasma levels *decrease.* Replacement of plasma bicarbonate and excretion of hydrogen ions may cease, with consequent metabolic acidosis. Impaired excretion of inorganic acids such as *sulfates* and *phosphates* prevails, as in acute renal failure, contributing to the acidosis. The diagnosis is established by repeated high blood urea nitrogens and serum creatinine with a normal retrograde pyelogram to exclude obstructive uropathy.

Common causes of chronic renal failure are pyelonephritis, glomerulonephritis, nephrosclerosis, polycystic kidneys, and obstructive uropathy, but collagen diseases may also be the etiology.

Summary of Laboratory Findings:

Serum sodium: Decreased
Serum potassium: Normal or decreased
Serum bicarbonate: Decreased
Serum chloride: Normal or decreased
Blood volume: Variable
Urine sodium: Increased
Urine potassium: Increased
Urine pH: Increased
Urine volume: Variable but usually increased

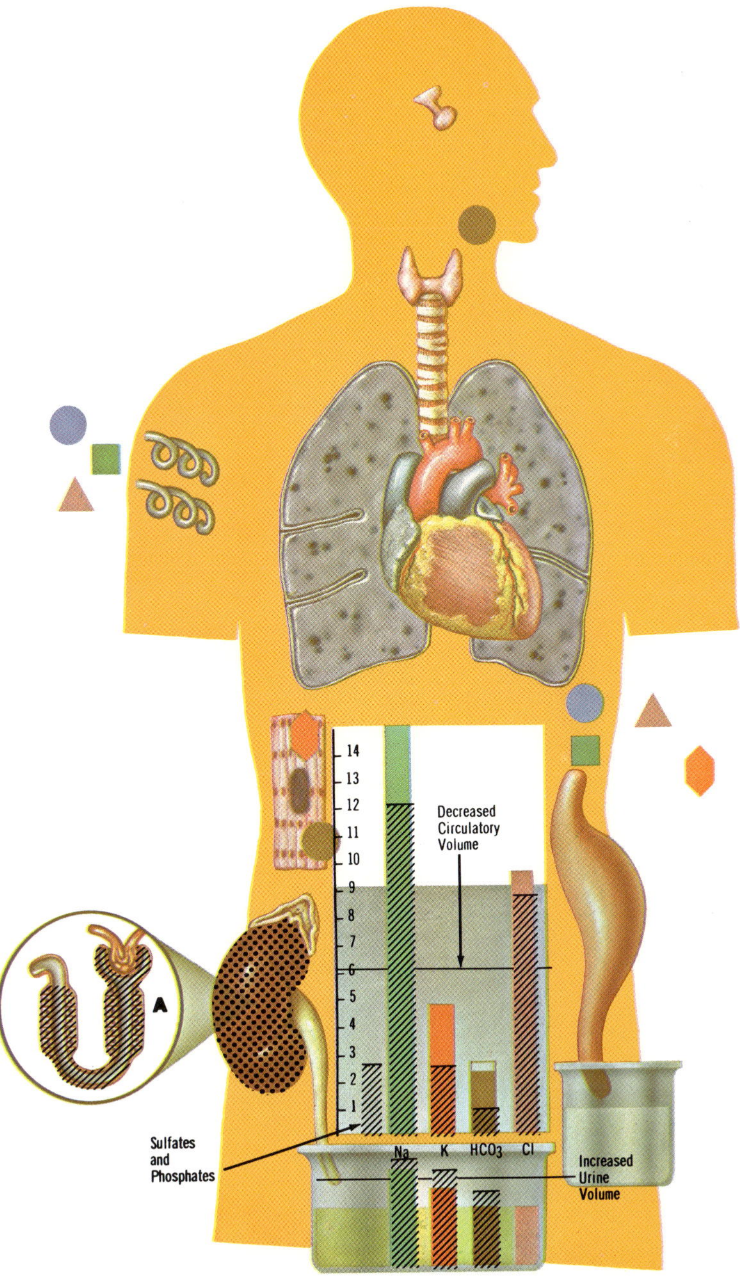

DIABETIC ACIDOSIS

In diabetic acidosis the concentration of most of the *serum electrolytes* is *reduced,* and *body water* is *depleted* (A). This eventuality follows a fascinating sequence of deviations from normal metabolism.

With an insufficient supply of insulin, the cells are unable to utilize glucose in metabolism. The blood sugar rises. Once the renal threshold is exceeded (170 mg.%), glucose spills into the urine and by its osmotic effect takes with it large amounts of water, sodium, chloride, and potassium. The cells must gain their energy from sources other than glucose. Therefore, large amounts of fat are mobilized and converted to ketones, such as acetoacetic acid and beta-hydroxybutyric acid, to meet this need. These strong acids are neutralized by the sodium bicarbonate, disodium phosphate, and other buffers to form organic salts, water, and carbon dioxide. The carbon dioxide is exhaled (B), whereas the sodium acetoacetate either is utilized by the cell or, if the rate of production of these ketones exceeds the ability of the cells to utilize them, is excreted in the urine. In the latter case they exert an osmotic effect as they pass through the kidney, taking with them sodium, potassium, and other electrolytes. When renal excretion of these *ketones* reaches its maximum, they *rise* in the blood.

The kidney attempts to maintain blood sodium bicarbonate by exchanging the sodium of the organic salts for hydrogen ion and ammonia, but its capacity to do this is limited. In like manner the sodium of sodium chloride is returned to the blood as bicarbonate, adding to blood chloride depletion.

Body potassium is depleted by three additional mechanisms. First, potassium moves out of the cell (C) to replace extracellular cation (sodium). Second, potassium moves out of the cell in exchange for hydrogen ion, "buffering" the acidosis. Finally, lack of insulin blocks an important avenue of potassium movement into the cell. Because of the decreased circulatory volume and consequent impairment in renal function, serum *potassium* is usually *normal* or *increased.*

Intracellular water moves extracellularly in an attempt to maintain a normal circulatory volume. The drop in pH stimulates respiration, and more carbon dioxide is exhaled to help to reduce the acidosis. The specific gravity of the urine is increased by the excessive solute, and the pH is usually low. Diabetics may develop lactic acidosis, especially while on phenformin or in hypoxic states, and this produces the same picture, except there are no ketones in the blood or urine.

Summary of Laboratory Findings:

Serum sodium: Decreased
Serum potassium: Normal, increased or decreased
Serum bicarbonate: Decreased
Serum chlorides: Decreased
Blood volume: Decreased
Urine sodium: Increased
Urine potassium: Increased
Urine pH: Decreased
Urine volume: Increased; ketones in the blood and urine

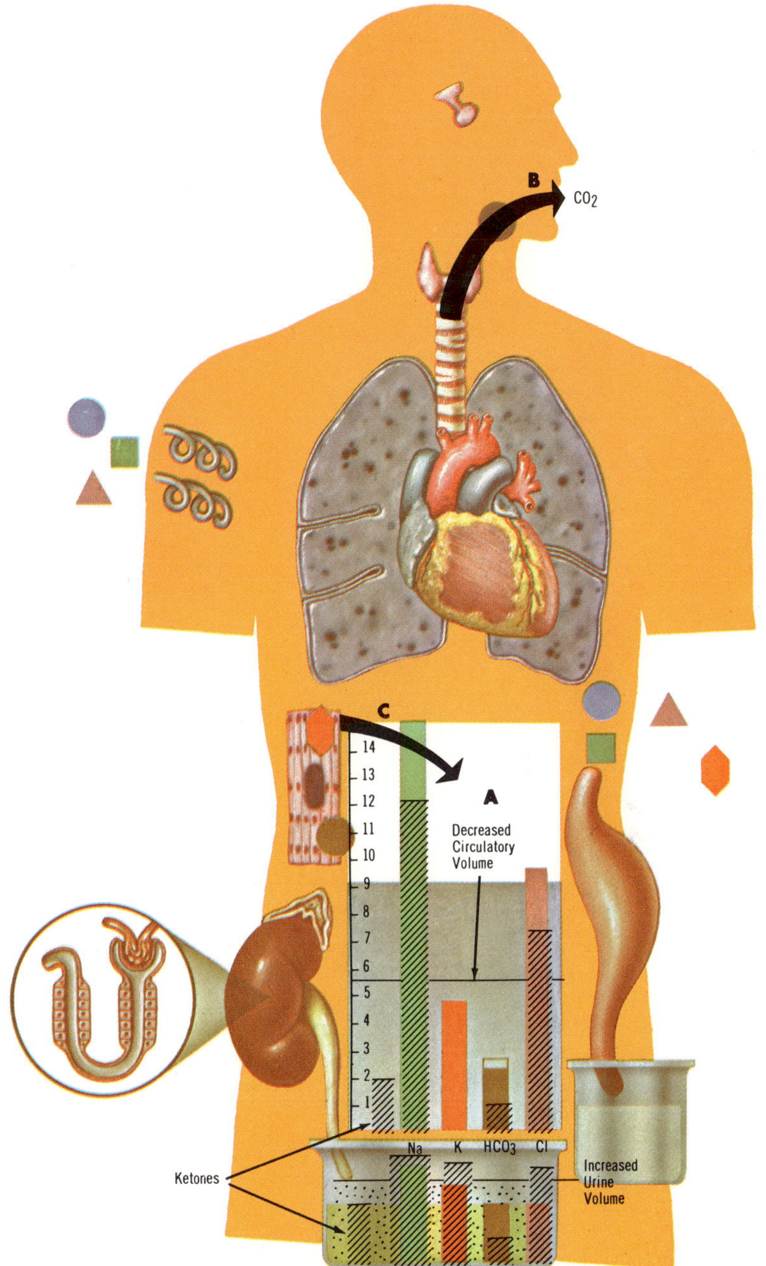

5 Disorders of Blood Glucose

Glucose is an important fuel for body metabolism. For some tissues (brain, etc.) it is almost the sole source of energy. The forces that maintain its blood level within a relatively narrow range are therefore of great interest.

NORMAL METABOLISM*

Intake. Glucose enters the body by way of the mouth in the form of starch, dextrin, or other carbohydrates. These constitute a good share of the average diet. In the gastrointestinal tract these substances are broken down by ptyalin, hydrochloric acid, pancreatic amylase, lactase, and other enzymes to glucose, fructose, and other sugars.

Absorption. Glucose is absorbed in the small intestine both by an active and a passive diffusion process. Normally, this absorption is virtually complete. The exact nature of the active diffusion process is uncertain. It is believed that glucose is phosphorylated by the intestinal cell and then discharged to the blood with the aid of a phosphatase (Grollman). Absorption seems to be favorably influenced by thyroid and adrenocortical hormones as well as vitamin B complex. Insulin is without influence on this process.

Transport. Glucose is transported by the blood, where its concentration is maintained within a relatively narrow range of 70 to 120 mg. per 100 ml. (Folin-Wu method) under fasting conditions. The Smogyi-Nelson method yields normal values of 70-110 mg. per 100 ml. This is somewhat less than the values for the Folin-Wu method, because the latter also measures other reducing substances (creatinine, glutathione, etc.).

Storage. Glucose is stored as glycogen primarily in the liver but also in muscle and to a lesser extent in other tissues of the body. Approximately 300 to 500 gm. are stored in this manner in the average adult. Although liver glycogen is readily returned to the blood as glucose by the action of hepatic phosphorylase and glucose-6-phosphatase according to body needs, peripheral stores of glucose may not be. Glucose may also be converted to fat and stored in this form. Free glucose exists extracellularly and may be considered to be stored there in this form.

Production. The liver is the primary site of glucose production. It converts other sugars such as galactose to glucose. It may convert lactic acid to glycogen and subsequently convert this to glucose under the influence of epinephrine. The liver may convert fat and protein to glucose (gluconeogenesis) by way of the Krebs cycle. This seems to be influenced by adrenocortical hormones.

Destruction. Almost all ingested glucose is eventually metabolized to carbon dioxide and water, and as it changes form in oxidation, it supplies energy for body needs. The breakdown, as already mentioned, may be postponed if it is stored as glycogen or converted to fat and protein. Many enzymes influence the anaerobic and the aerobic catabolism of glucose. Pertinent to this discussion are thiamine (vitamin B_1) and pantothenic acid. Thiamine is part of the enzyme cocarboxylase. For proper utilization it is essential that glucose be transferred into the cell. Apparently, insulin is responsible for this.

Excretion. Glucose is filtered through the glomeruli, but ordinarily almost all of this is reabsorbed by the proximal tubules. A 24-hour urine collection may contain as much as 0.5 to 0.75 gm. of glucose. The process of renal tubular reabsorption of glucose is not clear, but it is thought to be similar to intestinal absorption (phosphorylation). If the blood sugar exceeds 170 mg. per cent (the renal threshold), increasing amounts of sugar will appear in the urine.

Regulation. The remarkable constancy of the blood sugar in normal individuals depends on a number of homeostatic factors, the most important being the liver. In the fasting individual the liver is the primary source of blood glucose. When the blood sugar drops in the normal individual, the liver output of glucose increases. A rise in blood sugar, like that after a meal, causes the release of secretin which stimulates the islet cells and inhibits the liver output of glucose. This homeostatic mechanism of the liver is influenced by several hormones—notably insulin, thyroid, adrenocortical hormone, and epinephrine—and possibly by glycogen. The effects of these and other hormones on glucose metabolism will now be discussed.

Insulin. It is believed that insulin facilitates the transfer of extracellular free glucose across the cell membrane. The exact mechanism of this transfer is unknown. Insulin may also influence the deposition of glycogen in the liver and inhibit gluconeogenesis from protein.

Thyroid. Thyroid stimulates the intestinal and renal tubular absorption of glucose. It may indirectly cause liver glycogenolysis and deplete muscle glycogen. By elevating the metabolic rate it increases the peripheral utilization of glucose.

* See plate on p. 59.

Adrenocortical Hormone. The glucocorticoids mobilize protein and fat stores and in some way favorably influence hepatic gluconeogenesis. They may also diminish cellular capacity to utilize glucose.

Epinephrine. Either directly or indirectly, epinephrine provokes glycogenolysis in both liver and muscle. A rise in blood sugar is well documented after its administration. Vasopressin (Pitressin) may have a similar effect.

Glucagon. This hormone of the alpha cells of the pancreas promotes glycogenolysis in the liver.

Growth Hormone. This hormone of the anterior pituitary is believed to reduce the rate of glucose phosphorylation by the cell, to cause insulin resistance, and to lead to destruction of beta cells of the pancreas. The mechanism of these actions is not well understood.

Nervous excitement, exercise, and eating exert physiologic influences on the blood glucose.

THE APPROACH TO THE DIAGNOSIS

Urine Sugar. This is a poor test for hyperglycemia because the blood sugar must rise well above normal (170 mg. per 100 ml.) before it will show in the urine. Patients with severe diabetes and renal disease may not show glycosuria.

Fasting Blood Sugar. Only 30-40% of diabetics can be diagnosed with this method. Many early cases will be missed. Some conditions associated with hypoglycemia will also be missed.

Two-Hour Postprandial Blood Sugar. This is an excellent screening test for diabetes. Values above 160 mg. per 100 ml. are considered diagnostic. Between 140 mg. and 150 mg. per 100 ml. they are at least equivocal and warrant the use of the 5-hour glucose tolerance test. The test is not of much use in diagnosing cases of hypoglycemia.

Five-Hour Oral Glucose Tolerance Test. This is more definitive than the 2-hour postprandial blood sugar for detecting hyperglycemia and diagnosing its cause. It is also useful in diagnosing hypoglycemia, and its causes, and the malabsorption syndrome.

Insulin Radioimmunoassay. While this is commercially available it is not of much value in diagnosing diabetes mellitus because it may be high, low, or normal in this disease.

Other tests will be discussed where appropriate.

Abbreviations Used in Plates:

F.B.S. = Fasting blood sugar in mg. per 100 ml. of blood

2 hr. P.P. = Two-hour postprandial blood sugar in mg. per 100 ml. of blood

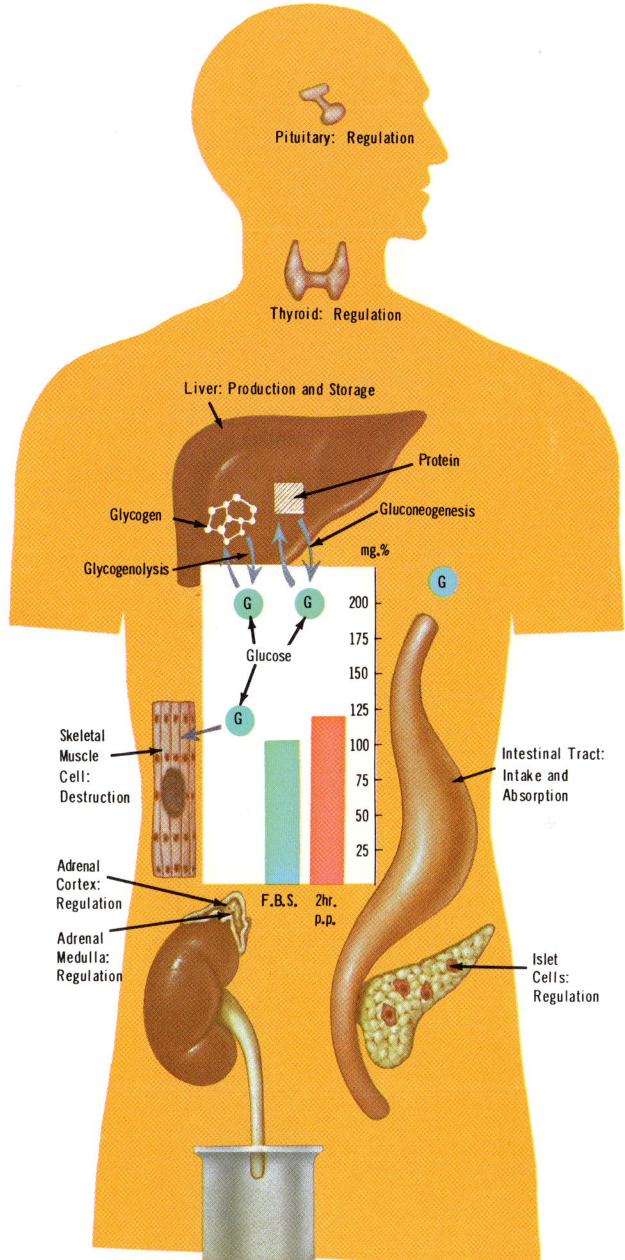

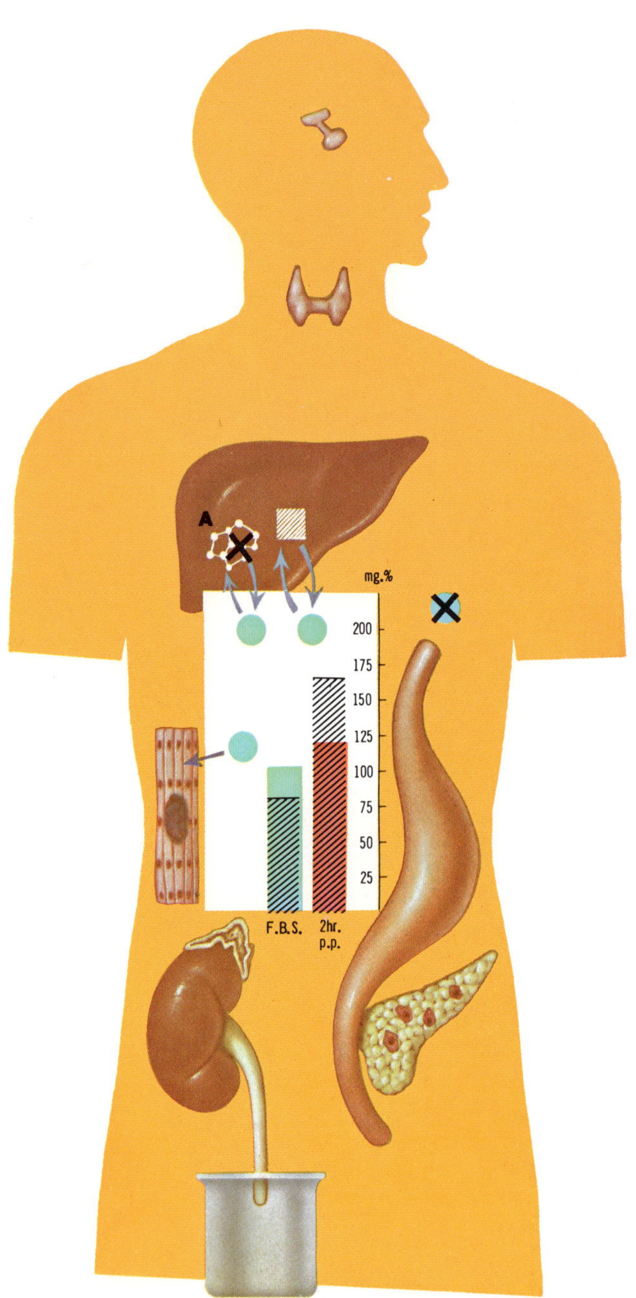

MALNUTRITION

In this disorder peripheral utilization of glucose continues despite decreased intake. Once hepatic glycogen stores are depleted (A), the *blood sugar falls* but is arrested before it reaches a critical level by gluconeogenesis from protein and fat. Following a carbohydrate meal the blood sugar will rise to abnormal levels and remain there, probably because the machinery of glycolysis has too long been at rest.

Summary of Laboratory Findings:

Fasting blood sugar: Decreased

Two-hour postprandial blood sugar: Increased

IDIOPATHIC STEATORRHEA

Although the *fasting blood sugar* is usually *normal* in this condition, the *blood sugar fails to rise* after a carbohydrate meal (there is a flat curve in the oral glucose tolerance test). The reason is that the intestinal absorption of glucose (A) is poor. The D-xylose absorption test (p. 26) is a much more sensitive indicator of this disorder. The oral glucose tolerance and D-xylose absorption tests are usually normal in pancreatic insufficiency and many other disorders that mimic idiopathic steatorrhea. Stool fat, serum carotene, and I^{131}-labeled triolein uptake will assist in the diagnosis of this disorder.

Summary of Laboratory Findings:

Fasting blood sugar: Normal

Two-hour postprandial blood sugar: Decreased

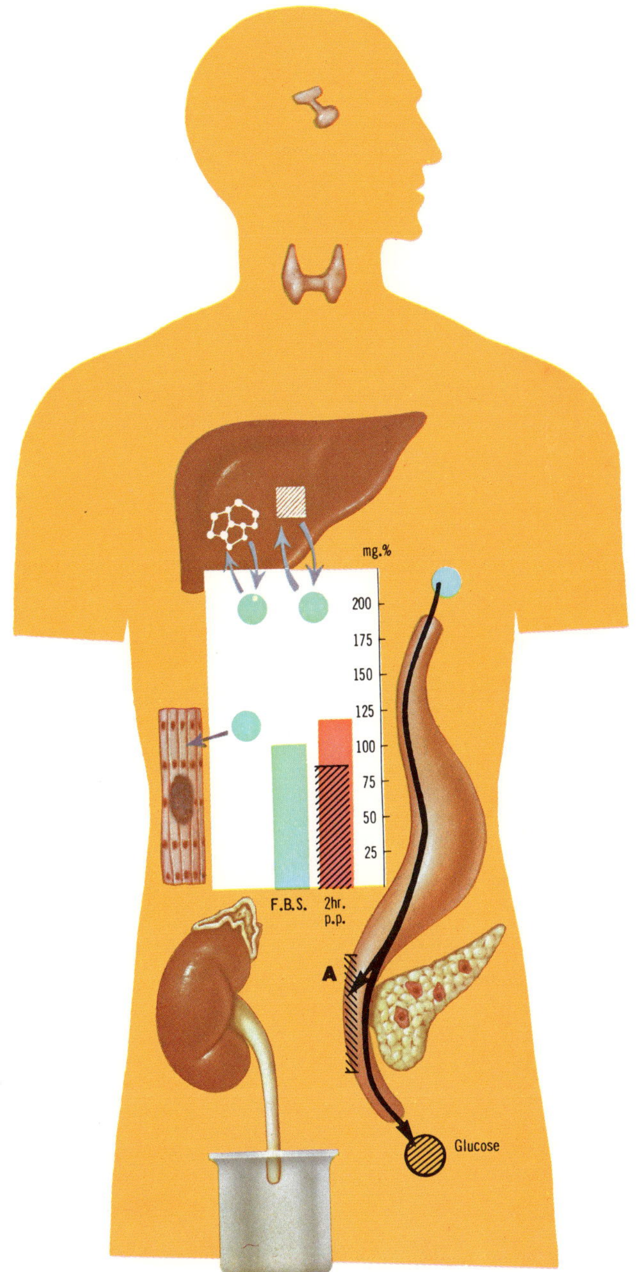

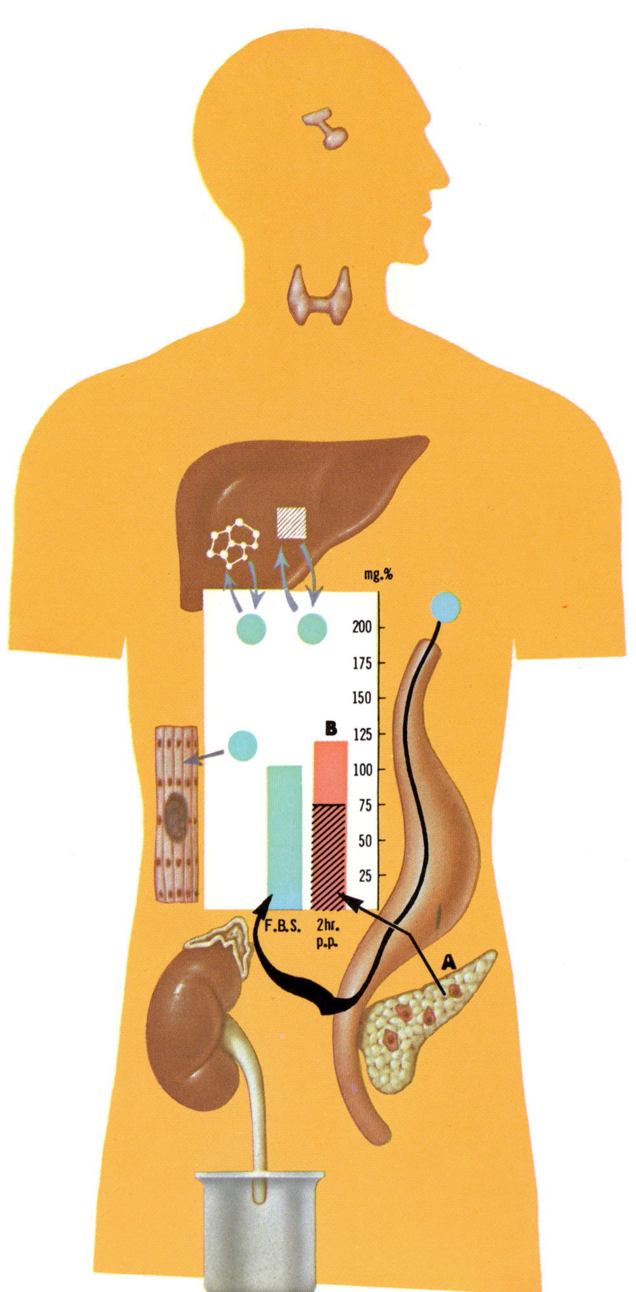

TACHYALIMENTATION HYPOGLYCEMIA

In gastrectomized patients ingested glucose may rapidly pass to the small intestine and be absorbed in increased amounts, producing a marked *hyperglycemia*. The beta cells are stimulated to produce insulin (A), and a *drop* in *blood sugar* may occur approximately 2 hours later (B). The 2-hour postprandial blood sugar will demonstrate this phenomena.

Summary of Laboratory Findings:

Fasting blood sugar: Normal

Two-hour postprandial blood sugar: Decreased

GALACTOSEMIA

As mentioned above under Normal Metabolism, sugars other than glucose such as galactose are converted to glucose by the liver. In congenital galactosemia, the absence of uridyldiphosphogalactose transferase prevents the liver conversion of galactose to glucose, and the level of *galactose rises in the blood and urine* (A).

Incomplete conversion of other carbohydrates is known to occur, resulting in pentosuria, fructosuria, lactosuria, maltosuria, or sucrosuria. None of these is of pathological significance.

Summary of Laboratory Findings:

Fasting blood sugar: Normal

Two-hour postprandial blood sugar: Normal

Galactose in blood and urine

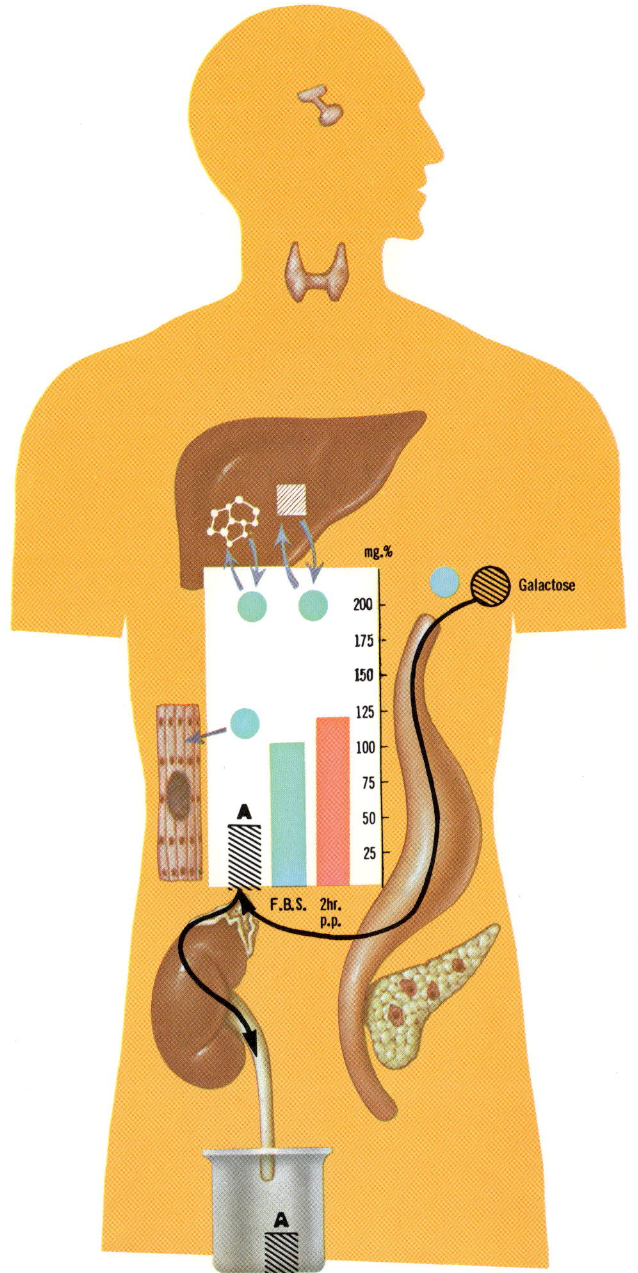

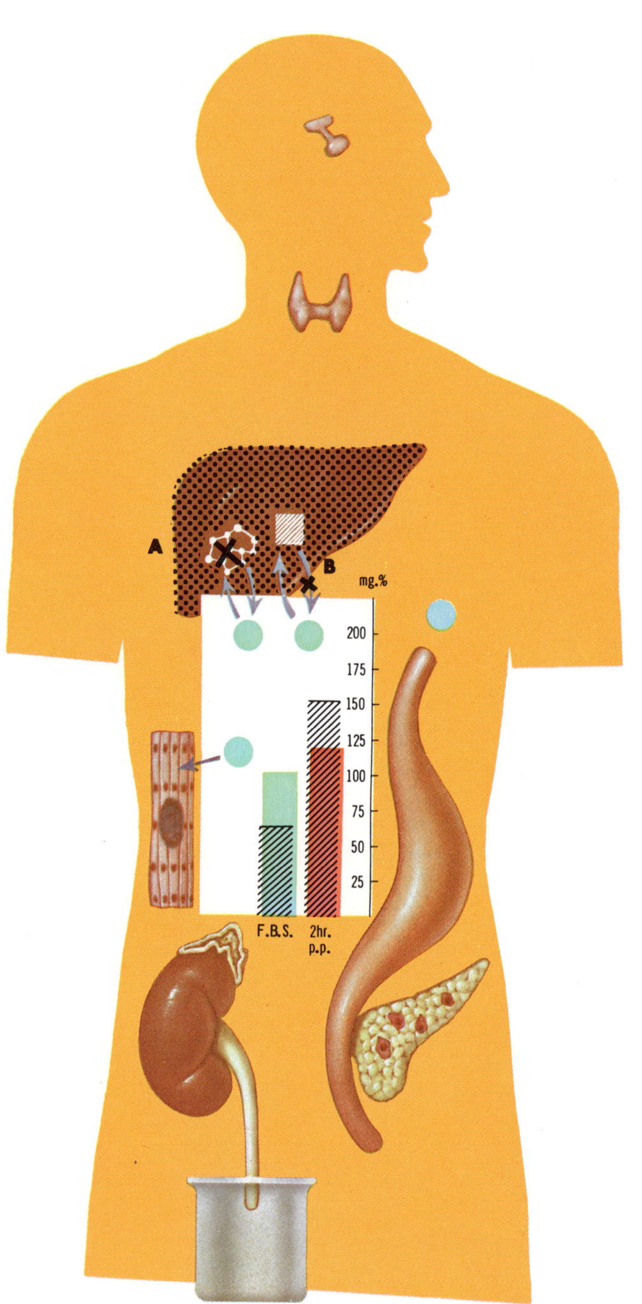

ADVANCED CIRRHOSIS OF THE LIVER

The *fasting blood sugar* in this disorder may be *decreased* because of depleted glycogen stores (A) or inadequate gluconeogenesis (B) in the diseased liver. The *2-hour postprandial blood sugar* may be *elevated,* because the liver removes sugar from the blood for storage poorly, and its influence on extrahepatic glycolysis is decreased. With severe liver disease the subject fails to manifest hyperglycemia in response to epinephrine. This diagnosis is best established by other tests of liver function and a liver biopsy. Carcinomatosis, severe hepatitis, obstructive jaundice, and other disorders of the liver may produce a similar picture.

Summary of Laboratory Findings:

Fasting blood sugar: Decreased

Two-hour postprandial blood sugar: Increased

GLYCOGEN-STORAGE DISEASE (von Gierke's Disease)

This condition is believed to be due to a deficiency of certain enzymes involved in glycogenolysis (Williams). In one variety there is a deficiency of glucose-6-phosphatase. Thus glucose may be stored, but it cannot return to the blood (A). The *blood sugar drops* under fasting conditions, and the liver enlarges (B) from the increasing stores of glycogen. There is a poor hyperglycemic response to epinephrine or glucagon. The *2-hour postprandial blood sugar* is often *decreased* as well.

Summary of Laboratory Findings:

Fasting blood sugar: Decreased

Two-hour postprandial blood sugar: Decreased

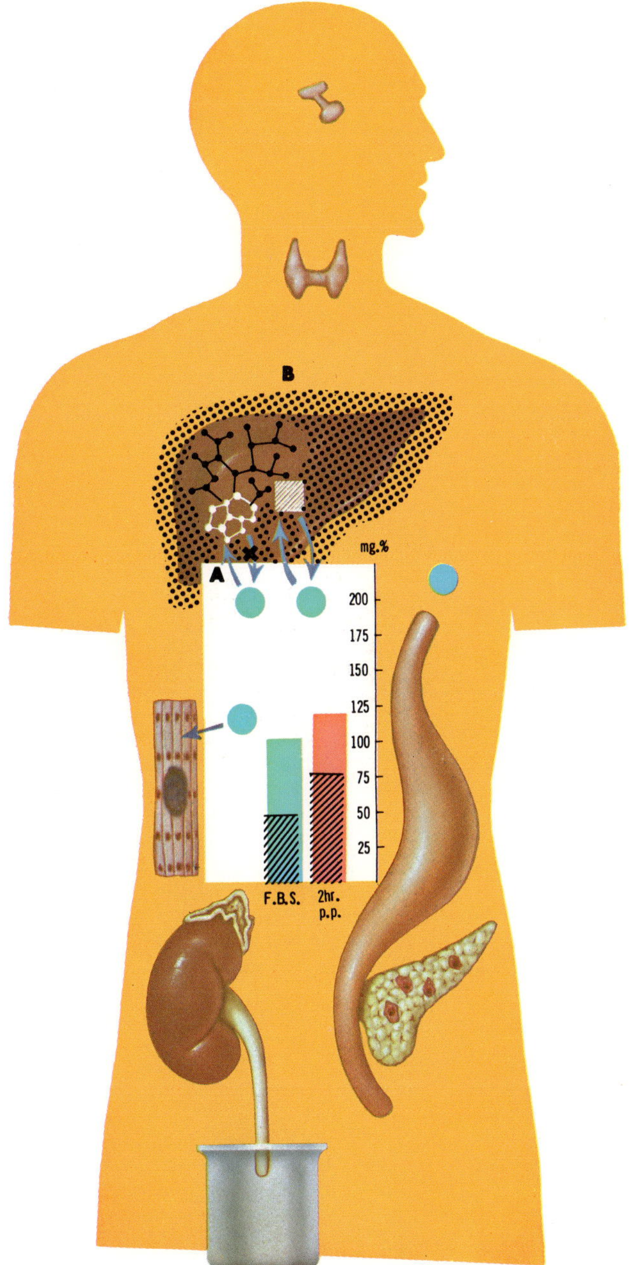

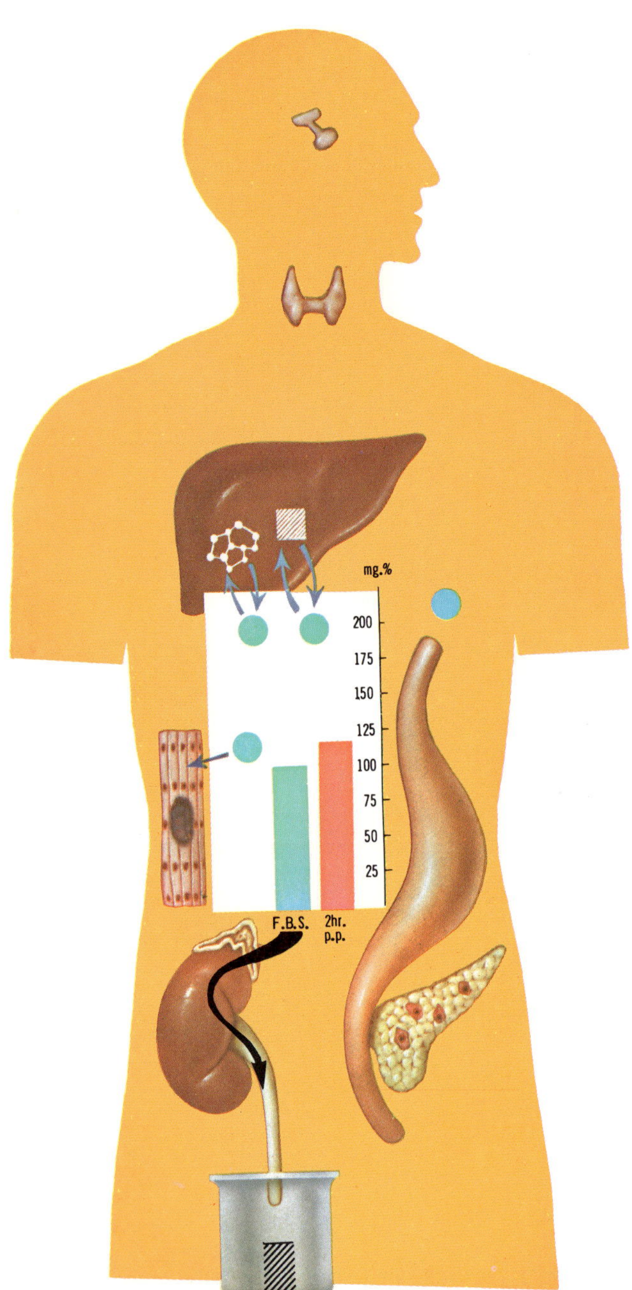

RENAL GLYCOSURIA

The lack of renal tubular reabsorptive capacity in this disorder leads to *glycosuria* in the presence of normal blood sugar values. Glycosuria of this nature may also occur in nephritis and de Toni-Fanconi syndrome. These disorders must be differentiated from other causes of melituria (p. 66).

Summary of Laboratory Findings:

Fasting blood sugar: Normal

Two-hour postprandial blood sugar: Normal

Urine sugar: Increased

ADDISON'S DISEASE

Lack of glucocorticoids in this disorder leads to decreased gluconeogenesis (A) and reduced intestinal absorption of glucose. The *fasting blood sugar* and *2-hour postprandial blood sugar* are often *decreased.* A 5–hour glucose tolerance test and insulin tolerance test help differentiate this condition from hypopituitarism and islet cell adenomas. This condition is best differentiated from other causes of hypoglycemia by measuring the urinary output of 17-hydroxycorticoids and 17-ketosteroids (p. 90).

Summary of Laboratory Findings:

Fasting blood sugar: Decreased

Two-hour postprandial blood sugar: Decreased

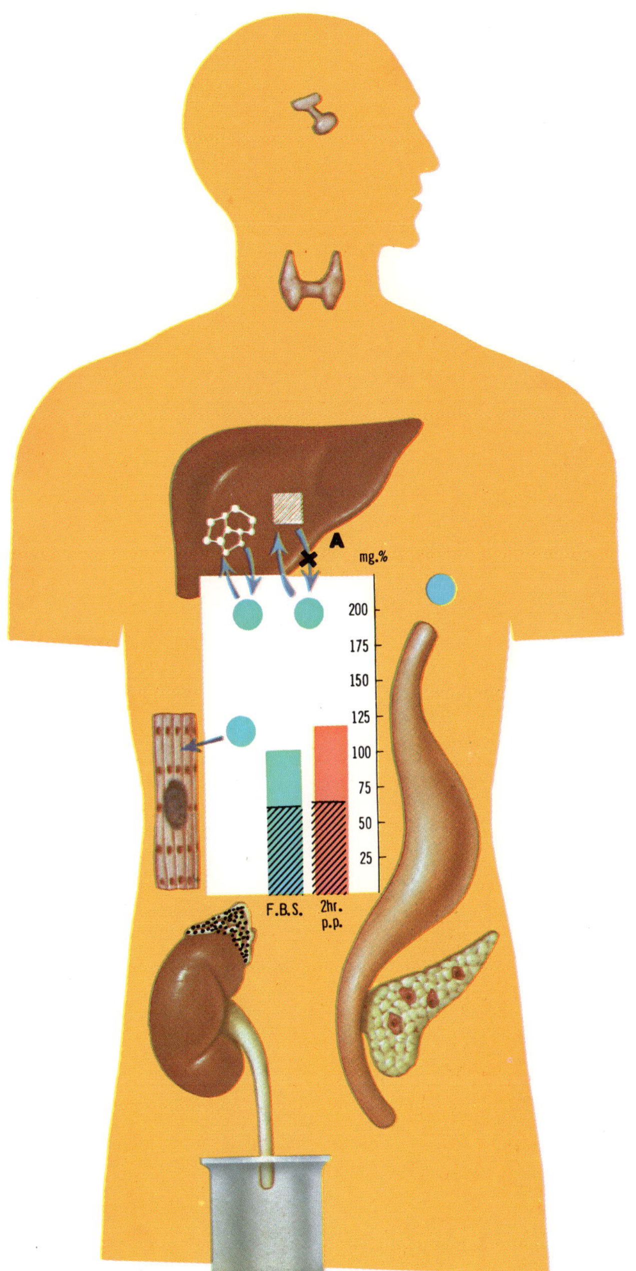

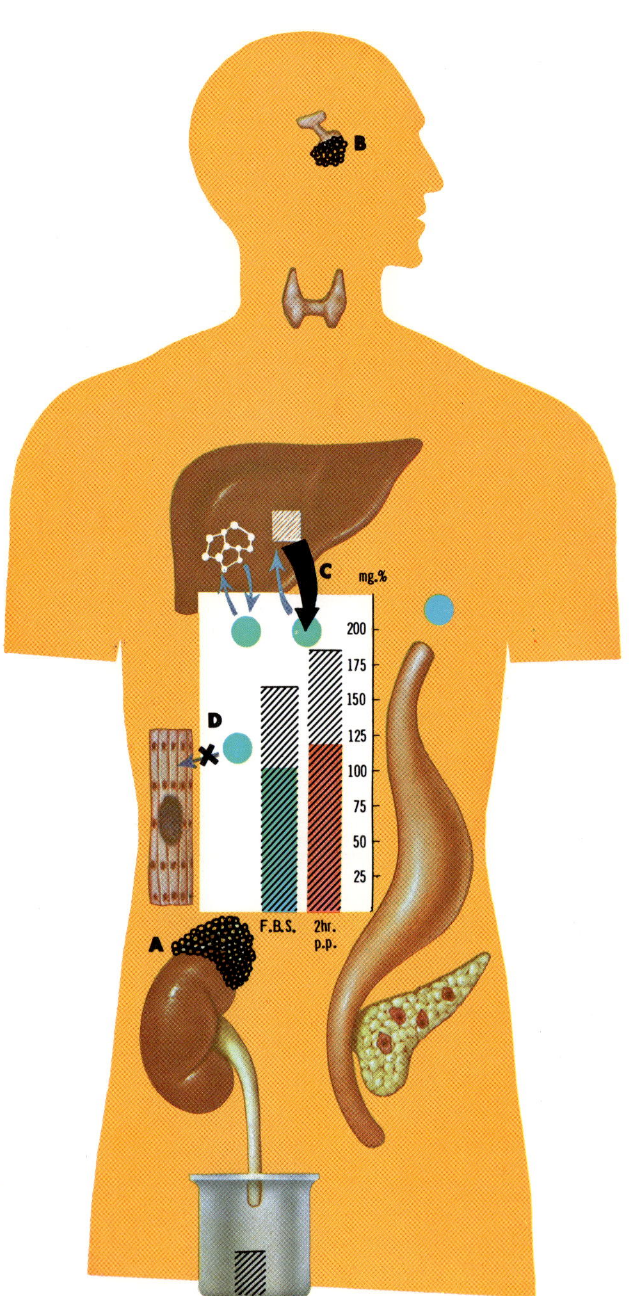

CUSHING'S SYNDROME

Whether caused by adrenocortical hyperplasia (A), adenoma, carcinoma, or basophilic adenoma of the pituitary (B), this syndrome may result in a *high fasting* and *2-hour postprandial blood sugar,* presumably by increasing gluconeogenesis (C) and decreasing peripheral utilization of glucose (D). *Glycosuria* is also manifested. These disorders are differentiated from other causes of hyperglycemia by urinary or blood ketogenic steroid determinations (p. 92).

Summary of Laboratory Findings:

Fasting blood sugar: Increased

Two-hour postprandial blood sugar: Increased

Urine sugar: Increased

ANTERIOR PITUITARY INSUFFICIENCY

The *low blood sugar* often associated with this disorder is the result of secondary adrenal insufficiency (A), hypothyroidism (B), and reduced growth hormone as well as malnutrition. Lack of glucocorticoids leads to deficient gluconeogenesis (C) and the unopposed action of insulin. The urinary 17-ketosteroids and 17-hydroxycorticosteroids, before and after ACTH, and the PBI (p. 85) are more useful in establishing this diagnosis than the blood sugar.

Summary of Laboratory Findings:

Fasting blood sugar: Decreased

Two-hour postprandial blood sugar: Decreased

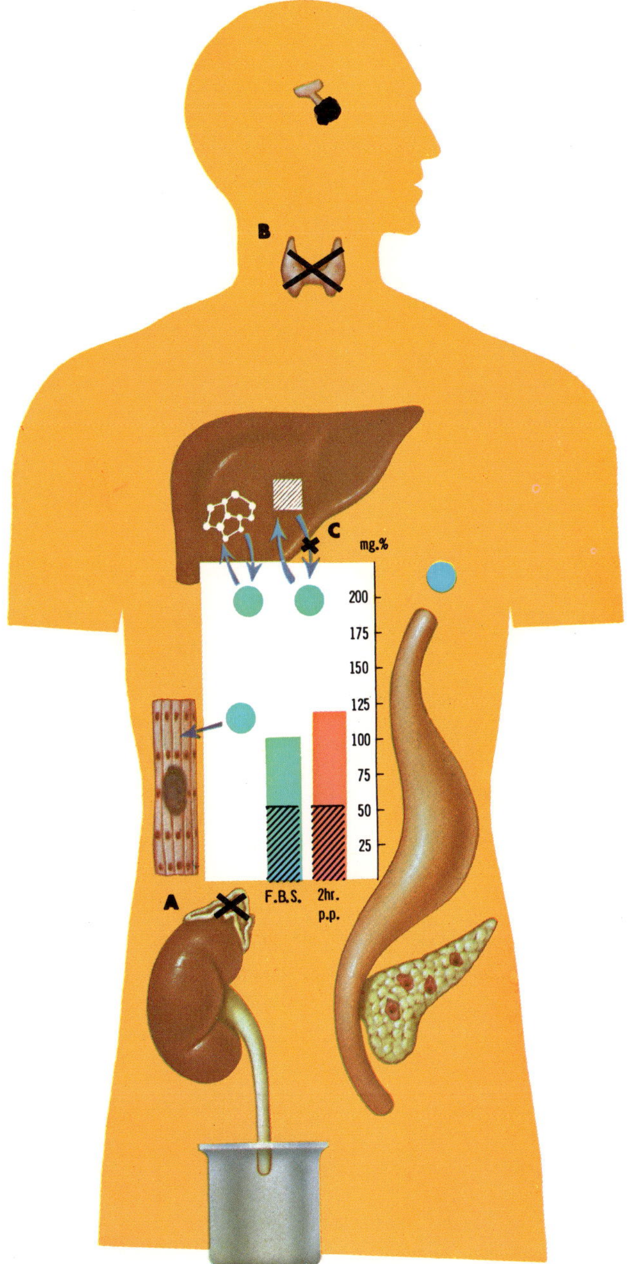

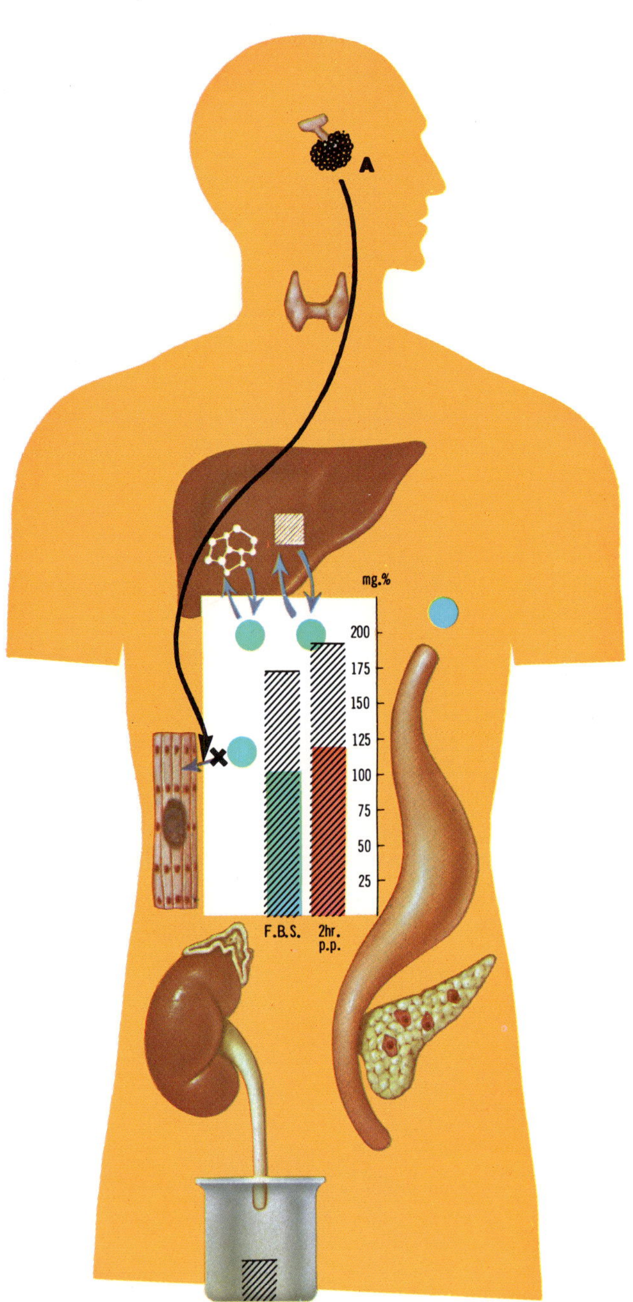

ACROMEGALY

Increased secretion of growth hormone (A) in this condition leads to insulin resistance and a reduced rate of glucose phosphorylation. There is also increased gluconeogenesis. Thus the *fasting* and *2-hour postprandial blood sugar* are usually *elevated*. Clinical and radiographic examinations and serum growth hormone assay after a glucose load establish the diagnosis.

Summary of Laboratory Findings:

Fasting blood sugar: Increased

Two-hour postprandial blood sugar: Increased

Urine sugar: Increased

HYPERTHYROIDISM

The secretion of excessive amounts of thyroid hormone increases intestinal absorption of glucose (A) and indirectly intensifies glycogenolysis (B). It also increases the peripheral utilization of glucose (C). If glycogenolysis is proceeding at a more rapid rate than peripheral glycolysis, an *increase* in the *fasting blood sugar* may be observed. More often the fasting blood sugar is normal, whereas the *2-hour postprandial blood sugar* is more regularly *increased*. Serum thyroxine, T_4 by column and T_4 by isotope, help establish the diagnosis.

Summary of Laboratory Findings:

Fasting blood sugar: Normal or increased

Two-hour postprandial blood sugar: Increased

Urine sugar: Increased

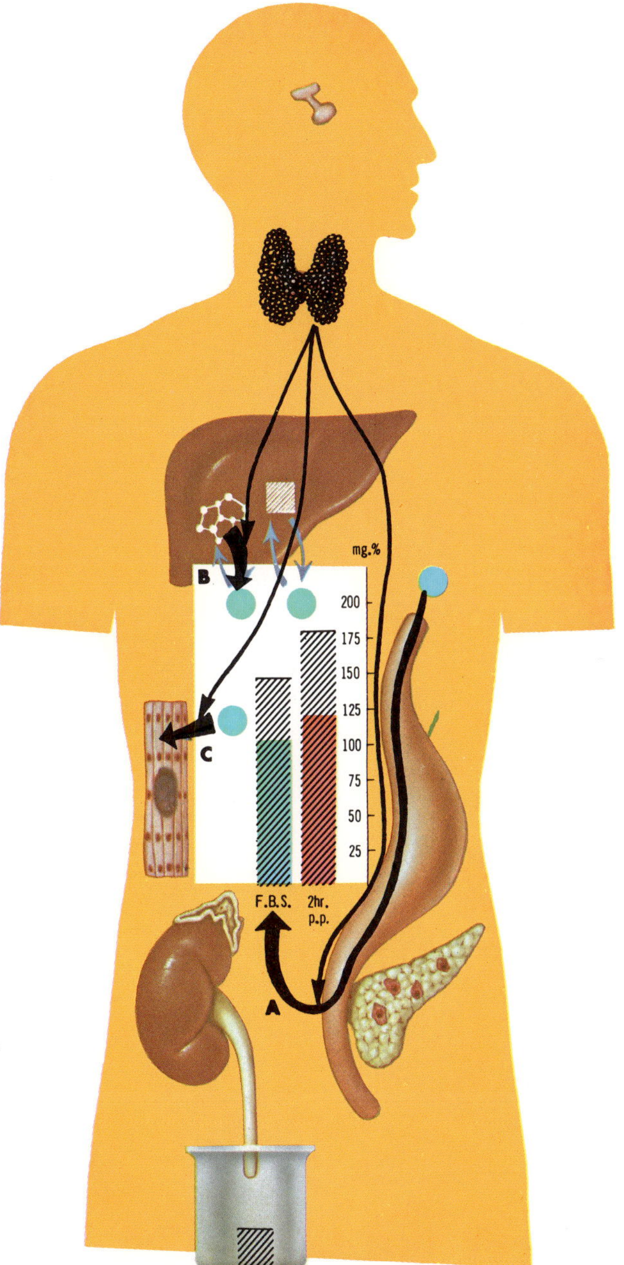

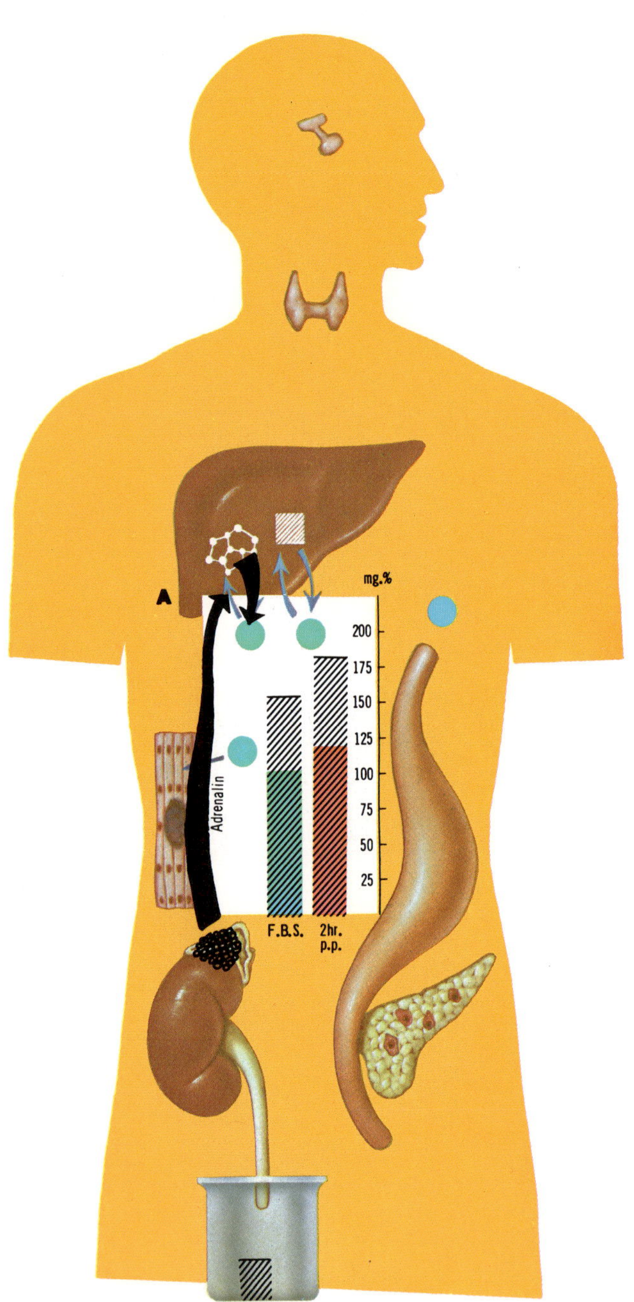

PHEOCHROMOCYTOMA

Increased secretion of epinephrine by these tumors directly or indirectly stimulates hepatic glycogenolysis (A). Epinephrine also blocks insulin release. Thus the *blood sugar* and the *urine sugar* have been found to be *elevated* in some cases. The presence of urinary catecholamines (p. 172) is of more assistance in the diagnosis.

Summary of Laboratory Findings:

Fasting blood sugar: Normal or increased

Two-hour postprandial blood sugar: Increased

Urine sugar: Normal or increased

CHRONIC PANCREATITIS

Hyperglycemia and glycosuria develop in this disorder from chronic inflammation and destruction of the islet cells of the pancreas (A), reducing insulin production. There is a decrease in hepatic uptake (B) and peripheral utilization (C) of glucose. The diagnosis is best determined by duodenal drainage, but it is suggested by elevation of serum lipase and amylase and calcifications of the pancreas seen on radiologic examination of the abdomen.

Deposit of iron in the pancreas in hemochromatosis also leads to islet cell destruction with hyperglycemia. Carcinoma of the pancreas produces hyperglycemia by a similar mechanism.

Summary of Laboratory Findings:

Fasting blood sugar: Normal or increased

Two-hour postprandial blood sugar: Increased

Urine sugar: Normal or increased

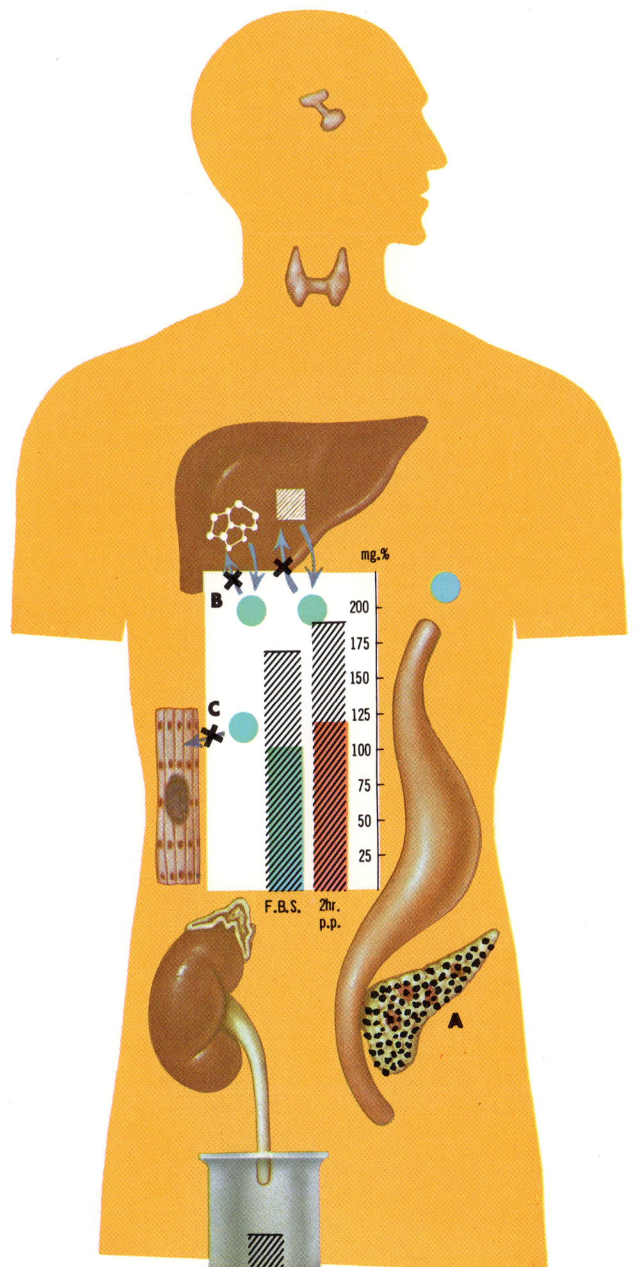

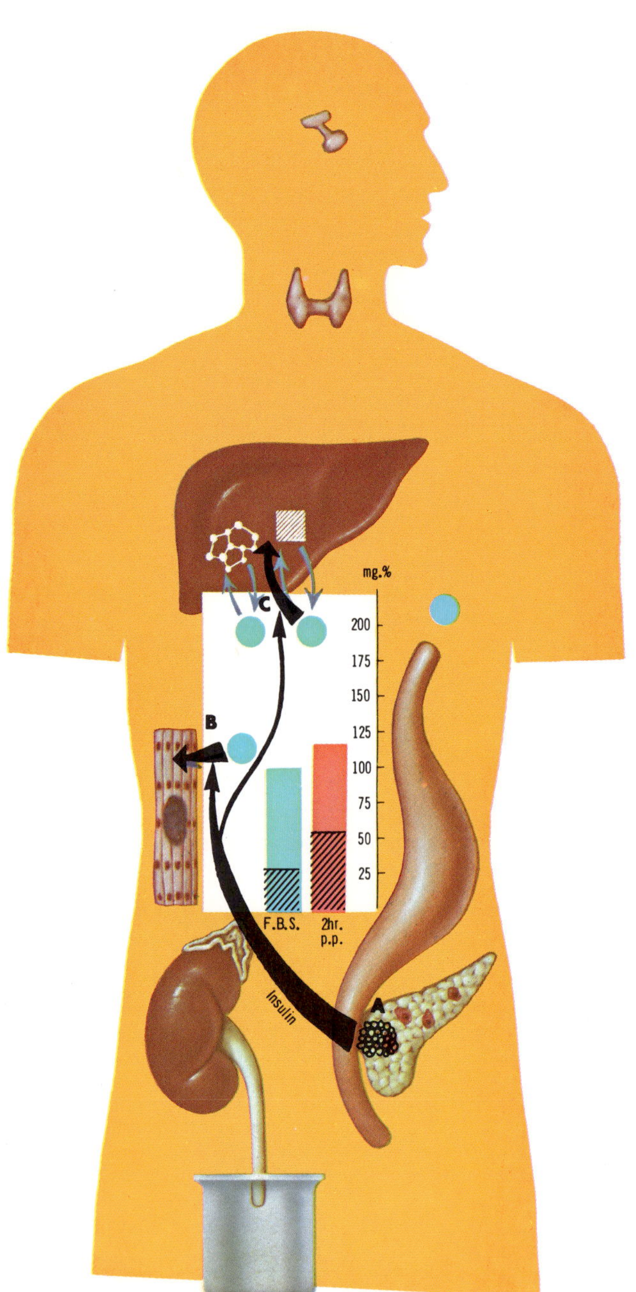

ISLET CELL ADENOMA

In this disorder a functioning adenoma (A) or carcinoma secretes large amounts of insulin, resulting in a *low fasting blood sugar* by increasing peripheral utilization (B) and hepatic storage (C) of sugar. Hyperglycemia is not usually manifested after a carbohydrate meal, and the *2-hour postprandial blood sugar is also low.*

Islet cell hyperplasia and carcinoma and retroperitoneal sarcomas may produce a similar picture. These conditions may be differentiated from functional hypoglycemia by a normal 48- or 72-hour fast and a return of the blood sugar to normal levels during a 6-hour glucose tolerance test in the latter condition.

A tolbutamide tolerance test may also assist the diagnosis.* After receiving 1 gm. of tolbutamide intravenously, subjects with an insulinoma experience a much greater and more prolonged hypoglycemia than those with functional hypoglycemia, Addison's disease, and other disorders. High plasma insulin levels are not found in sarcomas.

Summary of Laboratory Findings:

Fasting blood sugar: Decreased

Two-hour postprandial blood sugar: Decreased

* Fajans, S. S., *et al.:* The diagnostic value of sodium tolbutamide in hypoglycemic states. J. Clin. Endocr., *21*:371, 1961.

DIABETES MELLITUS

Although the many causes for the *elevated blood sugar* in this disorder are not all understood, it is safe to say that the condition results from a relative or absolute deficiency of insulin. Thus there is decreased hepatic (A) and extrahepatic (B) uptake of glucose. In many cases there is a reduced number of islet cells, often replaced with a hyaline substance or fibrosis (C). In those cases with normal islets the abnormality may be an overproduction of glucose by the liver, or an increase in insulin requirements by the tissue, or insulin antibody reaction.

Summary of Laboratory Findings:

Fasting blood sugar: Normal or increased

Two-hour postprandial blood sugar: Increased

Urine sugar: Increased

OTHER CAUSES OF HYPERGLYCEMIA

An elevated blood sugar is often associated with many stressful or serious conditions. Myocardial or cerebral infarction, certain malignancies, pregnancy, and anxiety states may induce hyperglycemia. Also hyperglycemia has been associated with the use of drugs such as chlorothiazide diuretics and Dilantin. The lipoproteinemias (page 118), especially Type V, are associated with hyperglycemia.

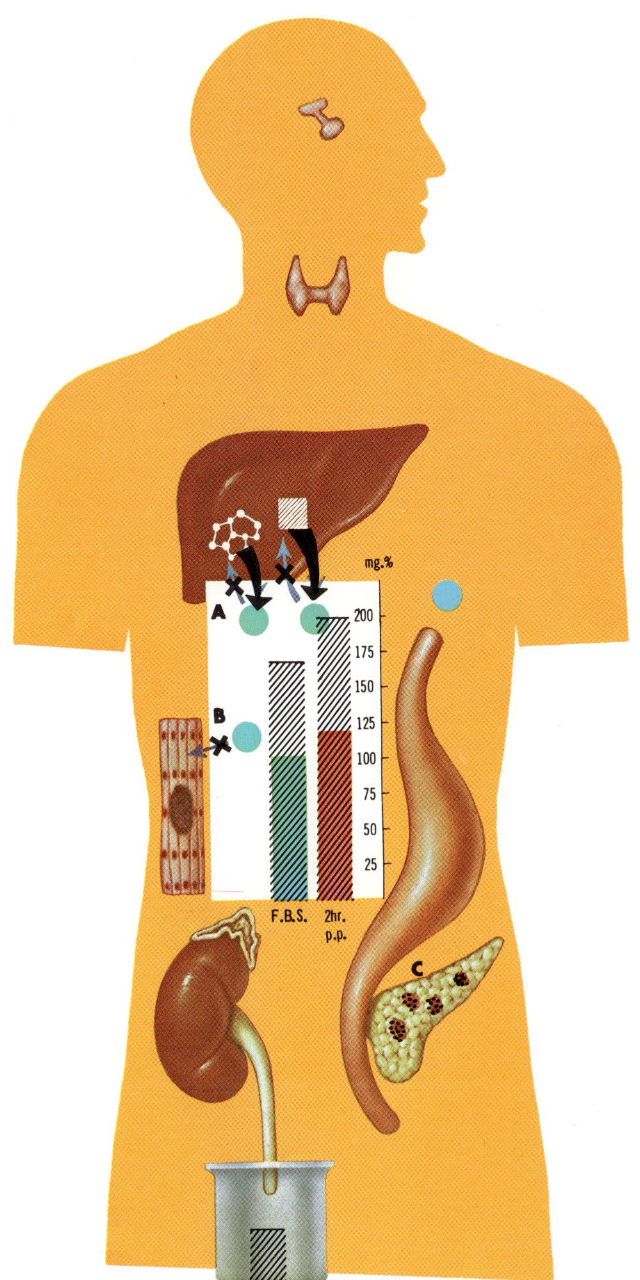

6 Disorders of the Hormones

The endocrine system is made up primarily of six important glands: the pituitary, thyroids, parathyroids, islet cells of the pancreas, adrenals, and gonads (ovaries in the female, testicles in the male). Altogether they secrete over 20 different hormones or types of hormones. This chapter is most concerned with those hormones that can be measured in the average clinical laboratory and/or those that are valuable indicators of endocrine diseases. These are the pituitary gonadotropins (FSH and LH), thyroxine, cortisol, the androgens, and aldosterone. Most of the hormones of the pituitary cannot be measured. However, disturbances of the secretion of some of them can be determined indirectly by measuring the level of target-organ hormone. They will therefore be included in this discussion. The metabolism of parathyroid hormone, insulin, and glucagon will not be discussed here. These hormones are measured by indirect methods (blood calcium, glucose, etc.), and the reader is referred to those sections of this text.

FUNCTIONS OF CERTAIN HORMONES

A brief description of each of the hormones to be discussed seems appropriate. *Follicle-stimulating hormone* (FSH) is a gonadotropin produced by the pituitary which influences spermatogenesis in the male and follicular growth and estrogen production and secretion in the female, provided that a small amount of luteinizing hormone is present with it. *Luteinizing hormone* (LH or ICSH) is a gonadotropin which stimulates testosterone secretion in the male and follicular growth, ovulation, luteinization, and estrogen and progesterone secretion in the female. To accomplish these functions in the female, a small amount of FSH is required. *Thyroid-stimulating hormone* (TSH) is the hormone of the pituitary which stimulates thyroxine secretion by the thyroid. The production and release of TSH by the pituitary is stimulated by thyrotropin releasing hormone (TRH), secreted by the hypothalamus into the hypothalamic-pituitary portal system. Both TSH and TRH release are inhibited by thyroid hormones. *Adrenocorticotropin (ACTH)* is the hormone of the pituitary which stimulates the production and/or secretion of adrenal cortical hormones (even aldosterone to a minor degree). There are probably releasing factors produced in the hypothalamus for all the pituitary hormones.

Thyroxine, the principal hormone of the thyroid gland, functions by increasing the rate of body metabolism and protein and fat catabolism.

Cortisol, the chief glucocorticoid of the adrenal gland, functions primarily by stimulating gluconeogenesis from protein and fat and controlling some adaptive changes of the cell in response to stress. *Aldosterone* is the chief mineralocorticoid of the adrenal gland which conserves certain electrolytes (sodium and chloride) and circulatory volume. The *androgens* of the adrenal cortex, principally dehydroepiandrosterone (DEA), are responsible for the development of the male and the formation of body protein in both growth in puberty and maintenance of body structure. *Testosterone,* secreted by the Leydig cells of the testicles, has primarily the same function. The *estrogens,* estradiol, etc., produced by the ovaries and to a minor extent by the adrenal cortex, are responsible for the sex characteristics of the female and stimulate anabolism of body protein and bone formation and growth of the female reproductive organs.

NORMAL METABOLISM

Production. *Thyroxine* is produced by the thyroid gland from tyrosine and iodide of the diet. The normal adult requires 15 to 25 mcg. of iodine a day. Over 50 per cent of ingested iodide is excreted by the kidney, and between 25 and 50 per cent is trapped by the thyroid gland. The amount of iodide concentrated by the thyroid gland is up to 25 times that of the plasma. The iodide is first oxidized to iodine and then combines with tyrosine to form monoiodotyrosine and diiodotyrosine. Finally, two molecules of these are coupled to form thyroxine or triiodothyronine. These compounds are then stored in the thyroid gland as thyroglobulin. Later they are secreted according to body needs. The average output is 2 gr. a day.

The *17-hydroxycorticosteroids* are produced by the adrenal cortex (presumably the zona fasciculata) from cholesterol. An outline of this synthesis is shown in Figure 6-1. The principal steroid in this fraction is cortisol. The average output of cortisol is 15 to 30 mg. a day.

Aldosterone is also produced in the adrenal cortex, probably by the glomerulosa layer. The gland produces 75 to 125 mcg. a day.

Two thirds of the *17-ketosteroids* are produced in the zona reticularis of the adrenal cortex from cholesterol; the other third is testicular in origin. The principal 17-ketosteroid of the adrenal cortex is dehydroepiandrosterone (DEA), 15 to 20 mg. being produced each day. The principal testicular hormone is testosterone.

The adrenal cortex also produces minimal amounts of progesterone and estradiol, but these are synthesized principally in the ovary and the placenta. Since a routine measurement of these hormones is impractical in clinical medicine, a detailed discussion will not be undertaken here.

FSH and LH (ICSH) are, of course, synthesized by the pituitary. Little is known about the details of this synthesis. They are measured collectively as *human pituitary gonadotropin* (HPG) in the urine by bioassay. In 24 hours 5 to 30 mouse units are excreted by the male, and 5 to 100 mouse units by the female.

Transport. All the hormones in this discussion are transported in the blood bound to proteins produced in the liver. *Thyroxine* is bound to an inter-alpha globulin, a prealbumin substance, and serum albumins. These are collectively called thyroxine-binding proteins (TBP). A small portion is free in plasma. The protein-bound iodine (PBI) consists almost entirely of thyroxine. Iodide normally accounts for 0.3 mcg. of it. The very small amounts of triiodothyronine present in the circulation are either free or loosely bound to albumin and do not account for significant portions of PBI.

Cortisol circulates in an unconjugated form bound to an alpha globulin (transcortin) and in a conjugated form with glucuronic acid or sulfates. Transcortin assures a ready source of circulating cortisol. Both transcortin and thyroxine-binding proteins are produced in the liver under the influence of estrogen.

Testosterone and *adrenal androgens* are also bound to plasma proteins.

Storage. Aside from thyroxine, none of the hormones is stored to any appreciable extent. Thyroxine is stored in the thyroid gland as thyroglobulin.

Excretion. The liver is involved in the excretion of thyroxine and the steroid hormones. *Thyroxine* is conjugated with glucuronate and excreted in the bile. However, much of this is reabsorbed after being freed from the glucuronate by bacterial enzymes in the intestines. Only 5 per cent is excreted in the feces and essentially none in the urine. Instead, thyroxine enters the cell, where it is enzymatically converted to pyruvic or acetic acid derivative, or deiodinated to triiodothyronine. *Cortisol, corticosterone, aldosterone, testosterone,* and other *androgens* and *estrogens* are also conjugated in the liver with glucuronate and, to a lesser extent, sulfates, but they are excreted in the urine. Five per cent or less of cortisol is excreted in the urine in the free (unconjugated) form. The average daily secretion of cortisol is 15 to 30 mg.

Regulation

The anterior pituitary under the influence of the hypothalamic nuclei is the master controller of most of the endocrine system. It secretes the so-called trophic hormones that stimulate the secretions of the thyroid, adrenal, and sex glands. Pertinent to this discussion are *thyroid-stimulating hormone* (TSH), which stimulates thyroxine secretion in the thyroid, *adrenocorticotropin* (ACTH), which stimulates glucocorticoid, androgen, and estrogen secretion by the adrenal gland, and the *gonadotropin hormones FSH* and *LH* (ICSH in the male), which stimulate estrogen and progesterone production and secretion in the female and *testosterone* production and secretion in the male. Some influence of ACTH on aldosterone secretion has been noted, but it is probably minimal.

The secretion of these trophic hormones by the pituitary is largely controlled by the feedback mechanism, whereby increased amounts of target-organ hormone (e.g., thyroxine, cortisol, etc.) inhibit their secretion, whereas a decrease in circulating target-organ hormones stimulates their secretion. This feedback action is mediated by the hypothalamic nuclei, which secrete releasing factors into the hypophyseal-portal system of blood vessels in response to decreasing blood levels of target-organ hormone, and in turn induce the pituitary to secrete trophic hormones.

In addition to the feedback mechanism, the pituitary may be influenced by central nervous system factors through the hypothal-

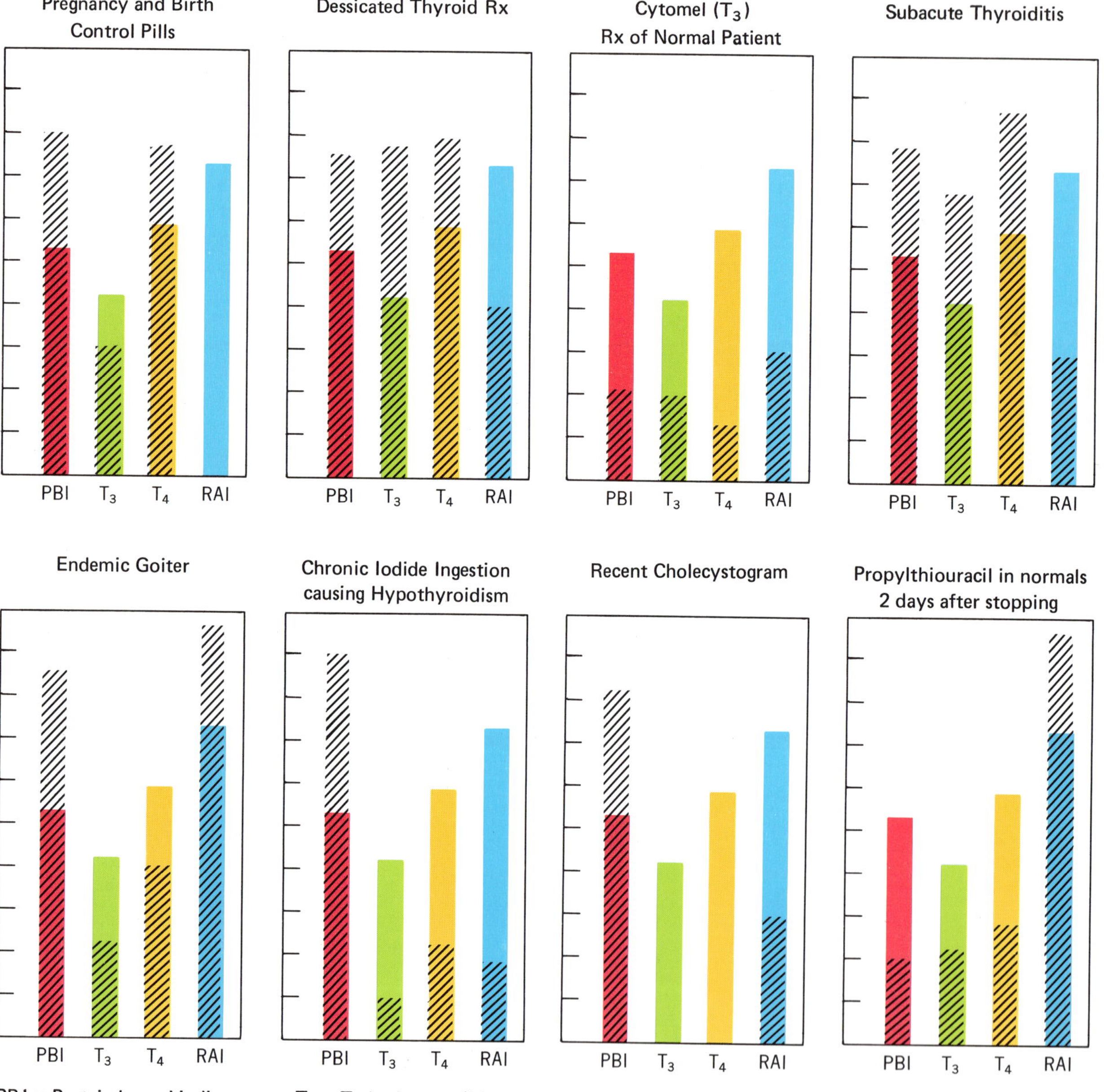

FIG. 6-1. Thyrograms of real and fictitious thyroid states.

amus. It is well known that stress will increase the output of ACTH and adrenocortical steroids. Other emotional and environmental stimuli may inhibit the secretion of the pituitary trophic hormones.

Several other less well understood factors seem to be involved in the regulation of hormones. For example, gonadotropin secretion may be increased by degeneration of the seminiferous tubules. Appropriate blood levels of estrogen may induce LH secretion. Thyroxine probably has some effect on adrenocortical secretion. Apparently, both ACTH and cortisol are necessary for normal thyroxine secretion. On the other hand, increased amounts of circulating cortisol may inhibit the release of thyroxine for 24 to 48 hours.

Aldosterone secretion may be controlled by a pineal extract, *adrenoglomerulotropin,* and by *angiotensin,* produced by the action of renin from the juxtaglomerular cells of the kidney on a precursor in the blood. Angiotensin production seems to be increased by a reduced circulatory volume and decreased by an increased circulatory volume.

Testosterone secretion in the male and *estrogen* and *progesterone* secretion in the female do not occur until puberty, at which time significant secretion of FSH and ICSH (LH) begins. Estrogen and progesterone secretion drop at the time of the menopause, whereas FSH and LH secretion continues, usually in increased amounts.

Cortisol is the most potent inhibitor of ACTH secretion, whereas adrenal androgens and estrogens have no measurable effect on ACTH secretion. On the other hand, triiodothyronine is a more potent TSH inhibitor than *thyroxine,* principal hormone of the thyroid gland.

THE APPROACH TO THE DIAGNOSIS

Clinical findings such as myxedema, tachycardia, high blood pressure, Cushingoid features, etc., will usually suggest which endocrine gland is involved. The appropriate tests that can be utilized to study each gland are now discussed.

Thyroid

The PBI, T_3-uptake, and radioactive iodine uptake are excellent tests of thyroid function but yield a significant number of false negatives and false positives. Thus the search for a more accurate test continues. In the past few years the T_4 by column, T_4 by isotope, free thyroxine, T_3 by radioimmunoassay, and the "corrected" T_4 by isotope have been made available. To date all of them have their drawbacks except perhaps the "corrected" T_4 by isotope (see Table 6-1), which is really too new to be relied upon.

Table 6-1. Effects of Various Substances and Conditions on Thyroid Tests

	Inorganic Iodine	Organic Iodine	Thyroid Hormone Therapy	Pregnancy and Estrogen Birth Control Pills	Increased Thyro-binding Protein	Drugs
PBI	↑	↑	↑	↑	↑	Usually ↓
BEI	0	↑	↑	↑	↑	Usually ↓
T_4 by Column	0	↑	↑	↑	↑	↑ ↓
T_3 Uptake	0	0	↑	↓	↓	
T_4 by Isotope	0	0	↑	↑	↑	↑ ↓
Corrected T_4 by Isotope	0	0	↑	0	0	(0)
Serum-free Thyroxine	0	0	↑	0	0	↑ ↓
T_3 by Radioimmuno-assay	0	0	0 or ↓	0	0	↑ ↓
RAI Uptake	↓	↓	↓	0	0	↓
Free Thyroxine Index	0	0	↑	0	0	(0)

Protein–Bound Iodine (PBI). This test has an accuracy of 90–95% but presents false elevations in patients exposed to inorganic iodides, organic iodides (Hypaque, Pantopaque, etc.), thyroid hormone, and estrogens and is altered up, and down by many drugs and diseases which affect the thyro-binding protein (TBP).

T_4 by Column. This test eliminates contamination from inorganic iodine, but contamination from organic iodides and the other disadvantages of the PBI are not eliminated.

Thyroxine by Isotope (Murphy-Pattee, T_4 by isotope). This test (see description on page 186) eliminates contamination from inorganic and organic iodides, but the other disadvantages of the PBI remain.

Serum–Free Thyroxine. This test is unaffected by contamination with inorganic and organic iodides and in addition is unaffected by alterations in the TBP. However, certain drugs and serious illnesses may affect it. It is done by only a few reference laboratories, and is very vulnerable to laboratory error because the amount of free thyroxine in the serum is normally infinitesimal.

Free Thyroxine Index (adjusted T_4, T_7). This test allows correction of the total serum thyroxine for any increase or decrease in thyrobinding protein (TBP). The results correlate very closely with the free thyroxine mentioned above but is less expensive. The following formula is used:

$$\text{Free thyroxine index} = T_4 \text{ (by Murphy-Pattee)} \times \frac{T_3 \text{ uptake of patient}}{\text{mean normal } T_3 \text{ uptake}}$$

T_3 by Radioimmunoassay. This test measures triiodothyronine by using antibodies against it. It is extremely valuable in diagnosing T_3 thyrotoxicosis in which the T_3 is elevated but the T_4 is normal. T_3 by radioimmunoassay is, however, affected by changes in TBP.

"Corrected" T_4 by Isotope. This test promises to be the best screening test for thyroid function in the near future. It is much like the T_7 (free thyroxine index). It is performed much like the usual T_4 by isotope, but in addition to using TBP from normal serum it uses the TBP from the patient's serum for comparison. Thus, not only are the effects of iodide contamination eliminated but also the effects of alterations of the TBP (estrogen, pregnancy, etc.).

Serum TSH (thyroid stimulating hormone). This is now available in many commercial laboratories and is pretty accurate. It is elevated in primary myxedema and reduced in pituitary myxedema. Normal value is below 10 microunits/ml.

Selection of Tests. The best combination of tests for the initial evaluation of thyroid dysfunction are the T_3 uptake, the T_4 by isotope, and the T_7 (free thyroxine index). If either one of these is abnormal the following tests should be done. If myxedema is suspected a serum TSH is ordered. If one suspects hyperthyroidism an RAI uptake and scan should be added. When the above tests are normal and hypothyroidism is still probable, a thyroid-stimulating hormone (TSH) test is done. An RAI is done before and after TSH. In myxedema it will not be increased. If the clinician suspects hyperthyroidism a PBI or RAI is done before and after 7 days therapy with 75 mcg. of T_3. Normally the PBI or RAI decreases, but in hyperthyroidism it will not. Figure 6-1 illustrates the changes of these tests in common conditions.

Indirect Tests. These have largely been replaced by the above, but a serum cholesterol (p. 113) and BMR may give support to the diagnosis in doubtful cases. The Achilles reflex test is very useful in diagnosing hypothyroidism but of little value in diagnosing hyperthyroidism. A special attachment for the Burdick electrocardiograph machine (called a Photomotograph) can be purchased. In hypothyroidism there is a delayed relaxation of the Achilles reflex while in hyperthyroidism the relaxation may be prompt.

Adrenal Cortex

Direct Tests. Hypersecretion or hyposecretion of *cortisol* and *adrenal androgens* are evaluated by serial determinations of the 24-hour urinary *17-hydroxycorticosteriods* and *17-ketosteroids*, respectively. Where available a plasma cortisol should be done. This test is gradually replacing urinary steroid determinations for the diagnosis of Addison's disease or Cushing's syndrome. In cases suspected of hyposecretion (Addison's disease, etc.) determinations after ACTH (the ACTH stimulation test) are done and will not show any appreciable increase. Differentiation of primary and secondary adrenal insufficiency are further discussed on page 90.

In cases suspected of hypersecretion (Cushing's syndrome, adrenogenital syndrome), an ACTH test and dexamethasone suppression test may be helpful in differentiating adrenocortical adenomas and hyperplasia from carcinomas (p. 92). Note the similarity of these accessory tests to those used in evaluating thryoid dysfunction.

Hypersecretion or hyposecretion of *aldosterone* is evaluated by determining the 24-hour urinary levels of this hormone or the plasma aldosterone level where available. The test is not widely available and is subject to considerable variations under normal conditions. Thus, in evaluating disordered secretion of this hormone, heavy reliance still is placed on indirect tests.

Indirect Tests. With the exception of disorders of aldosterone secretion, these tests have largely been replaced by direct tests. Cortisol secretion may be indirectly evaluated by the eosinophil count and Thorn test (p. 247) and glucose tolerance test (p. 68), but these are often normal in disorders of the adrenal cortex. Aldosterone secretion is evaluated by *serial blood electrolytes, plasma renin* (p. 91) and the *water-load test.* The last of these tests is especially valuable in diagnosing cases of adrenal cortical insufficiency in which the secretion of aldosterone is reduced. Following a period of fluid restriction, a water load is administered (20 ml./kg.), and hourly urine volumes are recorded. Normally, the patient will excrete at least 1,000 ml. of urine in the 4 hours after the water load. In adrenal insufficiency less will be excreted.

Testicles

Since over two thirds of the urinary 17-ketosteroids come from the adrenal cortex, this test is unreliable in assessing *testosterone* secretion. Plasma testosterone is useful in diagnosing cases of hirsutism, virilization, and suspected hypogonadism. Hyposecretion and hypersecretion of this hormone may be determined indirectly by the *24-hour urinary gonadotropins* (HPG). In accordance with the feedback mechanism described above, decreased secretion of testosterone leads to increased pituitary secretions of ICSH (LH) and thus increased levels of urinary HPG. In cases of increased testosterone production the reverse is true. A decrease in testosterone secretion is often associated with reduced spermatogenesis. Thus *semen analysis* may also be a useful adjunct in diagnosing disorders of secretion of this hormone.

Ovaries

Urinary *estrogen* and *progesterone* determinations are too expensive for routine use in diagnosis. As with testosterone, secretion of these hormones may be evaluated indirectly by measuring the *urinary gonadotropins.* The *vaginal smear* provides an indirect test of estrogen secretion. If adequate amounts of estrogen are being secreted, the vaginal epithelial cells are polygonal in shape and contain small pyknotic nuclei and orange-red-staining cytoplasm with the Shorr trichrome technique. If estrogen secretion is inadequate, the cells are small and round and contain large nuclei and blue- or violet-staining cytoplasm (basal cells).

Pituitary

FSH and LH secretion, as mentioned above, may be measured collectively by the *24-hour urinary gonadotropins.* TSH and ACTH secretion may be determined indirectly by the *PBI* and *urinary 17-hydroxycorticosteroids* and *17-ketosteroids,* respectively. However, measurement of plasma ACTH and TSH is now becoming possible. When TSH secretion is decreased, the PBI is also decreased. Likewise, when ACTH secretion is increased, the urinary steroids will increase. Diminished ACTH secretion will be associated with a decrease in the urinary steroids. Diminished TSH secretion is further substantiated by the *TSH stimulation test.* If there truly is diminished TSH secretion (as in hypopituitarism), the PBI will rise to normal levels after TSH administration. Diminished ACTH secretion is determined in an analogous fashion by the *ACTH stimulation test.*

Growth hormone is now measured directly by radioimmunoassay (p. 83). Growth hormone can also be measured indirectly (glucose tolerance test and serum phosphate). ADH (antidiuretic hormone) is also determined indirectly (see p. 50). The recent development of a radioimmunoassay for serum arginine vasopressin (ADH) will probably replace the indirect tests.

Placenta

One of the many functions of the placenta is to act as an endocrine gland. In early pregnancy it secretes *chorionic gonadotropin,* which maintains *estrogen* and *progesterone* secretion by the corpus luteum. The chorionic gonadotropin can be measured in the urine and constitutes a useful diagnostic test of pregnancy. In the absence of pregnancy, a high urinary chorionic gonadotropin suggests a hydatidiform mole or chorioepithelioma. In males the presence of chorionic gonadotropin in the urine is diagnostic of testicular neoplasms (chorioepithelioma, etc.)

Later on in pregnancy the placenta produces estrogen, progesterone, and other steroids. However, determinations of these do not constitute useful diagnostic procedures in placental disorders.

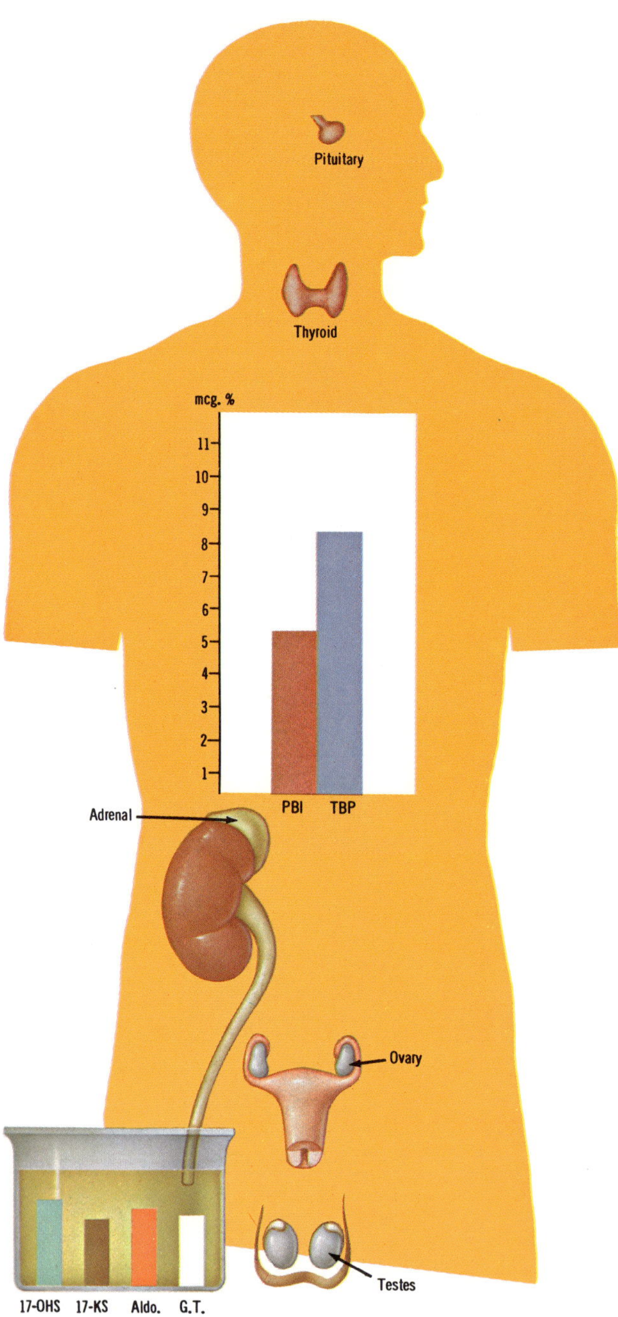

Abbreviations Used in Plates:

17-OHS	= 17-hydroxycorticosteroids, 24-hr. urine
17-KS	= 17-ketosteroids, 24-hr. urine
Aldo.	= Aldosterone, 24-hr. urine
G.T.	= 24-hr. urine gonadotropins
PBI	= Serum protein-bound iodine
TBP	= Thyrobinding protein

ACROMEGALY

Although the increased output of somatotropin hormone in this disorder leads to alterations in carbohydrate metabolism (p. 70) and elevated blood phosphorus, *PBI* and *urinary steroid* levels are usually *not disturbed.* However, in advanced cases the tumor compresses and destroys the basophilic cells of the pituitary, occasionally leading to a drop in urinary steroids. Roentgenograms of the skull and hands are the most useful adjunct in diagnosis. An x-ray of the foot may show a heel pad greater than 13 mm. that is diagnostic. Growth hormone assay reveals an increase. This is confirmed by observing the effect of intravenous glucose on the blood level of growth hormone. Normal persons demonstrate a decrease while acromegalics usually do not.

Summary of Laboratory Findings:

Serum PBI: Normal

Serum thyrobinding protein: Normal

Urine 17-hydroxycorticosteroids: Normal

Urine 17-ketosteroids: Normal

Urine aldosterone: Normal

Urine gonadotropins: Normal

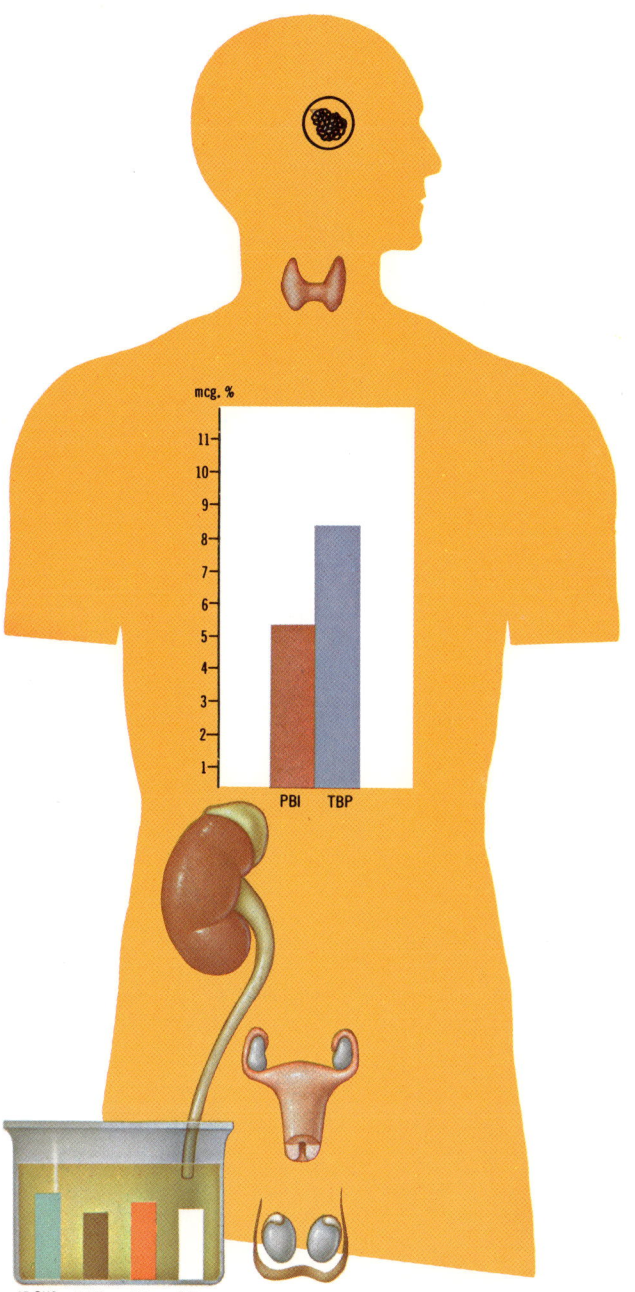

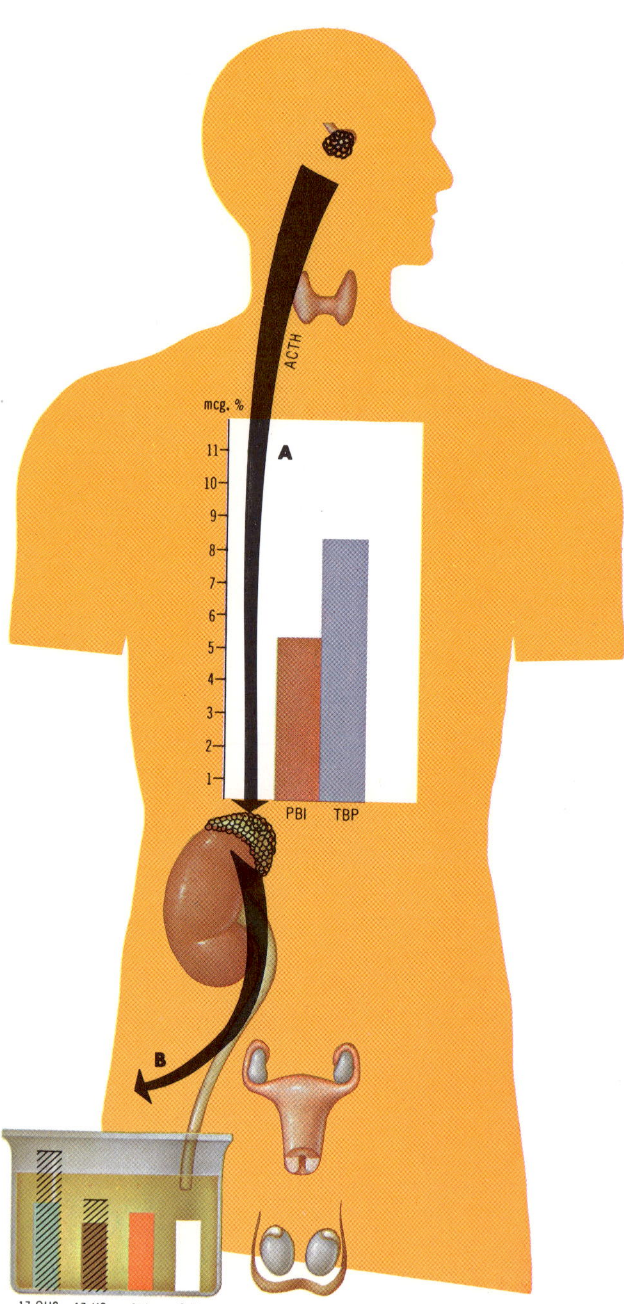

BASOPHILIC ADENOMA OF THE PITUITARY

Increased secretion of ACTH (A) in this disorder leads to adrenal cortical hyperplasia (B) and increased output of corticosteroids. *Urinary 17-hydroxycorticosteroids* and *17-ketosteroids rise.*Plasma cortisol will also be increased. A dexamethasone suppression test (p. 92) will differentiate this condition from adrenal cortical adenomas and carcinomas.

Pituitary tumors associated with hypersecretion of TSH have also been reported recently.* Chromophobe adenomas occasionally secrete an excess of one or more pituitary hormones (ACTH, growth hormone, etc.).

Summary of Laboratory Findings:

Serum PBI: Normal

Serum thyrobinding protein: Normal

Urine 17-hydroxycorticosteroids: Increased

Urine 17-ketosteroids: Increased

Urine aldosterone: Normal

Urine gonadotropins: Normal

* Jailer, J. W., and Holuh, D. A.: Remission of Graves' disease following radiotherapy of a pituitary neoplasm. Am. J. Med., *28*:497, 1960.

PANHYPOPITUITARISM

Whether due to a pituitary neoplasm (A), postpartum necrosis, or other etiologies, the secretion of all the trophic hormones of the pituitary are usually decreased in this disorder. Plasma ACTH, TSH, and growth hormone are all decreased. The *PBI* and *urinary 17-hydroxycorticosteroids, 17-ketosteroids,* and *HPG* drop accordingly. The PBI and urinary steroids increase after TSH and ACTH administration, respectively. Blood levels of TSH will not increase after administering TRH (thyrotrophin releasing hormone). Further confirmation of diminished pituitary ACTH reserve may be had by the *metyrapone* (formerly methopyrapone) (SU-4885) *test.* Since this substance inhibits the 11-beta-hydroxylation of steroids, circulating cortisol is decreased after its administration. This indirectly increases ACTH secretion in the normal adult, with a corresponding increase in urinary steroids. In hypopituitarism such an increase does not occur. Further confirmation of the reduced growth hormone can be obtained by inducing hypoglycemia with insulin or arginine. Growth hormone levels will not increase in true pituitary insufficiency under these conditions.

Rarely, the secretion of only one of the trophic hormones is diminished in this disorder (pituitary myxedema, pituitary adrenal insufficiency, etc).

Skull roentgenograms are useful in diagnosing pituitary neoplasms.

Summary of Laboratory Findings:

Serum PBI: Decreased

Serum thyrobinding protein: Normal

Urine 17-hydroxycorticosteroids: Decreased

Urine 17-ketosteroids: Decreased

Urine aldosterone: Normal

Urine gonadotropins: Decreased

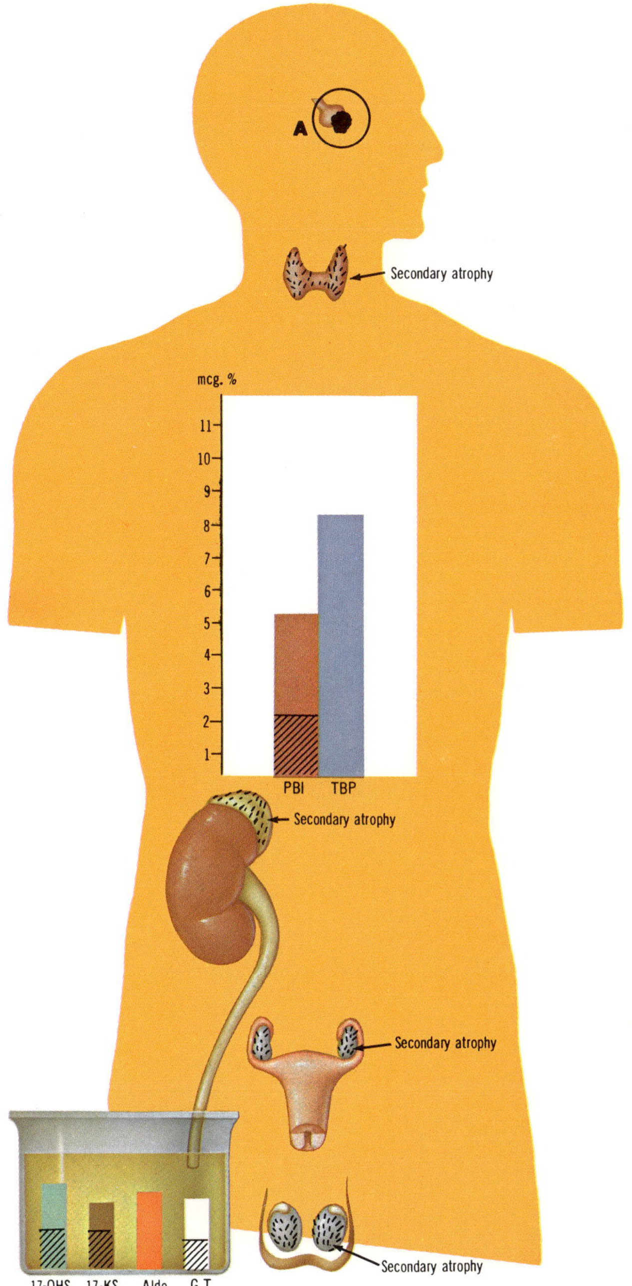

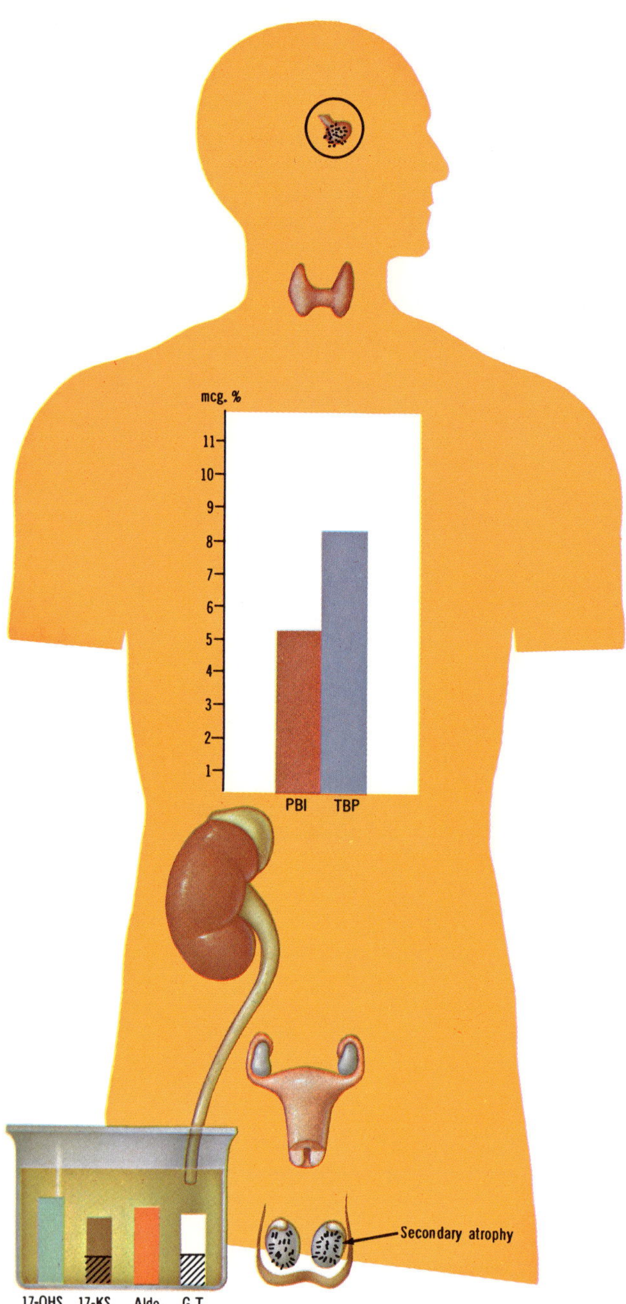

PITUITARY HYPOGONADISM

This rare condition is characterized by a selective drop in pituitary FSH and LH (ICSH) secretion. *Urinary gonadotropins* are diminished. In addition, *urinary 17-ketosteroids* are often decreased in males as a result of reduced testosterone secretion. Plasma testosterone levels are reduced. Anorexia nervosa may produce a similar picture. Semen analysis reveals oligospermia or azoospermia. This disorder must be differentiated from panhypopituitarism (p. 85), in which other hormones are depressed as well.

Summary of Laboratory Findings:

Serum PBI: Normal
Serum thyrobinding protein: Normal
Urine 17-hydroxycorticosteroids: Normal
Urine 17-ketosteroids: Decreased
Urine aldosterone: Normal
Urine gonadotropins: Decreased

HYPERTHYROIDISM

Increased production of thyroxine (A) in this disorder leads to an *elevated PBI* and increased radioactive iodine uptake (50% or more in 24 hours). A triiodothyronine suppression test is of value when the levels are borderline.

The PBI may be increased also in normal subjects who have ingested excessive thyroxine or inorganic iodides and in those who have had radiocontrast studies. In these cases the RAI will be normal or low, and a red cell radioactive T_3 uptake will be normal. The T_4 by column and T_4 by isotope will also usually help to distinguish this condition and other false positives. Another test to distinguish Grave's disease and mild hyperthyroidism will soon be available. TRH (thyrotropin releasing hormone) is injected intravenously and TSH determinations are made. Normally the TSH rises markedly, but in Grave's disease this does not occur.

Toxic adenomas of the thyroid may be differentiated from diffuse hyperplasia by a thyroid scan using radioactive I^{131}. In adenomas there is a localized accumulation of radioactivity, whereas in hyperplasia the increased radioactivity is diffuse. Toxic adenomas may display a normal PBI because they are manufacturing triiodothyronine principally. A radioimmunoassay of T_3 will help diagnose these cases.Thyroid carcinomas do not usually alter the PBI or RAI but may be detected by a localized reduction in radioactivity on the scan (p. 186).

Summary of Laboratory Findings:

Serum PBI: Increased

Serum thyrobinding protein: Normal

Urine 17-hydroxycorticosteroids: Normal

Urine 17-ketosteroids: Normal

Urine aldosterone: Normal

Urine gonadotropins: Normal

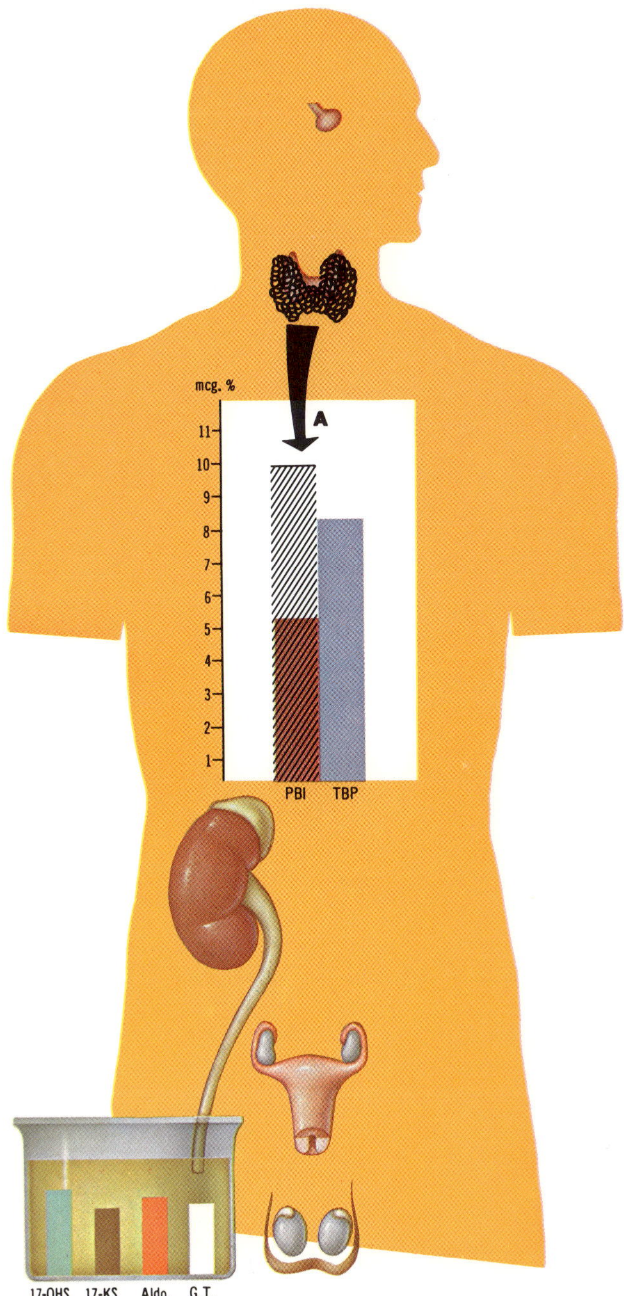

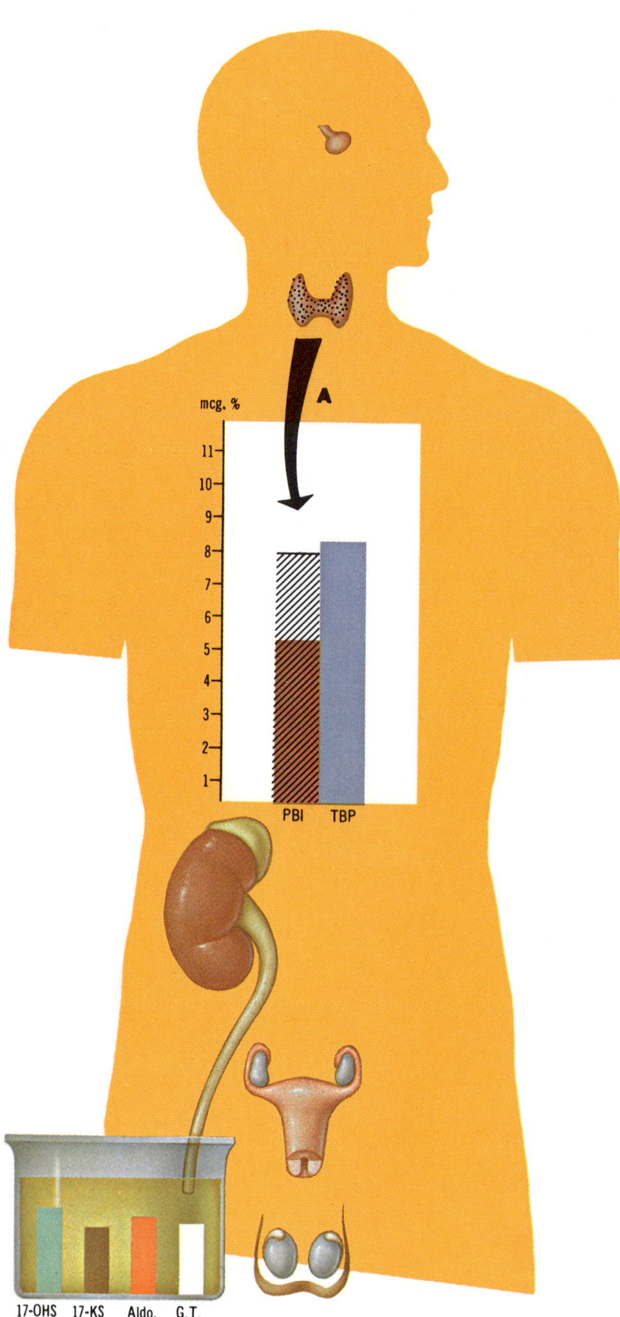

SUBACUTE THYROIDITIS

Thyroxine output is often increased (A) in this inflammatory disorder of the thyroid, with a corresponding *rise* in the *PBI*. On the other hand, the inflammation reduces the RAI uptake by the gland. Continued and extensive damage to the gland may lead to a drop in the PBI and subsequent myxedema. At least half of these patients show positive serologic tests for thyroid antibodies.

Summary of Laboratory Findings:

Serum PBI: Increased
Serum thyrobinding protein: Normal
Urine 17-hydroxycorticosteroids: Normal
Urine 17-ketosteroids: Normal
Urine aldosterone: Normal
Urine gonadotropins: Normal

MYXEDEMA

An atrophied thyroid is unable to produce sufficient thyroxine for body needs, and the *PBI drops*. The gland also fails to trap iodides, and the RAI uptake is diminished (less than 15% in 24 hours).

Subjects with myxedema who have received inorganic or organic iodide compounds may have normal PBI's. However, neither their PBI's nor their RAI's will rise after TSH (TSH stimulation test). Also the T_4 by column and the T_4 by isotope will be diminished in these cases. Elevated thyroid antibodies are often found in cases of myxedema associated with Hashimoto's thyroiditis.

The PBI is also low in pituitary myxedema, but it returns to normal or near normal after TSH. Serum TSH levels will be low in pituitary myxedema.

Summary of Laboratory Findings:

Serum PBI: Decreased

Serum thyrobinding protein: Normal

Urine 17-hydroxycorticosteroids: Normal

Urine 17-ketosteroids: Normal

Urine aldosterone: Normal

Urine gonadotropins: Normal

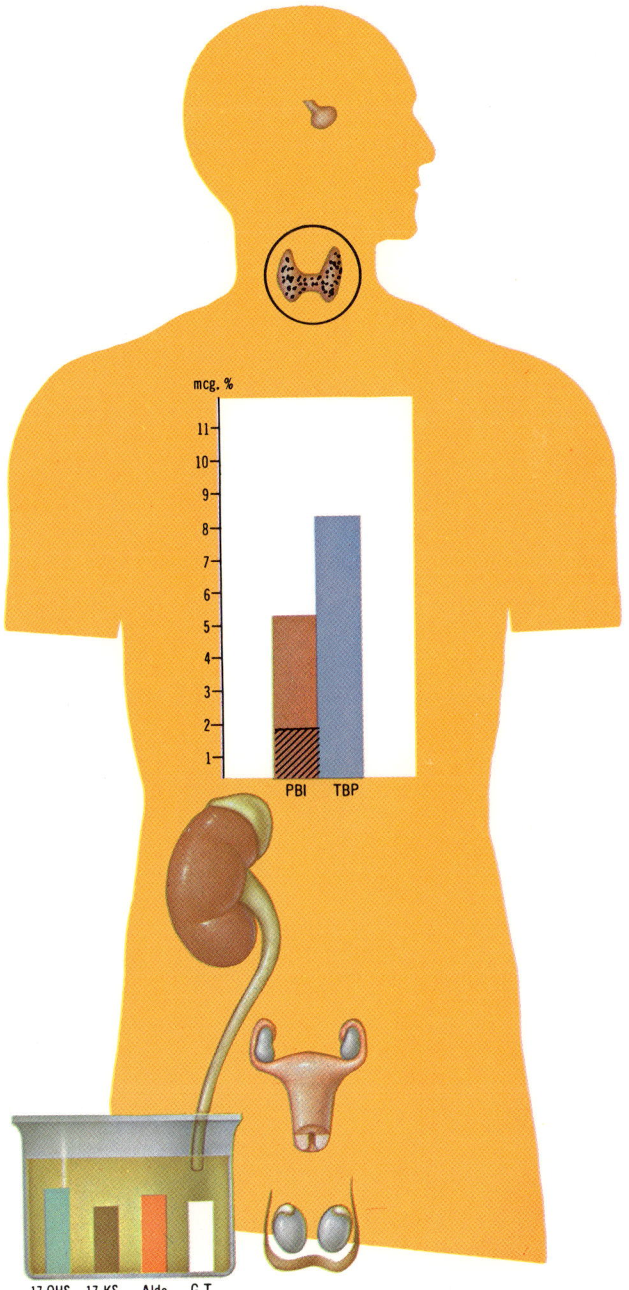

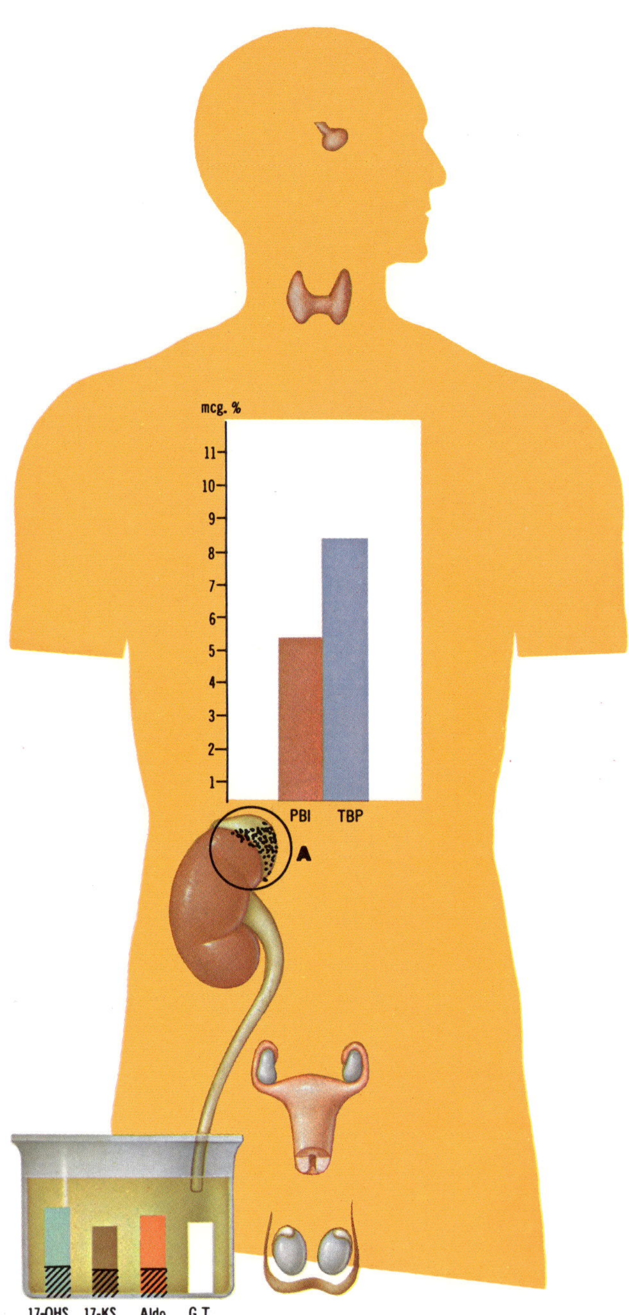

ADDISON'S DISEASE

Atrophy or tuberculosis of the adrenal cortex (A) leads to diminished secretion of mineralocorticoids, glucocorticoids, and androgens, with a corresponding *drop* in the plasma and *urinary aldosterone, 17-hydroxycorticosteroids,* and *17-ketosteroids.* These remain low after ACTH administration in contrast with the steroid levels in "pituitary" adrenal insufficiency. Less specific tests such as the serum sodium-potassium ratio (p. 49), the eosinophil count (p. 247), and the water-load test heretofore mentioned are useful in diagnosing this disorder. The water-load test is particularly useful as a screening test.

Summary of Laboratory Findings:

Serum PBI: Normal

Serum thyrobinding protein: Normal

Urine 17-hydroxycorticosteroids: Decreased

Urine 17-ketosteroids: Decreased

Urine aldosterone: Decreased

Urine gonadotropins: Normal

PRIMARY ALDOSTERONISM

Adrenocortical hyperplasia or adenomas (A), particularly of the glomerulosa cell layer, may produce excessive amounts of *aldosterone,* a potent mineralocorticoid. *Urinary and plasma levels* of *aldosterone* are *increased,* but these are difficult to measure accurately even in the best laboratories. The plasma renin is usually diminished but this test is non-specific unless it remains low after sodium depletion and attaining an upright posture. In screening for this disorder, indirect tests are best. A consistently *low serum potassium* and other electrolyte abnormalities (p. 49) are very suggestive of this disorder. The serum potassium will promptly rise after 300 mg. of Aldactone (spironolactone test) is administered.

Aldosteronism secondary to nephrosis, cirrhosis, or congestive heart failure must be differentiated by other means (pp. 42, 55). Renovascular hypertension is differentiated by an angiotensin infusion test or plasma renin. The plasma renin will be elevated in this condition. At least eight cases of renin-secreting tumors of the kidney have been reported. Both plasma renin and aldosterone are elevated in this disorder.

Summary of Laboratory Findings:

Serum PBI: Normal
Serum thyrobinding protein: Normal
Urine 17-hydroxycorticosteroids: Normal
Urine 17-ketosteroids: Normal
Urine aldosterone: Increased
Urine gonadotropins: Normal

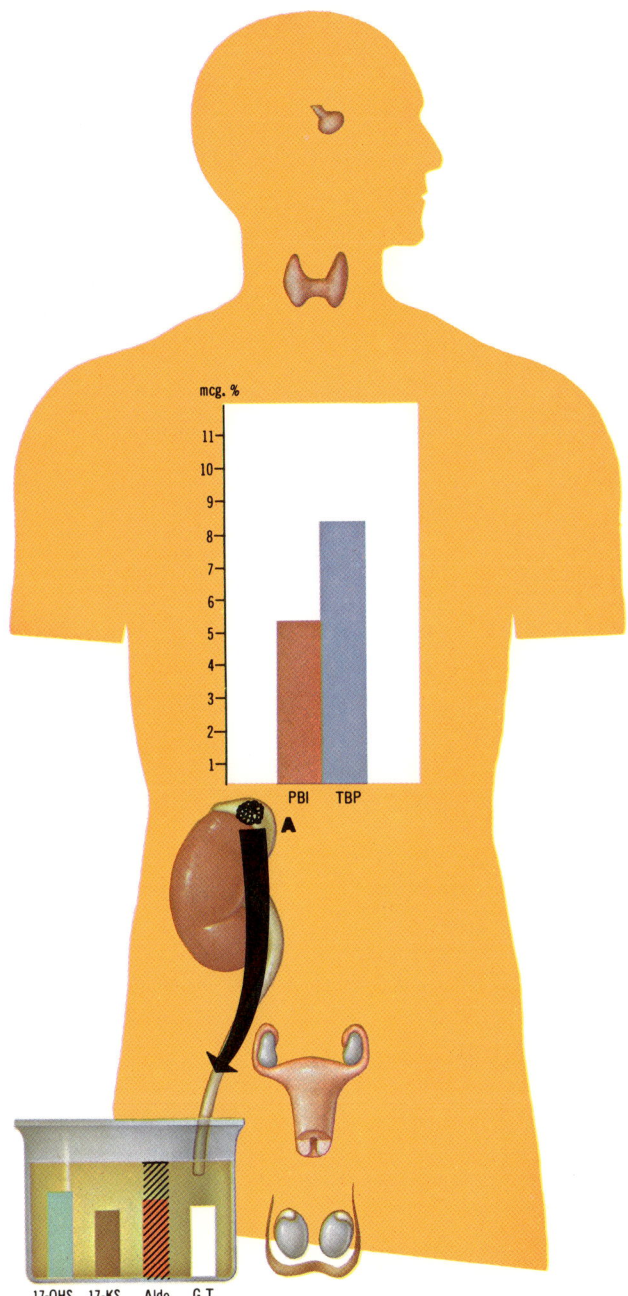

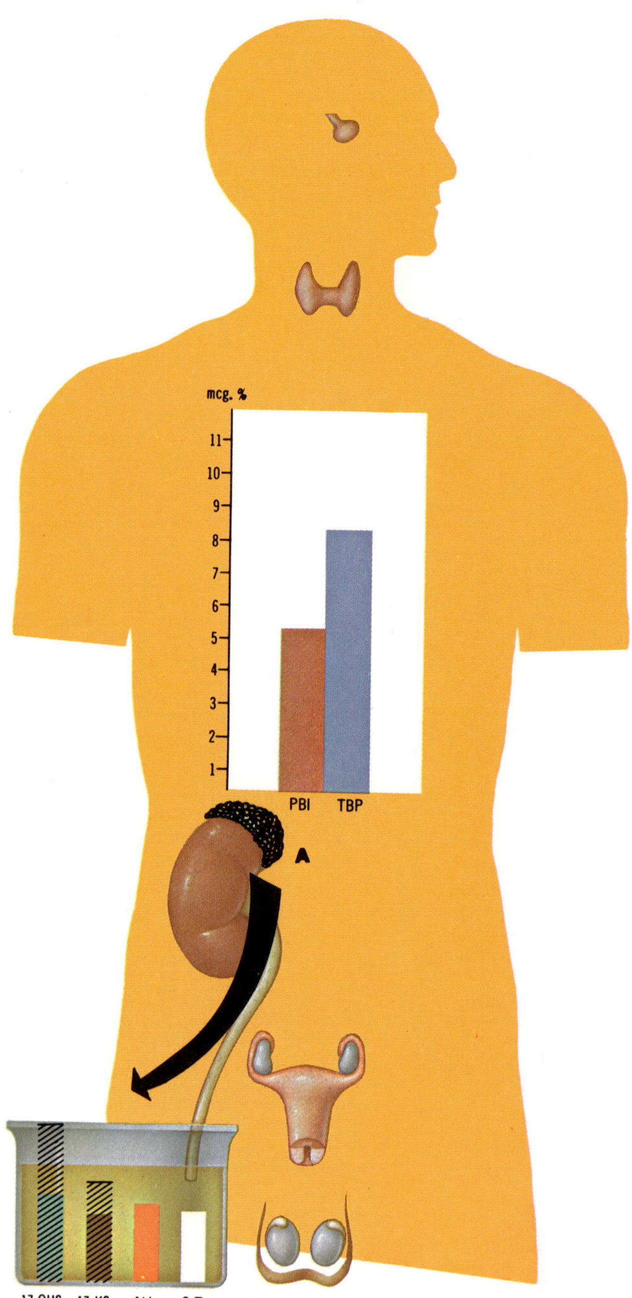

CUSHING'S SYNDROME

In Cushing's syndrome, whether due to adrenocortical hyperplasia (A), adenoma, or carcinoma, or a pituitary adenoma (p. 84), the secretion of glucocorticoids and, to a lesser extent, androgens and estrogens is increased. Therefore, plasma cortisol and urinary *17-hydroxycorticoids* and *17-ketosteroids* are *elevated.* Associated increased aldosterone secretion is rarely seen. Alterations in the white count (p. 248), electrolytes (p. 51), and blood sugar (p. 68) are suggestive but not diagnostic of this condition.

Additional tests are used to determine whether this syndrome is due to an adenoma, carcinoma, or hyperplasia of the adrenal cortex. In cases of adenoma or hyperplasia, the urinary steroids rise markedly after intravenous ACTH, whereas they do not change appreciably in cases of carcinoma. Furthermore, the secretion of corticosteroids, and thus the urinary output of corticosteroids, can be inhibited by administering dexamethasone (8 mg. or more/day) in patients with hyperplasia, but not in those with carcinoma or adenoma. Finally, adrenocortical carcinomas are associated with higher levels of urinary 17-ketosteroids, and their glucocorticoids are more primitive (e.g., dehydroisoandrosterone, etc.).

Summary of Laboratory Findings:

Serum PBI: Normal

Serum thyrobinding protein: Normal

Urine 17-hydroxycorticosteroids: Increased

Urine 17-ketosteroids: Increased

Urine aldosterone: Normal

Urine gonadotropins: Normal

ADRENOGENITAL SYNDROME

This disorder is most commonly caused by adrenocortical hyperplasia (A). A block in the synthesis of cortisol and related glucocorticoids leads to the accumulation of 17-hydroxyprogesterone and other precursors of cortisol. Much of the 17-hydroxyprogesterone is transformed to a number of *17-ketosteroids,* and the *level* of these *rises* in the *urine.* There is an elevation of pregnanetriol in the blood and urine. Blood progesterone can now be measured, and this is also elevated.

This reaction is intensified by an associated increased ACTH secretion by the pituitary (B), induced by the low plasma cortisol levels (see p. 77).

The adrenogenital syndrome is also associated with adenomas and carcinomas of the adrenal cortex and with arrhenoblastomas of the ovary. Differentiation depends on the *dexamethasone suppression test* and *ACTH stimulation test* (p. 92).

One third of patients with the Stein-Leventhal syndrome (polycystic ovaries) have adrenal androgenic hypersecretion with increased urinary 17-ketosteroids.

Summary of Laboratory Findings:

Serum PBI: Normal

Serum thyrobinding protein: Normal

Urine 17-hydroxycorticosteroids: Normal

Urine 17-ketosteroids: Increased

Urine aldosterone: Normal

Urine gonadotropins: Normal

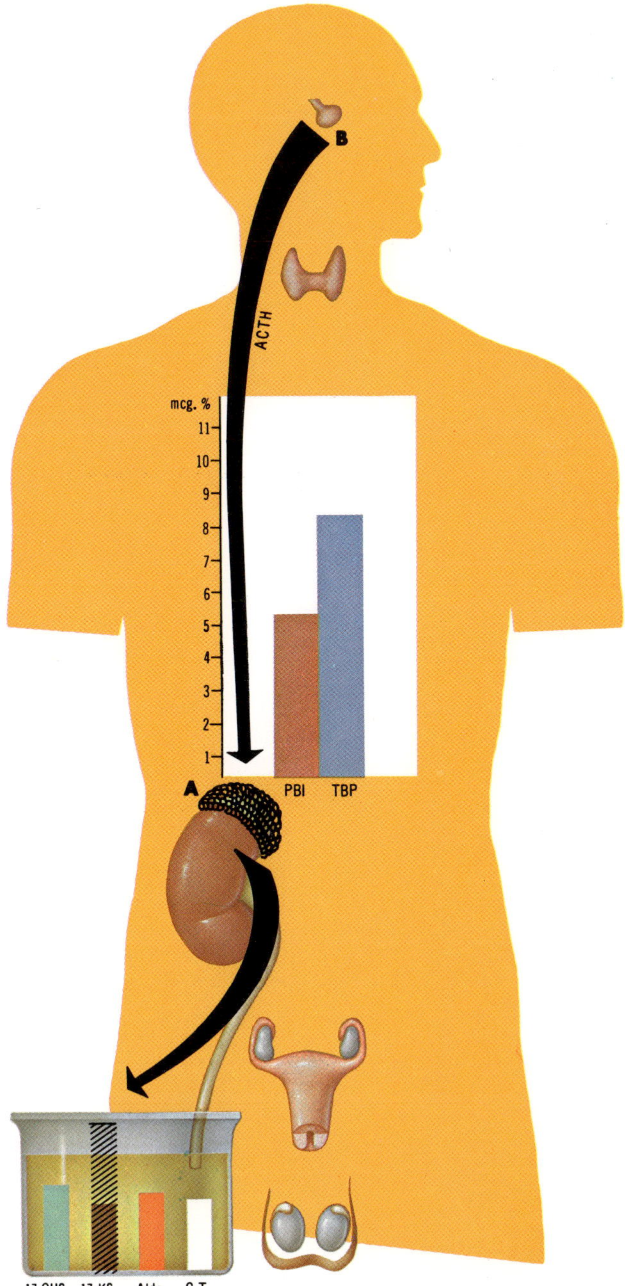

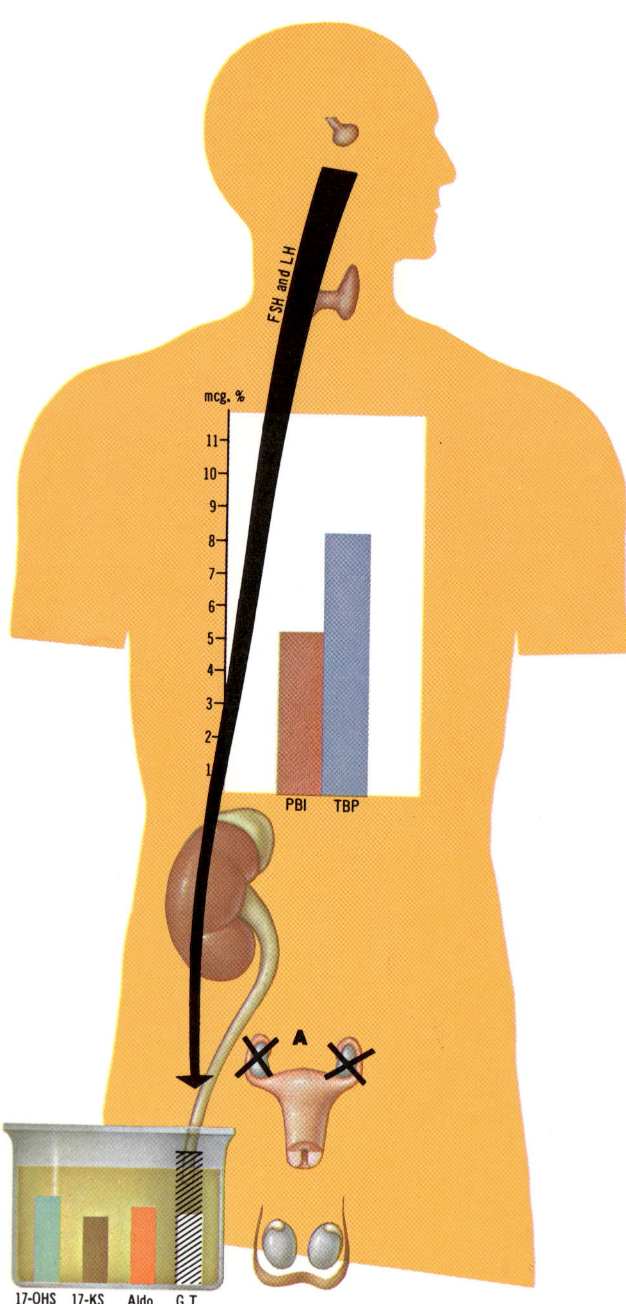

TURNER'S SYNDROME

In this disorder there are no true ovaries present (A). Thus pituitary production of FSH and LH is uninhibited, and *urinary gonadotropins increase* some time after 9 years of age (expected age of puberty). The diagnosis is substantiated by performing a sex chromatin test (Barr). These subjects are chromatin-negative, indicating an XO sex chromosome constitution and a chromosome number of 45. Other sex chromosomal aberrations have been reported (XO/XX, etc.). A cytological study for fluorescent Y should be done to exclude mosaicism and gonadoblastomas. Vaginal smears reveal a predominance of the *basal cells* typical of reduced estrogen secretion.

Summary of Laboratory Findings:

Serum PBI: Normal
Serum thyrobinding protein: Normal
Urine 17-hydroxycorticosteroids: Normal
Urine 17-ketosteroids: Normal
Urine aldosterone: Normal
Urine gonadotropins: Increased

POLYCYSTIC OVARIES (STEIN-LEVENTHAL SYNDROME)

Although many of these patients have no alterations in hormone secretion, most have *increased urinary 17-ketosteroids* secondary to adrenocortical hyperplasia or ovarian secretion. Serum testosterone and total androgens may also be elevated. Plasma LH is high, while plasma FSH is low.

Arrhenoblastomas of the ovary may also lead to increased urinary 17-ketosteroids but the chief characteristic is a high plasma testosterone. However, the urinary levels do not drop after corticosteroid therapy, a test which will distinguish this condition from polycystic ovaries.

Summary of Laboratory Findings:

Serum PBI: Normal
Serum thyrobinding protein: Normal
Urine 17-hydroxycorticosteroids: Normal
Urine 17-ketosteroids: Increased
Urine aldosterone: Normal
Urine gonadotropins: Normal

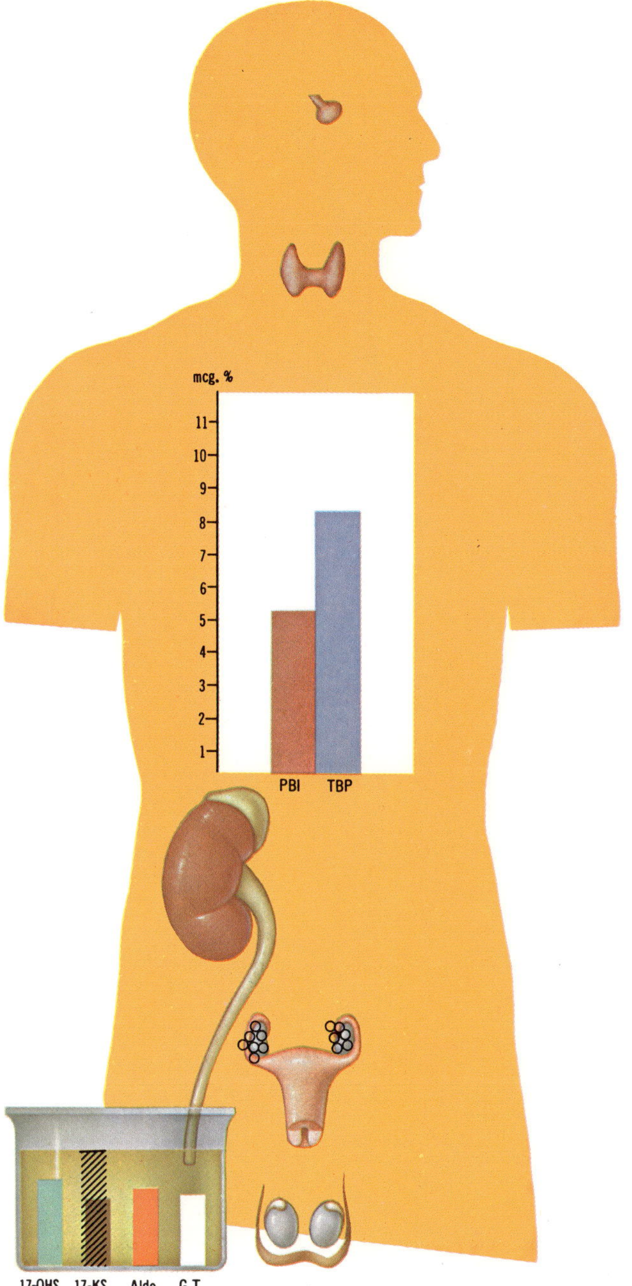

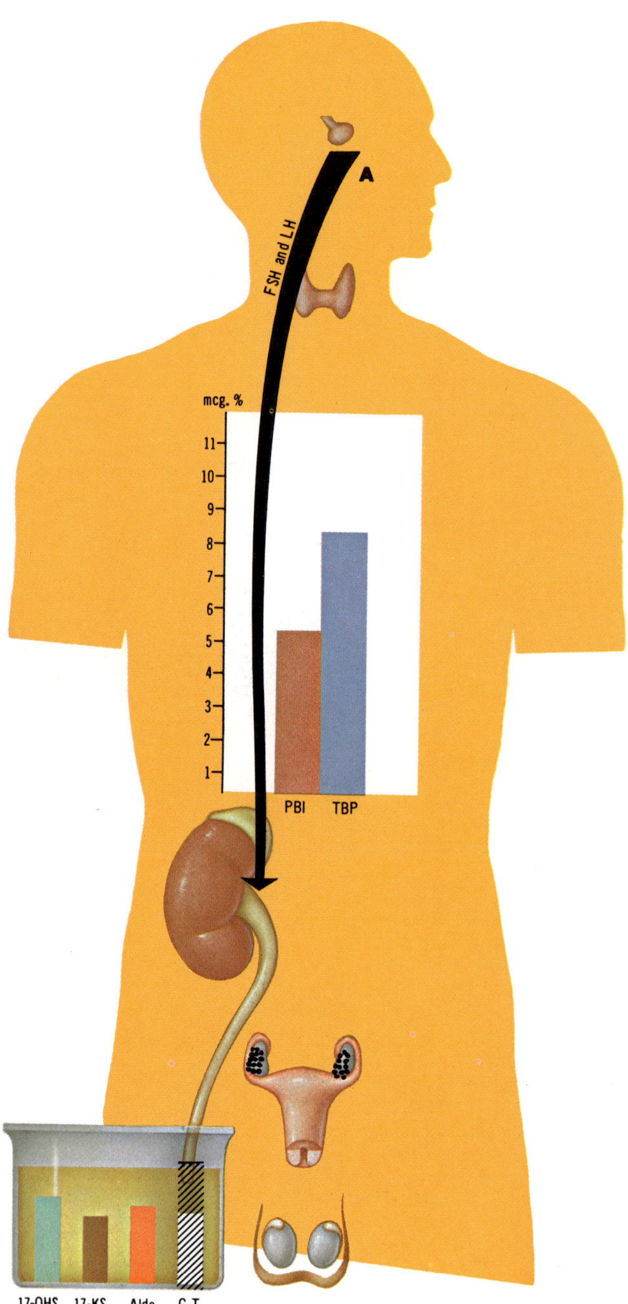

MENOPAUSAL SYNDROME

Progressive atrophy of the ovaries in middle-aged women leads to a reduced ovarian secretion of estrogen and progesterone. The uninhibited pituitary secretes increasing amounts of FSH and LH (A). Consequently, *urinary gonadotropins* are *elevated.* Vaginal smears reveal the *basal cells* and *precornified cells* typical of diminished estrogen secretion. Roentgenograms of the spine may reveal osteoporosis.

Summary of Laboratory Findings:

Serum PBI: Normal

Serum thyrobinding protein: Normal

Urine 17-hydroxycorticosteroids: Normal

Urine 17-ketosteroids: Normal

Urine aldosterone: Normal

Urine gonadotropins: Increased

PREGNANCY

During the first trimester of pregnancy the Langhans cells of the placenta secrete *chorionic gonadotropin,* which *increases* in the *urine.* The chorionic gonadotropin maintains the output of estrogen and progesterone by the corpus luteum and is the basis of most of the diagnostic tests of pregnancy. After the first trimester the level of chorionic gonadotropin decreases. Consequently, pregnancy tests which measure this substance are negative between the 14th and the 32nd week of gestation. In the latter part of pregnancy the placenta itself secretes estrogen, progesterone, and glucocorticoids, all of which increase in the blood and the urine. The *urinary 17-hydroxycorticosteroids* are elevated. The increased estrogen induces the liver to produce *thyroxine-binding protein* with a corresponding *rise* in the PBI. Thus pregnancy is associated with increased levels of all the commonly measured hormones in the blood and urine except the 17-ketosteroids. Such levels might be expected with a "panhyperpituitarism," if such a condition were to exist.

Summary of Laboratory Findings:

Serum PBI: Increased

Serum thyrobinding protein: Increased

Urine 17-hydroxycorticosteroids: Increased

Urine 17-ketosteroids: Normal

Urine aldosterone: Normal

Urine gonadotropins: Increased

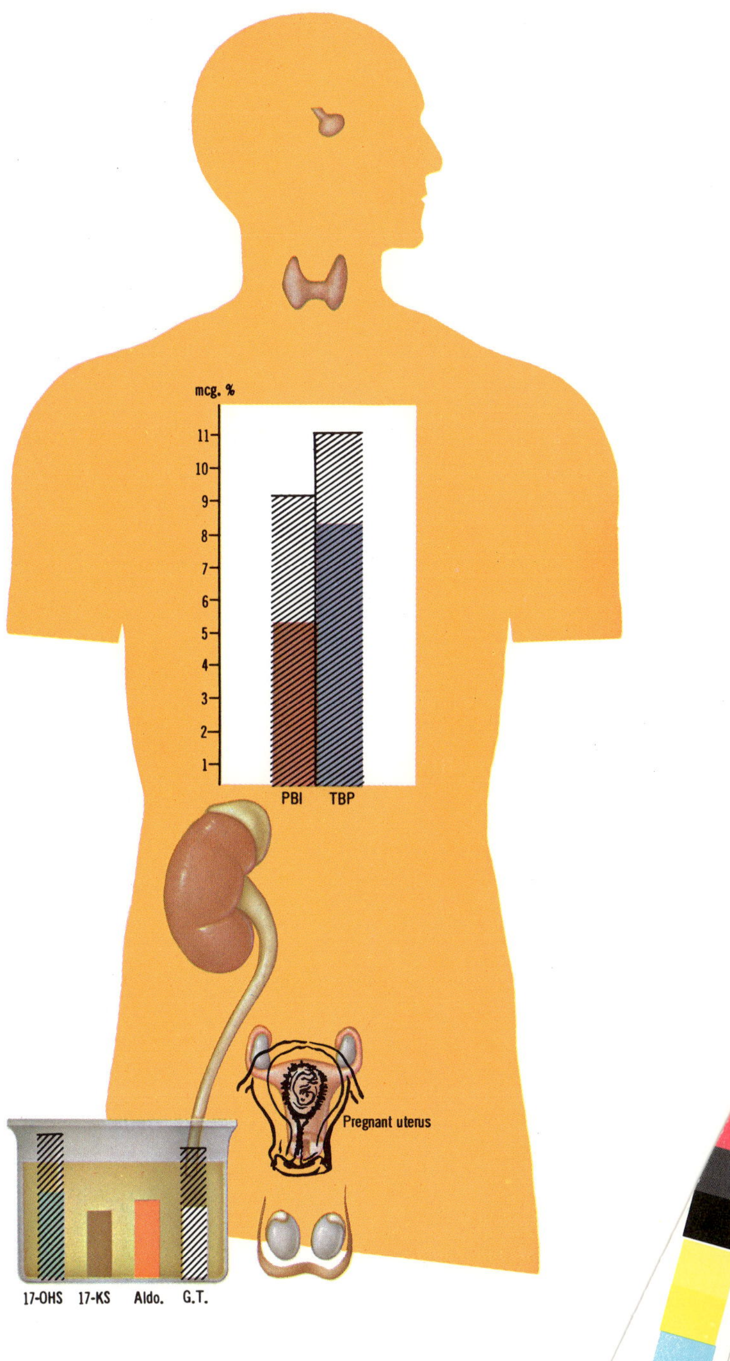

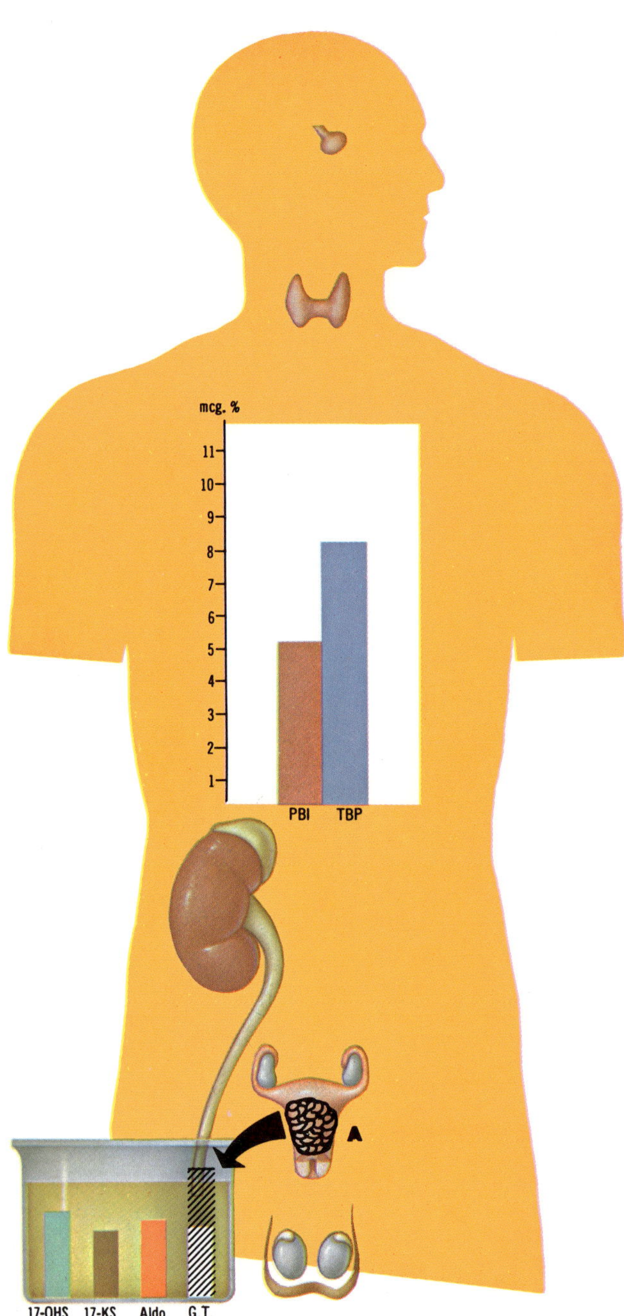

CHORIONEPITHELIOMA

This neoplasm of the placenta (A) secretes enormous amounts of chorionic gonadotropin, and its level rises in the urine. (Chorionic gonadotropin is indistinguishable from HPG by routine bio-assay). The diagnosis is confirmed by curettage. Continuing high levels after hysterectomy usually indicate distant metastasis. Hydatidiform mole produces a similar laboratory picture.

Summary of Laboratory Findings:

Serum PBI: Normal

Serum thyrobinding protein: Normal

Urine 17-hydroxycorticosteroids: Normal

Urine 17-ketosteroids: Normal

Urine aldosterone: Normal

Urine gonadotropins: Increased

SEMINOMA

This neoplasm of the seminiferous tubules does not secrete any known hormone, and yet *urinary gonadotropin* is *increased*. This is a result primarily of increased pituitary secretion of FSH for some unknown reason.

Embryonal tumors of the testes, particularly chorionepitheliomas, are also associated with *increased urinary gonadotropin*, but in these cases it is primarily chorionic gonadotropin produced by the tumor cells.

Summary of Laboratory Findings:

Serum PBI: Normal
Serum thyrobinding protein: Normal
Urine 17-hydroxycorticosteroids: Normal
Urine 17-ketosteroids: Normal
Urine aldosterone: Normal
Urine gonadotropins: Increased

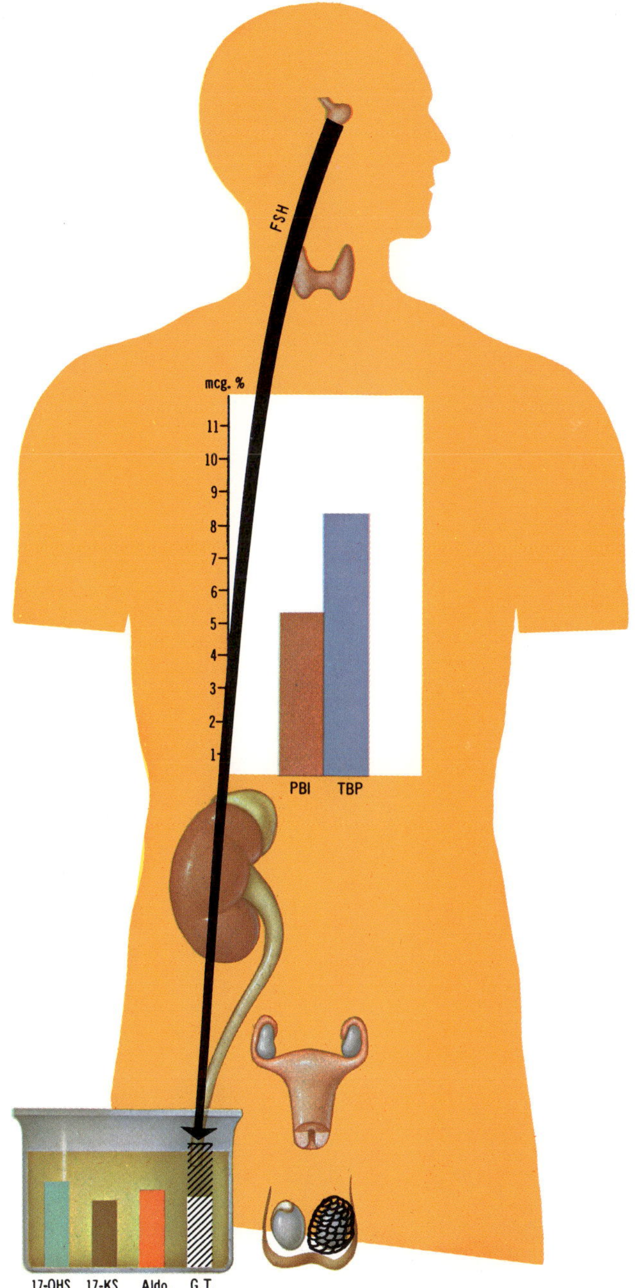

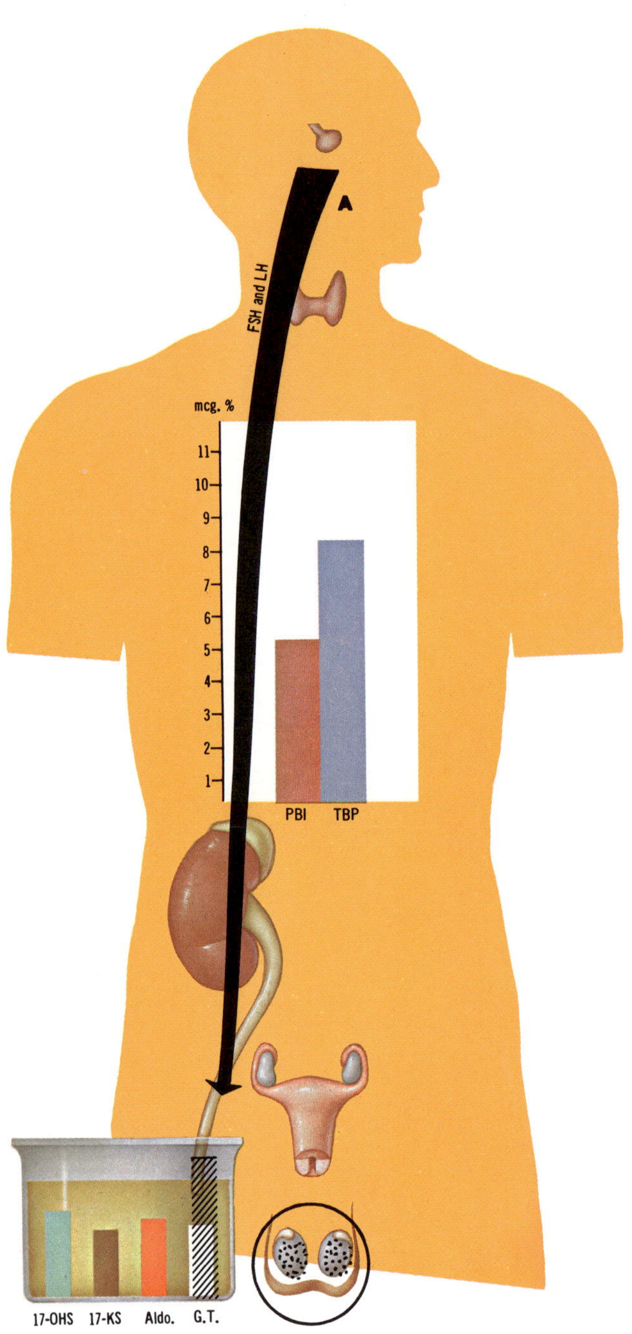

KLINEFELTER'S SYNDROME

This disorder is characterized by atrophy and hyalinization of the seminiferous tubules, but the Leydig cells are usually preserved although decreased in number. Nevertheless, the *urinary gonadotropins* are *increased,* an indication of increased FSH and/or LH secretion by the pituitary (A). Plasma testosterone levels are often decreased. Urinary 17-ketosteroid levels are normal. Semen analysis reveals azoospermia. Rarely is testicular biopsy needed to establish the diagnosis. More significant in diagnosis is a buccal smear for chromatin analysis. This reveals an XXY sex chromosome constitution and a chromosome number of 47. The extra X seems to "inhibit" normal spermatogenesis. Other sex chromosomal abnormalities have been reported (XXYY, XXXY, and XXXXY). The hormone changes are somewhat analogous to those in Turner's syndrome in the female.

Summary of Laboratory Findings:

Serum PBI: Normal

Serum thyrobinding protein: Normal

Urine 17-hydroxycorticosteroids: Normal

Urine 17-ketosteroids: Normal or decreased

Urine aldosterone: Normal

Urine gonadotropins: Increased

* McCullough, D. R.: Dual endocrine activity of the testis. Science, *76*:19, 1932.

7 Disorders of Serum Lipids

Body lipids serve primarily as a source of energy for metabolism. Perhaps foremost among their many other important functions is their integral part in the make-up of cell membranes. Moreover, they are precursors of steroid hormones and bile acids. The measurement of the blood lipids is very useful in the diagnosis of certain metabolic diseases.

NATURE OF BODY LIPIDS

Cholesterol is an alcohol of the large group of compounds containing a cyclopentenophenanthrene nucleus. It has an OH-group at the C_3 carbon in the phenanthrene nucleus and a long carbon chain at C_{17}. The corticosteroids, vitamin D, bile acids, and many other compounds with biological activity have a similar structure. Cholesterol exists in the body in both the free and the *esterified form* (combined with a fatty acid at C_3).

Phospholipids are nitrogenous lipids that contain phosphoric acid. They are divided into *phosphatides,* which are triglycerides with one fatty acid replaced by a phosphoric acid ester, and *sphingomyelins,* which are nitrogenous lipids with only one molecule of fatty acid to each molecule of phosphoric acid attached to the unusual basic alcohol, sphingosine. Lecithin, sphingomyelins, and cephalin are the major phospholipids of the serum. Sphingomyelins are also widely distributed in the tissues, particularly the nervous system and the lung.

Triglycerides are esters of glycerol and fatty acids. If only one or two of the OH-groups of glycerol are combined with a fatty acid, the substances are called monoglycerides and diglycerides, respectively. Triglycerides of fatty acids with less than 12 carbons are rare in mammalian tissues. The major fatty acids of the body are palmitic and palmitoleic acids (containing 16 carbons) and stearic and oleic acids (containing 18 carbons). Palmitoleic and oleic acid are monounsaturated fatty acids (i.e., with one double bond). Three other fatty acids, linoleic acid (18 carbons and 3 unsaturated bonds), linolenic acid (18 carbons and 3 unsaturated bonds), and arachidonic acid (20 carbons and 4 unsaturated bonds), are present in the body and seem to be essential for life. There are apparently no appreciable quantities of free fatty acids in the body.

Another group of lipids, the cerebrosides, are not present in the blood, but are widely distributed in the cells of the body, especially the nervous system. These are nitrogen-containing lipids composed of fatty acids and galactose but no phosphoric acid.

NORMAL METABOLISM

Intake. Lipids constitute 40 per cent of the calories in the average American diet. After ingestion the lipids pass to the duodenum, where digestion takes place. The majority of the triglycerides are emulsified by bile and hydrolyzed to fatty acids and glycerol by pancreatic lipase. Serum *cholesterol* and *phospholipids* are similarly hydrolyzed.

Absorption. Absorption of fat is facilitated by bile, pancreatic lipase, and phospholipids. The diffusion across the intestinal mucosa into the blood or lymph is an active process. The exact nature of this process is not clear. *Cholesterol* is absorbed into the lymph in both the free and the esterified form. Most of the cholesterol esters are first hydrolyzed to the free form before absorption by the intestinal cells. The intestinal cells subsequently esterize some of the free cholesterol before releasing it into the lymph. Most vegetable sterols are not well absorbed and, in fact, may inhibit the absorption of cholesterol. Intestinal synthesis and absorption of cholesterol are related to the absorption of other lipids.

That portion of the phospholipids which is not broken down by digestion is actively absorbed by the intestinal mucosa and delivered into the lymphatics. However, the majority of phospholipids, as well as triglycerides, are broken down to fatty acids and glycerol. The fatty acids are actively absorbed by the intestinal cells, where they are reconverted into triglycerides and then discharged into the lymphatics (long-chain fatty acids) or portal blood (short-chain fatty acids).

Under normal conditions 95 to 98 per cent of ingested fat is absorbed. The rest is excreted in the feces. Fecal fat is not all residua from ingestion. Some is from intestinal secretion. Fat absorption is enhanced by the administration of lecithin, choline, or glycerophosphate.

Transport. Lipids are transported in both the blood and the lymphatics. The chief lipids of the blood are cholesterol, phospholipids, and the triglycerides. The normal serum total *cholesterol* ranges from 150 to 250 mg. per 100 ml. but is remarkably constant from day to day in a healthy individual. Recently it has been described that normal values vary with age. Normal values are 120-230 mg. per 100 ml. below age 20 and rise to 160-330 mg. above age 50. From 68 to 76 per cent of the total cholesterol is esterized. The serum *phospholipid* ranges from 230 to 300 mg. per 100 ml. This is made up of lecithin, sphingomyelin, and cephalin. The serum *triglycerides* do not normally exceed 150 to 300 mg. per 100 ml. but are variable even in the same individual. The amount of free fatty acid is normally negligible, although this is the most important form in which lipids are mobilized from fatty tissues.

Almost all the plasma lipids are bound to protein except after a meal. These lipid-binding proteins or lipoproteins are in the alpha-2, prebeta, and beta fractions of globulin. The very-low-density lipoproteins (as determined by ultracentrifuge) contain predominantly triglycerides, whereas the low-density lipoproteins contain predominantly cholesterol.

After a meal much of the lipids absorbed by the intestinal mucosa is transferred into the lymphatics and travels up the thoracic duct and hence into the blood stream. Because the triglyceride portion (chylomicrons) does not readily dissolve in the serum, the serum has a lactescent appearance.

Storage. The stored fat that is available for fuel is chiefly the *triglycerides* (see Triglycerides under Production, this chapter). This is stored in adipose tissue throughout the body and the liver. *Cholesterol* exists free in muscle and blood cells. It is also a part of all cell membranes. Cholesterol esters are present in the intestinal mucosa, liver, adrenal cortex, and genital organs. The cholesterol in the adrenal cortex is diminished by stimulation of that gland. *Phospholipids* are contained in all the cells of the body. In the majority of the tissues they are the only vehicle for fatty acids. They, too, are a part of the cell membranes. The phospholipids lecithin and cephalin are required by all types of living cells, whereas sphingomyelin is found most in the brain and the lungs.

Production. *Cholesterol* is synthesized in the reticulum cells and the histiocytes throughout the body but chiefly in those of the liver. Cholesterol formed by the liver is discharged into the blood and bile. Although many steps of cholesterol synthesis are not known, the raw materials are undoubtedly acetate fragments that are linked by coenzyme A. Carbohydrate, amino acids and other fats can be converted to cholesterol through this (acetate) common denominator. Thus it is not surprising that cholesterol-free diets are relatively ineffective in lowering serum cholesterol if the diet contains a surplus of protein and carbohydrate. *Cholesterol esters* are formed chiefly in the liver. Limited amounts are also formed by the intestinal mucosa, adrenal cortex, testes, and ovaries. The formation of cholesterol esters is probably the first step in steroid hormone synthesis.

Phospholipids are synthesized by all tissues from fatty acids, inorganic phosphorus, and choline, or some other nitrogenous base. Choline may be supplied by the diet or produced in the liver by the transfer of a methyl group from methionine to ethanolamine. Methionine must be supplied in the diet. Plasma phospholipid is produced almost solely by the liver.

Triglycerides are produced from glycerol and fatty acids in the liver and adipose tissue of the body. The major raw material for triglyceride synthesis is carbohydrate, although protein and other fats can be utilized. The carbohydrate is split into the acetate fragments necessary for fatty acid synthesis by glycolysis. In addition, carbohydrate supplies glycerol by the production of L-alpha-glycerophosphate in anaerobic glycolysis. The biosynthesis of triglyceride is probably dependent on carbohydrate metabolism for additional reasons. Two other essentials for lipogenesis, DPNH and TPNH, are produced in the breakdown of glucose to pyruvate.*

Most body cells can also change one saturated fatty acid to another by adding or subtracting one or more 2-carbon groups. They may saturate bonds or unsaturate single bonds, but this is limited to one bond per fatty acid. Thus compounds with more than one double bond, linoleic acid, linolenic acid, and arachidonic acid, must be

* Masoro, E. J., *et al.*: Previous nutritional state and glucose conversion to fatty acids in liver slices. J. Biol. Chem., *185*:845-856, 1950.

supplied by the diet and are called essential fatty acids. Dietary deficiencies of these acids result in fatty livers in animals.

Utilization. *Cholesterol* is utilized by the body to form steroid hormones, bile acids, and cell membranes. For the most part it is not metabolized, since the body is unable to disintegrate the sterol ring. *Triglycerides* and *phospholipids,* on the other hand, are important sources of energy. They may be utilized directly after absorption or stored for later use. Their breakdown products, glycerol and fatty acid, may be burned to carbon dioxide and water by way of the Krebs cycle. The fatty acids are first broken down to acetoacetic acid, beta-hydroxybutyric acid, and acetone.

Excretion. *Cholesterol* is the only lipid with appreciable excretion. The other lipids are metabolized, stored, or utilized in body anabolism. 1 to 2 gm. of free cholesterol pass into the intestinal tract daily through the biliary tree. A small amount is secreted by the mucosal cells. Most of this is reabsorbed, but approximately 500 mg. is excreted in the feces. Most of the cholesterol excreted in the bile is produced from acetate by the liver. Only minute amounts of *fatty acids* appear in the feces unless there is defective absorption.

Regulation. The serum levels of the various lipids depend on an equilibrium between intake and production, on the one hand, and excretion, storage, or utilization, on the other. The various factors controlling this equilibrium are not well understood. Neither quality nor quantity of fats in the diet seems to have any effect on the serum lipids except immediately after a meal. The liver is the main organ of regulation of the blood lipids. For example, an increase of dietary cholesterol may lead to a decreased liver synthesis of cholesterol and an increased biliary excretion of cholic acid.†

† Tomkins, G. M., Sheppard, H., and Bennett, I. L.: Cholesterol synthesis by liver; IV. Its regulation by ingested cholesterol. J. Biol. Chem., *201*:137-141, 1953.

Insulin increases the synthesis of fatty acid in the liver and adipose tissue, whereas *cortisol* probably contributes to a breakdown of fatty acids and mobilization of fats from fat depots. *Growth hormone* seems to have a similar effect. *Epinephrine* apparently mobilizes fatty acids from adipose tissue indirectly by inducing adrenocortical hormone secretion. *Estrogen* decreases the half-life of plasma cholesterol, whereas ovariectomy increases it. *Heparin* apparently increases protein-bound lipid and thus decreases the emulsified fraction following a meal. *Thyroxine* induces a reduction in plasma cholesterol and phospholipids by some unknown mechanism.

THE APPROACH TO THE DIAGNOSIS

The preliminary steps in the diagnosis of a disorder of blood lipids are a serum total cholesterol and esters, a careful family history, and tests of protein and carbohydrate metabolism (blood sugar, urine acetone, and serum protein and A/G ratio). Lipoprotein electrophoresis has now become popular, as it allows for the separation of the 5 distinct types of familial hyperlipemia. This is important, because the treatment of each type is different. The procedure is similar to protein electrophoresis except that fat-soluble dyes such as sudan black B and oil red O are used to stain for lipoproteins. This divides the lipoproteins into 4 classes—alpha-lipoproteins, beta-lipoproteins, prebeta-lipoproteins, and chylomicrons. The normal electrophoretic pattern is shown below. Determination of serum triglycerides and phospholipids is also being done routinely today. A PBI is usually indicated to exclude hyper- and hypothyroidism.

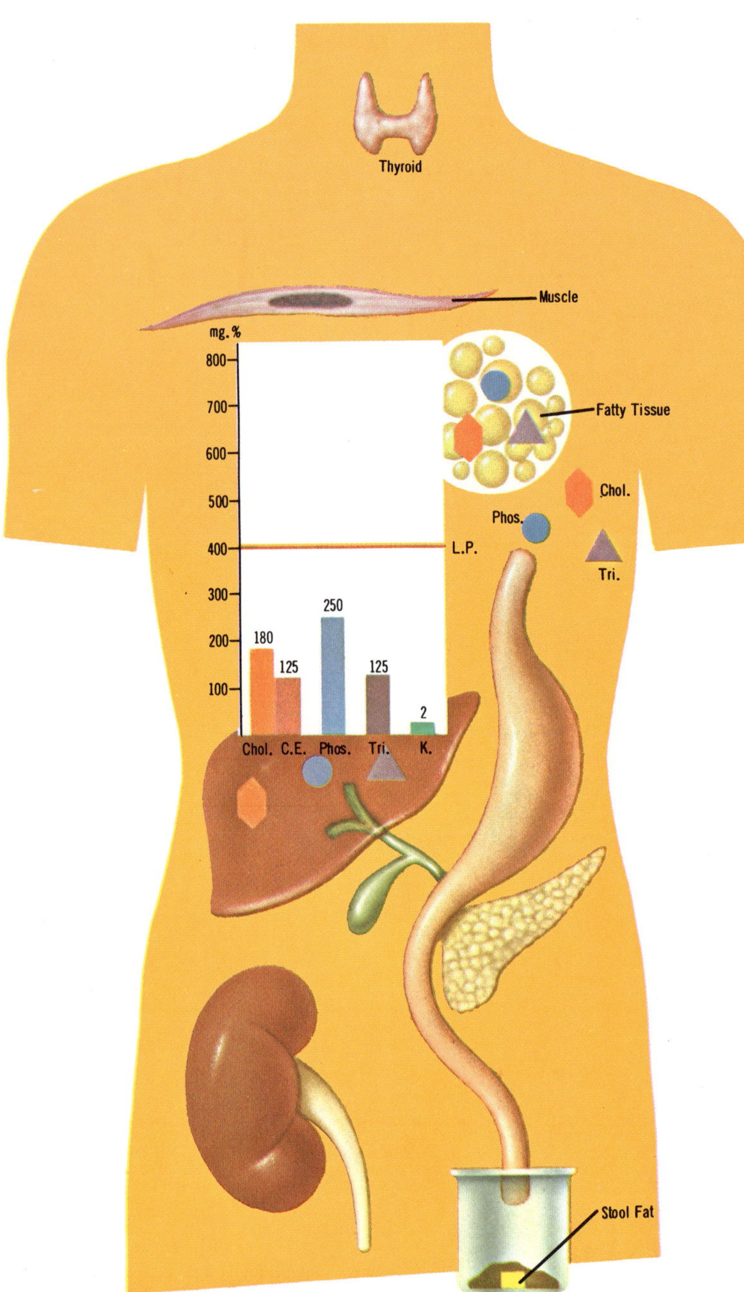

Abbreviations Used in Plates:

Chol.	= Serum total cholesterol
C.E.	= Cholesterol esters
Phos.	= Serum phospholipids
Tri.	= Serum triglycerides
K.	= Ketones
L.P.	= Serum lipoproteins
Chylo.	= Chylomicrons
β	= Beta lipoproteins
Pre-β	= Prebeta lipoproteins
α	= Alpha lipoproteins

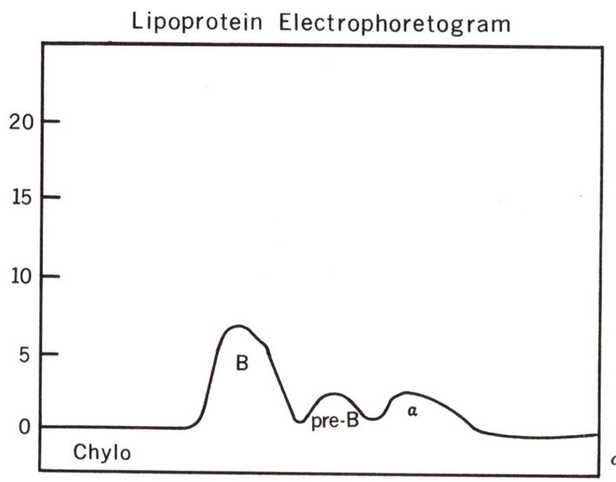

EARLY STARVATION

Although there may be a decreased hepatic synthesis of lipids in this disorder (A), fats are mobilized from peripheral depots (B) (as in diabetes mellitus), and consequently *serum cholesterol, triglycerides,* and *phospholipids increase*. Breakdown of these lipids to ketones by the liver may exceed peripheral utilization. Thus blood *ketones* may also *increase*.

Summary of Laboratory Findings:

Serum cholesterol: Increased

Serum cholesterol esters: Increased

Serum phospholipids: Increased

Serum triglycerides: Increased

Plasma ketones: Increased

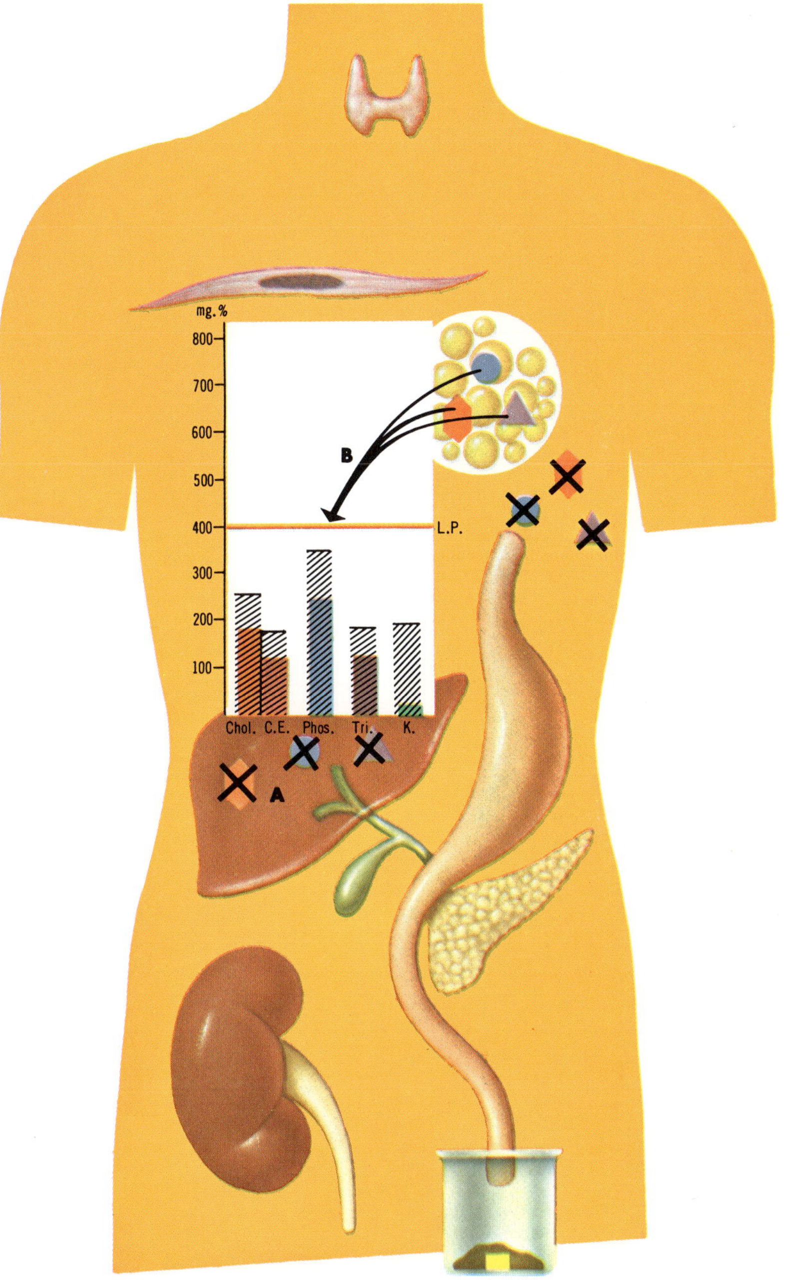

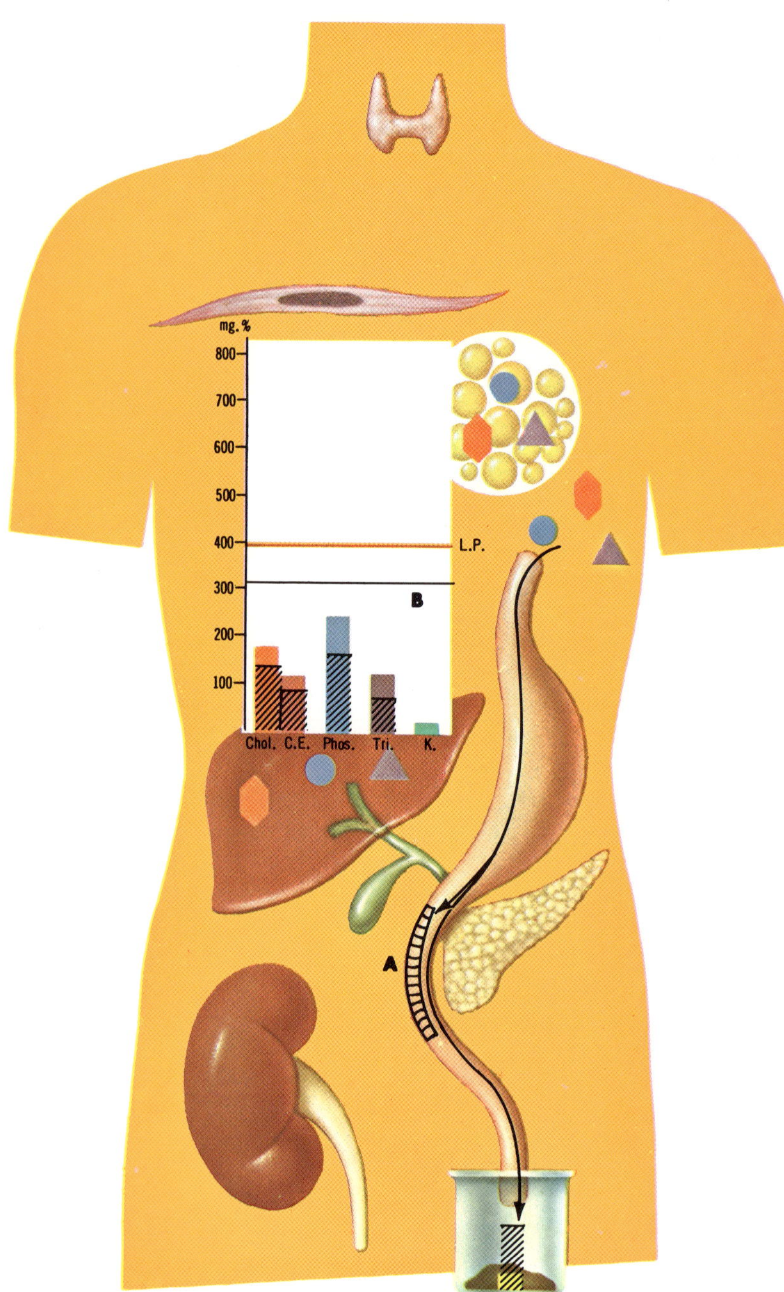

IDIOPATHIC STEATORRHEA

The inability of the small intestine to absorb amino acids (A) leads to a decreased hepatic synthesis of lipoprotein (B) in this disorder. Thus the *serum concentration* of all the *blood lipids drops*. There is no doubt that the block in lipid and carbohydrate absorption also contributes to these alterations. A small bowel series, urinary 5-HIAA, radioactive triolein uptake, and mucosal biopsy are all useful in establishing the diagnosis. Malabsorption syndromes related to bacterial overgrowth can now be diagnosed with a breath test measuring the rate of excretion of $^{14}CO_2$ following the ingestion of ^{14}C-glycine labeled glycocholic acid (a bile acid). Increased excretion of $^{14}CO_2$ indicates excessive breakdown of bile acid by excessive bacteria.*

Summary of Laboratory Findings:

Serum cholesterol: Decreased
Serum cholesterol esters: Decreased
Serum phospholipids: Decreased
Serum triglycerides: Decreased
Serum lipoproteins: Decreased
Plasma ketones: Normal

* Wilson, F.A., and Dietschy, J.M.: Differential diagnostic approach to clinical problems of malabsorption. Gastroenterology 61:911-931, 1972.

MALNUTRITION

In malnutrition caloric intake may be sufficient to prevent mobilization of lipid stores, but the amount of dietary protein (A) may be insufficient for liver synthesis of lipoproteins. Under these circumstances serum *cholesterol* and *phospholipids* will *decrease* along with the *lipoproteins*.

Summary of Laboratory Findings:

Serum cholesterol: Decreased
Serum cholesterol esters: Decreased
Serum phospholipids: Decreased
Serum triglycerides: Normal
Serum lipoproteins: Decreased
Plasma ketones: Normal or increased

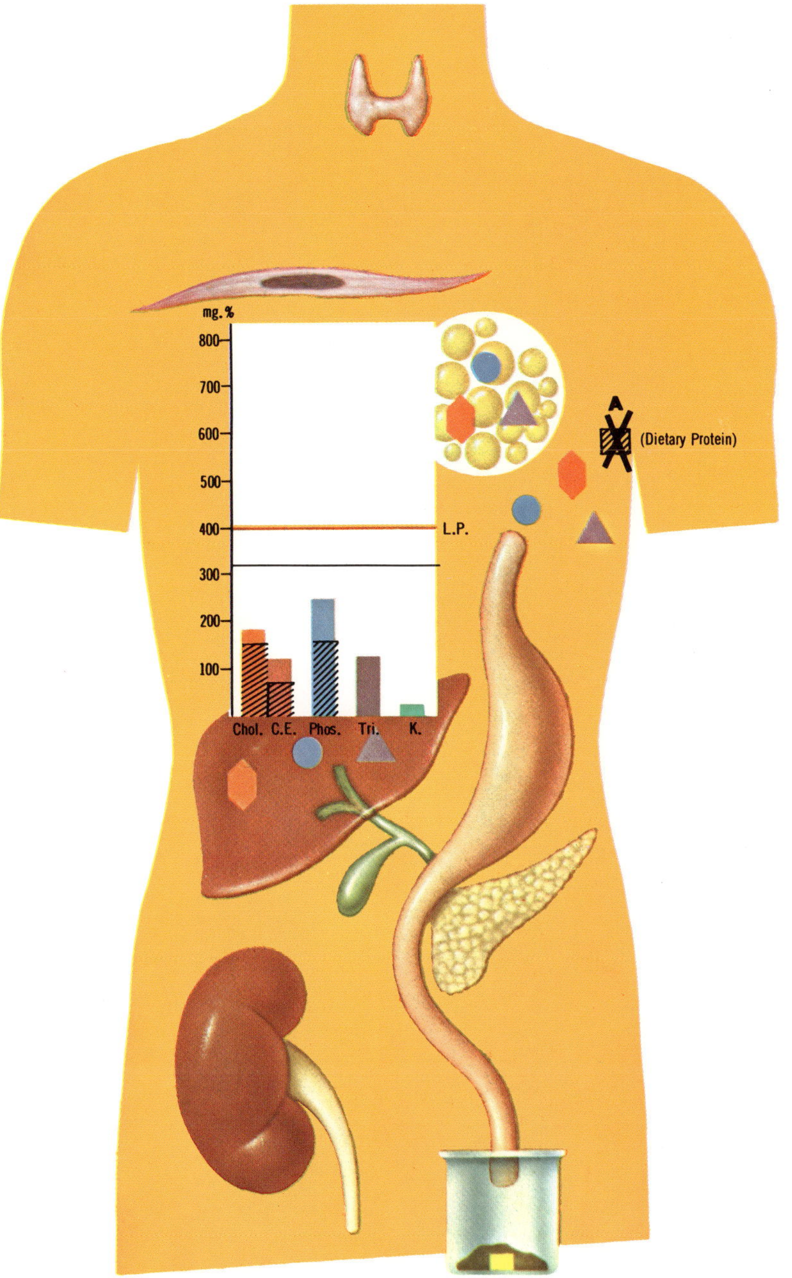

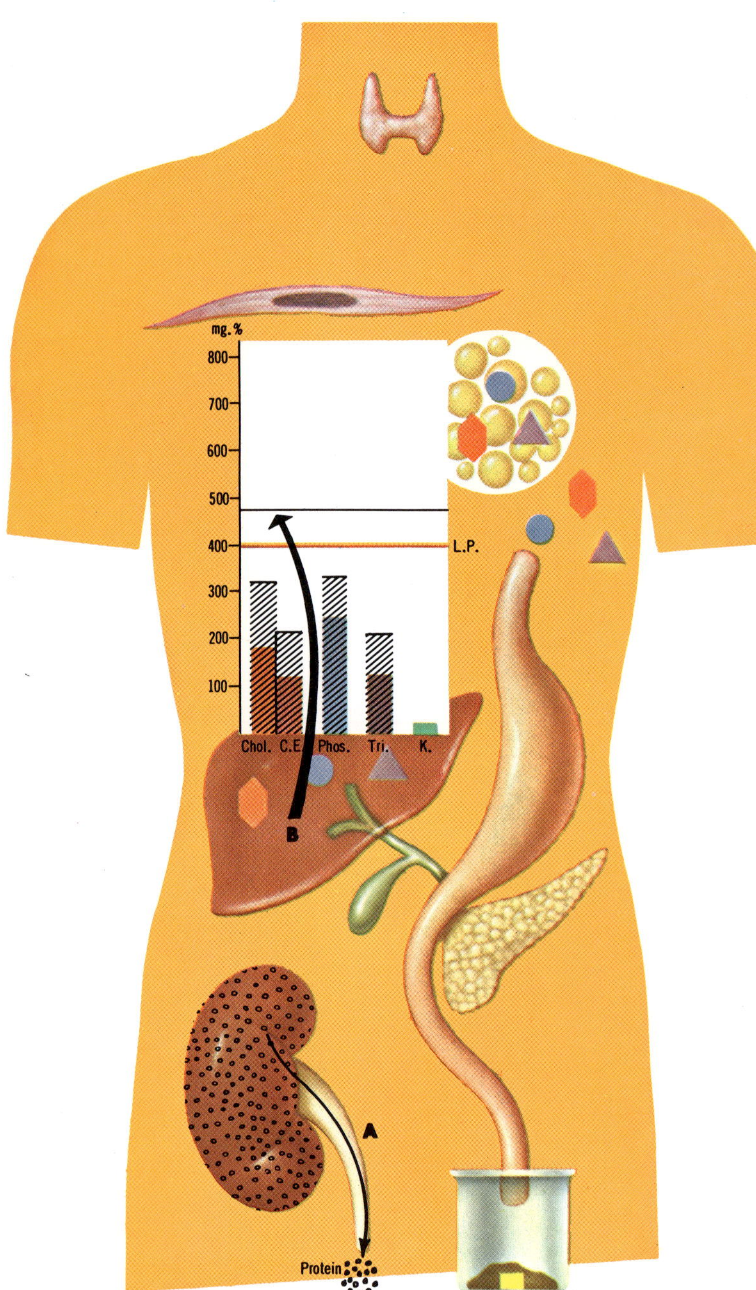

NEPHROTIC SYNDROME

Loss of protein through the diseased glomeruli (A) in this disorder leads to a drop in the level of most plasma proteins. To compensate for this, hepatic synthesis of all plasma proteins including lipoproteins increases (B). It is believed that much of the lipid-binding proteins do not pass into the urine,* and consequently they accumulate in the blood, with a resulting *increase* in the *serum cholesterol, phospholipid,* and *triglyceride*. However, this is only one theory. The finding of doubly refractile bodies in the urine and abnormal renal function tests confirm the diagnosis. In doubtful cases renal biopsy may be employed.

Summary of Laboratory Findings:

Serum cholesterol: Increased
Serum cholesterol esters: Increased
Serum phospholipids: Increased
Serum triglycerides: Increased
Serum lipoproteins: Increased
Plasma ketones: Normal

* Marsh, G. B., and Drablein, D. L.: Experimental reconstruction of metabolic pattern of lipid nephrosis: Key role of hepatic protein synthesis in hyperlipemia. Metabolism, *9*:946-955, 1960.

PORTAL CIRRHOSIS

The damaged liver cells are unable to convert protein and carbohydrate to fat in this condition (A), and thus *serum cholesterol* (particularly the esters) and other *lipids decrease. Decreased serum lipoproteins* may also contribute to these alterations. Other liver function tests and liver biopsy may be used to confirm the diagnosis.

Summary of Laboratory Findings:

Serum cholesterol: Decreased
Serum cholesterol esters: Markedly decreased
Serum phospholipids: Decreased
Serum triglycerides: Decreased
Plasma ketones: Normal

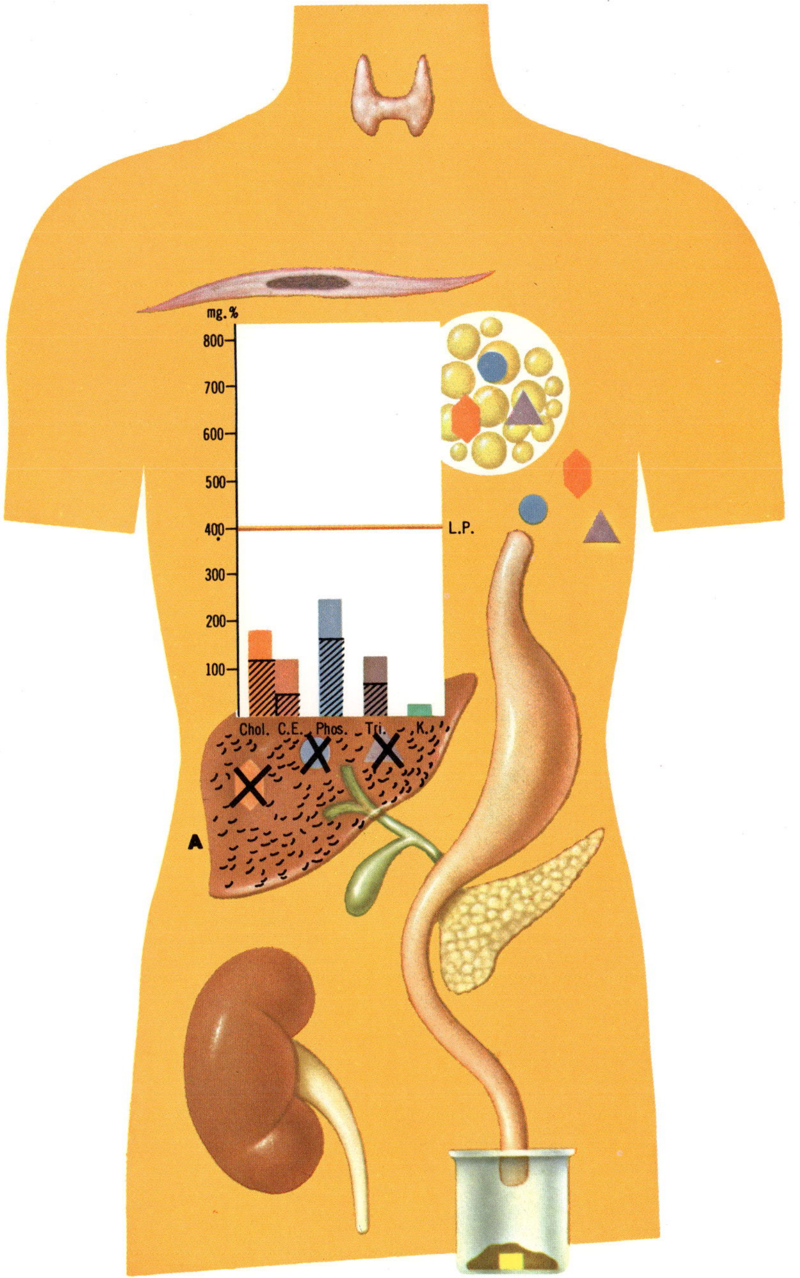

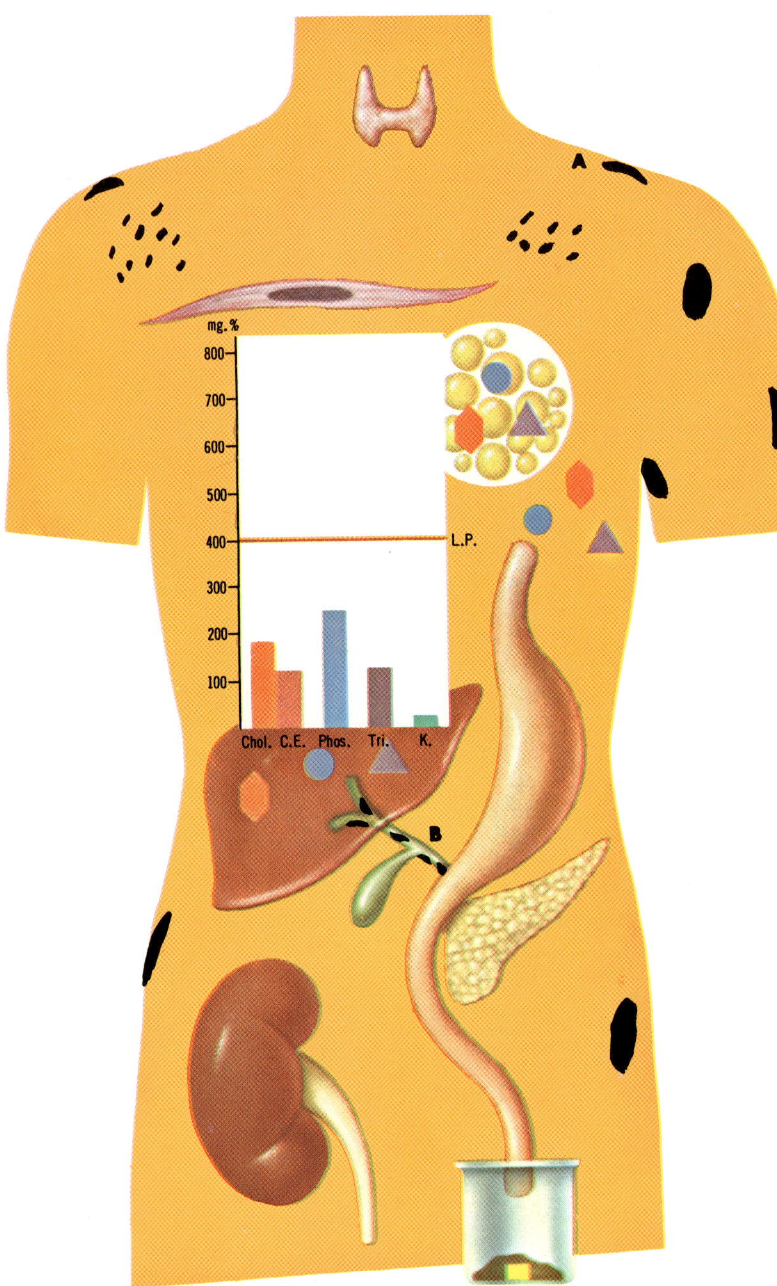

XANTHOMA DISSEMINATUM

This is an example of a disorder in which the serum lipids are usually *normal,* but fat deposits are found in the skin (A) and other body tissues. When they occur in the biliary tree (B), there may be obstructive jaundice.

Other disorders of lipid metabolism with normal blood lipids are *Gaucher's disease,* in which the cerebroside kerasin infiltrates the visceral organs, *Hand-Schüller-Christian disease,* in which lipid deposits in the membranous bones of the skull, and *Tay-Sachs disease,* in which a galactoside (neuraminic acid) is deposited in the brain.

Summary of Laboratory Findings:

Serum cholesterol: Normal
Serum phospholipids: Normal
Serum triglycerides: Normal
Plasma ketones: Normal

DIABETES MELLITUS

Because carbohydrate utilization is often decreased in this disorder, there is increased utilization of lipids for body metabolism. *Lipids* are mobilized from body stores (A), and the *blood levels* of all of them *increase* on their way to the liver, where they are broken down to ketones, which may be metabolized through the Krebs cycle. In diabetic acidosis these *ketones* may *accumulate in the blood* because the liver produces them (B) more rapidly than the cells can utilize them.

The blood lipids are elevated in glycogen-storage disease (von Gierke) for the same reason (i.e., inability to utilize carbohydrate for energy).

Summary of Laboratory Findings:

Serum cholesterol: Increased
Serum phospholipids: Increased
Serum triglycerides: Increased
Plasma ketones: Markedly increased at times

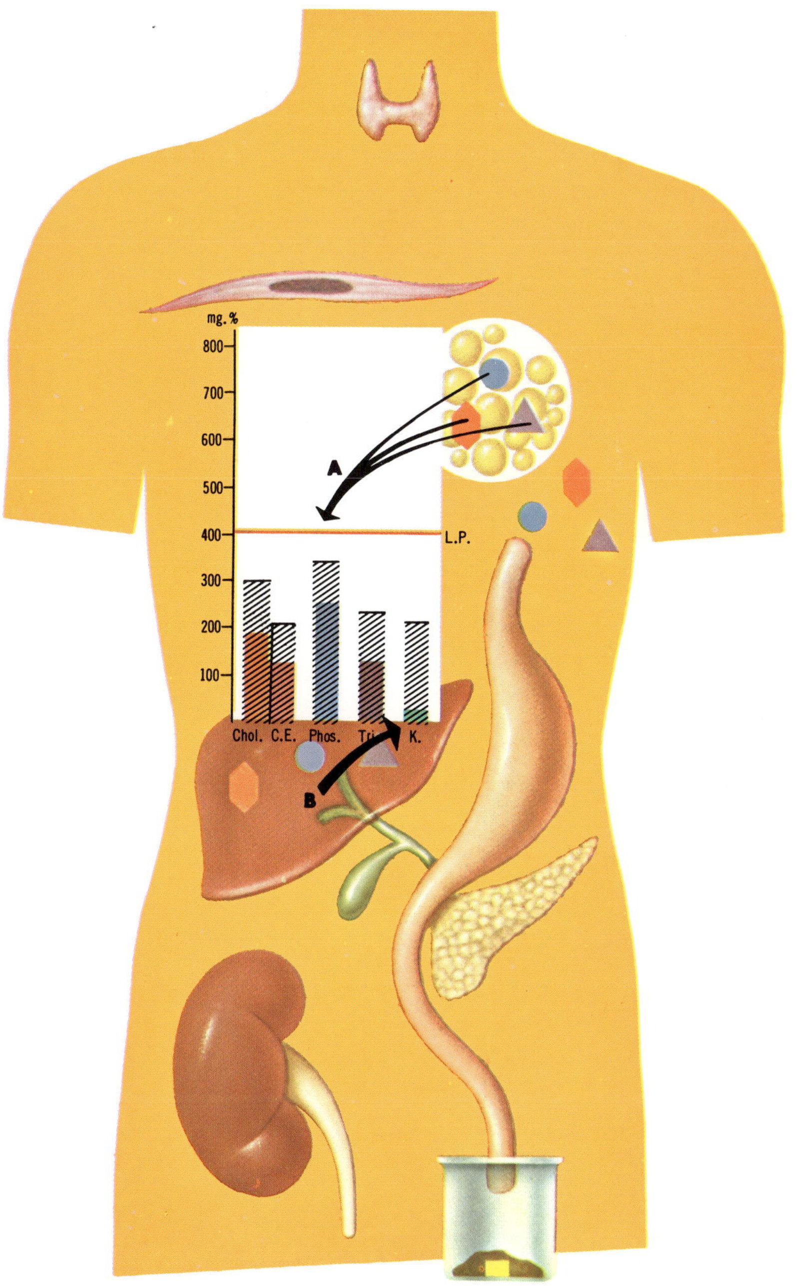

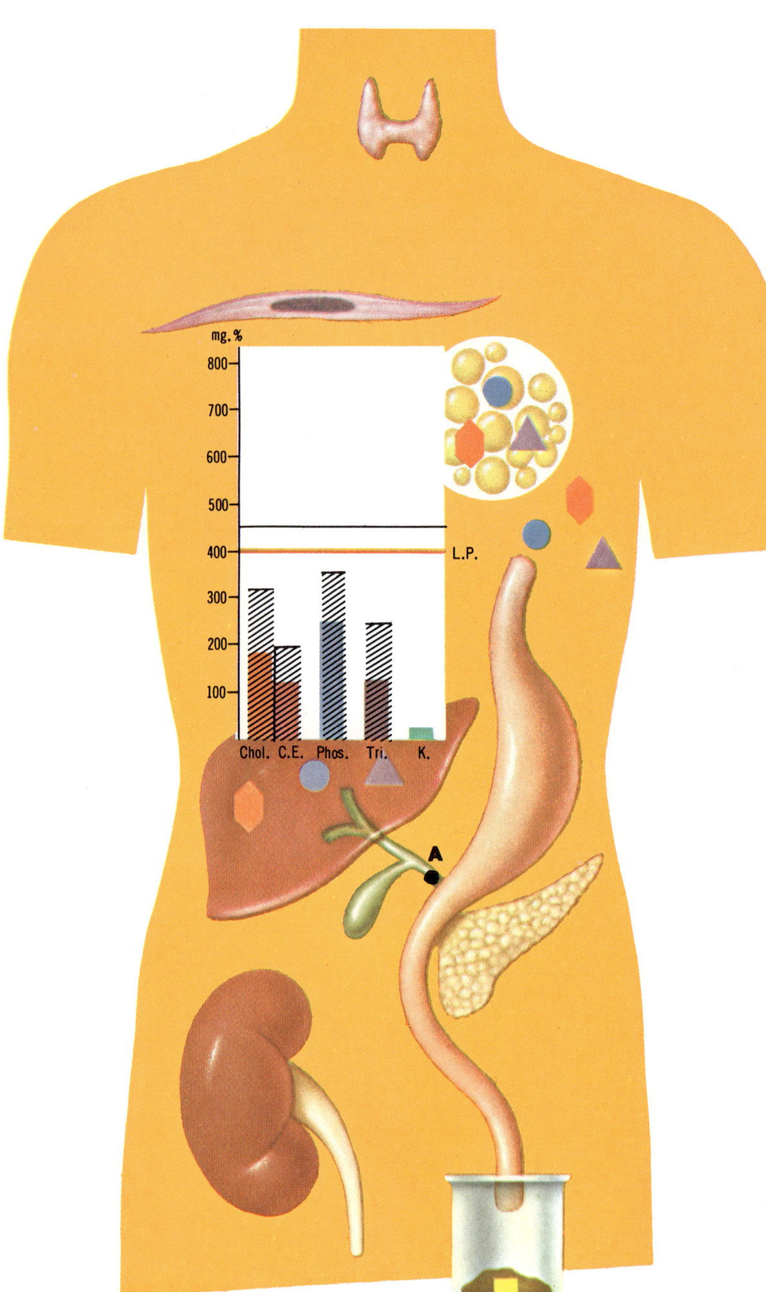

OBSTRUCTIVE JAUNDICE

It has been thought that the *serum cholesterol* level *rises* in this disorder because of impaired excretion through the obstructed bile ducts (A). However, recent evidence suggests that the rise is related to the increased bile acids in the blood stream. Serum *triglycerides* and *phospholipids* may also be *increased*. This is particularly true of primary biliary cirrhosis, in which abnormal lipoproteins and an overall increase of *lipoproteins* are found. The diagnosis will be supported by other liver function tests and radiocontrast studies of the biliary tree, if the jaundice subsides, but usually an exploratory laparotomy is needed to confirm the diagnosis.

Summary of Laboratory Findings:

Serum cholesterol: Increased

Serum phospholipids: Increased

Serum triglycerides: Increased

Serum lipoproteins: Increased or normal

Plasma ketones: Normal

HYPOTHYROIDISM

Hepatic synthesis of cholesterol is decreased in this disorder. Nevertheless, the serum *free* and *esterified cholesterol* rises because its tissue utilization, storage, and excretion are decreased. The serum *phospholipids* and *triglycerides* are also usually *increased.* A PBI or RAI uptake will usually establish the diagnosis, but a trial of thyroid extract is sometimes helpful. The picture is similar to Type IV lipoproteinemia.

Summary of Laboratory Findings:

Serum cholesterol: Increased

Serum phospholipids: Increased

Serum triglycerides: Increased

Plasma ketones: Normal

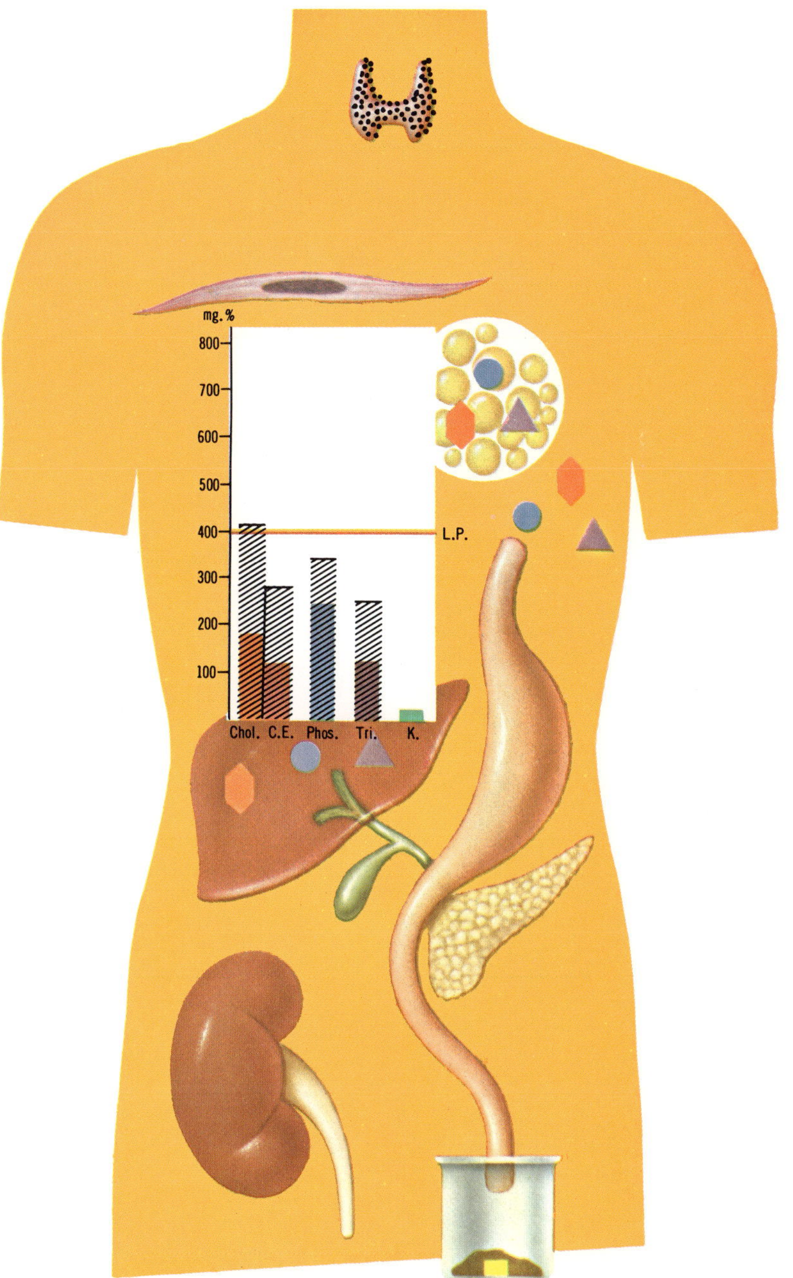

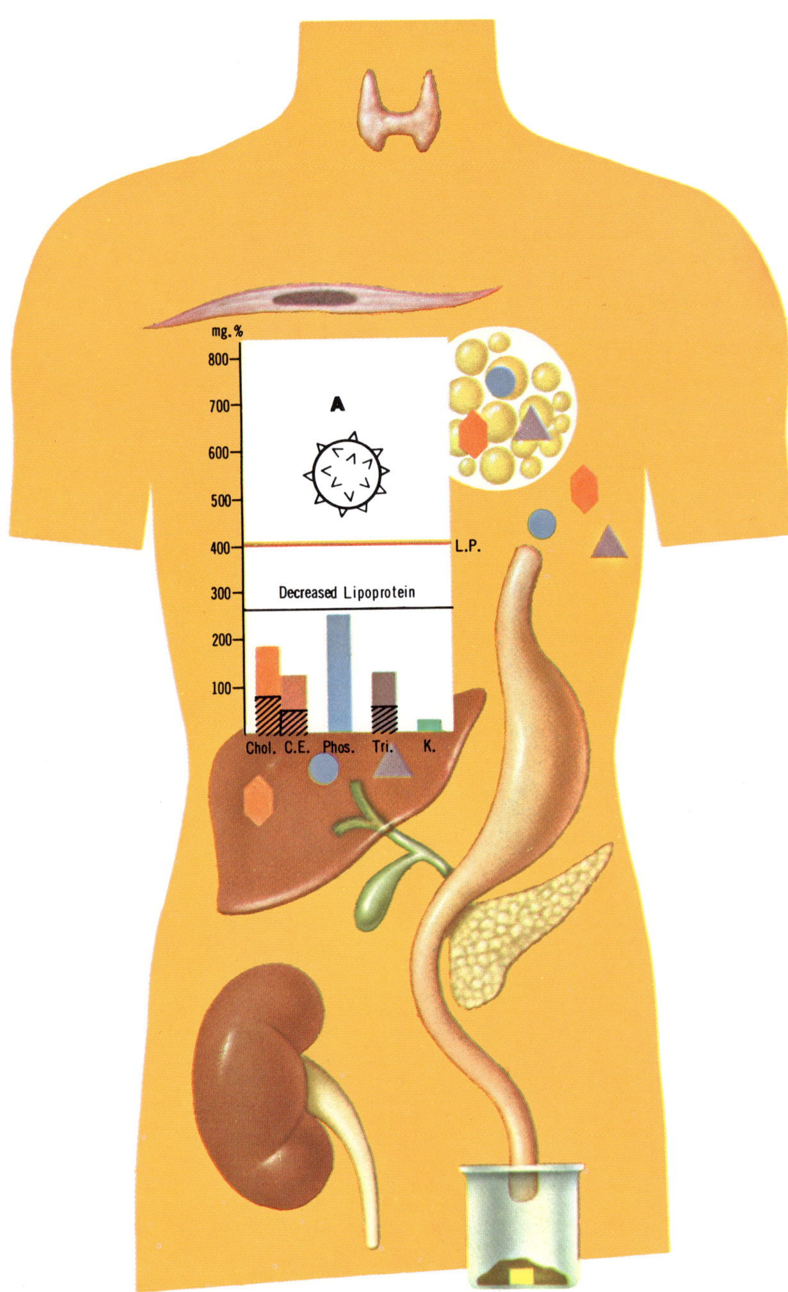

ACANTHOCYTOSIS

In this disorder a *deficiency* of *low-density* and *very-low-density lipoproteins* leads to a corresponding *drop* in *serum cholesterol* and *triglycerides*. The latter may drop to zero. The diagnosis is supported by the finding of spherical erythrocytes with numerous projecting spines and spicules, called acanthocytes (A).

Summary of Laboratory Findings:

Serum cholesterol: Decreased

Serum phospholipids: Normal

Serum triglycerides: Decreased

Serum lipoproteins: Decrease in low-density and very-low-density fraction

Plasma ketones: Normal

TYPE I HYPERLIPOPROTEINEMIA

Probably because of a deficiency of lipoprotein lipase, there is deficient removal of dietary triglycerides. There is a marked *elevation* of the serum *triglycerides,* and chylomicrons are found in the blood even after fasting. These separate to form a creamy layer over clear serum after overnight refrigeration. On lipoprotein electrophoresis there is a marked elevation of the chylomicron fraction, while the other fractions are usually normal. *Cholesterol* is only *mildly increased.* Xanthomata develop on the skin (A), and splenomegaly is a frequent finding. Atherosclerosis is less common. The diagnosis is established by the clinical findings, skin biopsy, and the finding of elevated triglycerides in blood relatives.

Summary of Laboratory Findings:

Serum cholesterol: Normal or increased
Serum phospholipids: Normal or increased
Serum triglycerides: Increased markedly
Serum lipoproteins: Increased very-low-density fraction
Plasma ketones: Normal

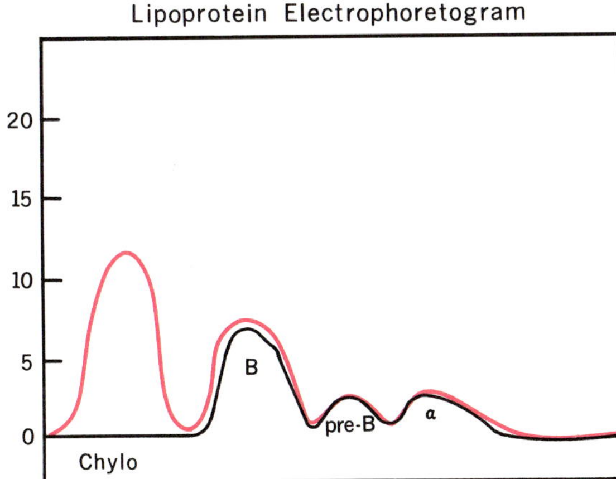

Type I Hyperlipoproteinemia

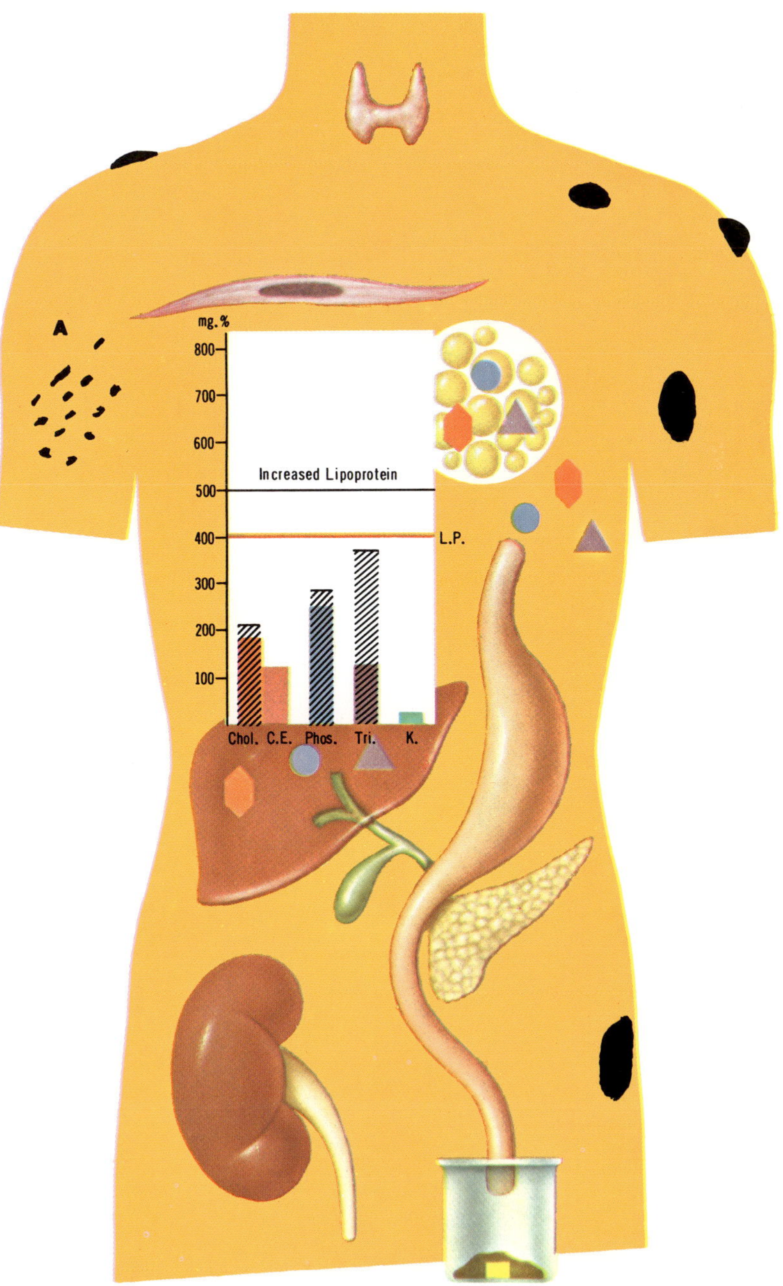

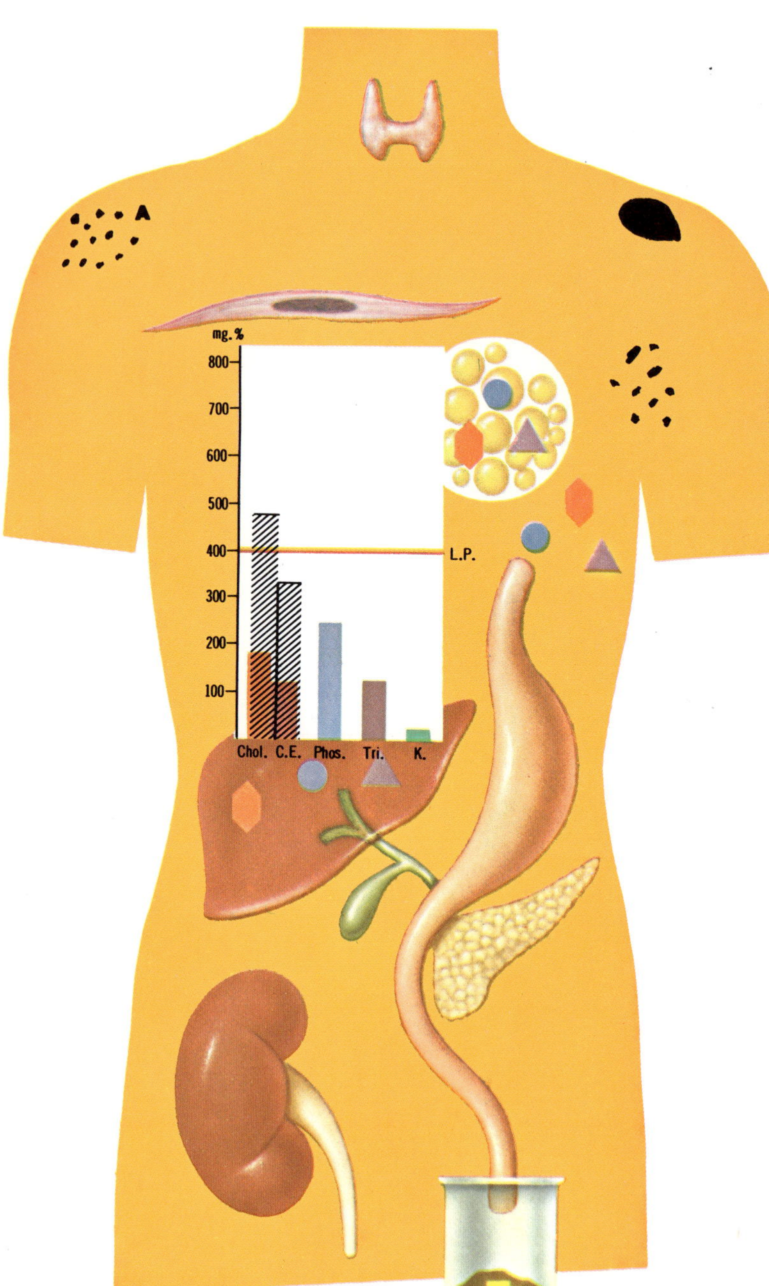

TYPE II HYPERLIPOPROTEINEMIA

For unknown reasons the *serum cholesterol* is *increased* in this hereditary disorder, usually without a concomittant rise in triglycerides. Lipoprotein electrophoresis shows a marked increase in the beta fraction, and occasionally some increase in the prebeta fraction. The serum is not lactescent and there is no creamy layer on top. As the disease progresses, xanthomata develop on the skin (A), subcutaneous tissue, and joints. The metabolic derangement is not yet known. There is an increased incidence of atherosclerosis and its complications. Tendon xanthoma, skin biopsy, and the finding of blood relatives with hypercholesterolemia establish the diagnosis.

Summary of Laboratory Findings:

Serum cholesterol: Increased

Serum phospholipids: Normal

Serum triglycerides: Normal

Plasma ketones: Normal

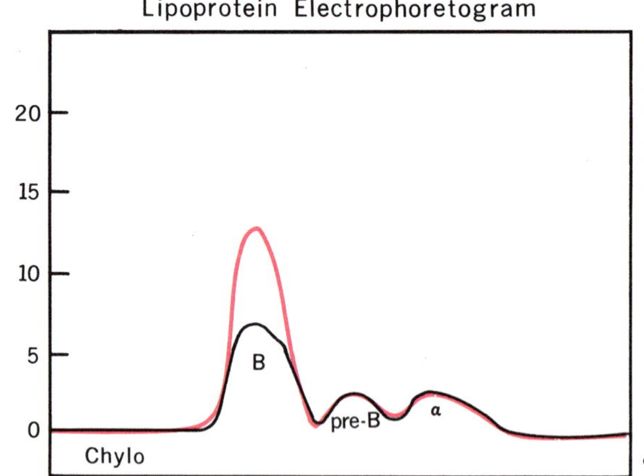

Type II Hyperlipoproteinemia

TYPE III HYPERLIPOPROTEINEMIA

In this hereditary disorder the cholesterol, esters, and triglycerides are increased. Lipoprotein electrophoresis shows an increased beta fraction which widens to encompass the prebeta fraction. The alpha fraction and chylomicrons are normal. The serum is usually uniformly lactescent. Clinically there are palmar xanthomas, a distinctive feature, and tendon xanthomas do not occur.

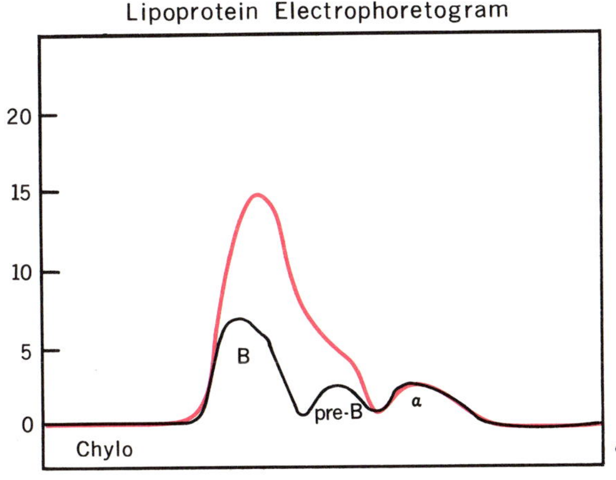

Type III Hyperlipoproteinemia

TYPE IV HYPERLIPOPROTEINEMIA

Probably due to impaired catabolism and increased secretion of very low density lipoprotein-triglycerides there is an *increase* of the *tryglycerides* in this disorder. The cholesterol may be increased also but not markedly. Lipoprotein electrophoresis shows a moderate or marked increase in the prebeta fraction. The beta and alpha fraction occasionally are decreased. The serum is lactescent but does not form a creamy layer on standing. There usually are not xanthoma unless the hyperlipemia is severe. Clinical diabetes or decreased glucose tolerance is common in this disorder.

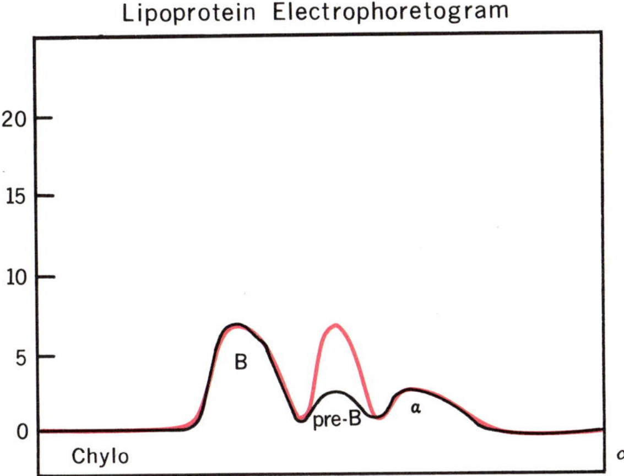

Type IV Hyperlipoproteinemia

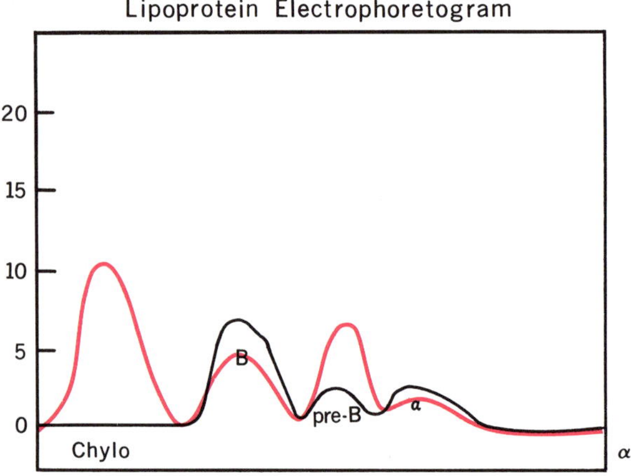

Type V Hyperlipoproteinemia

TYPE V HYPERLIPOPROTEINEMIA

In this disorder of multiple genetic defects there usually is an *increase* of both the *triglycerides* and *cholesterol*. The cholesterol is only slightly elevated in most cases and is completely normal in 40 per cent. Lipoprotein electrophoresis shows an increase of both the chylomicron and prebeta fraction with a decrease in the beta and alpha fraction. On standing a thick creamy layer forms over the serum, but the underlying serum remains lactescent. Clinically there are often diabetes mellitus, hepatosplenomegaly, and recurrent pancreatitis.

8 Disorders of Blood Nonprotein Nitrogen Substances

The blood nonprotein nitrogenous elements include urea nitrogen, uric acid, creatinine, creatine, ammonia, and amino acids as well as a residue of undetermined composition. In this chapter *urea nitrogen, creatine* and *creatinine,* and *ammonia* will be considered.

NORMAL METABOLISM

Production. *Urea* is produced in the process of protein degradation. The amino groups (NH_2) are released from the amino acids and transformed to ammonia by oxidative deamination, and the ammonia is subsequently transformed to urea in the "ornithine cycle." In this cycle the amino acid ornithine combines with ammonia to form urea. The liver is the sole site of this cycle, and urea is the chief nitrogenous end-product of amino acid metabolism.

Ammonia, as mentioned above, is produced by the liver in the process of protein degradation. In addition, some ammonia is formed in the colon by bacterial action on the amides of protein digestion and excreted urea. Finally, ammonia is produced in the renal tubules by the deamination of glutamic acid in the tubular cells and is secreted into the urine; in the process the base is conserved.

Creatine production occurs in two steps, the first mainly in the kidney and the second in the liver. In the kidney the amidine group of the amino acid arginine reacts with glycine to form guanidinoacetic acid. This passes through the blood into the liver, where it is methylated to creatine, which passes back into the blood and is transported to muscle.

Creatinine is produced from creatine in muscle. Here creatine is first phosphorylated to phosphocreatine, an important compound for storing muscular energy. When energy is needed for metabolic processes, phosphocreatine is broken down to creatinine. There is an interesting constancy in the quantity of creatine converted to creatinine, for the amount is related directly to the total body muscle mass.

Transportation. All of the above nonprotein nitrogenous substances are transported by the blood, where they exist in the following concentrations: *urea nitrogen,* 10 to 20 mg. per 100 ml.; *creatine,* 2 to 7 mg. per 100 ml.; *creatinine,* 1 to 2 mg. per 100 ml.; and ammonia, 40 to 70 mcg. per 100 ml.

Utilization. Of these nonprotein nitrogenous substances, only creatine is utilized by the body. In the form of phosphocreatine it is stored as energy for muscle metabolism.

Detoxification and Excretion. Both *urea* and *creatinine* are excreted in the urine. The quantity of urea excreted is variable, being proportional to the amount of protein in the diet. On an average diet, the normal adult excretes approximately 20 to 35 gm. of urea in 24 hours. The amount of creatinine excreted each day, however, is very constant, being proportional to the muscle mass and independent of any exogenous source of nitrogen. Normally, adult males excrete 1.5 to 2.0 gm. in 24 hours, and females excrete 0.8 to 2.5 gm. in 24 hours.

Creatine is normally present only in very small amounts in the male urine but is found in substantial amounts in the urine of prepubertal children (4.2 mg. per kilogram daily) and pregnant women. Blood *ammonia* is detoxified in the liver by urea formation and transamination in amino acid synthesis. Nevertheless, from 0.5 to 1.0 gm. is present in a 24-hour urine. This is derived from the renal tubules in the excretion of acid, as mentioned above.

Regulation. The blood and urine *urea nitrogen* vary directly with dietary protein intake and indirectly with the rate of tissue anabolism in pregnancy, growth, convalescence, etc. On the other hand, blood and urine *creatinine* are independent of any exogenous source of nitrogen and are proportional to total body muscle mass. Urine *ammonia* is proportional to the amount of acid in the diet.

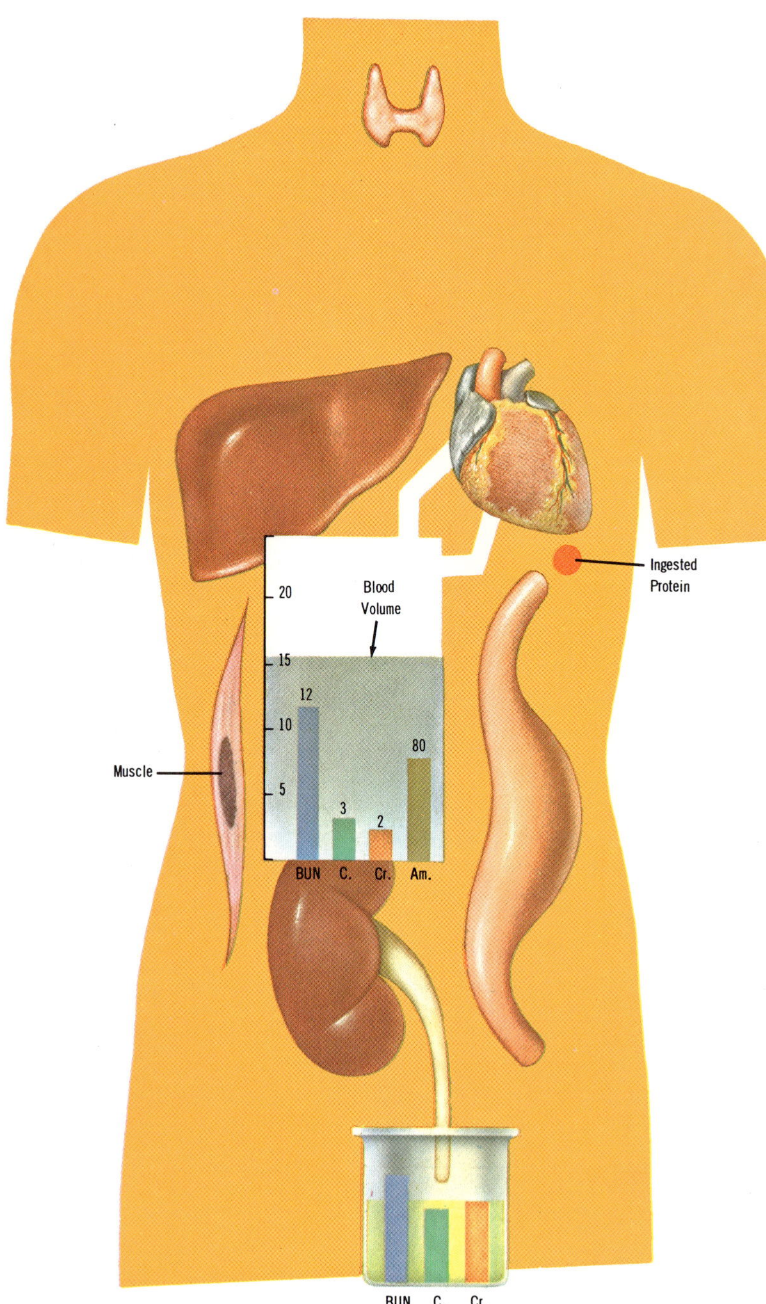

Abbreviations Used in Plates:

BUN = Blood urea nitrogen in mg. per 100 ml. of blood

C. = Creatine in mg. per 100 ml. of blood

Cr. = Creatinine in mg. per 100 ml. of blood

Am. = Blood ammonia in mcg. per 100 ml. of blood × 10

(Note: This increase in BUN is almost always higher than that noted in plates, but scale cannot be extended enough.)

STARVATION

Under the conditions of reduced protein intake (A), the organism must get food for metabolism from its tissues. Thus there is protein catabolism, and with it the *blood* and *urine urea nitrogen* and *creatine increase*.

Febrile diseases and diabetes mellitus may produce a similar picture.

Summary of Laboratory Findings:

Blood urea nitrogen: Increased

Blood creatine: Increased

Urine urea: Increased

Urine creatine: Increased

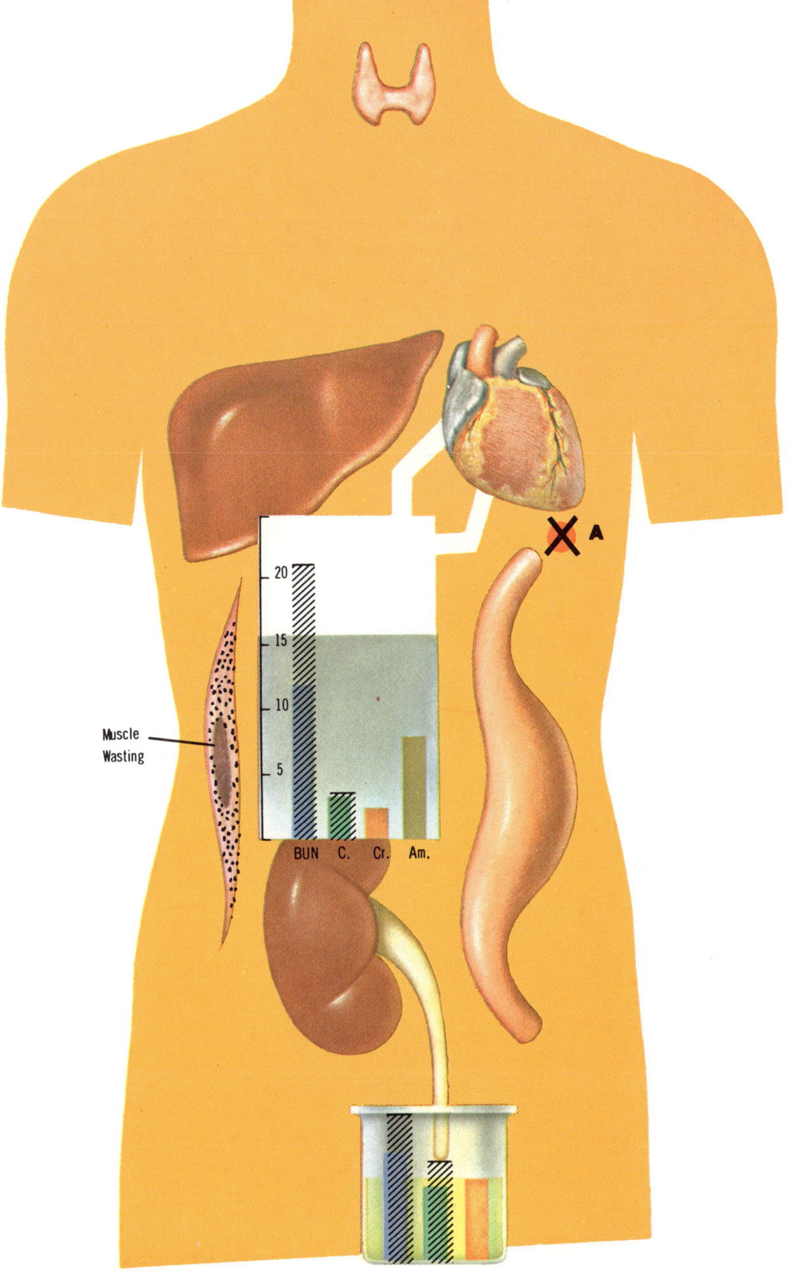

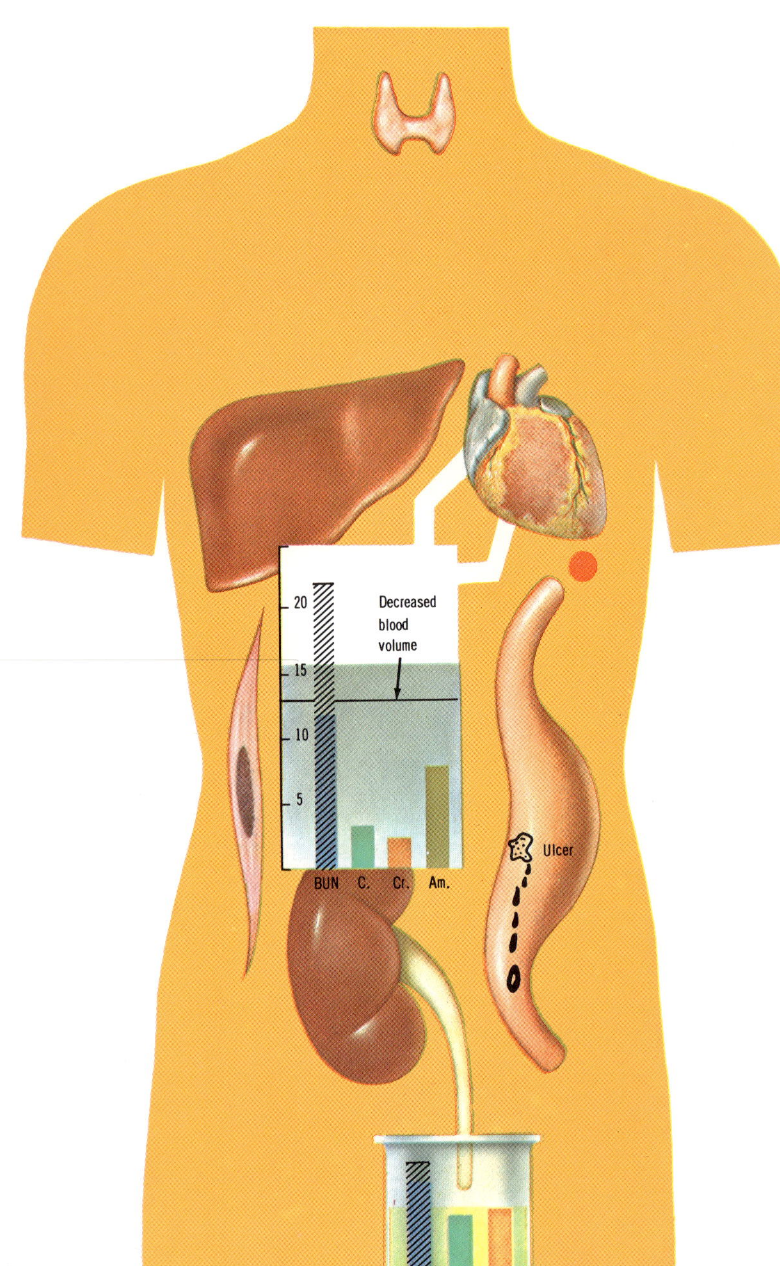

BLEEDING GASTRIC ULCER

In this disorder the rise in the *blood urea nitrogen* may be due to an increased production of urea from the breakdown of blood in the gastrointestinal tract as well as from the factors discussed under Shock (see p. 125). The diagnosis is confirmed by examining stools for occult blood, an upper gastrointestinal series, and gastroscopy.

Summary of Laboratory Findings:

Blood urea nitrogen: Increased

Urine urea nitrogen: Increased

CIRRHOSIS OF THE LIVER

In severe cases of cirrhosis, the liver is unable to convert ammonia to urea. Thus the *blood urea nitrogen drops,* whereas the *blood ammonia rises.* The changes here are analogous to the rise in blood creatine and fall of creatinine in muscle-wasting disease. Liver function studies and liver biopsy usually establish the diagnosis.

Summary of Laboratory Findings:

Blood urea nitrogen: Decreased

Blood ammonia: Increased

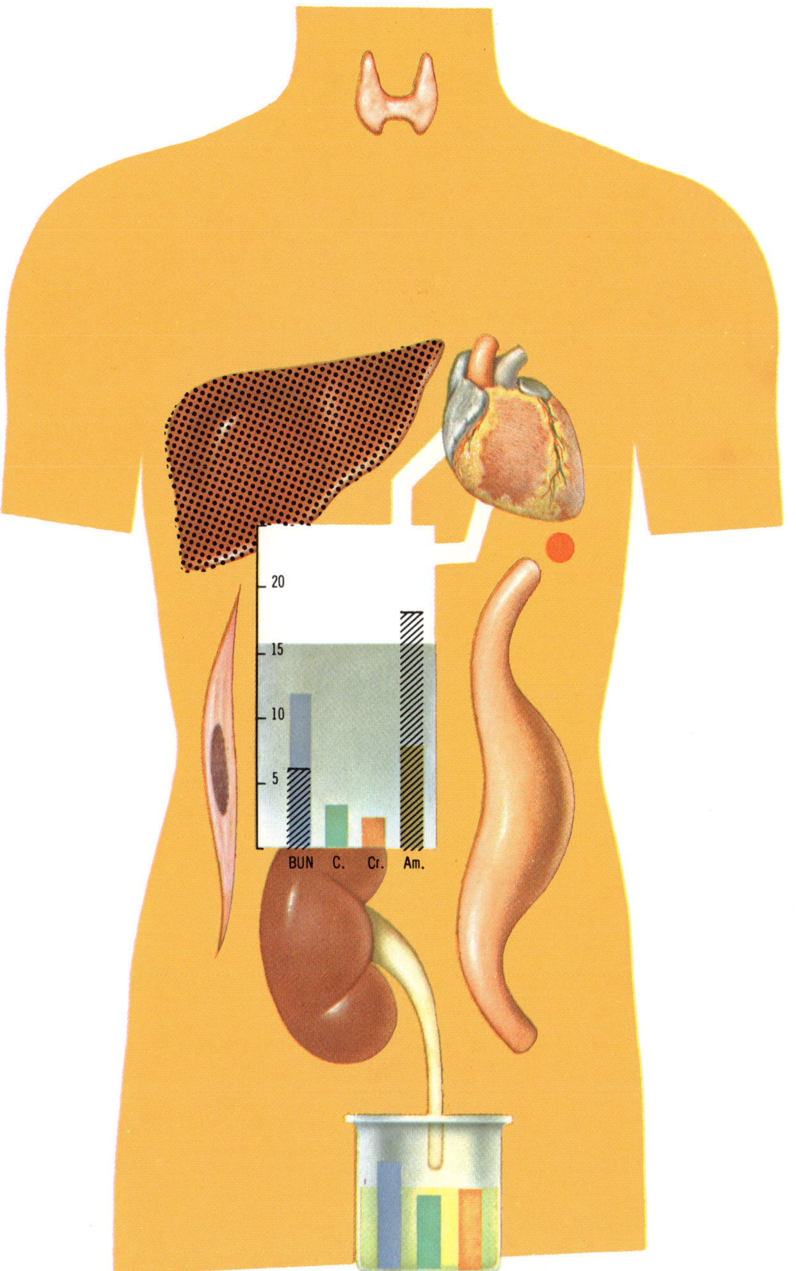

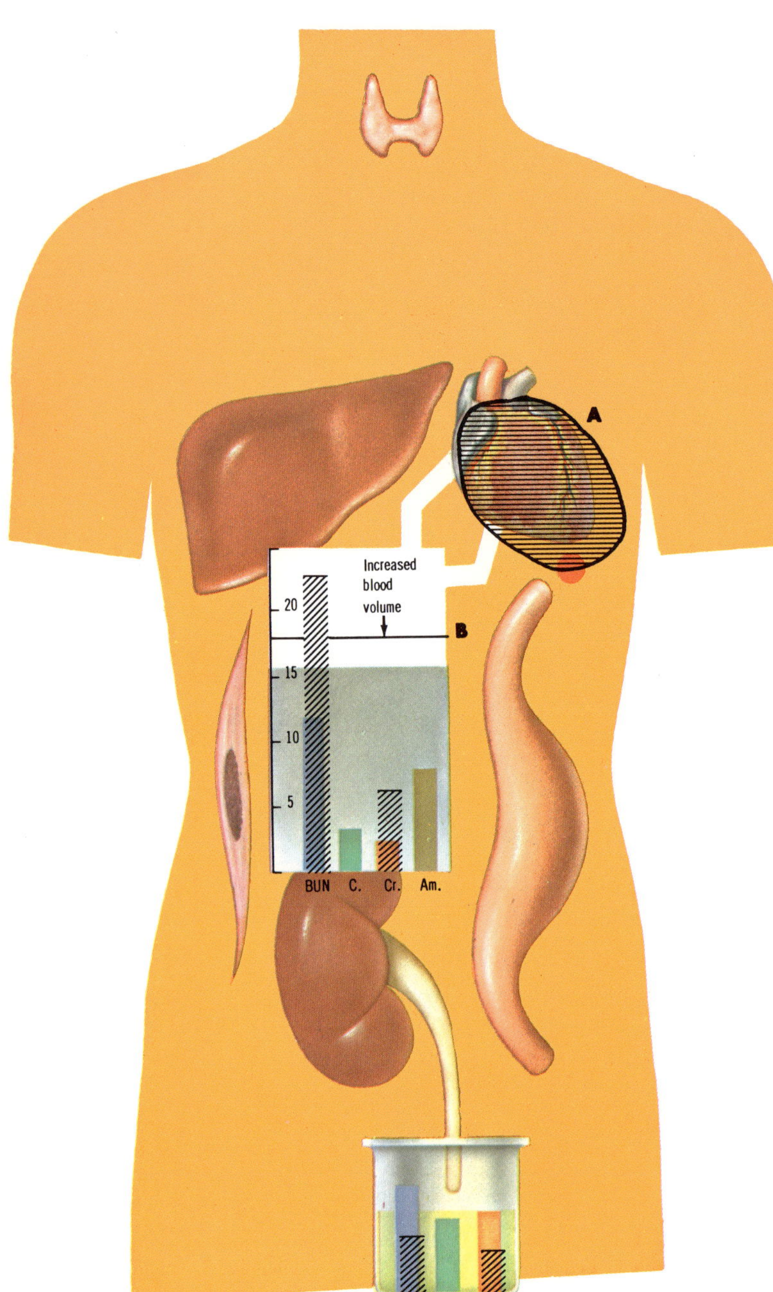

CONGESTIVE HEART FAILURE

In congestive heart failure (A) the decreased cardiac output results in a considerable decrease in the renal blood flow. A decreased glomerular filtration rate follows, with a concomitant *rise* in *blood urea* and *creatinine* and blood volume (B). The diagnosis is assisted by a venous pressure and circulation time, ECG, pulmonary function studies, and a chest roentgenogram.

Bilateral renal artery thrombosis and dissecting aneurysm of the abdominal aorta will produce a similar picture.

Summary of Laboratory Findings:

Blood urea nitrogen: Increased

Blood creatinine: Increased

HYPOVOLEMIC SHOCK

Mandatory for renal excretion of urea and creatinine is an adequate perfusion of the kidneys with blood. In this disorder blood volume and hence renal blood flow decreases, and there is a consequent rise in the *blood urea nitrogen* and *creatinine,* with an associated *drop* in *urine urea* and *creatinine.*

Hypovolemic shock, cardiogenic shock, and vasomotor collapse may all produce a similar picture.

The diagnosis is confirmed by repeated hematocrits, blood volumes, a study of venous pressure and circulation time, and determining the urine output.

Summary of Laboratory Findings:

Blood urea nitrogen: Increased

Blood creatinine: Increased

Urine urea: Decreased

Urine creatinine: Decreased

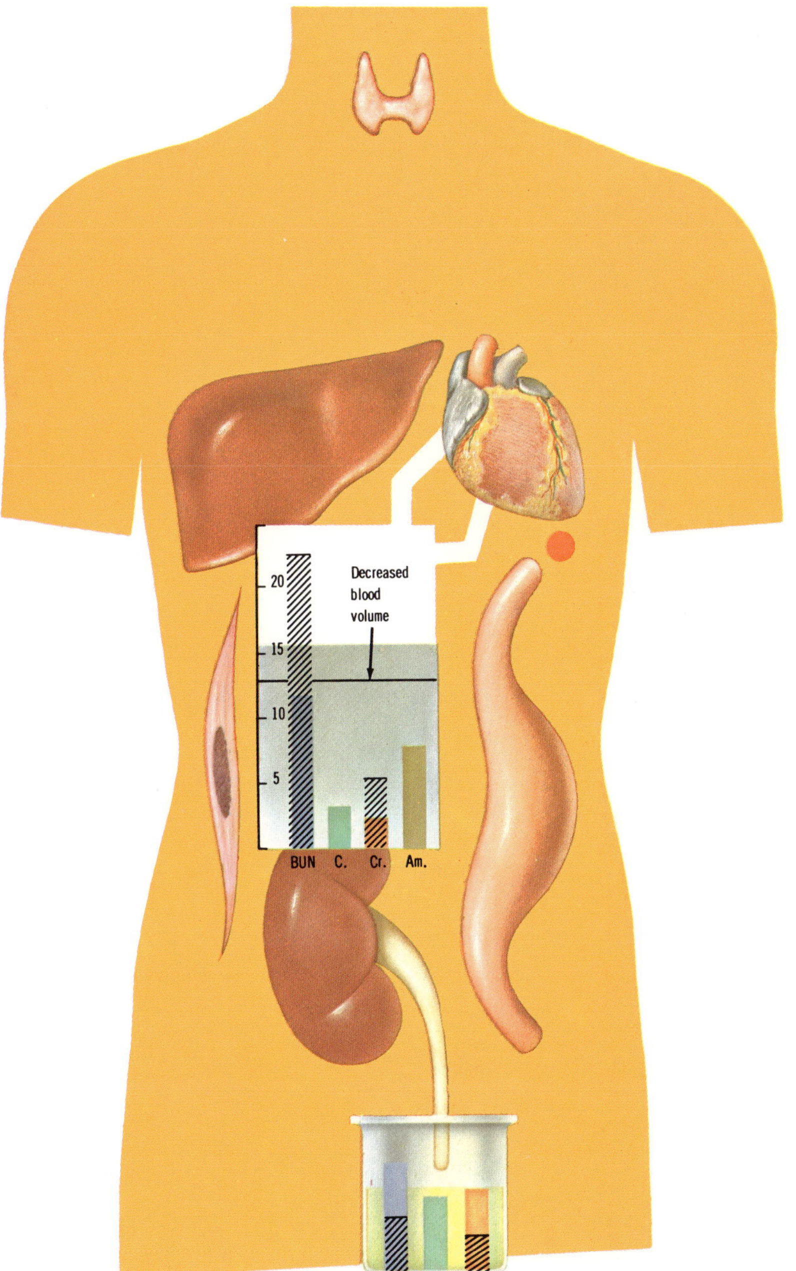

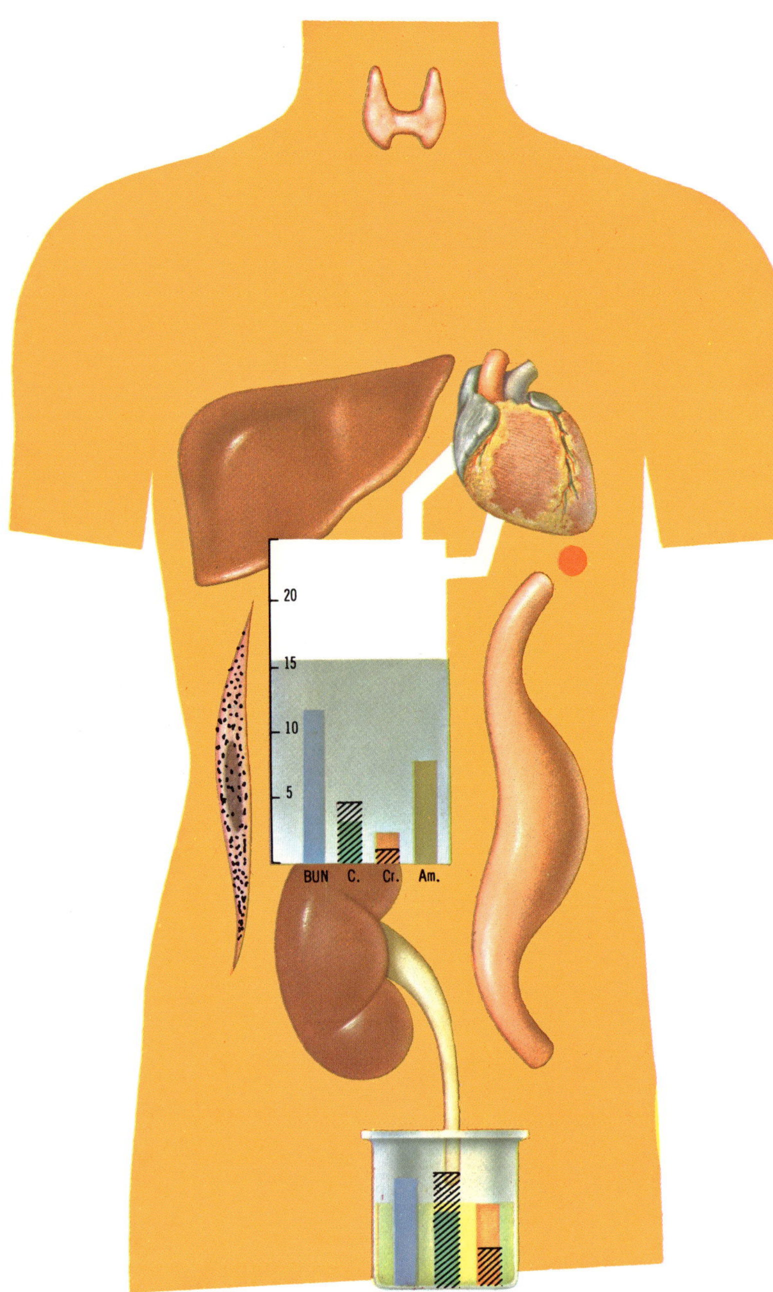

MUSCULAR DYSTROPHIES

These disorders are associated with a reduction in total body muscle mass, and therefore the amount of creatine converted to creatinine each day will be reduced. Thus *creatine builds up* in the *blood* and is excreted in the *urine,* whereas *blood* and *urine creatinine* drop.

Progressive muscular dystrophy, amyotonia congenita, myotonic muscular dystrophy, and myasthenia gravis may all produce this picture. The diagnosis is established by muscle biopsy and electromyography.

Summary of Laboratory Findings:

Blood creatine: Increased

Blood creatinine: Decreased

Urine creatine: Increased

Urine creatinine: Decreased

OBSTRUCTIVE UROPATHY

Obstruction of the urogenital tree compromises the free flow of urine and glomerular filtration. If this is bilateral and severe, the renal clearance of urea and creatinine is depressed, and the *blood urea nitrogen* and *creatinine rise*. Prostatic hypertrophy, bilateral ureteral stricture, and renal calculi may all produce this picture. The diagnosis is confirmed by cystoscopy and retrograde pyelography.

Summary of Laboratory Findings:

Blood urea nitrogen: Increased

Blood creatinine: Increased

Urine urea nitrogen: Decreased

Urine creatinine: Decreased

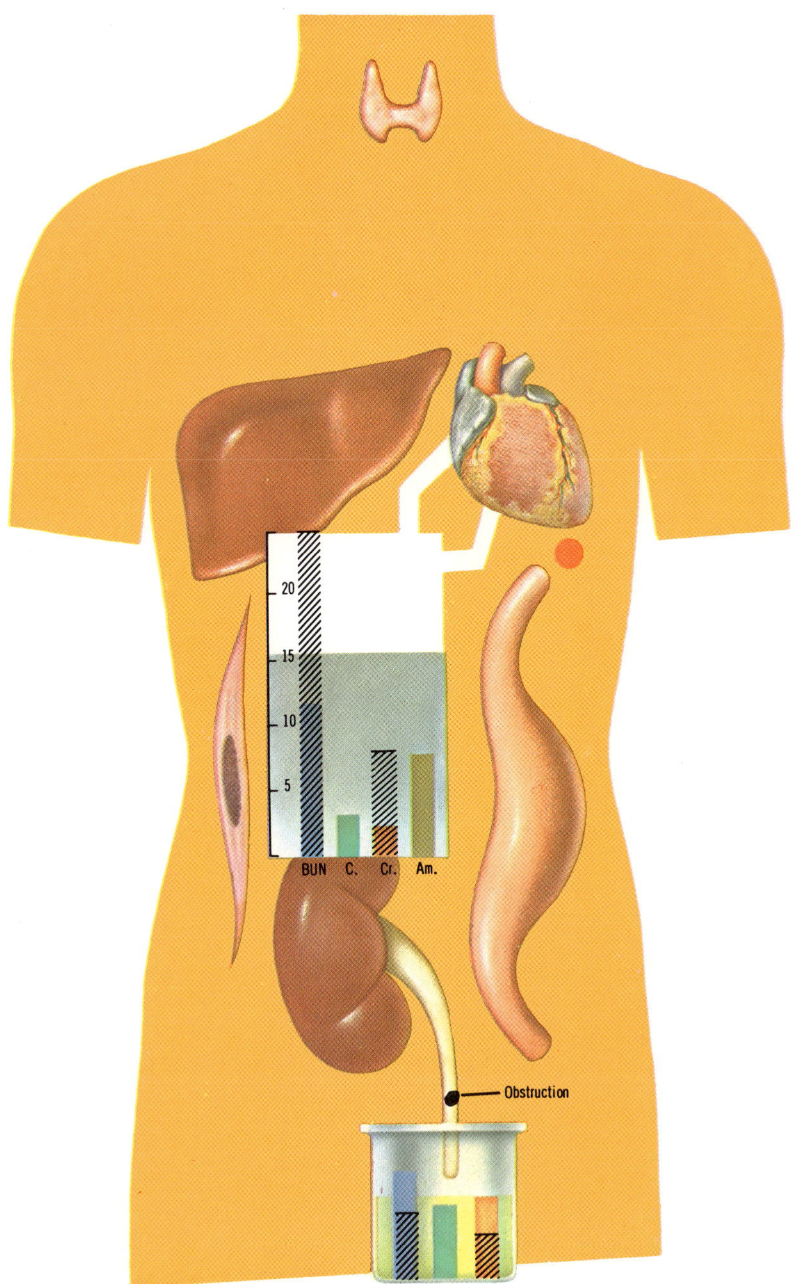

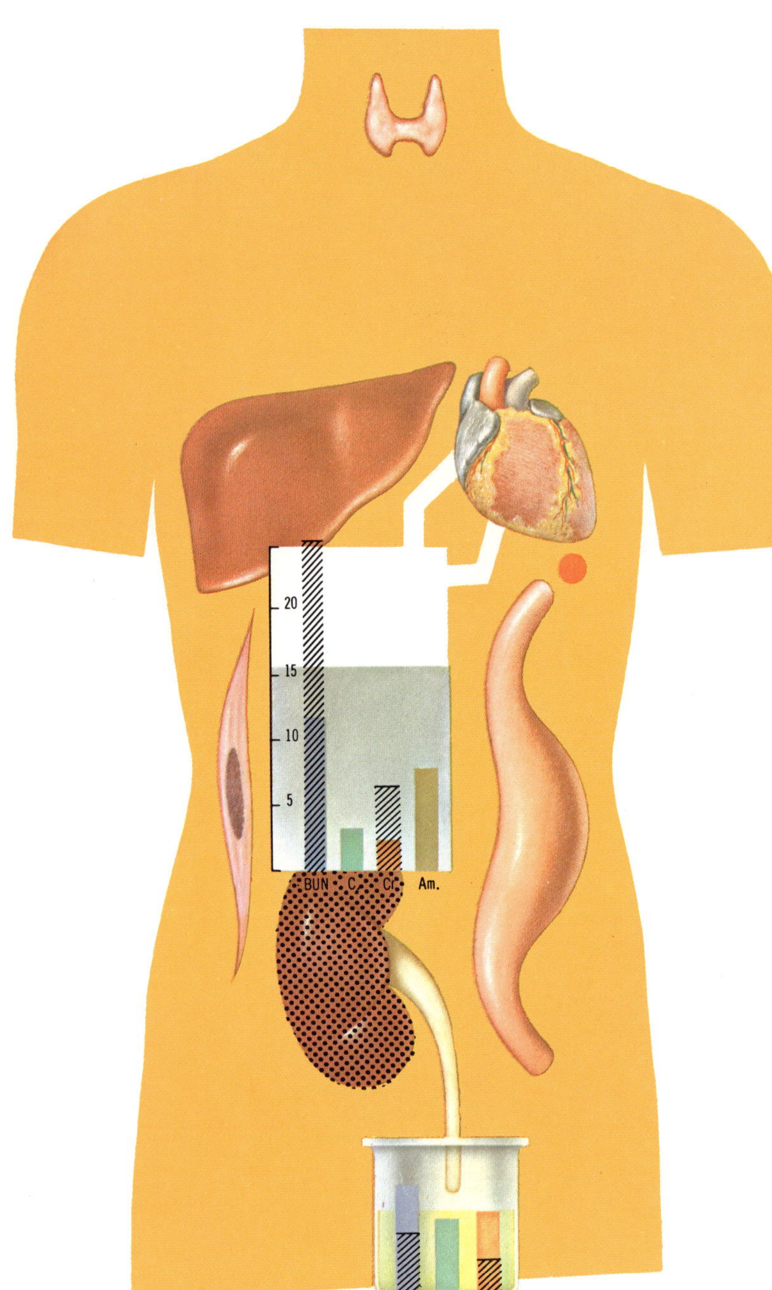

CHRONIC GLOMERULONEPHRITIS

The diseased kidneys in chronic glomerulonephritis are unable to excrete *urea* and *creatinine,* and the level of both of these *rises* in the *blood.* At the same time they *decrease* in the urine. The all-important exclusion of obstructive uropathy by retrograde pyelograms and by cystoscopy assists in this diagnosis, but Addis counts and renal biopsy are more conclusive.

Other parenchymal diseases of the kidney such as diabetic nephrosis, polycystic kidney disease, gout, nephrosclerosis, and chronic pyelonephritis may produce a similar picture.

Summary of Laboratory Findings:

Blood urea nitrogen: Increased

Blood creatinine: Increased

Urine urea nitrogen: Decreased

Urine creatinine: Decreased

HYPERTHYROIDISM

Because of a decreased total body muscle mass produced by the muscle catabolism in this disorder, less creatine is converted to creatinine. Thus serum *creatine increases* slightly, and *large amounts appear* in the *urine*, whereas *urinary creatinine drops*. It is also probable that excess thyroid hormone inhibits the conversion of creatine to creatinine in the remaining muscle. The diagnosis is established by a T_4 or a RAI uptake.

Many other endocrine disorders are marked by excessive protein catabolism. Acromegaly in its late stages causes muscle weakness and catabolism. Addison's disease, gonadal dysfunction such as that in castration, eunuchoidism, postmenopausal disturbances in women, etc., are all associated with protein catabolism and thus creatinemia and creatinuria. Replacement of the appropriate hormone will abolish the abnormal muscle and creatine metabolism, thus returning the serum and urine levels to normal in most cases.

Summary of Laboratory Findings:

Urine creatine: Increased

Urine creatinine: Decreased

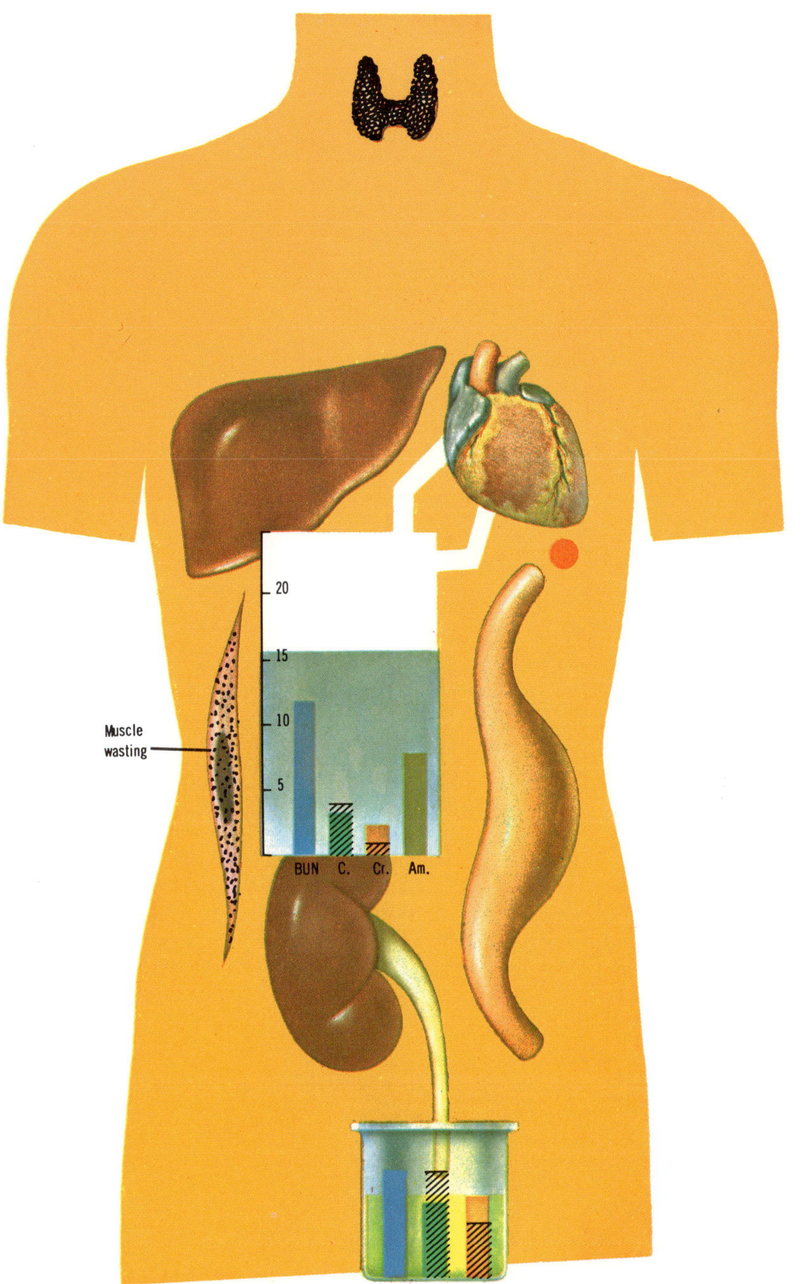

9 Disorders of Blood Oxygen Content

The process that involves the delivery of oxygen to the cells of the organism and the removal of carbon dioxide from them is called respiration. According to Fulton, this function is performed by a system composed of four important components. These are: (1) an *air pump* (the lungs, thoracic cage, and respiratory muscles), which brings oxygen into the body from the atmosphere, where it can be absorbed into the blood; (2) *diffusion surfaces* (the lung alveoli and capillaries), by which means the oxygen is absorbed into the blood; (3) a *transport system* (the blood, the heart, and circulation), which transfers the oxygen from the pulmonary capillaries to the other tissues of the body; and (4) a *regulating center* (the central nervous system together with various chemoreceptors), which adjusts the function of the other components of the system to meet body demands under a variety of conditions. The role of each of these components in relation to the metabolism of oxygen will now be discussed in detail.

NORMAL METABOLISM

Intake. Oxygen intake may be considered the most important part of ventilation. Oxygen enters the body through the nose or mouth and travels through the pharynx, larynx, trachea, bronchi, bronchioles, and alveolar ducts to the alveoli, where it may be absorbed into the blood stream. Because very little oxygen can be absorbed in the respiratory passages (the larynx, trachea, etc.), these are called "the anatomic dead air spaces" (in extent, approximately 150 cubic centimeters).

The amount of oxygen that might reach the alveoli by simple diffusion down the air passages would be inadequate to sustain life. Thus nature has developed an "air pump" made up of the thoracic cage, the diaphragm, and the elastic tissue in the walls of the lungs. Just as the heart pumps blood through the circulatory system, this mechanism pumps air in and out of the lungs under the influence of the respiratory centers in the brain stem. During *inspiration* the external intercostal muscles contract, pulling the ribs upward and increasing the volume of the thorax. At the same time the diaphragmatic muscles may contract, lowering the level of the diaphragm and increasing the volume of the thorax. In this fashion air is drawn into the lungs. In *expiration* the recoil ("resistance") of the elastic tissues of the lungs and thorax presses air out of the lungs. This elastic resistance is called "compliance" and may be measured. Ordinarily, this is a passive process. However, active expiration may be accomplished by contraction of the abdominal muscles, forcing the diaphragm up against the lungs and expressing more air.

Thus the intake of oxygen depends on patent respiratory passages, good neuromuscular function, a mobile and elastic thoracic cage, elastic lungs, and the rate and depth of respirations, determined by an intact respiratory center in the brain stem. It also depends on how much air the lungs can hold (total lung capacity). As will be discussed subsequently, each of these capacities can be measured.

Absorption. Oxygen is absorbed in the alveoli, which under normal conditions are richly supplied with capillaries. Collectively, the alveoli constitute an absorbing surface of 50 to 100 sq. m. To get to the blood, the oxygen molecules must diffuse across a surface film (covering the alveolar membrane), the alveolar membrane, the interstitial fluid, and a capillary membrane. Any of these layers may be thickened in disease states and prevent the absorption of oxygen.

From the above it is evident that oxygen absorption may be influenced by the total surface area of the alveoli and the character of the alveolar-capillary membranes. It is also influenced by the partial pressure of oxygen in the alveolar air (and thus the atmosphere). Normally, this must be greater than the partial pressure of oxygen in pulmonary capillary blood.

Oxygen absorption is also influenced by the partial pressure of carbon dioxide in the alveolar air and blood. High concentrations of carbon dioxide in the blood tend to inhibit the uptake of oxygen. Low concentrations of carbon dioxide in the blood have a reverse effect.

Furthermore, for adequate absorption to take place, the alveoli must be well ventilated and well supplied with pulmonary capillary blood. One is no good without the other. If an alveolus is well ventilated but has no functioning capillaries (as in a pulmonary embolus), there will be no absorption of oxygen. Likewise, if an alveolus is well supplied with functioning capillaries but is inadequately ventilated (as in atelectasis), there will be no oxygen absorption.

When some alveoli are better ventilated than others, there is said to be an uneven distribution of inspired gas. Such a situation occurs in many pulmonary diseases. The tests that have been developed to measure this will be discussed below. The distribution of pulmonary capillary blood flow may also be uneven. Direct measurement of this is more difficult. It should be emphasized that overall alveolar ventilation and pulmonary capillary blood flow may be adequate, and yet there may be anoxemia and carbon dioxide retention if alveoli that are ventilated are not well perfused, and if those that are well perfused are not well ventilated.

Transport. Following absorption, oxygen is carried to the tissues by the blood in the circulatory system under the force of the heart. The rate and stroke volume of the heart are adjusted to meet the oxygen needs of the body. Most of the oxygen is carried by the hemoglobin of the red cells. One gram of hemoglobin can hold 1.34 ml. of oxygen.

Thus, transport of oxygen will be inadequate if there is inadequate hemoglobin (e.g., in anemia); if some of the hemoglobin is altered in such a way that it cannot carry oxygen (e.g., in methemoglobinemia); or if the heart is not capable of pumping the blood to the tissues (e.g., in heart failure). Finally, some tissues may not receive adequate oxygen when blood is temporarily shunted to more vital tissues (e.g., in shock).

Utilization. Oxygen is utilized by the tissues in the aerobic catabolism of carbohydrate, fat, and protein, with the formation of carbon dioxide, water, and other waste products. Adequate utilization depends on many cellular enzymes.

Excretion. Oxygen, following its utilization, is excreted in the form of carbon dioxide and water. Water may be excreted in a variety of ways (kidney, lungs, skin, etc.). Although some carbon dioxide is excreted as bicarbonate in the urine, most of the carbon dioxide is excreted by way of the lungs.

Carbon dioxide is transported to the lungs in the blood as free carbon dioxide, bicarbonate, in combination with plasma proteins, or as carboxyhemoglobin. In the lungs it diffuses from the blood through the alveolar-capillary membrane into the alveoli. The rate of diffusion depends on a low partial pressure of carbon dioxide in the alveoli. Normally, carbon dioxide makes up 0.04 per cent of inspired air, and carbon dioxide from this source is also present in the alveoli. Poorly ventilated alveoli do not have this low partial pressure of carbon dioxide. Carbon dioxide diffusion does not seem to be influenced by the thickness of the alveolar-capillary membrane, probably because carbon dioxide has 10 to 20 times the diffusing capacity of oxygen. On the other hand, unless a large number of alveoli are adequately ventilated, there will be overall carbon dioxide retention.

Regulation. Normally, blood oxygen and carbon dioxide content are maintained in a relatively narrow range by adjusting the rate and depth of respiration according to body requirements for intake of oxygen and excretion of carbon dioxide. This is very similar to the way in which the rate and stroke volume of the heart are adjusted to meet the oxygen requirements of the tissues. Thus, respirations are increased by a low blood oxygen saturation and a high carbon dioxide content acting on the chemoreceptors in the carotid and aortic bodies and the respiratory center in the brain stem. Anoxemia is not as good a stimulus for respiration as a high carbon dioxide content (hypercapnia). Respirations may also be increased by acidosis (also acting through the carotid and aortic bodies and the respiratory center), impulses from higher cortical centers, painful stimulation of the peripheral nerves, and hypotension. Respirations may be depressed by a prolonged elevation of blood carbon dioxide, prolonged anoxia, or hypertension.

THE APPROACH TO THE DIAGNOSIS

In disease states the arterial and venous blood oxygen content may decrease, or, less commonly, the venous blood oxygen content may increase. A low arterial blood oxygen content is called *anoxemia.* This is usually expressed in terms of *arterial blood oxygen saturation* and is normally 95 to 97 per cent or above. Arterial blood is obtained with special needles inserted in the brachial or femoral arteries.

Anoxemia may result from decreased oxygen intake (as in severe pulmonary emphysema), from impaired absorption (as in sarcoidosis), or inadequate perfusion, as when pulmonary arterial blood bypasses the lungs (e.g., in hemangiomas of the lung). There may be an inadequate supply of oxygen to the tissues without anoxemia in anemia (anemic anoxia), heart failure, shock (stagnant anoxia), or disorders that block the uptake of oxygen by the tissue enzymes (histotoxic anoxia), as in cyanide poisoning.

In many of the disorders associated with anoxemia, the blood oxygen saturation does not drop until the disease process is advanced. Thus more sensitive tests have been developed for diagnosing these conditions. These will be discussed according to the use to which these tests have been put in evaluating a particular part of oxygen metabolism.

Disorders of Intake and Excretion

Information regarding the adequacy of the chest and lungs as an air pump may be obtained from spirometric studies. (Only a brief description of these will be given here. For a detailed account of the performance of these tests and the calculation of the results, the reader is referred to one of the many texts on pulmonary physiology.*) The most practical of these studies are the *vital capacity,* the *timed vital capacity,* and the *maximum breathing capacity* (MBC).

The *vital capacity* is the maximum amount of air that may be exhaled after a maximum inspiration. In the normal adult male this is usually 2½ times the body surface and is expressed in liters. The vital capacity is decreased in restrictive disease of the lung. The *timed vital capacity* is the volume of air that may be expired in 1, 2, or 3 seconds after a maximum inspiration.

Normally, 72 to 92 per cent of the vital capacity may be expired in 1 second, 85 to 100 per cent in 2 seconds, and 92 to 100 per cent in 3 seconds (McCombs). This test is most valuable in diagnosing obstructive disease of the lung. The test may be repeated after administering a bronchodilator to determine the part played by bronchospasm in the obstruction.

The *maximum breathing capacity* (MBC) (not illustrated in the Plate on p. 134) is the maximum amount of air that can be ventilated over a given interval (usually 15 seconds). It is influenced by the rate of respiration and the vital capacity. It is important that the patient be encouraged to exert his maximum effort. The maximum breathing capacity is normally 58 to 169 L. per minute in adult males but is dependent on age and size. This volume may be decreased in both restrictive and obstructive diseases of the lung.

* Comroe, J. H., Jr., *et al.*: The Lung. ed. 2. Chicago, Year Book Medical Publishers, 1962.

The *residual volume* would be a useful test of pulmonary function if its measurement were practical. This is the amount of air remaining in the lungs after a forced expiration or, in other words, the total lung capacity minus the vital capacity. Normally, this is about 25 per cent of the total lung capacity. The residual volume may be measured by the oxygen open circuit method or the closed circuit method, in which helium is used. Since these procedures are beyond the capability of the average hospital laboratory, they will not be discussed here. For a description of the performance of these tests as well as other useful tests in evaluating ventilatory function, the reader is referred to *The Lung* by J. H. Comroe, Jr., *et al.* (ed. 2, Chicago, Year Book Medical Publishers, 1962).

Ventilatory function may also be evaluated by fluoroscopy. Since carbon dioxide excretion is often affected in many diseases of the lung, measurement of its level in the blood provides a useful test of ventilatory function. The partial pressure of carbon dioxide may be measured in arterial or venous blood. It is normally 46 mm. Hg in venous blood and 40 mm. in arterial blood. In chronic respiratory failure, arterial carbon dioxide pressure may rise to 60 mm. Hg or more. The partial pressure of carbon dioxide is not the same as the carbon dioxide content of blood. The latter includes bicarbonate and is measured in milliequivalents per liter. Although less sensitive, this test along with the blood pH is a more practical method of measuring blood carbon dioxide content, since it can be performed on venous blood.

Disorders of Absorption

Absorption is influenced, as already discussed, by the distribution of inspired air, the distribution of the pulmonary circulation, the area of the absorbing surface, and the character of the alveolar-capillary membrane.

The *distribution* of *inspired air* may be evaluated by determining the *nitrogen-emptying rate* or by the single-breath oxygen test, in which a nitrogen flow meter is used. The latter test will be explained even though it is not practical for the average laboratory. This is a continuous measurement of the nitrogen content of expired air following a single breath of pure oxygen. Normally, after the first 750 ml. of expired air, the nitrogen content does not rise more than 1.5 per cent because the oxygen has been evenly distributed and mixed throughout the lungs. In patients with uneven distribution (e.g., in pulmonary emphysema), it may rise as much as 16 per cent. The distribution of inspired air may also be measured by inhalation of radioactive xenon and subsequent scanning (p. 189).

The *distribution* of *pulmonary capillary blood flow* can now be measured by radioactive xenon scanning. It may be disturbed by an anatomic venous-to-arterial shunt (e.g., hemangioma of the lung, p. 139), pulmonary emboli, compression of the pulmonary vessels by tumors or pneumothorax, and other less common conditions. It is practical to differentiate the first of these (shunt) from other causes of anoxemia. This can be done by measuring the *arterial oxygen saturation* before and after breathing pure oxygen. In those cases in which a significant shunt exists, the arterial oxygen will not increase appreciably after pure oxygen. When the anoxemia is due to hypoventilation or alveolar-capillary block, the arterial oxygen will approach normal after pure oxygen. It should be noted that smaller amounts may not be differentiated by this means unless oxygen tension is measured by an oxygen electrode. Cardiac catheterization may be employed to help to determine the location of the shunt if a congenital heart lesion is suspected.

When both the distribution of inspired air and the pulmonary capillary blood flow are disturbed, arterial oxygen saturation decreases, whereas carbon dioxide content increases. This results primarily from either a decreased ventilation in proportion to perfusion of an area or decreased perfusion in proportion to ventilation. However, this may not be the case if those areas that are well ventilated are also well perfused. Even under normal circumstances the ventilation and perfusion may be somewhat disproportionate in various parts of the lung.

The *overall area* and *character of the alveolar-capillary membrane* is best evaluated by measuring with carbon monoxide or oxygen the pulmonary diffusing capacity. Again, since these tests are not performed in the average hospital laboratory, a detailed discussion of them is omitted. However, disorders of impaired diffusing capacity (alveolar-capillary block) may be differentiated from other causes of anoxemia simply by utilizing the tests already discussed above, namely, spirometric tests and arterial oxygen and carbon dioxide determinations. When alveolar-capillary block is the principal disorder, anoxemia occurs without carbon dioxide retention in contrast with disorders producing hypoventilation. The anoxemia is corrected by breathing pure oxygen in contrast with pulmonary venous-to-arterial shunts. However, the anoxemia is not corrected by intermittent positive pressure breathing (IPPB) of atmospheric air, as it is in patients with hypoventilation. Finally, spirometric tests reveal very little obstructive disease even though the vital capacity is reduced.

Alveolar-capillary block may be diagnosed before permanent anoxemia develops if an exercise test is employed. Arterial oxygen saturation and tension are decreased by exercise, because the increase in velocity of pulmonary blood flow shortens the time that blood remains in contact with the alveolocapillary membranes, where diffusion takes place.

In practice, most chronic pulmonary diseases affect both ventilation (oxygen intake) and diffusing capacity (oxygen absorption), and therefore the studies will yield a mixed picture.

Disorders of Transport

The adequacy of the blood as a carrier may be determined simply by a hemoglobin and hematocrit test in most cases. When further study is indicated, diluted blood may be examined spectroscopically for methemoglobin or sulfhemoglobin. It is easier to shake a sample of venous blood vigorously with air for 15 minutes. If the blood retains a brownish hue, methemoglobinemia or sulfhemoglobinemia should be suspected. Cardiac function is easily evaluated by a venous pressure and circulation time. More sophisticated methods of determining the cardiac output and catheterization studies may be employed as needed.

Disorders of Utilization

Impaired oxygen uptake by the tissues (e.g., in cyanide poisoning) may be diagnosed by determining the oxygen saturation of venous blood. This is characteristically high in these disorders.

Summary

In summary, the vast majority of disorders of blood oxygen content may be diagnosed by a good clinical history, fluoroscopy, spirometry, arterial oxygen saturation, carbon dioxide content, and pH.

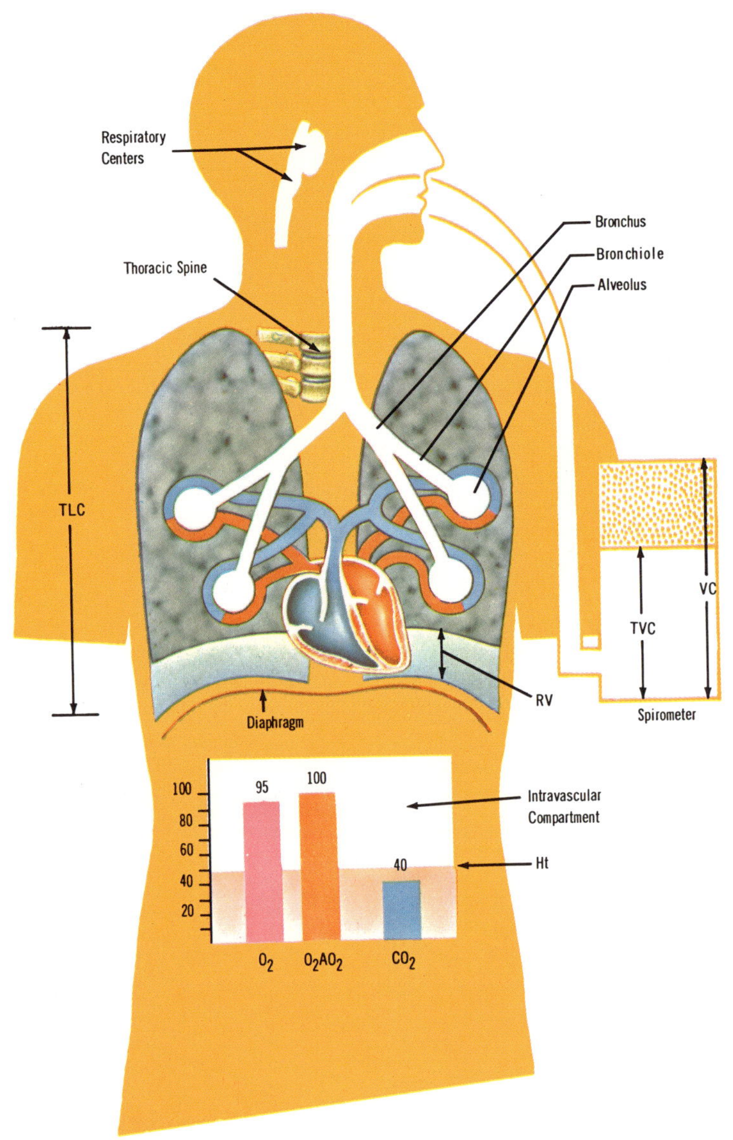

Abbreviations Used in Plates:

O_2 = Arterial oxygen saturation in per cent
O_2AO_2 = Oxygen saturation after pure oxygen (in per cent)
CO_2 = Arterial carbon dioxide in mm. Hg of partial pressure
Ht = Hematocrit in per cent of whole blood
RV = Residual volume
TVC = One second timed vital capacity
VC = Vital capacity
TLC = Total lung capacity

ASTHMATIC BRONCHITIS

In this condition, bronchospasm (A), along with mucosal congestion and edema, obstructs the respiratory passages, causing overall alveolar hypoventilation. *Vital capacity* and *timed vital capacity* are *decreased,* with a proportionate *increase* in *residual volume.* Isoproterenol and other bronchodilators may relieve the obstruction and correct these abnormal pulmonary functions. *Total lung capacity* is *normal* or *increased.* During an asthmatic attack *arterial oxygen saturation* is often *decreased,* whereas *carbon dioxide content* is *increased.* Examination of the sputum for eosinophils and allergic skin testing are additional diagnostic aids.

Summary of Laboratory Findings:

Vital capacity: Decreased
Timed vital capacity: Decreased
Residual volume: Increased
Total lung capacity: Normal
Arterial oxygen saturation: Decreased during attack
Carbon dioxide content: Increased

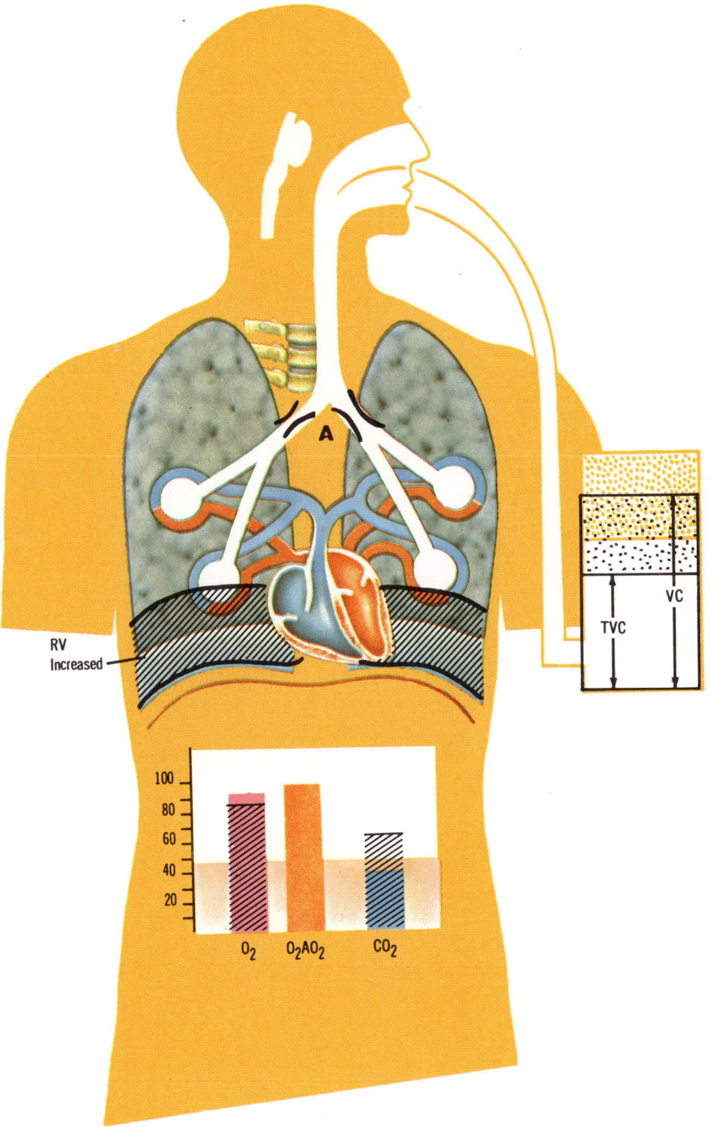

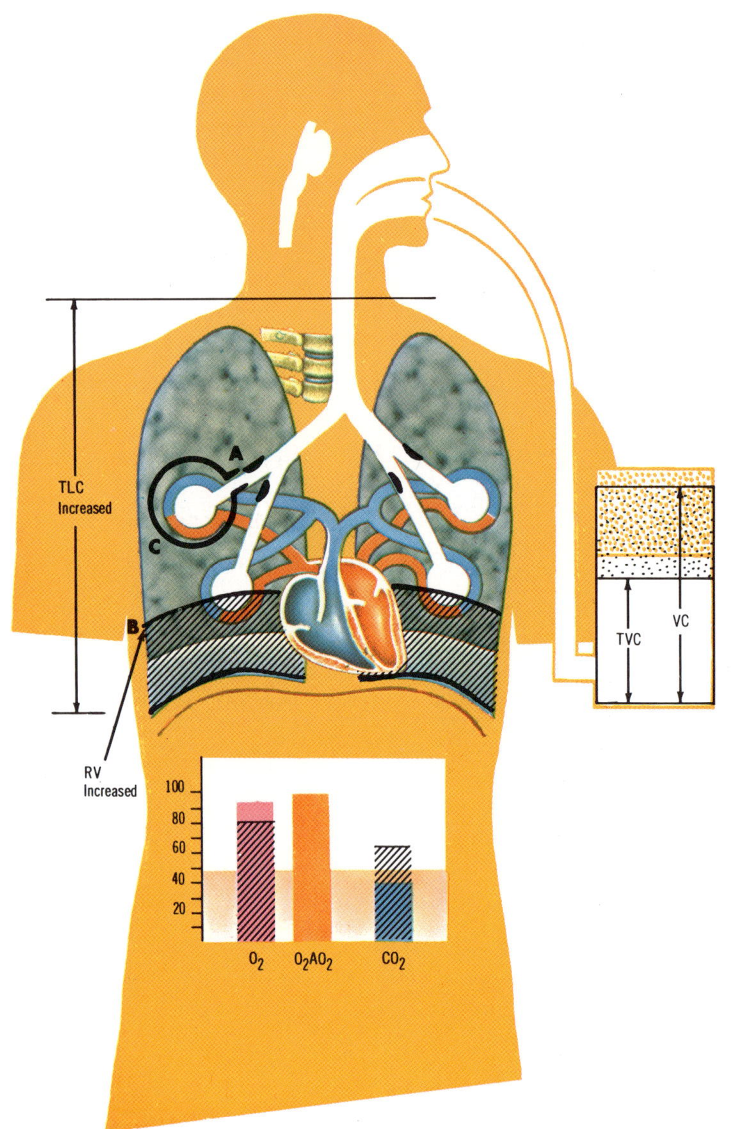

PULMONARY EMPHYSEMA

In this disorder there are expiratory obstruction (A), which may be due to weakening of the bronchial walls, causing them to collapse during expiration; closure of the smaller air passages because of poor elasticity of the surrounding tissues; and/or plugging of the respiratory passages with thick mucus. There is also destruction of the walls of the alveoli, which are replaced by larger air spaces of various sizes (C) (bullae, etc.).

The obstruction and air trapping *reduce* the *vital capacity* and the *timed vital capacity,* with a proportionate *increase* in the *residual volume* (B). These abnormalities are not usually altered by bronchodilators. On the other hand, the *total lung capacity* is *unchanged or increased* unless there is associated pulmonary fibrosis, in which case it would be decreased.

Arterial oxygen saturation is characteristically *reduced* but will return to normal after pure oxygen has been breathed. Before anoxemia occurs, there is usually significant *carbon dioxide retention* from the impaired ventilation and uneven distribution of inspired gas and pulmonary blood flow. Fluoroscopic and radiologic examination of the chest are further aids to diagnosis.

Summary of Laboratory Findings:

Vital capacity: Decreased

Timed vital capacity: Decreased

Residual volume: Increased

Total lung capacity: Increased

Arterial oxygen saturation: Decreased

Carbon dioxide content: Increased

ANKYLOSING SPONDYLITIS

Ankylosing spondylitis may cause fixation of the costovertebral joints (A), with restriction of inspiration and expiration. *Vital capacity* and *total lung capacity* are *decreased,* with some *increase* in *residual volume.* Arterial oxygen and carbon dioxide content are not altered unless thoracic excursions are so minimal that diaphragmatic breathing cannot compensate for it. Roentgenograms of the spine establish the diagnosis in most cases.

Kyphoscoliosis and neuromuscular diseases such as poliomyelitis are associated with a similar picture.

Summary of Laboratory Findings:

Vital capacity: Decreased

Residual volume: Increased

Total lung capacity: Decreased

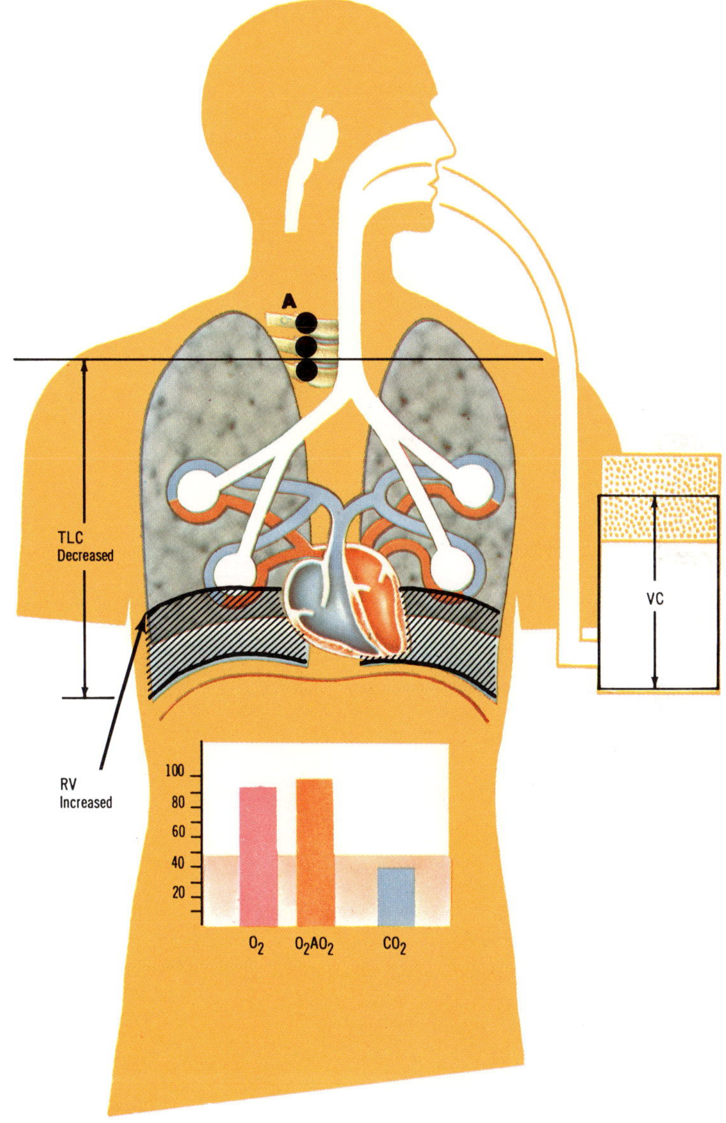

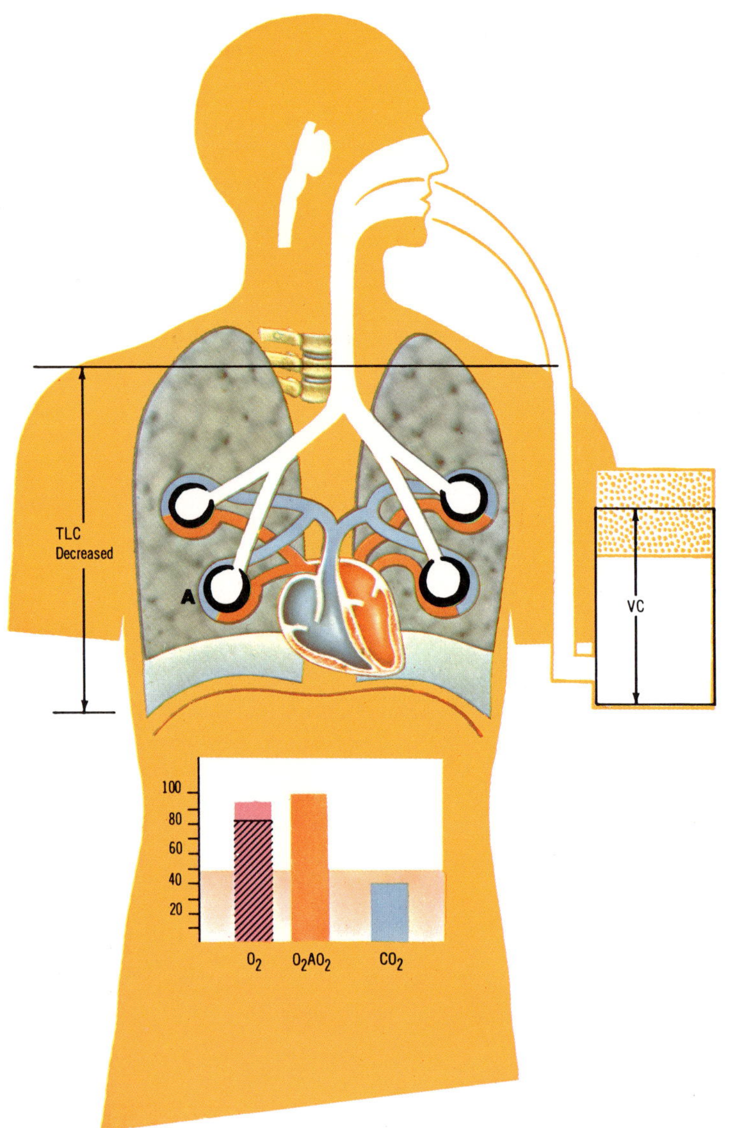

SARCOIDOSIS

The chronic granulomatous process in this disorder causes a thickening of the alveolar-capillary membranes (A) and a block in oxygen diffusion and absorption. This is in effect a "malabsorption syndrome" of the lung. The diffusing capacity of oxygen and carbon monoxide is decreased. Thus *arterial oxygen saturation drops* but may be returned to normal by inhalation of pure oxygen. Since the solubility of carbon dioxide is much greater than that of oxygen, its diffusion is not greatly impaired. Consequently, there is *no carbon dioxide retention.*

Vital capacity and *total lung capacity* are often decreased because of fibrosis and loss of elasticity of the lung. However, the *timed vital capacity* (1 sec. and 2 sec.) is often *normal* because there is no obstruction of the major respiratory passages. Gas distribution is unequal because the granulomatous process is rarely uniform. In the late stages diffuse pulmonary fibrosis leads to increased resistance to pulmonary blood flow and pulmonary hypertension. Roentgenograms of the hands, scalene node biopsy, and the Kveim skin test may assist in establishing this diagnosis.

The Hamman-Rich syndrome, miliary tuberculosis, anthrosilicosis, scleroderma of the lung, and beryllium poisoning may produce a similar picture.

Summary of Laboratory Findings:

Vital capacity: Decreased
Timed vital capacity: Normal
Total lung capacity: Decreased
Arterial oxygen saturation: Decreased
Carbon dioxide content: Normal

PULMONARY HEMANGIOMA

In pulmonary hemangioma a part of the venous blood from the right side of the heart is short-circuited to the pulmonary veins and left atrium, bypassing the alveoli (A). This blood does not become oxygenated. Hence, overall *arterial oxygen saturation* is *reduced.* This condition is not improved by breathing pure oxygen. Spirometric studies are usually normal, since the alveolar tissue is not diseased. Angiography will often establish this diagnosis. Ventricular septal defects and other congenital anomalies of the heart may produce the same picture.

Summary of Laboratory Findings:

Arterial oxygen saturation: Decreased

Arterial oxygen after pure oxygen: Decreased

Spirometric studies: Normal

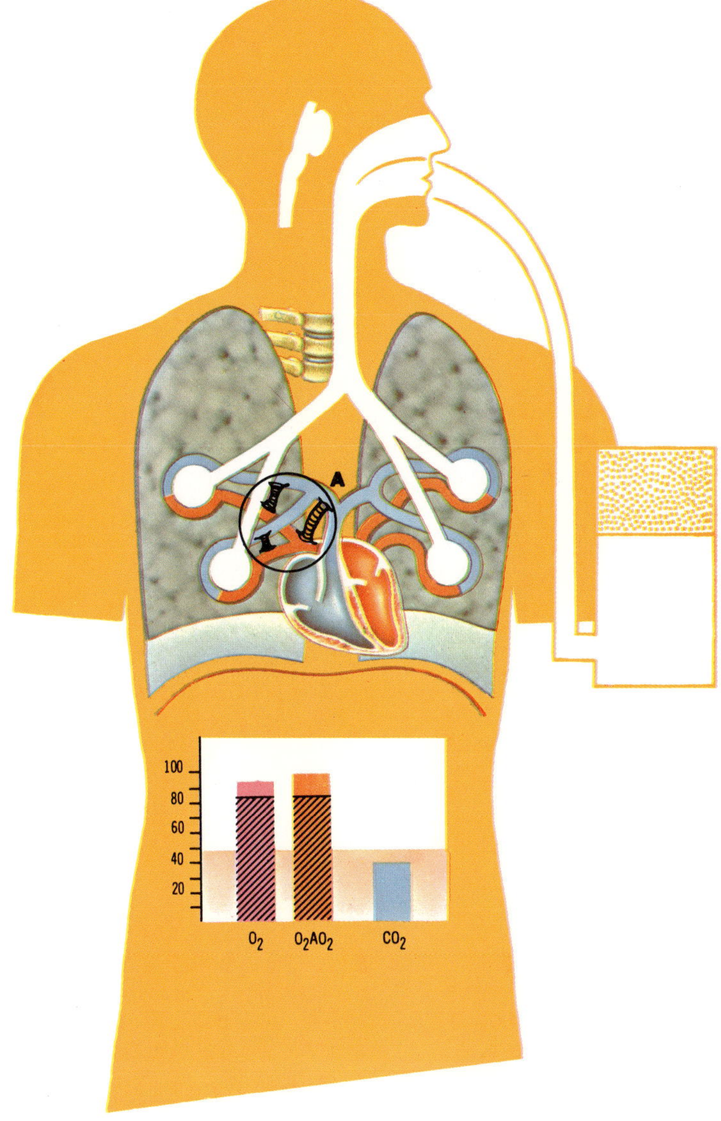

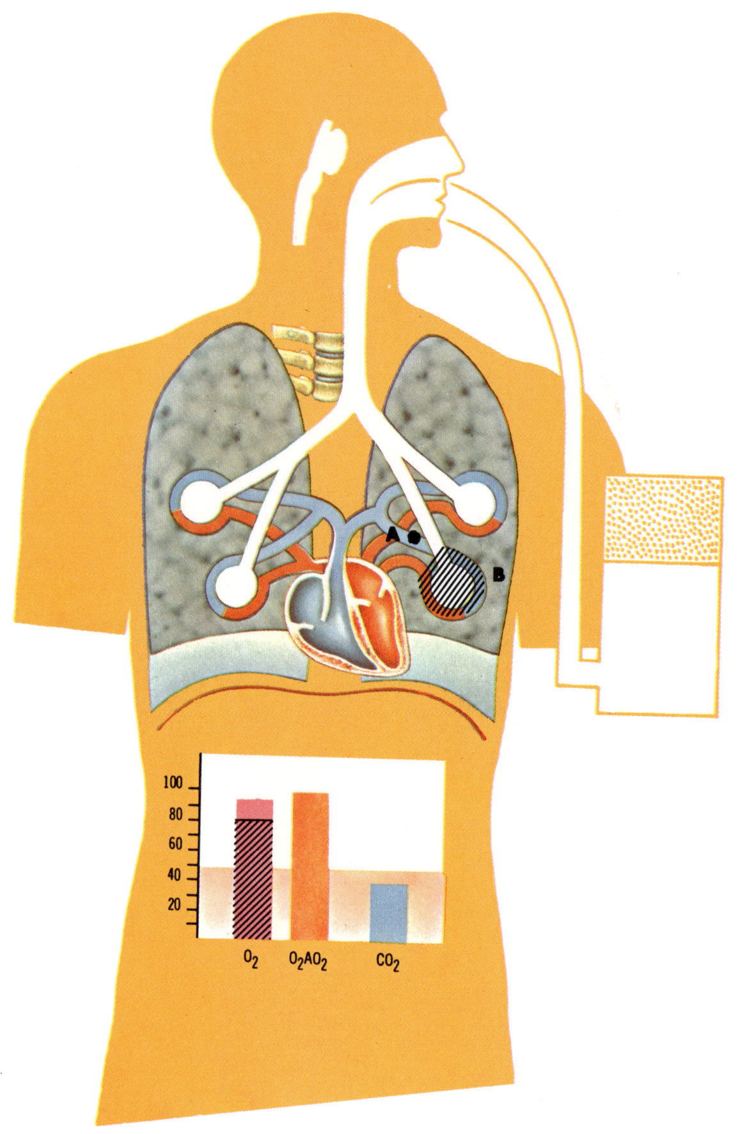

PULMONARY EMBOLISM

In this condition clots obstruct the pulmonary arteries (A) and/or arterioles, decreasing the blood supply to large areas of ventilated alveoli. Thus the amount of effectively functioning lung tissue is reduced (B), even though *vital capacity* and *total lung capacity* are usually *normal*. *Arterial oxygen saturation* is often decreased but is corrected by the inhalation of pure oxygen, thus distinguishing this condition from a venous-to-arterial shunt. Carbon dioxide content is not altered, since there is no impairment of ventilation. Roentgenograms of the chest, enzyme studies (p. 162), and electrocardiograms will assist in diagnosis. Frequently arteriograms and lung scans are needed.

Summary of Laboratory Findings:

Arterial oxygen saturation: Decreased

Arterial oxygen after pure oxygen: Normal

Carbon dioxide content: Normal

Spirometric studies: Normal

CONGESTIVE HEART FAILURE

Cardiac output in this disorder decreases, and the volume and the speed of blood flow through the tissues are decreased. As a result, there is diminished oxygen supply to the tissues (stagnant anoxia). Blood accumulates in the left side of the heart and backs up into the pulmonary circulation. The pressure in the pulmonary veins and capillaries increases, and pulmonary edema develops. *Vital capacity* and *total lung capacity* are *somewhat reduced,* whereas *residual volume* is usually *normal. Arterial oxygen saturation* is *reduced* by the impaired diffusion of oxygen through the pulmonary edema (A). This diagnosis may be further substantiated by a venous pressure and circulation time and improvement on digitalis therapy.

Summary of Laboratory Findings:

Vital capacity: Decreased
Timed vital capacity: Normal
Total lung capacity: Decreased
Arterial oxygen saturation: Decreased
Carbon dioxide content: Normal

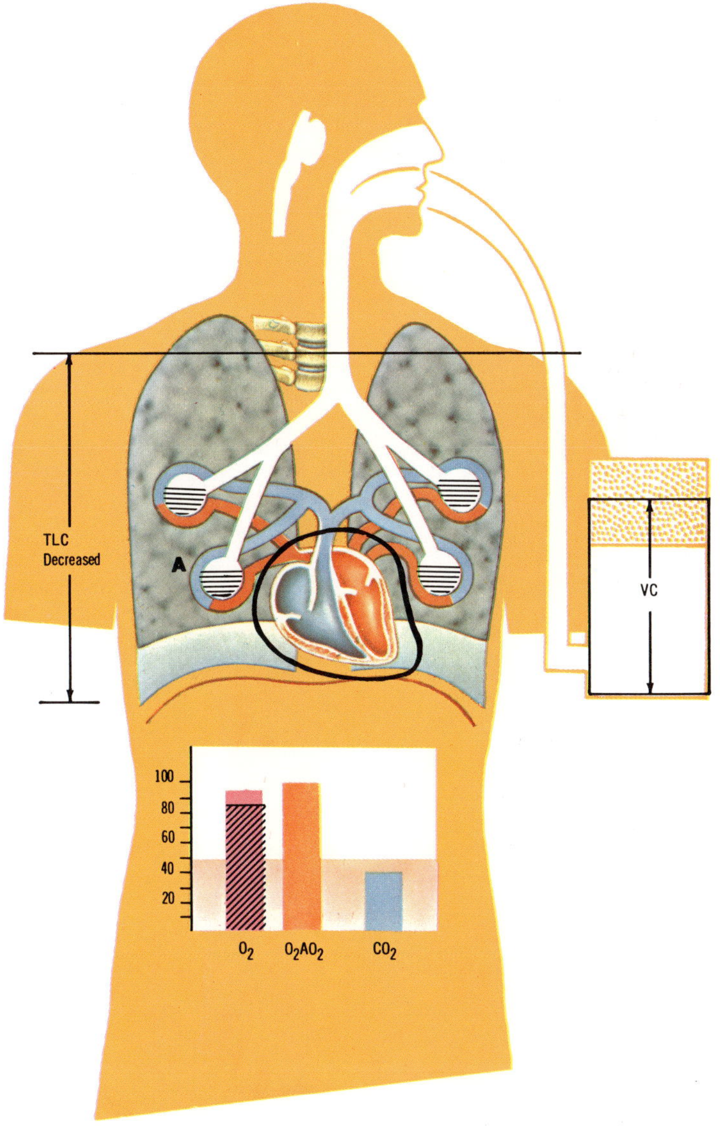

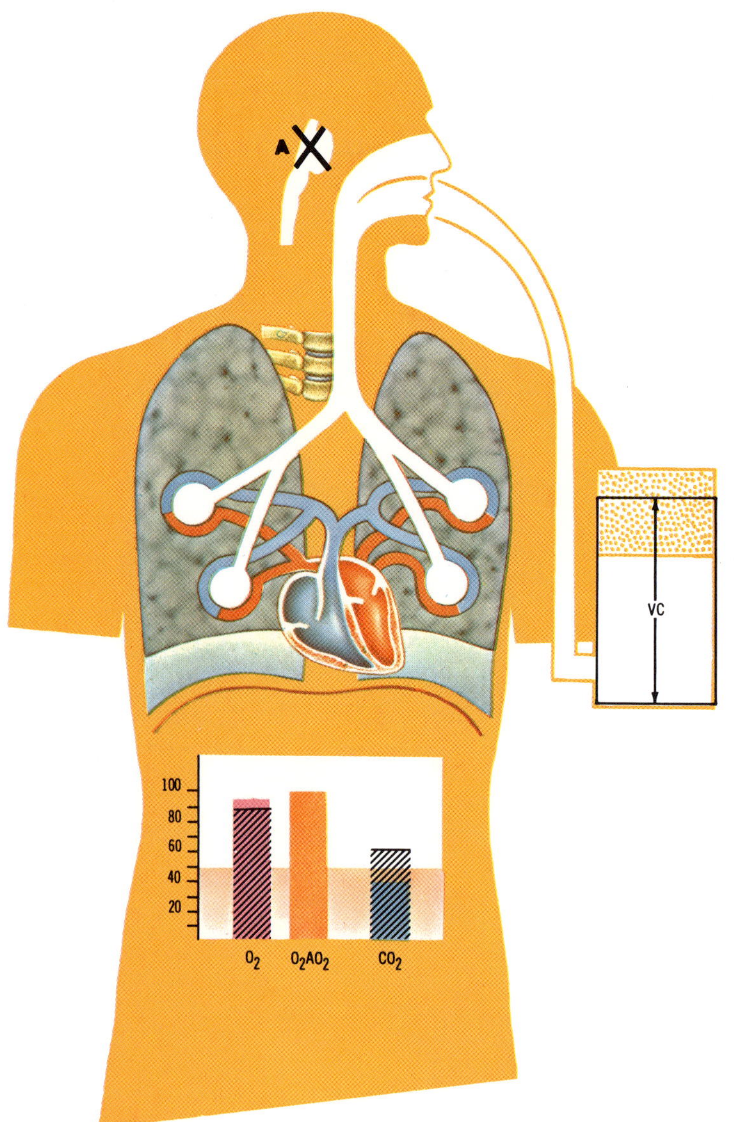

BARBITURATE INTOXICATION

Barbiturates in sufficient quantity depress the respiratory center in the brain stem (A), with a consequent decrease in the respiratory rate and alveolar hypoventilation. *Vital capacity* and maximum breathing capacity would be *decreased* if they could be measured; but, of course, the patient cannot cooperate in tests. Total lung capacity is normal. The rate and depth of respirations are often depressed to the point that *arterial oxygen saturation* is *reduced*, and *carbon dioxide* is *retained*. This state can be corrected by breathing pure oxygen or intermittent positive pressure breathing (IPPB). High levels of barbiturates will be found in the urine.

Similar respiratory depression may result from other toxic, inflammatory, vascular, or neoplastic diseases of the nervous system.

Summary of Laboratory Findings:

Vital capacity: Decreased
Timed vital capacity: Normal
Total lung capacity: Normal
Arterial oxygen saturation: Decreased
Carbon dioxide content: Increased

10 Disorders of Plasma Proteins

NORMAL METABOLISM

Intake. Proteins enter the body through the alimentary canal and undergo hydrolysis to amino acids in the stomach and the small intestine. They are acted on by hydrochloric acid and pepsin in the stomach and by trypsin, chymotrypsin, and carboxypeptidase (pancreatic enzymes) as well as aminopeptidase (intestinal enzymes) in the intestinal lumen. Approximately 95 per cent of the proteins in the diet are fully digested to amino acids in this manner, only a small amount of the intermediate polypeptides being available for absorption or excretion in the feces.

Absorption. The amino acids are promptly and actively absorbed by the small intestine, virtually none passing into the feces normally.

Production. Following their absorption, the amino acids are transported by the blood to the liver, the reticuloendothelial system, and all the other body cells in which formation of proteins takes place. Of the proteins circulating in the blood, albumin, the alpha and beta globulins, prothrombin, and fibrinogen are all formed in the liver. The gamma globulins are not exclusively of hepatic origin but are synthesized in all the reticuloendothelial tissues of the body. A 70-kg. man produces and degrades about 15 to 20 gm. of plasma protein a day, maintaining a dynamic equilibrium.

The average adult requires 0.5 gm. of protein per kg. per day, including certain essential amino acids.

Transport and Functions. Once synthesized, the plasma proteins are released into the blood stream to assume their various metabolic roles. Normally, there is 6 to 8 gm. of plasma protein per 100 ml. of blood. Electrophoretic analysis has shown that 100 ml. of blood contains 4.0 to 5.1 gm. of albumin, 0.7 to 1.5 gm. of alpha globulin, 0.7 to 1.5 gm. of beta globulin, and 0.7 to 1.3 gm. of gamma globulin.

These proteins have many useful functions in the body. They serve as a source of protein nutrition for the tissues during protein deprivation. They serve as buffers for acid-base balance. One of their most important roles is maintaining the normal distribution of water in the organism. This function is performed primarily by the albumin fraction, which is responsible for about 80 per cent of the oncotic pressure of human plasma.

Equally important is their role in transporting other constituents of the blood. Thus plasma lipids, vitamins, steroid and thyroid hormones, metals (iron, copper, etc.), and certain enzymes are carried by the blood proteins.

The gamma globulins contain the all-important antibodies (to typhoid, mumps, poliomyelitis, etc.). Fibrinogen, prothrombin, and a number of the plasma proteins participate in coagulation.

Storage. Unlike fat, stored protein cannot be assigned to any particular cell. However, all body cells, particularly those of the liver, kidney, and intestines, possess labile proteins that can be metabolized during starvation to meet the body's caloric requirements of the organism.*

Destruction. The plasma proteins, as indicated above, may be broken down to amino acids by the liver and utilized by the body either as energy or in the formation of substances essential to the body such as enzymes, hormones (insulin, etc.), and purines or pyrimidines for the production of new cells. Amino acids are utilized for energy by deamination to such substances as pyruvic acid (formed from alanine), alpha-ketoglutaric acid (formed from glutamic acid), and aspartic acid and introduced into the Krebs cycle. The end-products of protein catabolism are urea, carbon dioxide, water, uric acid, phosphates, and creatinine.

Excretion. Only minimal amounts of protein and amino acids are excreted normally. The quantities that are filtered through the glomeruli are almost completely reabsorbed. However, both amino acids and protein appear in the urine in a variety of pathologic conditions. The degradation products of protein (urea, carbon dioxide, water, etc.) are, of course, excreted in the urine and through the lungs. These are discussed elsewhere.

Regulation. The plasma proteins, and in fact all the body proteins, are constantly being broken down to amino acids and then resynthesized. All the factors influencing this equilibrium are not known, but among them are the quantity and the quality of amino acids in the diet, the metabolic rate, and certain hormones, the most important of which are growth hormone, corticosteroids, androgens, thyroid hormone, and insulin. Growth hormone, androgens, and

* Duncan, G. G. (ed.): Diseases of Metabolism. ed. 5, p. 15. Philadelphia, W. B. Saunders, 1964.

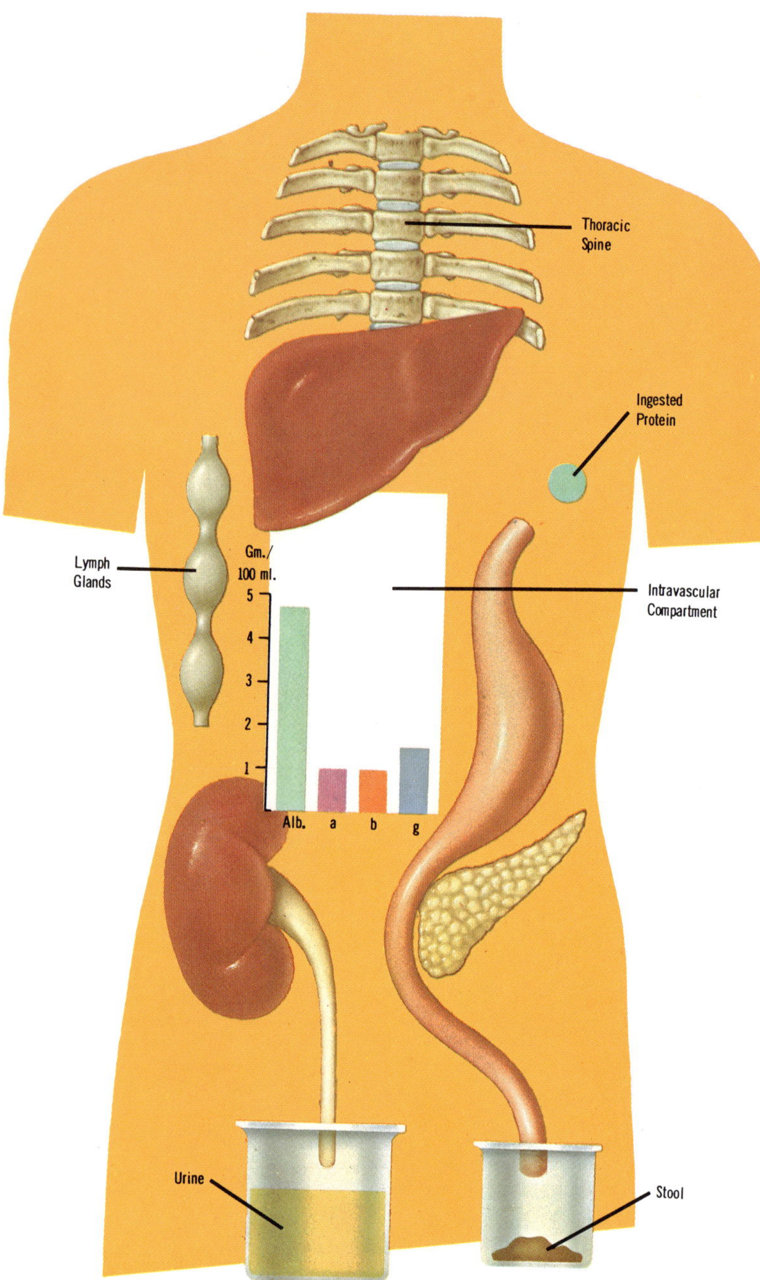

insulin increase protein synthesis, whereas glucocorticoids and large amounts of thyroid increase protein catabolism. There is some evidence that growth hormone and insulin act synergistically in promoting protein synthesis. Physiologic amounts of both corticosteroids and thyroid hormone exert an anabolic effect on protein metabolism.

METHODS OF STUDY

Paper electrophoresis has virtually replaced the older salting-out methods of fractionation as described by Howe and Milne. The basic principle of electrophoretic analysis depends on differences in migratory velocities of charged amino acids in an electric field. The migration rate of any one amino acid group is directly proportional to the magnitude of its surface electrical charge. If the pH of the protein-containing solution is controlled, a negative charge may be imparted to all of the amino acids (zwitterion effect), and thus a standard direction of migration. The rate of migration varies with the type of protein. By using this technique a mixture of proteins may be separated, and each fraction may be quantitated. Paper electrophoresis is also useful in distinguishing the types of lipoproteinemias. This technique will be discussed further on page 103.

Immunoelectrophoresis has made it possible to separate the gamma globulins into antigenically distinct groups, which may support the diagnosis of various collagen diseases, multiple myeloma, etc.

Ultracentrifugation is another method by which the proteins may be separated, in this case according to their relative densities (Svedberg units). This method is not practical for the average hospital laboratory but may be necessary to detect macroglobulins.

The sedimentation rate is a crude method of estimating changes in plasma proteins. It is elevated by increased plasma fibrinogen, as in hepatitis and pregnancy, and by increases in gamma globulins, as in multiple myeloma.

The *thymol turbidity* and *cephalin-cholesterol flocculation* tests are very useful in detecting alterations in the serum albumin and globulin, particularly those that occur in hepatic disease and jaundice. These tests are usually abnormal when either the gamma globulin increases or the albumin decreases. The cephalin-cholesterol flocculation is also increased in diseases associated with lipemic serum, such as diabetes mellitus and nephrosis. These are further discussed in Chapter 7, Disorders of Serum Lipids, pages 101–118.

Abbreviations Used in Plates:

Alb. = Albumin
a = Alpha globulin
b = Beta globulin
g = Gamma globulin

STARVATION

The intake of protein (A) and other nutrients is inadequate in this disorder. Thus the synthesis of plasma proteins is decreased, and plasma proteins are utilized for energy. The concentrations of both *albumin* and *globulins decrease.*

Other simple studies that provide general knowledge of the nutrition of the patient are the complete blood count, urinalysis, blood sugar, blood cholesterol, BUN, uric acid, and creatinine. In special centers serum carotene, B_{12}, and folic acid levels may be determined, as well as the evaluation of vitamin excretion in the urine after a loading dose.

Summary of Laboratory Findings:

Albumin: Decreased
Alpha globulin: Decreased
Beta globulin: Decreased
Gamma globulins: Decreased

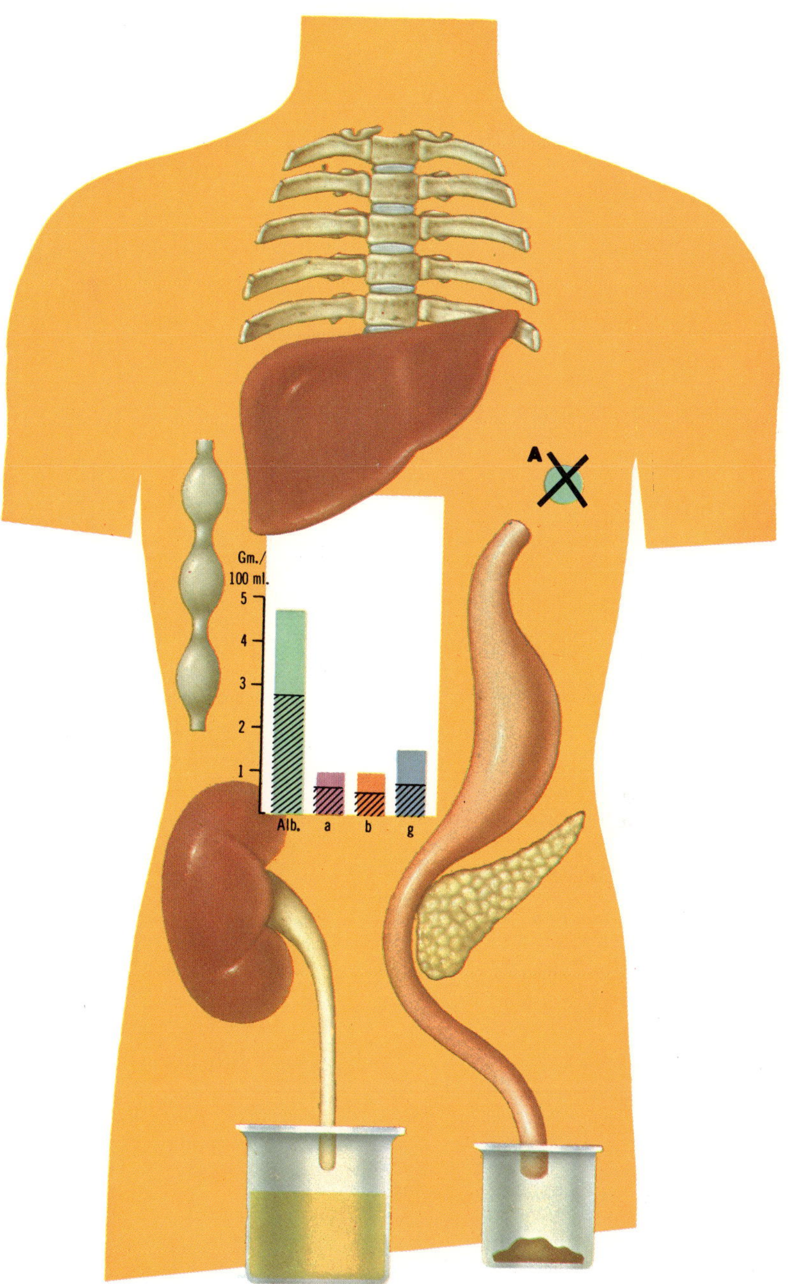

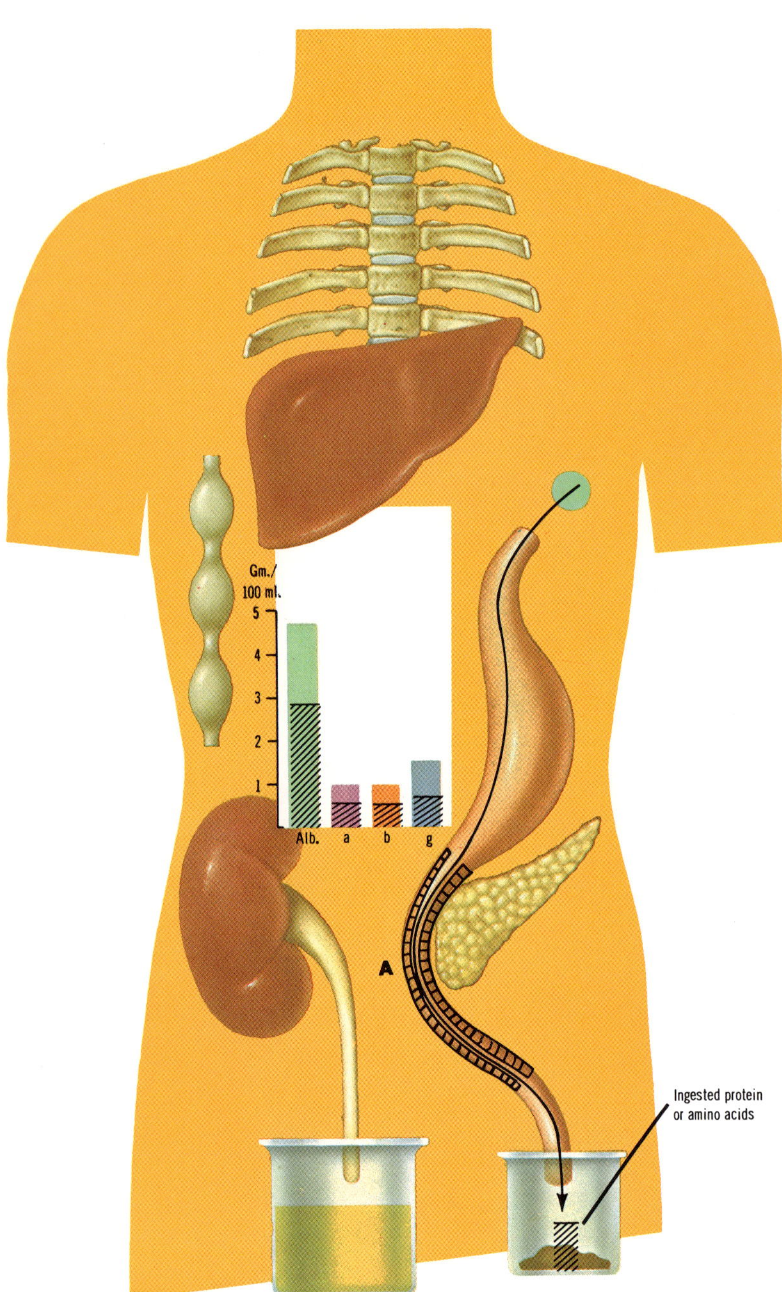

IDIOPATHIC STEATORRHEA

In this condition absorption of amino acids by the diseased bowel (A) is impaired. As a result, production of both albumin and globulin drop, and there is a *decrease* in all the fractions of the *plasma protein*. Because the absorption of carbohydrate and fat is also impaired, plasma proteins are utilized for energy, and thus their concentration is further diminished. The diagnosis is assisted by the D-xylose absorption test, urine 5-HIAA, mucosal biopsy, and many other tests (p. 61).

Chronic pancreatitis, tropical sprue, Whipple's disease, and other causes of the malabsorption syndrome may produce a similar picture.

Summary of Laboratory Findings:

Albumin: Decreased

Alpha globulin: Decreased

Beta globulins: Decreased

Gamma globulins: Decreased

PORTAL CIRRHOSIS

Characteristically, a *decrease* in *plasma albumin* occurs in this disorder because of a decrease in the functioning hepatic cell mass, the *plasma gamma globulin increases* due to overactivity of the reticuloendothelial system manifested by hepatic lymphoid and plasma cell metaplasia and hyperplasia. These changes in the plasma proteins result in increased cephalin-cholesterol flocculation and thymol turbidity. Empirical studies have shown that the cephalin-cholesterol flocculation is correlated with hepatic cell damage, and the thymol turbidity is most closely correlated with proliferation of the supporting tissues of the liver. There may be variable degrees of incorporation of the beta globulins in the gamma globulin peak resulting in a slurring effect on the electrophoretic pattern. The diagnosis is supported by other liver function tests (p. 17) and liver biopsy.

Postnecrotic cirrhosis produces a similar picture, but hypocholesterolemia is more common. In biliary cirrhosis, on the other hand, albumin remains normal in the early stages despite marked hypergammaglobulinemia and hyperbetaglobulinemia.

Summary of Laboratory Findings:

Albumin: Decreased

Gamma globulins: Increased

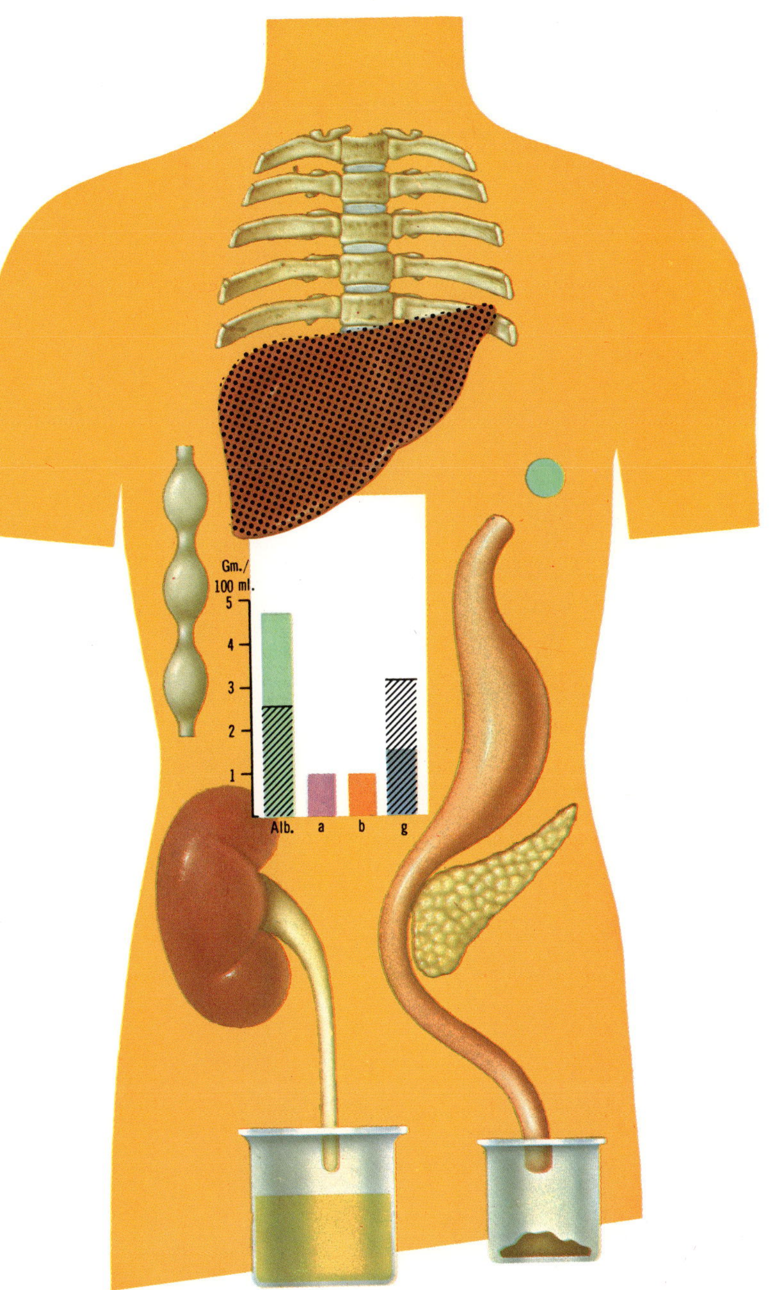

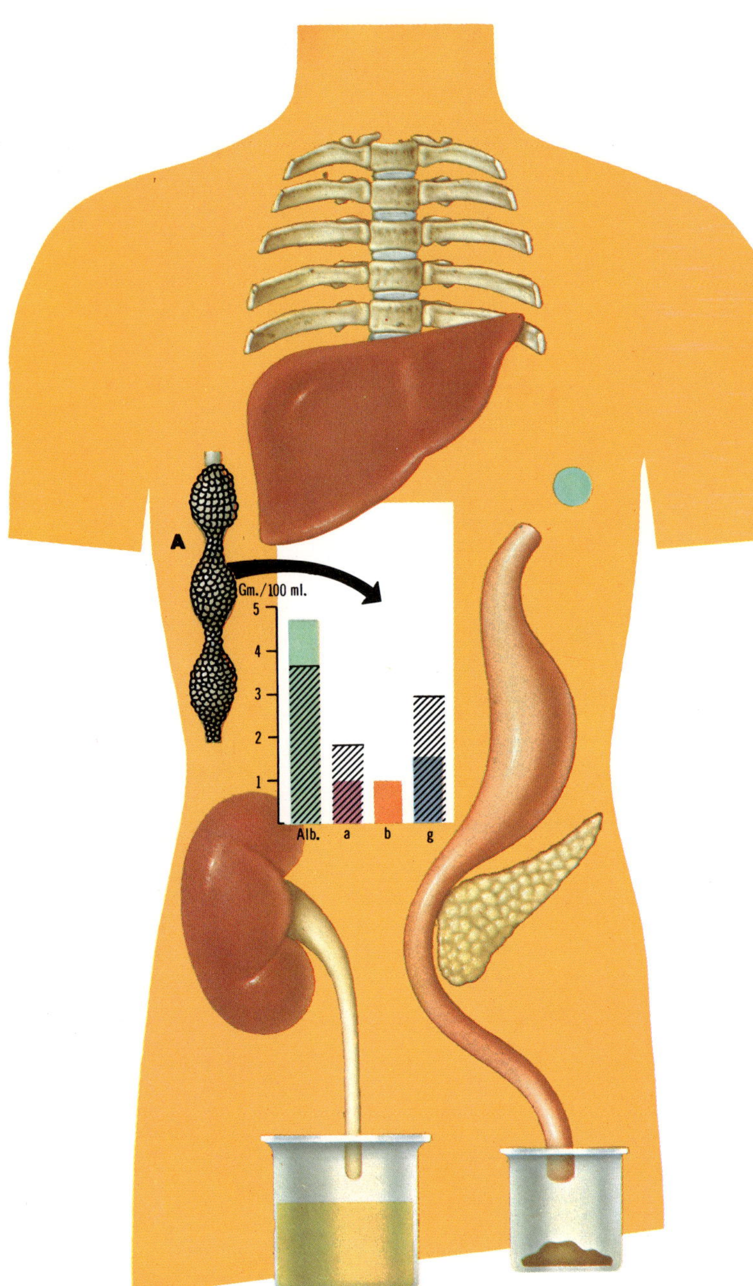

ACUTE AND CHRONIC BACTERIAL INFECTIONS

In these disorders there is an *increased* production of the *alpha* and *gamma globulins* from the hypertrophied lymph tissue (A), with an associated *decrease* in *plasma albumin*. Occasionally, the beta globulins are increased. Diagnosis is established by cultures of the appropriate body fluids, serologic tests, and skin tests.

Viral, protozoal, and parasitic disease may produce a similar picture, but the increase in globulin may be more marked, particularly in infectious hepatitis, kala-azar, typhus, and lymphogranuloma venereum.

Summary of Laboratory Findings:

Albumin: Decreased or normal

Alpha globulins: Increased

Gamma globulins: Increased

FAMILIAL IDIOPATHIC DYSPROTEINEMIA

In this condition there is a marked *decrease* in the serum *albumin* with a compensatory *increase* in all the globulin fractions due to a genetic defect in albumin production.

Summary of Laboratory Findings:

Albumin: Decreased
Alpha globulin: Increased
Beta globulin: Increased
Gamma globulin: Increased

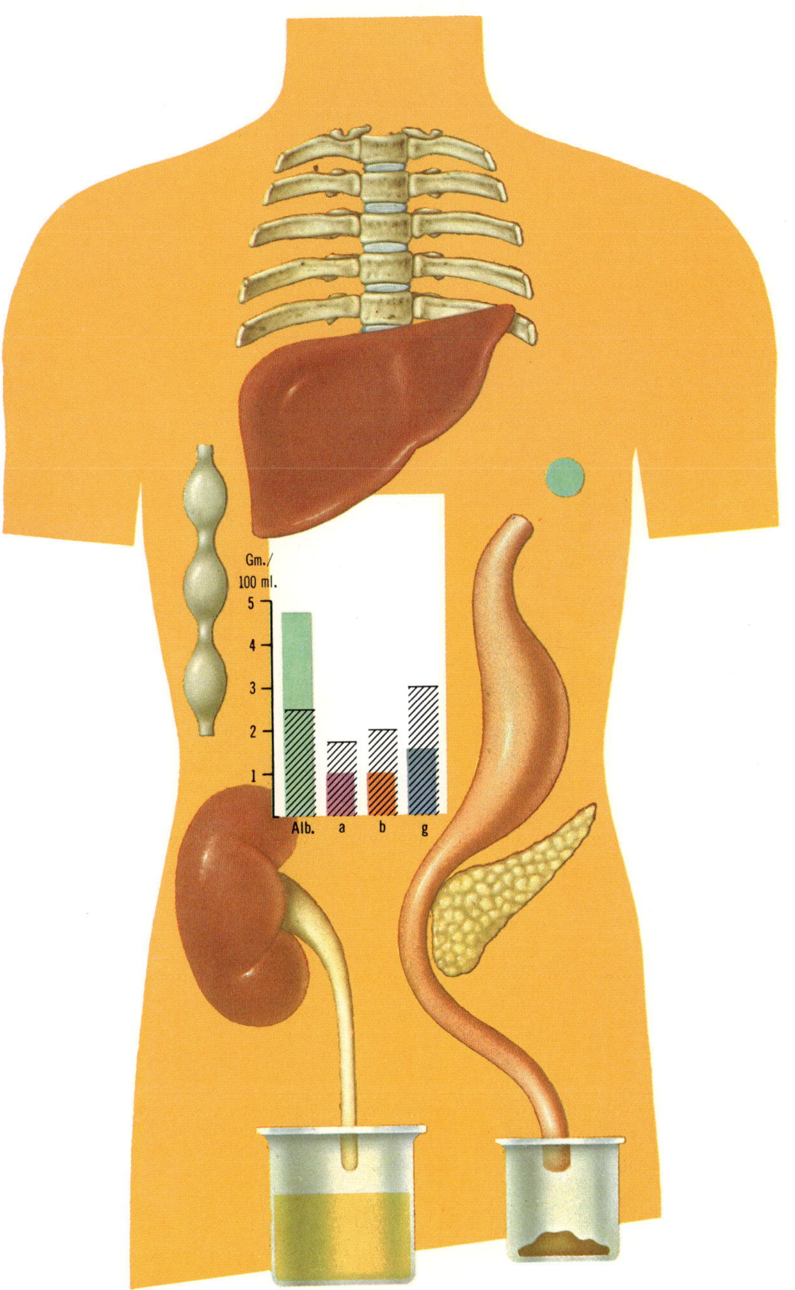

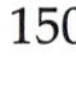

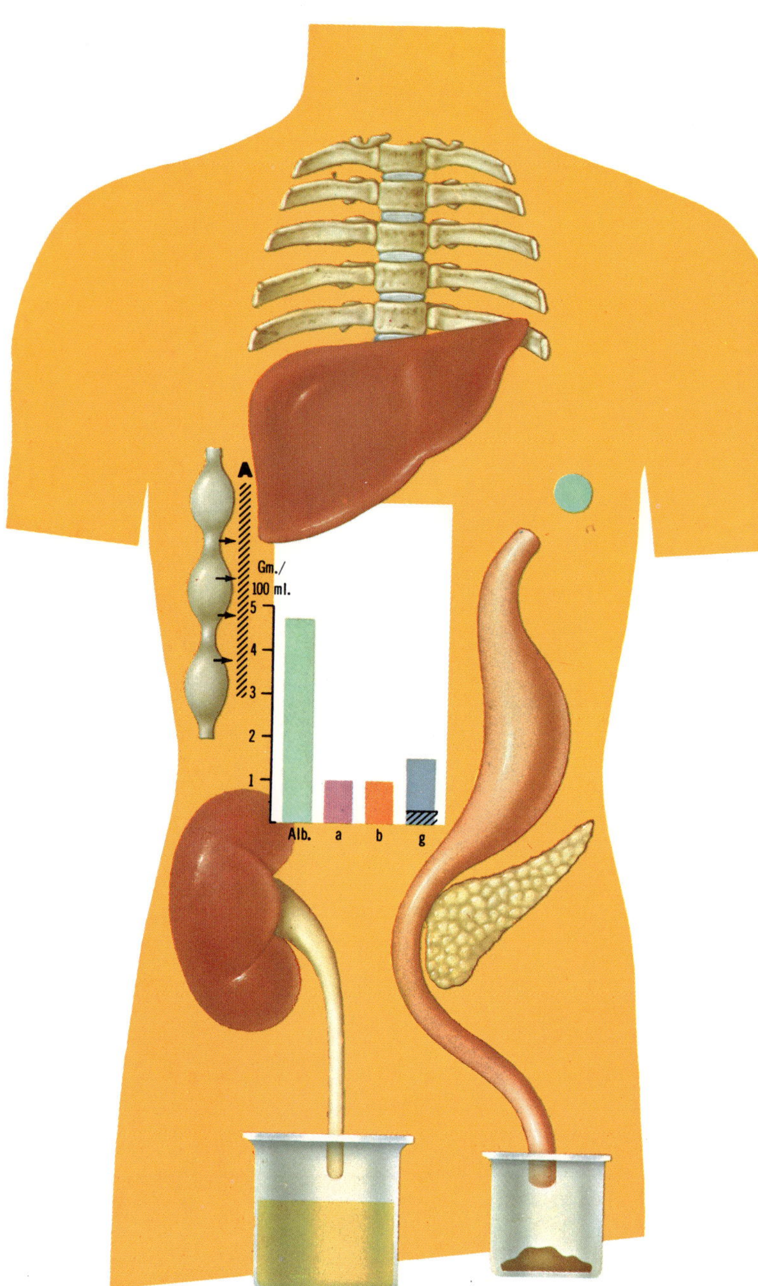

HYPOGAMMAGLOBULINEMIA

This condition, whether congenital, physiological, idiopathic, or secondary to multiple myeloma, leukemia, or Hodgkin's disease, is due to a decreased production of gamma globulin (A), often *less* than 0.1 gm. of *globulin* per 100 ml. In subjects with blood type O there is an absence of anti-A and anti-B isoagglutinins. These subjects do not develop significant antibody titers to various vaccines (diphtheria, etc.). These subjects respond poorly to bacterial infections but usually maintain a good resistance to viruses.

Summary of Laboratory Findings:

Albumin: Normal

Gamma globulins: Markedly decreased

ALPHA-1 ANTITRYPSIN DEFICIENCY

In this condition the alpha-1 globulin is entirely absent and emphysema develops. Therefore serum protein electrophoresis is extremely valuable in diagnosing this condition.

Summary of Laboratory Findings:

Albumin: Normal

Alpha-1 globulin: Absent

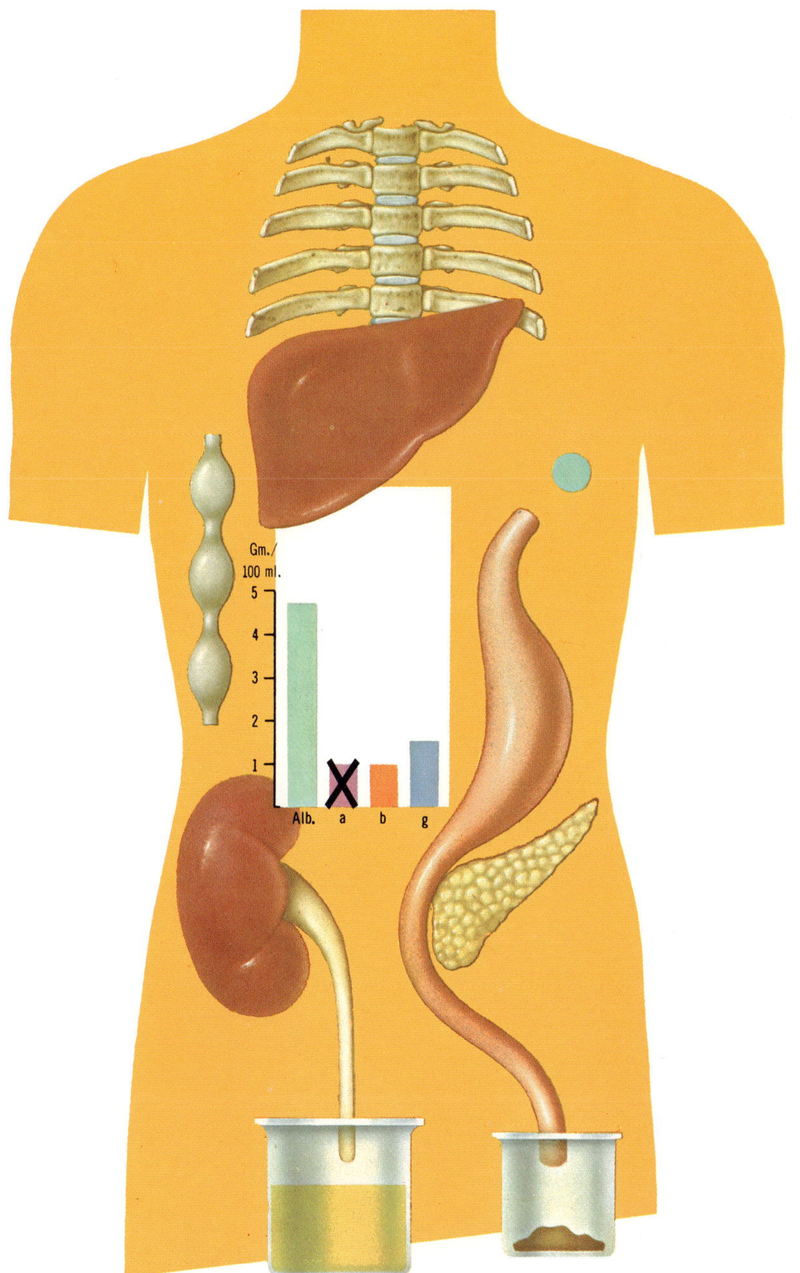

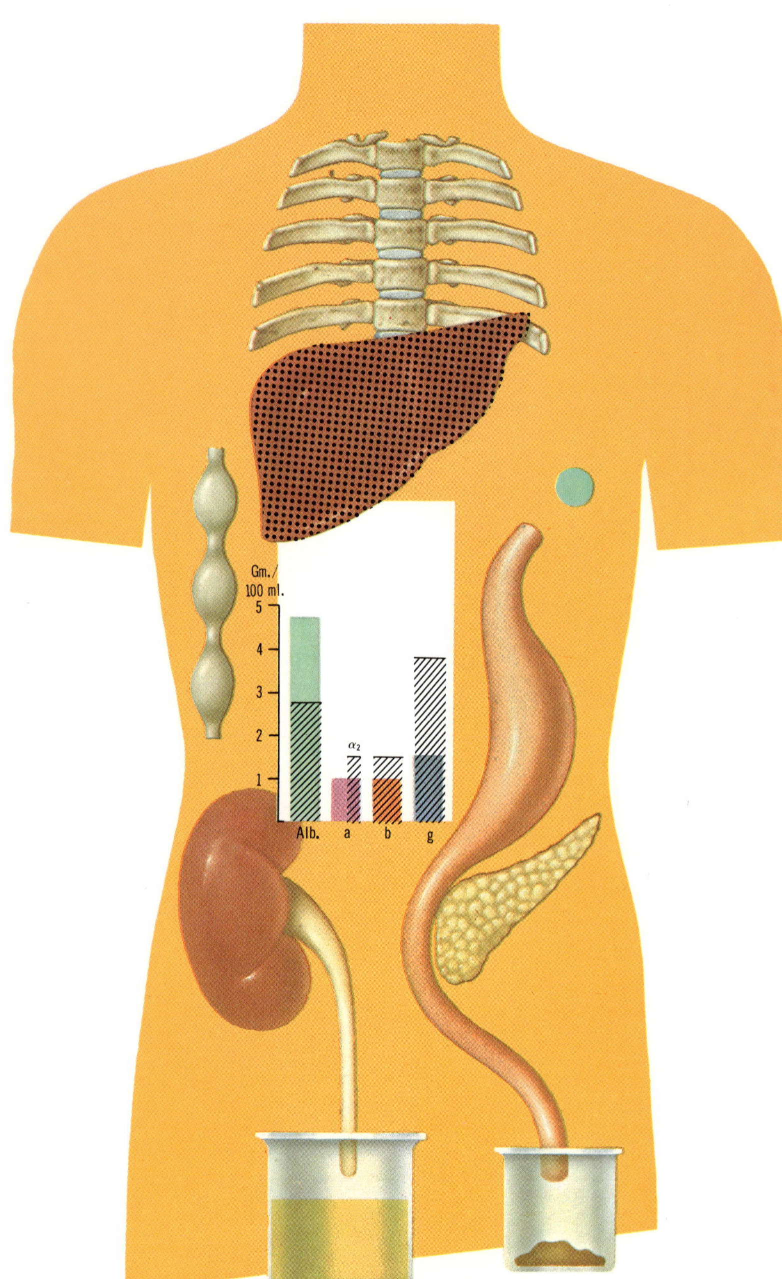

VIRAL HEPATITIS

The necrotic hepatic cells are unable to produce albumin in this disorder, and consequently the *serum* level of *albumin drops*. At the same time there is an *elevation* of the *serum gamma globulin* because of the immunologic response to the virus and to the necrotic hepatic cells, and because of the swollen and proliferating reticuloendothelial cells. The alpha-2 globulin and beta globulin may also increase.

The albumin changes, if present, occur usually early in the icteric stage or late in the preicteric stage, reaching a maximum level in 8 to 16 days. A return to normal levels is anticipated in 5 to 6 weeks. Prolongation of the hypoalbuminemia suggests massive necrosis, chronic hepatitis, or postnecrotic cirrhosis. With these complications the plasma albumin levels assume prognostic significance, since they parallel the extent of the destructive process. Hypergammaglobulinemia occurs frequently before the onset of jaundice and approaches maximal levels in 8 to 10 days. Its return to normal is more prolonged, taking often 3 to 4 months to reach basal levels.

The gamma globulin concentration is an excellent guide to the severity and progression of the disease. Another laboratory study that is of immeasurable value in diagnosis is the serum transaminase level. These reach their highest levels in this disease. Serum and urinary bilirubin determinations, flocculation studies, and sedimentation rate are likewise helpful, not only in diagnosis but also in following the course of the disease (p. 16).

Summary of Laboratory Findings:

Albumin: Decreased

Gamma globulin: Increased

Alpha-2 globulin: Increased

Beta globulin: Increased

MULTIPLE MYELOMA

In this disorder an *abnormal globulin appears in the serum* and usually migrates in the *gamma-globulin range* (A). Occasionally, it may migrate in the beta- or alpha-2 globulin range. It may be necessary to perform immunoelectrophoresis to distinguish this type from macroglobulinemia. Three immunoglobulins are distinguished: IgG (which migrates in the gamma region on electrophoresis); IgA (which migrates in the pregamma region on electrophoresis); and IgM (which migrates in the prebeta or beta region on electrophoresis). If immunoelectrophoresis shows an IgM peak, multiple myeloma is ruled out. On the other hand, if the peak is not IgM, macroglobulinemia is ruled out. Ultracentrifugation shows the abnormal proteins of macroglobulinemia to have high molecular weights (1,000,000 or 19-S) even though they migrate on electrophoresis just like myeloma proteins. There is an overall increase in the plasma protein, but *serum albumin* is often *decreased*. In addition, an abnormal globulin (Bence-Jones protein) appears in the urine (p. 197). Other abnormal proteins found less frequently are paramyloid and the cryoglobulins. Roentgenograms of the skull, spine, and the long bones and bone marrow aspiration assist in the diagnosis.

Summary of Laboratory Findings:

Albumin: Decreased

Gamma globulin: Increased

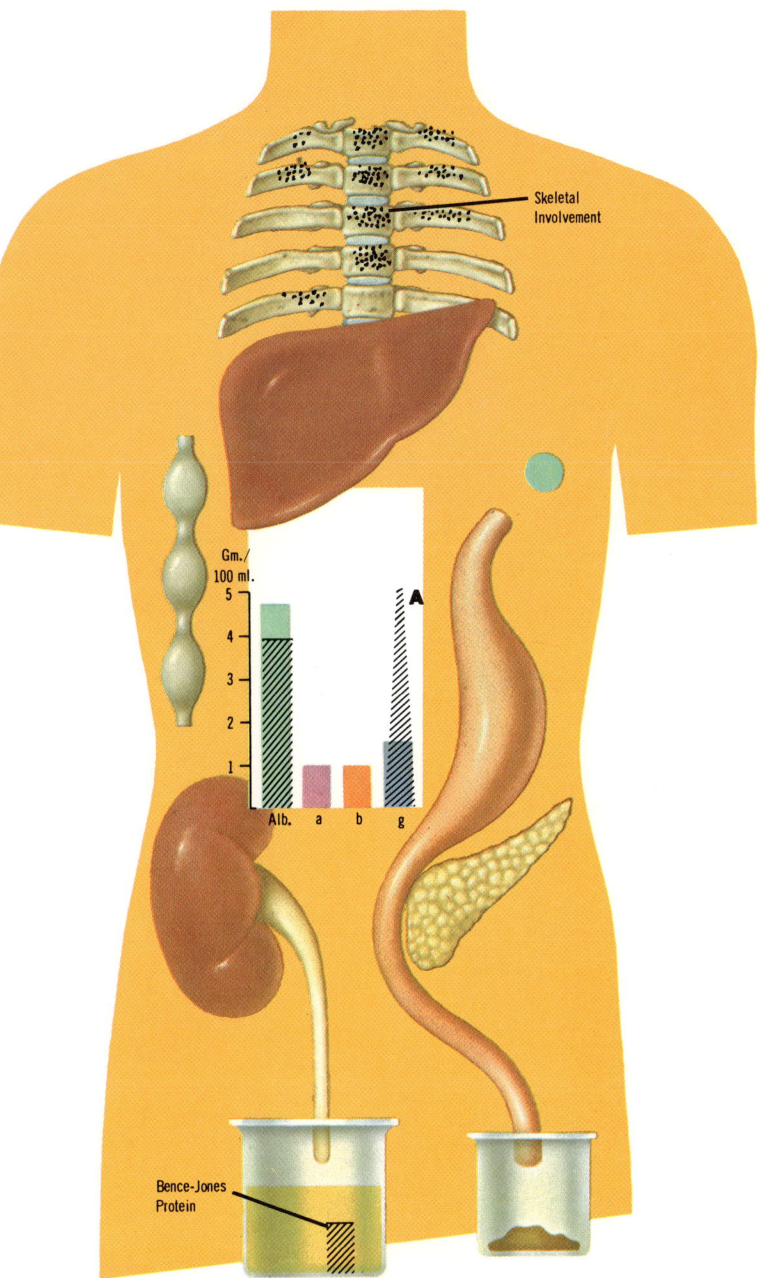

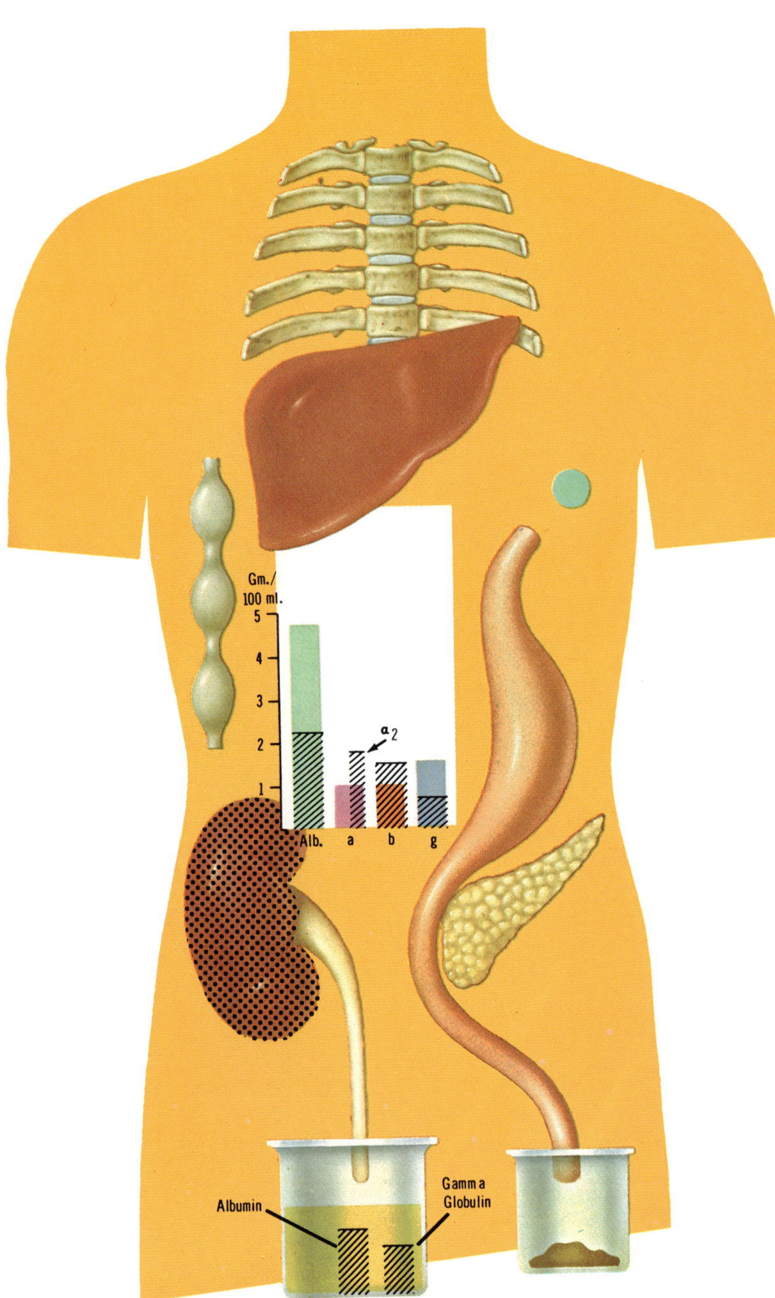

NEPHROTIC SYNDROME

Whether caused by Kimmelstiel-Wilson's disease, glomerulonephritis, amyloidosis, or lupus erythematosus, this condition is associated with a *low serum albumin* and *gamma globulin*. These proteins are lost in the urine due to an increased permeability of the glomeruli. The alpha-2 and beta globulins are usually increased, the latter being related to the coexisting hyperlipemia. The diagnosis is confirmed by the finding of doubly refractile fat bodies in the urine and by renal biopsy.

Summary of Laboratory Findings:

Albumin: Decreased

Alpha-2 globulins: Increased

Beta globulins: Increased

Gamma globulin: Decreased

11 Disorders of Serum Creatine Phosphokinase, Transaminases, and Lactic Dehydrogenases

NORMAL METABOLISM

It is known that virtually every chemical reaction in the body is influenced by special proteins called enzymes. Research has now made available practical means by which many of these can be measured. Of particular value in clinical diagnosis is the measurement of serum creatine phosphokinase, transaminases, and lactic dehydrogenases.

Transaminases. These enzymes catalyze the transfer of the amino group from one amino acid to a keto acid, so that another amino acid is formed. Two of these, the glutamic-oxalacetic transaminase (GOT) and the glutamic-pyruvic transaminase (GPT), are practical for clinical use and are measured by the average clinical laboratory. They are widely distributed in the tissues, particularly in those of high metabolic activity, the heart, liver, and muscle. Even the tissues of the brain produce significant quantities. Small amounts spill over into the serum, where 5 to 40 Karmen units per 100 ml. are found normally. Because of the blood-bile barrier, very little of the transaminases is excreted by the bile, but whether what is present in the bile all comes from the liver or some from the blood is uncertain.

Lactic Dehydrogenases. This group of enzymes catalyzes the end reaction of the anaerobic phase of carbohydrate metabolism. They influence the reduction of pyruvic acid to lactic acid in the relative absence of oxygen and the reverse reaction, lactic acid to pyruvic acid, in the presence of adequate oxygen. Like the transaminases, these enzymes are widely distributed in the tissues of the body, particularly in the kidney, liver, heart, and skeletal muscle. Again, a small amount spills over into the serum, possibly because of normal cellular death or catabolism. Various values have been given as normal, most laboratories considering 50 to 200 units per 100 ml. as normal. Recent investigation has demonstrated that five different LDH fractions can be isolated and measured.* These have been called isoenzymes. Different tissues have been found to contain large amounts of specific isoenzymes. The isoenzymes are separated by electrophoresis and then made visible with nitroblue tetrazolium. Their value in diagnosis will be discussed subsequently.

Creatine Phosphokinase. Tests for this enzyme are extremely useful in diagnosing diseases of the heart and skeletal muscle, because there is very little activity of this enzyme in other tissues aside from the brain. It is more specific for myocardial infarction and is the first to be elevated (3 to 4 hours postinfarction). The liver contains no CPK activity, so that elevation in patients not suspected of having a myocardial infarct is a strong indication of muscle disease (muscular dystrophy, etc.).

Other Cellular Enzymes. *Aldolase* exists in muscle liver and myocardium but has not become widely used because it is elevated in the same conditions as CPK. It is very high in pseudohypertrophic muscular dystrophy (as is the CPK). Leucine aminopeptidase (LAP) was hoped to be a useful test in diagnosing carcinoma of the pancreas, but it has been found to be elevated in many diseases of the liver and pancreas. Serum glutamic pyruvic transaminase (SGPT) was felt to be more specific than the SGOT for liver disease; but this has been found not to be the case, as some cases of myocardial infarction are associated with elevated SGPT.

* Wrablewski, F., Ross, C., and Gregory, K.: Isoenzymes and myocardial infarction. New Eng. J. Med., *263*:531, 1960.

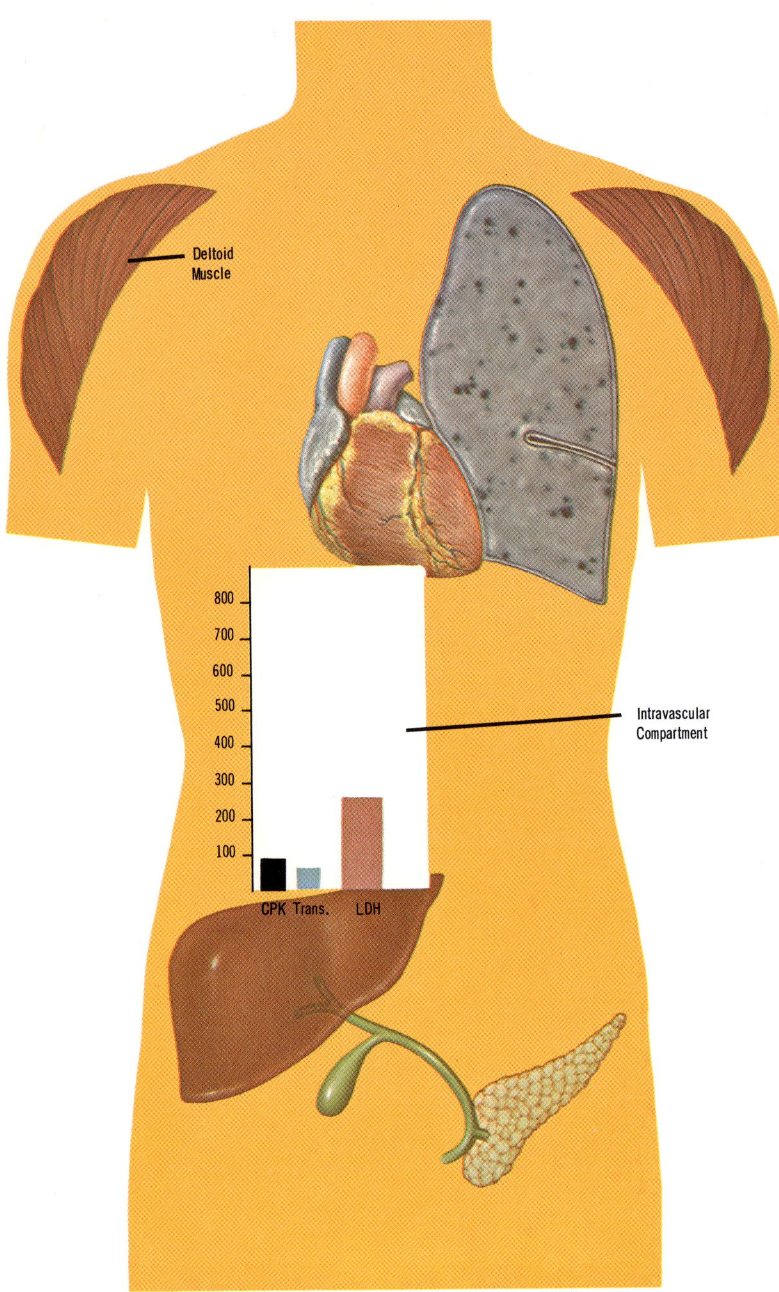

Abbreviations Used in Plates:

CPK = Creatine phosphokinase
Trans. = Transaminase in Karmen units per 100 ml. of blood
LDH = Lactic dehydrogenase in units per 100 ml. of blood

MYOCARDIAL INFARCTION

Cellular injury and necrosis in myocardial infarction (A) leads to the outpouring of intracellular transaminases and dehydrogenases into the blood. As a result, the *serum creatine phosphokinase* (CPK), *transaminases* (SGOT), and *lactic dehydrogenases* (LDH) *rise*. There is a high correlation between the size of the infarct and the degree of enzyme elevation. The CPK rises within the first 4–6 hours and is more specific, as it does not rise in liver disease. The SGOT rises early (6 to 12 hours after the infarction) and drops to normal within 4 to 7 days, whereas the LDH rises later (12 to 24 hours afterward) and falls gradually over a 1- to 2-week period. Electrophoretic analysis has shown that the first and second isoenzymes of LDH account for the bulk of the elevation. These isoenzymes are also heat stable. This is the basis of another differential test, as liver isoenzymes are heat labile. Serial electrocardiograms help to substantiate the diagnosis.

Summary of Laboratory Findings:

Transaminases: Increased
Lactic dehydrogenases: Increased

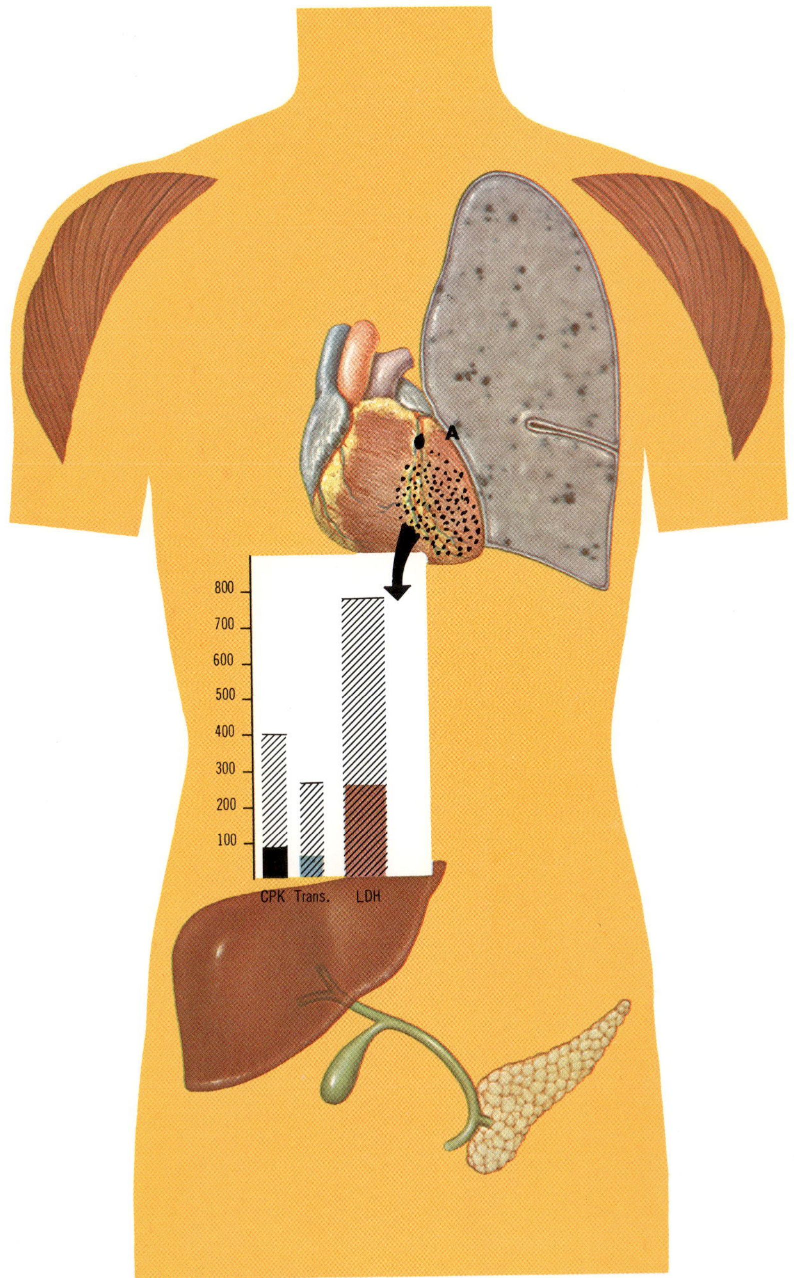

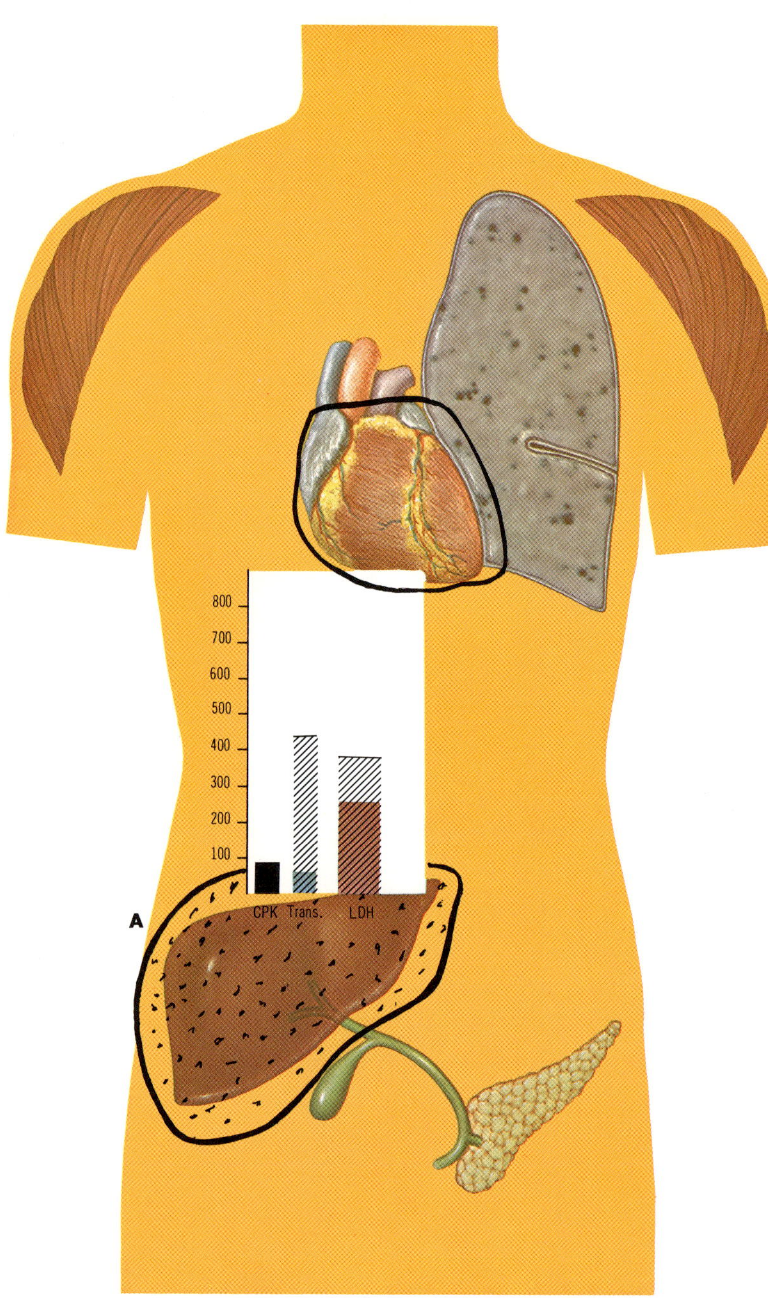

CARDIAC FAILURE

This disorder is associated with an *elevation* of the *serum transaminase* that occasionally is as high as 1,000 units. This is apparently due to congestion and central necrosis of the liver* (A). The LDH is increased in many cases, but the CPK is normal, distinguishing this from myocardial infarction. Electrophoresis shows that it is the 5th isoenzyme fraction of LDH that is elevated rather than the 1st and 2nd, as in myocardial infarction. A venous pressure and circulation time and serial electrocardiograms help to differentiate this condition from myocardial infarction.

Summary of Laboratory Findings:

CPK: Normal

Transaminases: Increased

Lactic dehydrogenases: Normal or increased

* Logan, R. G., Mowry, F. M., and Judge, R. D.: Cardiac failure simulating viral hepatitis. Ann. Intern. Med., *56*:784-788, May 1962.

VIRAL HEPATITIS

In hepatitis the necrotic liver cells release large amounts of intracellular transaminase into the blood. As a result, the *serum transaminases rise*. Serum levels of *lactic dehydrogenases and creatine phosphokinase do not usually increase*. The rise is more marked than that in myocardial infarction. Levels of 2,000 units/ml. are common in viral hepatitis, and in carbon tetrachloride poisoning they may reach as high as 30,000 units/ml.

The enzyme levels do not reflect liver cell function per se, but they are believed to represent the cells' reaction to injury. Thus in viral hepatitis they rise in the prodromal phase of the disease and fall later than the values for hepatic function tests. Functional changes occur only after necrosis has occurred. Transaminase levels may be used to follow the course of the disease process, since serial alterations occur in the course of the acute process and follow a characteristic pattern. Deviation, such as a sudden elevation superimposed on a falling curve, or a persistently high level when the level should be falling, suggests the development of a relapse, a complication, or postnecrotic cirrhosis. Diagnosis is supported by other tests of liver function (pp. 11, 16) and liver biopsy. Viral hepatitis B ("serum" hepatitis) can be differentiated by finding HAA ("Australian antigen") in the serum.

Other liver diseases associated with hepatic necrosis, e.g., cirrhosis, metastatic malignancy, hepatomas, etc., will produce a similar picture. These can be differentiated by liver scans, liver biopsy, or exploratory laparotomy.

Summary of Laboratory Findings:

CPK: Normal

Transaminases: Increased

Lactic dehydrogenases: Normal or increased

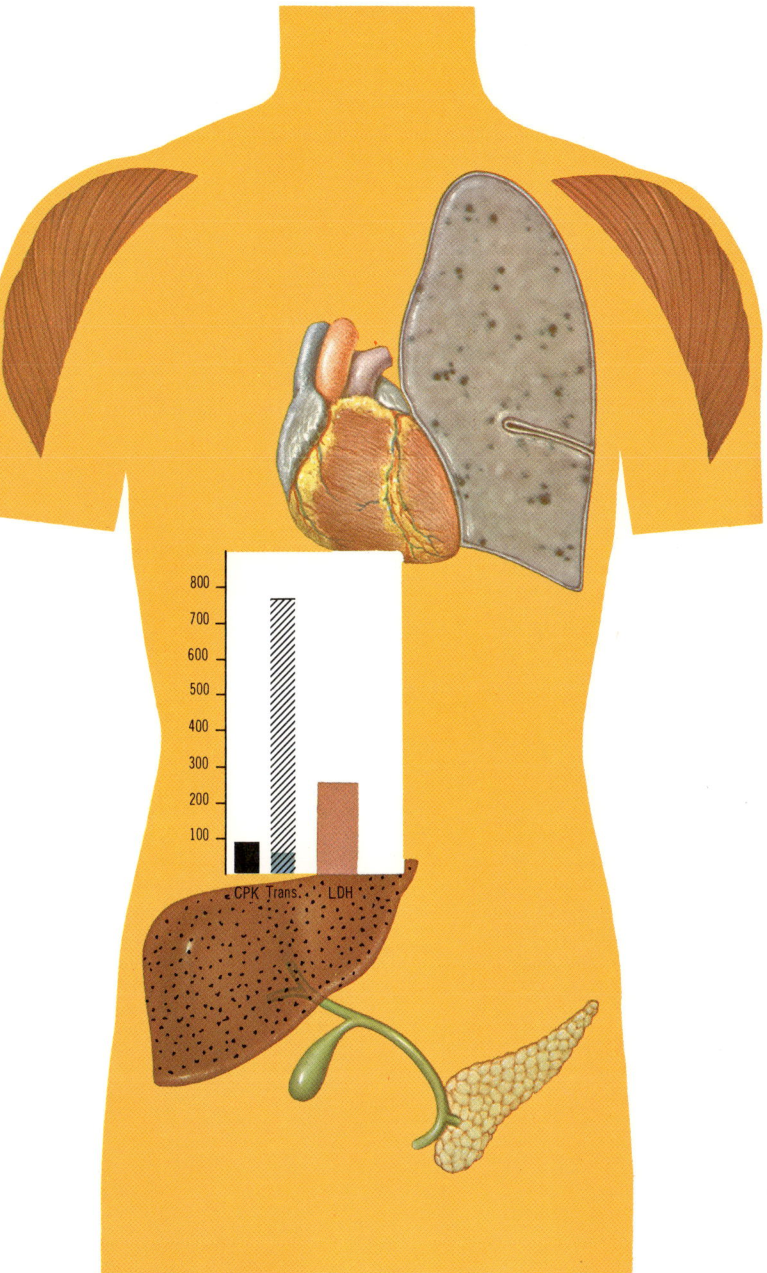

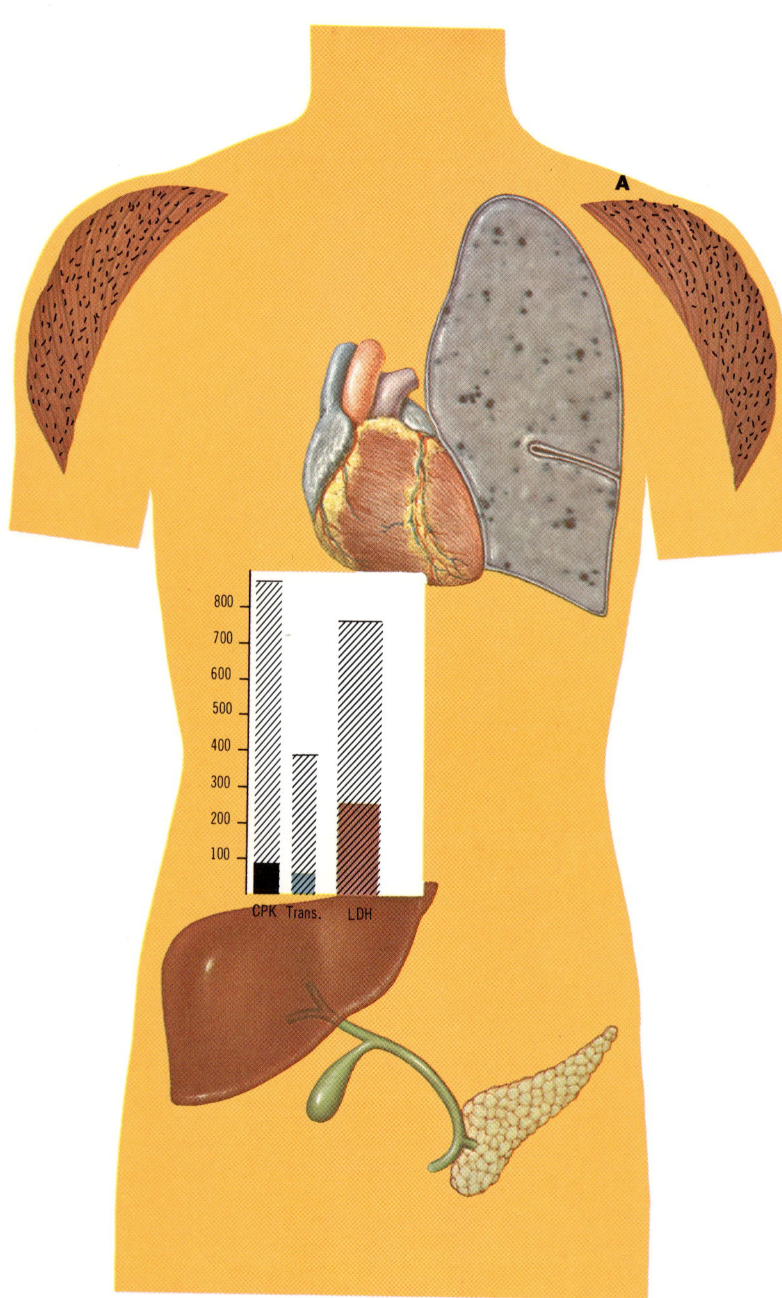

DERMATOMYOSITIS

The muscle inflammation and necrosis (A) associated with this disorder leads to *elevated serum transaminases* and *lactic dehydrogenases* and marked elevations of creatine phosphokinase. The diagnosis is established by muscle biopsy.

Progressive muscular dystrophy, muscular trauma, and trichinosis may produce a similar picture. Serum aldolase is also significantly elevated in these disorders.

Summary of Laboratory Findings:

CPK: Increased

Transaminases: Increased

Lactic dehydrogenases: Increased

EXTRAHEPATIC BILIARY OBSTRUCTIONS

Whether due to carcinoma of the pancreas (A) or ampulla of Vater or a common duct stone (B), these disorders are associated with a *rise* in *serum transaminases,* without a rise in serum lactic dehydrogenases or creatine phosphokinase. The LDH may be elevated, however, if there is an associated malignancy. This is apparently due to blockage of the excretion of transaminase through the bile ducts. The levels are not nearly as high as those in hepatitis and are stable despite the increasing hyperbilirubinemia frequently seen in complete biliary obstructions. The diagnosis is established by global liver function tests, percutaneous cholangiography, gastrointestinal roentgenograms, and exploratory laparotomy.

Acute pancreatitis and morphine administration are associated with elevated transaminases on the same basis.

Summary of Laboratory Findings:

CPK: Normal

Transaminases: Increased

Lactic dehydrogenases: Normal

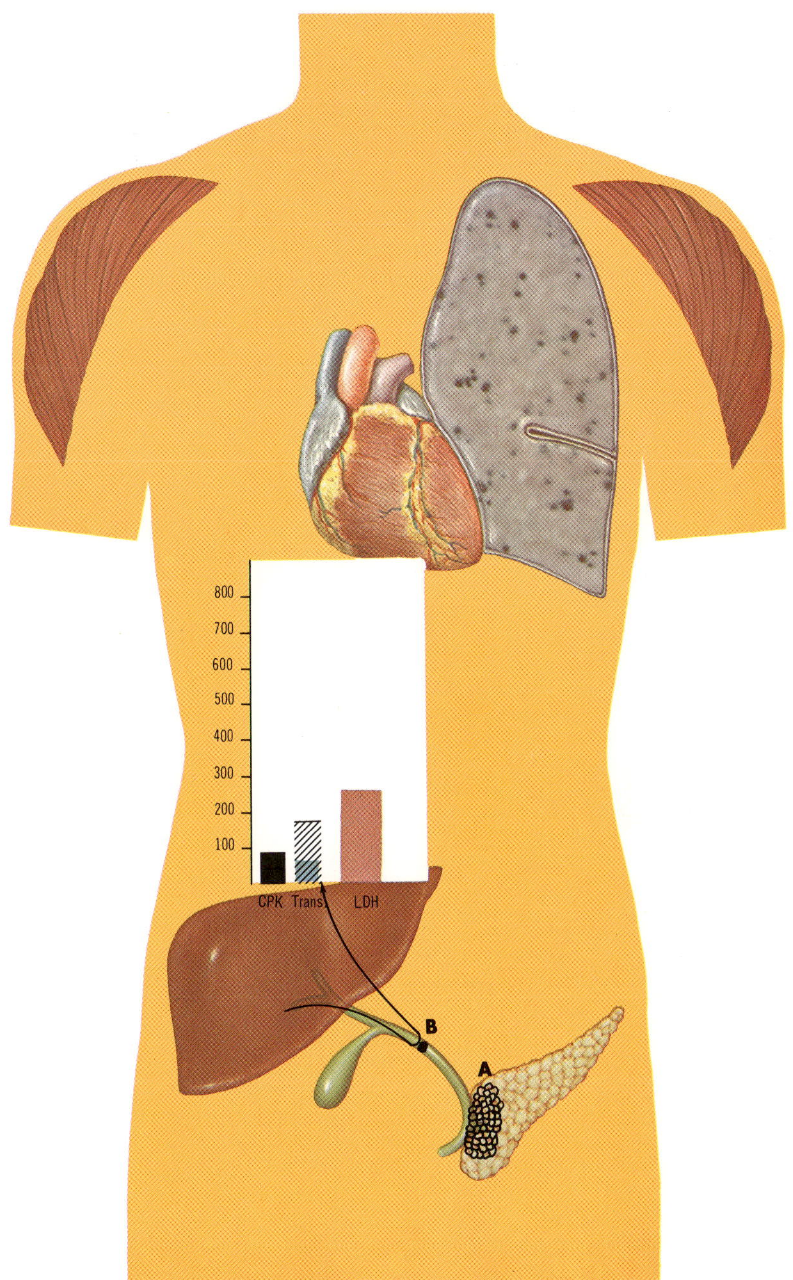

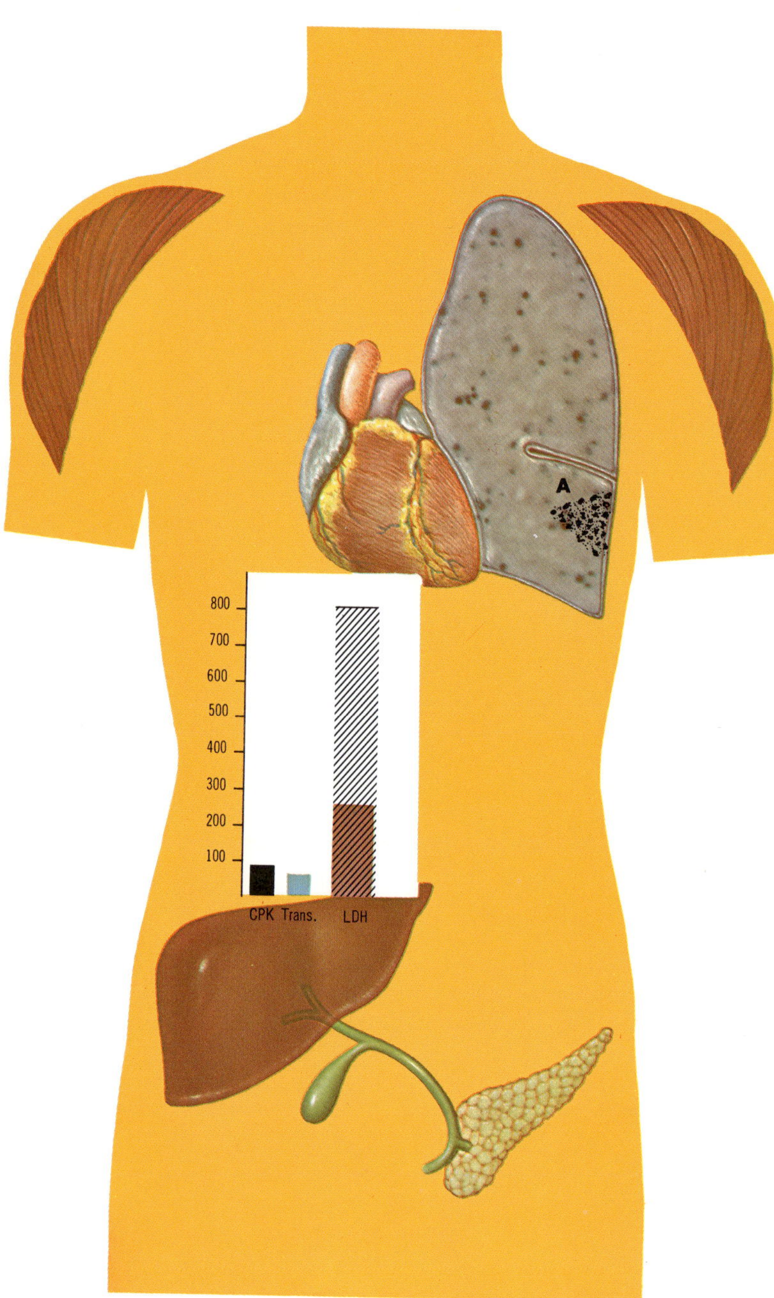

PULMONARY INFARCTION

For unknown reasons the *serum lactic dehydrogenases rise* in pulmonary infarction (A), whereas the serum transaminases remain normal unless there is associated congestive heart failure. The creatine phosphokinase is normal. This is in distinct contrast with hepatic and cardiac necrosis. The diagnosis is supported by chest roentgenogram, lung scans, electrocardiogram, and thoracentesis. Electrophoretic analysis has shown that isoenzymes L.D.2 and L.D.3 account for the bulk of the elevation.

Summary of Laboratory Findings:

CPK: Normal

Transaminases: Normal

Lactic dehydrogenases: Increased

12 Disorders of Serum Uric Acid

Uric acid is unique in that it is a metabolite of nucleic acid degradation, and as such it affords a means of quantitating disorders in nucleic acid metabolism. It is the end-product of purine metabolism, is represented in certain quantities in the serum, and is excreted mainly in the urine, a minor amount being secreted into the gastrointestinal lumen. Uric acid is a simple determination and can be helpful not only in the identification of certain diseases but also occasionally in differentiating among several diseases.

NORMAL METABOLISM

Production. Uncertainty haunts present knowledge of uric acid formation, but a workable hypothesis has been formulated. Purines (adenine and guanine, etc.) are believed to be the parent compounds from which uric acid is derived, the production occurring in organs of high metabolic turnover such as the liver, bone marrow, and perhaps muscle. Exogenous purines are absorbed in the form of nucleotides from the intestinal lumen, after enzymatic degradation has separated them from the larger, more complex nucleoproteins that are incorporated in the foods of the mammalian diet. This purine fraction is thought to be mainly catabolized directly to waste products, i.e., uric acid. The rest of the body's purine fraction is synthesized from small fragments (CO_2, NH_3, formate, and glycine), and this is utilized anabolically for the production of nucleic acid, vital for tissue reproduction. Uric acid is, of course, formed from purines of both sources by way of a series of enzymatic-controlled reactions, after which it is passed into the blood for general circulation. If the diet is moderately restricted, approximately 750 mg. of uric acid is produced daily.

Transport. After formation uric acid passes into the blood stream. The serum concentration is approximately 3 to 6 mg. per 100 ml. of serum. There is a sexual difference, the levels in females being generally 15 to 20 per cent lower than the levels in males. The value in children is still lower and persists until the time of puberty. Average values for men, women, and children, respectively, are 5.1, 4.1, and 3.3 mg. per 100 ml. of serum. Ingestion of a diet high in purine-containing foods does affect the blood level of uric acid under normal conditions of excretion.

Storage. Uric acid, once formed by the metabolism of the purine bases adenine and guanine, is not metabolized by the body's tissues, but rather enters the "uric acid pool" (as determined by the extent of dilution of radioactive uric acid in the body). This normally contains approximately 1.2 gm. of uric acid. The pool is a dynamic one, 50 to 75 per cent of it being turned over each day for excretion.

Excretion. The main excretory pathway of uric acid is the kidney. Differential micropuncture studies have shown that there is initially total clearance of uric acid at the glomerular level. This is followed by almost total tubular reabsorption through an active transport mechanism. A comparison of urine levels of uric acid with serum levels in-

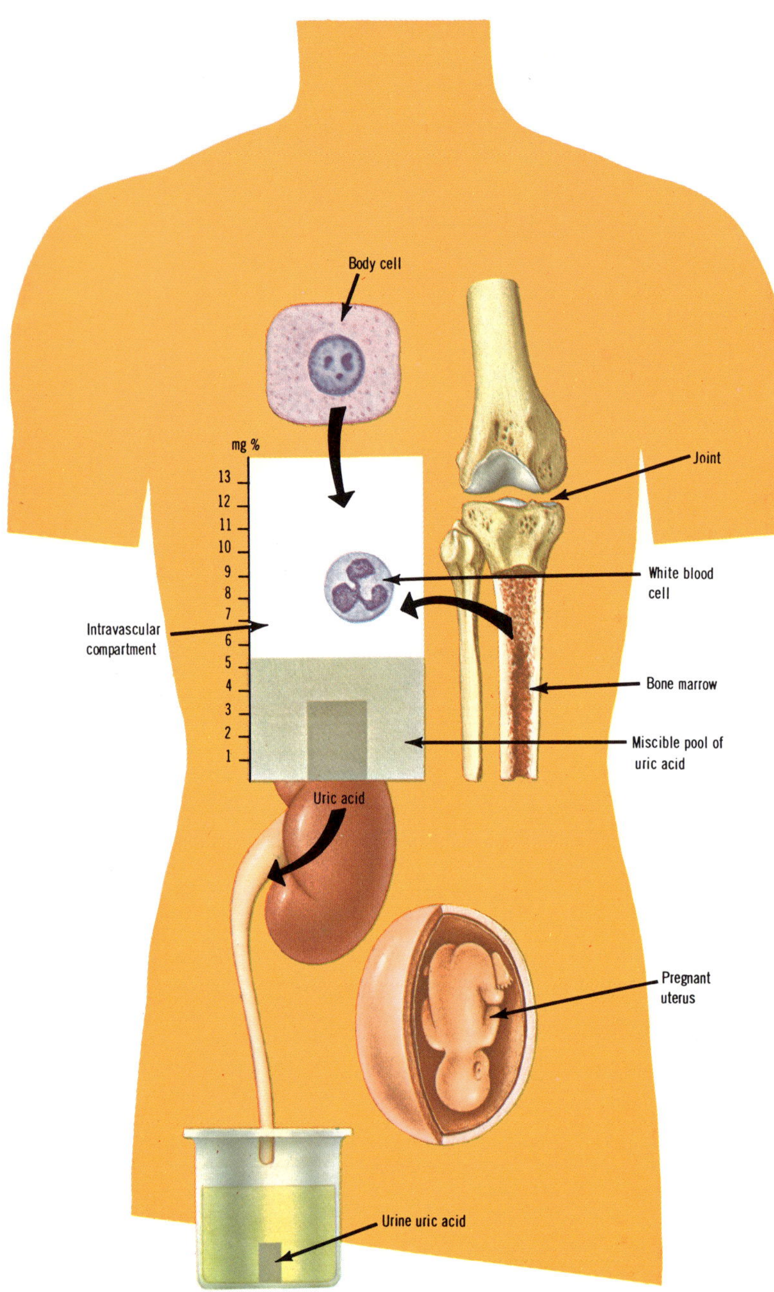

dicates that the amount excreted is equal to the amount filtered. This part is actively secreted by the tubules. Uricosuric agents are useful in promoting higher urinary levels of uric acid by their ability to block the tubular transport systems. The blood and urine uric acid concentrations vary directly with purine ingestion and also with protein and caloric intake. If the diet is a mixed normal one, the average daily excretion of uric acid is approximately 0.7 gm.

A second route of uric acid excretion is the gastrointestinal mucosa, where as much as one third of the total daily excretion may occur by secretion into the intestinal lumen.

GOUT

In most cases of primary gout there is an increased production of uric acid (A), with a concomitant rise in *serum* and *urine uric acid.* In a minority of cases, however, this mechanism has not been substantiated, and it is felt decreased urinary excretion of uric acid is responsible in these. These cases can be differentiated by doing a 24–hour urine uric acid. Cases of gout with a high 24–hour urine uric acid are due to an increased production, and those with low or normal 24–hour urine uric acids are due to diminished excretion. There is a tremendous *increase* in the size of the *uric acid pool* in all cases, and uric acid crystals are deposited in the joints (B). Diagnosis of gout depends on an adequate history, including a tedious family history, physical examination, synovianalysis, roentgenograms of the digits, and the dramatic response to colchicine therapy. The new drug allopurinol decreases serum uric acid by interfering with the production of uric acid from hypoxanthine. Recently cases of congenital gout associated with mental retardation, self-mutilation, and cerebral palsy have been reported and named the *Lesch-Nyhan syndrome,* after the discoverers. This is associated with an overproduction of uric acid because of a severe deficiency of hypoxanthine-guanine phosphoribosyl transferase.

Summary of Laboratory Findings:

Serum uric acid: Increased

Urine uric acid: Increased usually

Uric acid pool: Increased

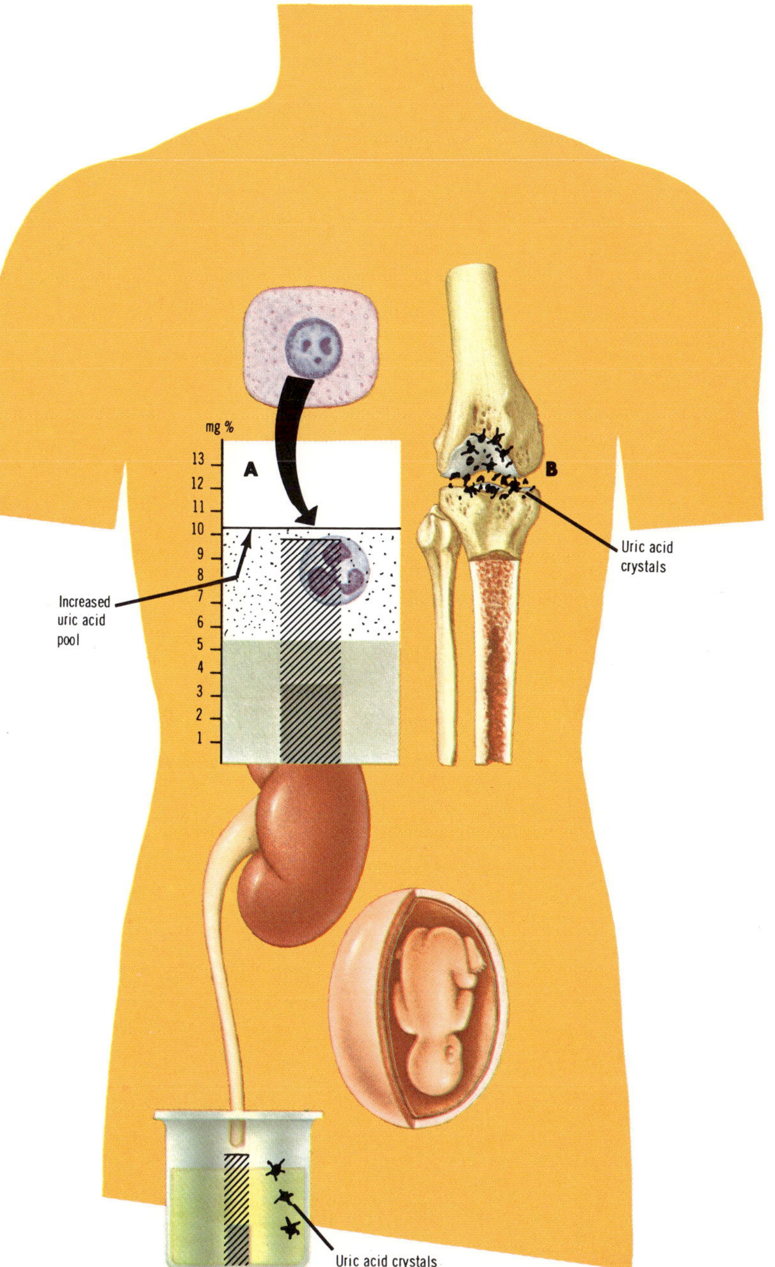

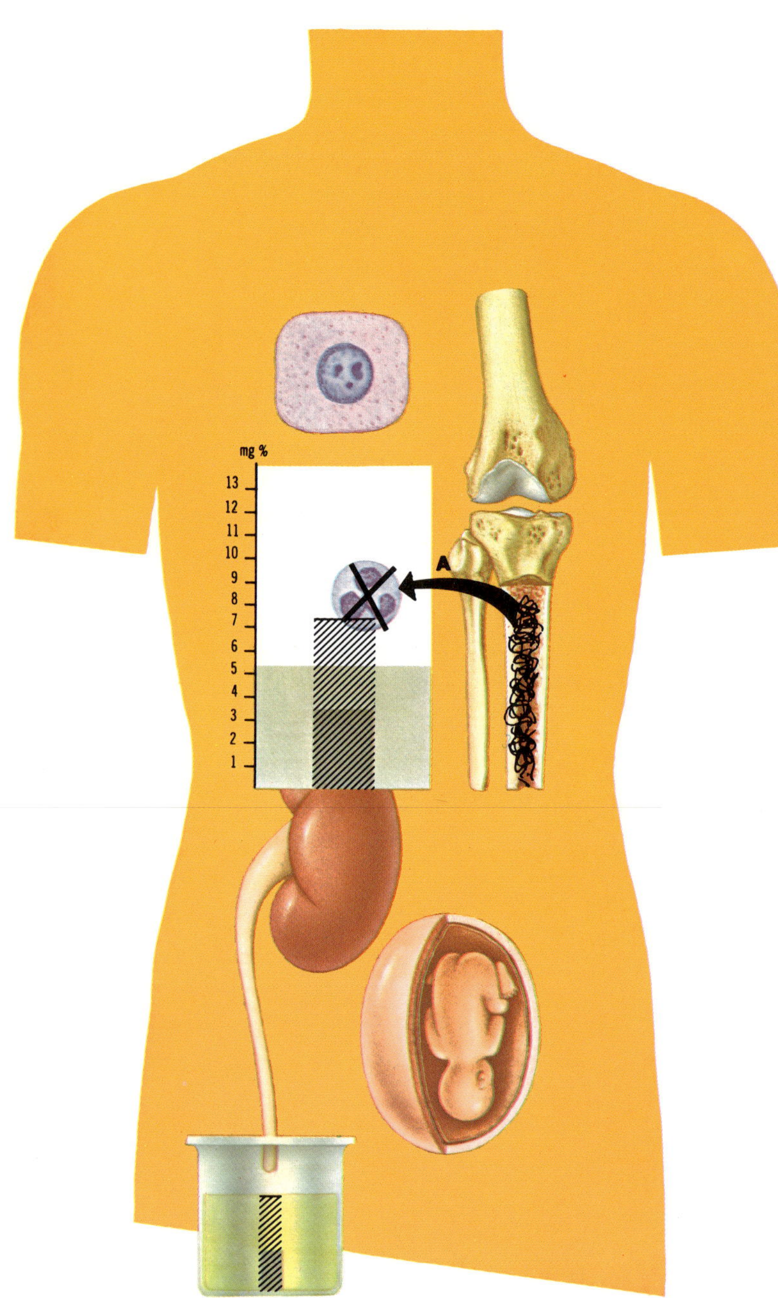

LEUKEMIA

The increased production and destruction of white cells (A) in leukemia leads to an increased rate of turnover of white cell nucleic acids, with an increased production of uric acid. The *serum and urine uric acid rises*. Blood and/or bone marrow smears are usually diagnostic.

Polycythemia vera, multiple myeloma, lymphoblastomas, and other malignancies may produce the same picture.

Summary of Laboratory Findings:

Serum uric acid: Increased

Urine uric acid: Increased

CHRONIC GLOMERULONEPHRITIS

In this disease the renal clearance and tubular secretion of uric acid are decreased, resulting in an *elevation* of the *serum uric acid.* At the same time the *urine uric acid decreases.* A BUN and creatinine and Addis count substantiate the diagnosis. Cystoscopy and retrograde pyelography help to distinguish this condition from obstructive uropathies, but a renal biopsy may clinch the diagnosis.

Toxic nephritis, collagen disease, and diabetic glomerulosclerosis can produce a similar picture. The retention of uric acid in patients on diuretics is probably related to inhibition of tubular secretion of uric acid.

Summary of Laboratory Findings:

Serum uric acid: Increased

Urine uric acid: Decreased

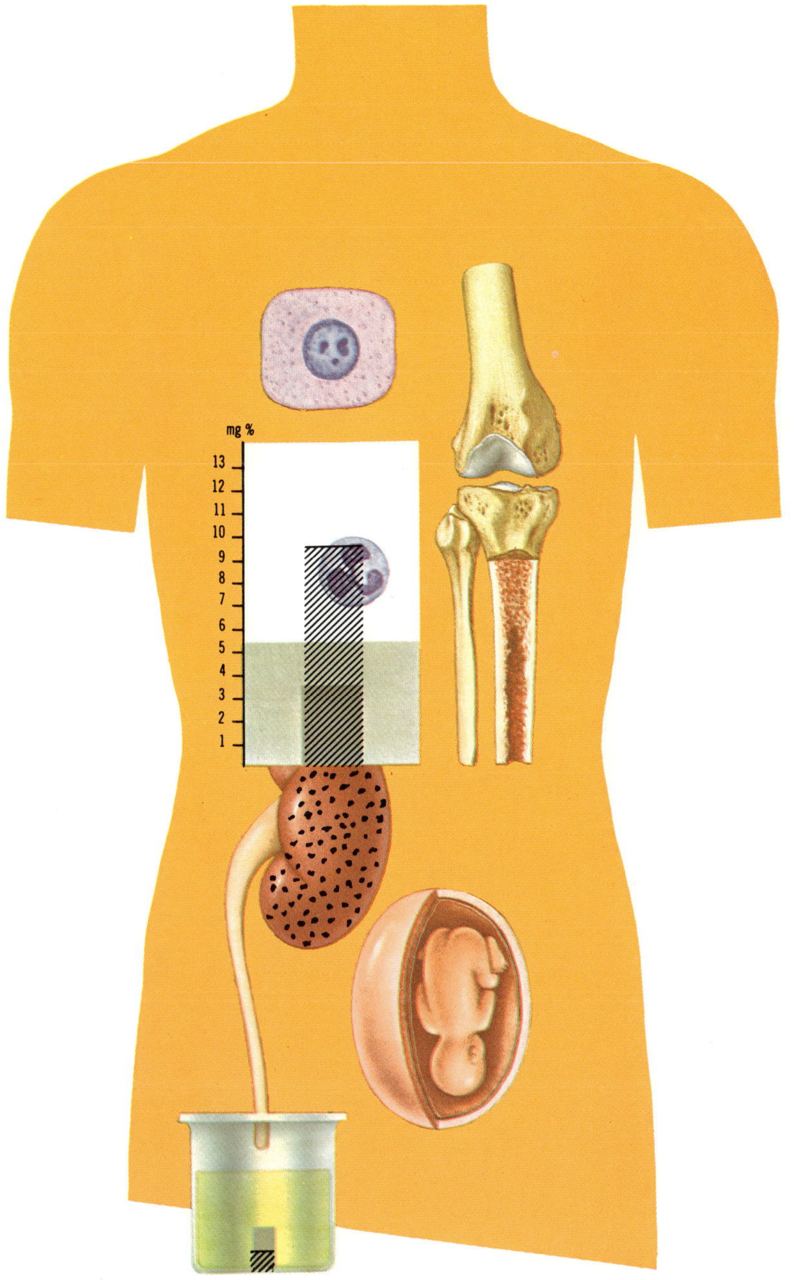

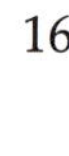

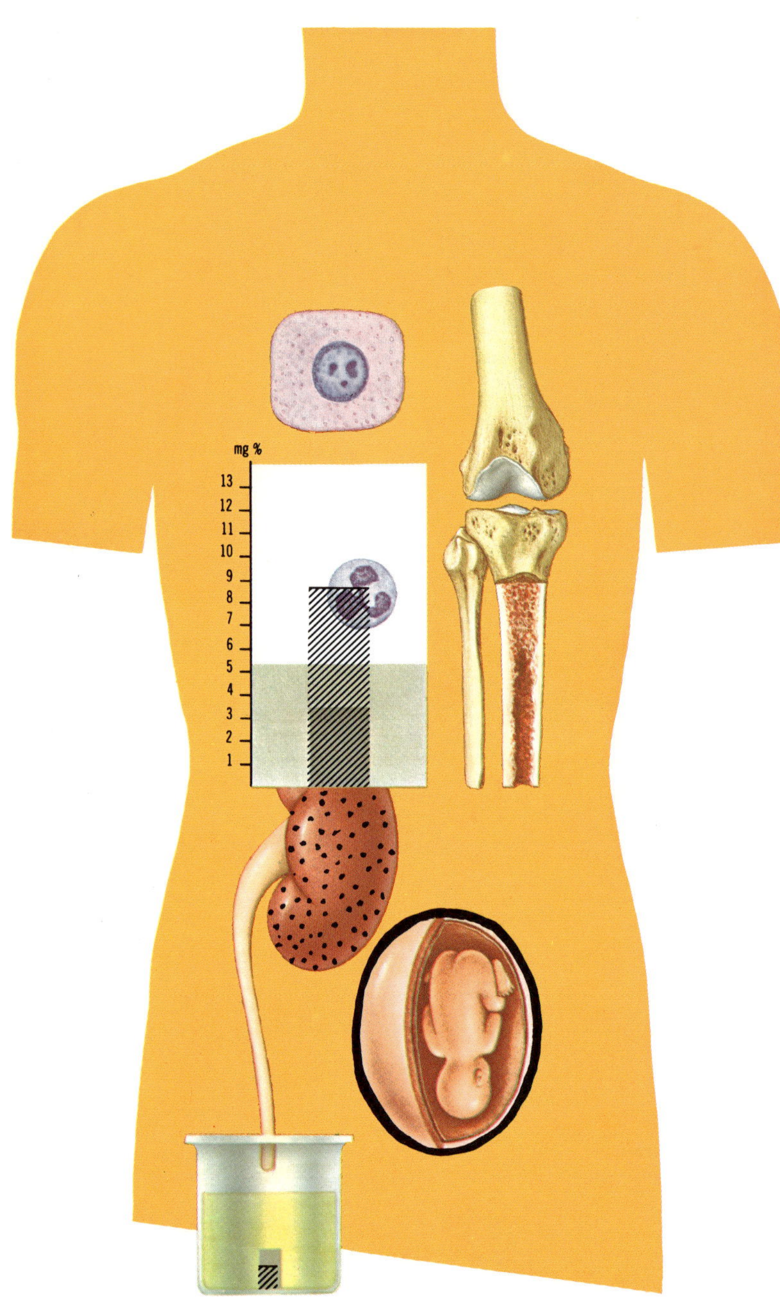

TOXEMIA OF PREGNANCY

In this disease the renal clearance of uric acid is decreased. Hence the blood *uric acid rises*. The blood urea nitrogen is usually normal, since urea clearance may not be altered. This helps to differentiate this condition from other toxic and inflammatory conditions of the kidney (glomerulonephritis, etc.).

Summary of Laboratory Findings:

Serum uric acid: Increased

Urine uric acid: Decreased

FANCONI SYNDROME

In this disorder a lack of tubular reabsorption of uric acid results in a *low serum uric acid* and a *high* output of *uric acid* (A) in the *urine*. The diagnosis is confirmed by the associated glycosuria, amino aciduria, and hyperphosphaturia.

Wilson's disease and uricosuric agents such as probenecid may produce a similar picture for similar reasons.

Summary of Laboratory Findings:

Serum uric acid: Decreased

Urine uric acid: Increased

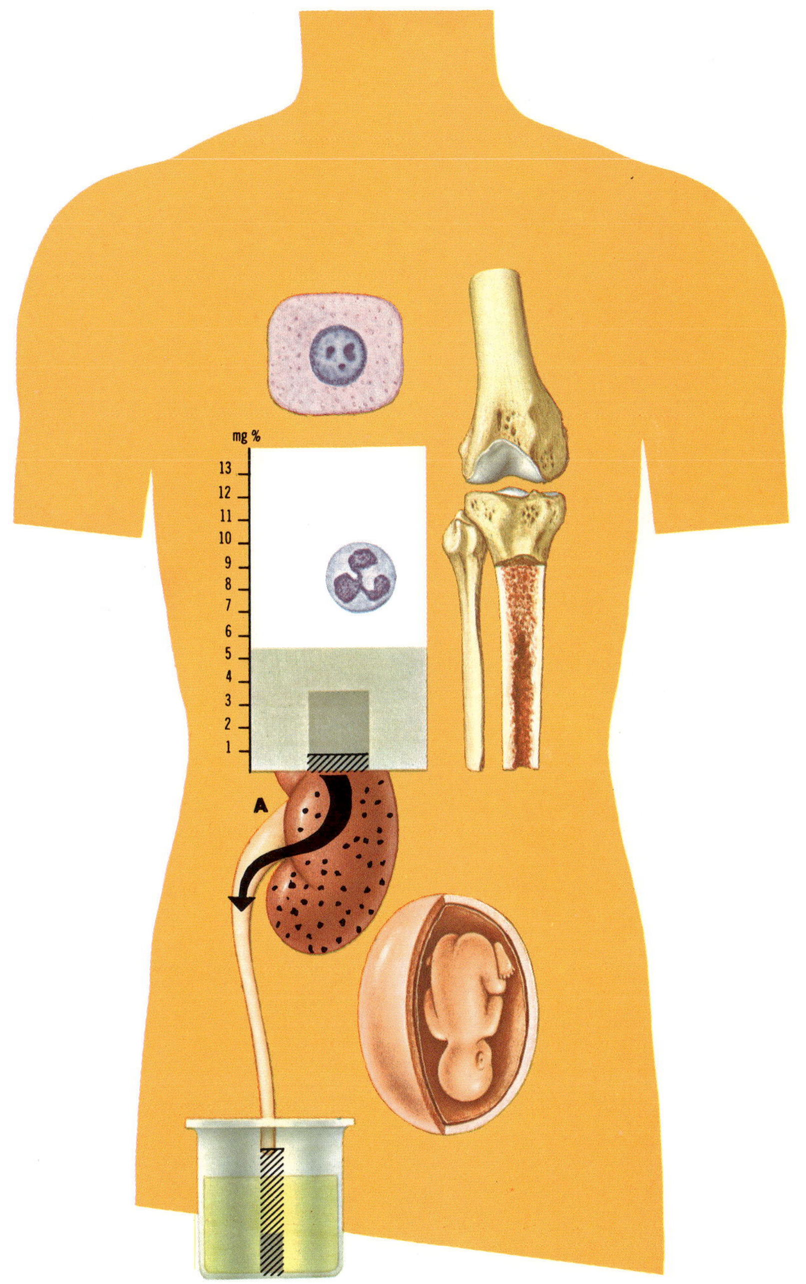

13 Miscellaneous Blood Chemistries

DISORDERS OF SERUM AMYLASE AND LIPASE

Normal Metabolism

Amylase. Serum amylase is composed of a group of enzymes that digest starch. Amylase is *produced* in the salivary gland, pancreas, liver, fallopian tubes, and possibly striated muscle. The amylase of normal serum varies between 80 and 150 Somogyi units per 100 ml. and is largely from the liver. The greater part of this is *transported* in association with the albumin fraction of serum. Smaller amounts of normal serum amylase are from the pancreas and salivary glands and are bound to gamma globulin. Serum amylase is *excreted* in the urine at the rate of 2,200 to 3,000 Somogyi units in 24 hours. By way of the pancreatic duct and common bile duct, pancreatic amylase is normally secreted into the duodenum, where it digests starch.

Lipase. The lipolytic activity of serum is contained in lipase. It splits triglyceride into glycerol and fatty acids. The acinar cells of the pancreas are the major source of lipase in the body. These cells, by way of the pancreatic duct and common bile duct, normally secrete the lipase into the duodenum, where fat digestion takes place. The lipase activity of normal serum varies between 0.2 and 1.5 Cherry-Crandall units. Like amylase, lipase is excreted in the urine, but no urine test has become popular.

Disorders

Acute Pancreatitis (Fig. 13-1A). In pancreatitis the acinar tissue of the pancreas is inflamed, and cell membranes rupture, allowing amylase and lipase to pass into the peritoneal cavity and the blood stream by way of the portal vein and the lymphatics. The serum levels of both *rise*. The amylase may rise to 3,000 Somogyi units in the first 24 hours, but usually it falls to normal within 48 hours of the onset of inflammation. Lipase also rises promptly, but the elevation will usually persist for 10 days or more. It may be necessary to take frequent blood samples during the first 48 hours of the illness to demonstrate these alterations. Only then can the diagnosis be safely excluded, should normal levels be obtained. Also, the amylase will be reduced by intravenous or oral intake of glucose; therefore other fluids should be given for 2 hours prior to drawing blood for the test. Occasionally, 24-hour urine amylases show marked elevation when the serum amylase is normal. Persistent elevations of the serum amylase for several days or months usually indicates a pancreatic pseudocyst has formed. Analysis of peritoneal fluid obtained in the early phases of illness may also reveal high amylase value. The serum transaminase (page 155) may be elevated in one half the cases of acute pancreatitis. Hyperglycemia and hypocalcemia are also frequent.

Chronic Pancreatitis (A). The amylase and lipase are not commonly elevated in this disorder except during relapse. Urinary amylase—1-hour, 2-hour, or 24-hour specimens—may be elevated. A provocative test with pancreozymin-secretin has been used but is not generally accepted. Duodenal drainage (p. 197) is a more accurate method of diagnosis in this disorder.

Pancreatic Carcinoma (B). This neoplasm may obstruct the pancreatic duct, with the result that amylase and lipase are backed up into the blood. Generally, the blood levels are normal.

Choledocholithiasis (C). Impaction of a gallstone at the sphincter of Oddi may also obstruct the pancreatic duct, and amylase backs up into the blood. This may result in acute inflammation of the gland, with a further *increase* in *serum* and *urinary amylase*.

Morphine and other opiates causing spasm of the sphincter of Oddi may produce a similar picture.

Intestinal Obstruction (D). High intestinal obstruction may distend the duodenum and lead to secondary obstruction of the pancreatic duct, backing amylase and lipase into the blood. This alone may explain the *rise* in *serum amylase* and *lipase*. If the duodenum becomes severely inflamed and necrotic, the enzymes may pass into the blood stream directly from the duodenal lumen. This constitutes another mechanism for the rise.

Duodenal Ulcer (E). A peptic ulcer in the duodenum may perforate the pancreas, causing a secondary pancreatitis. Thus the serum *lipase* and *amylase* may *rise*, as they do in primary pancreatitis.

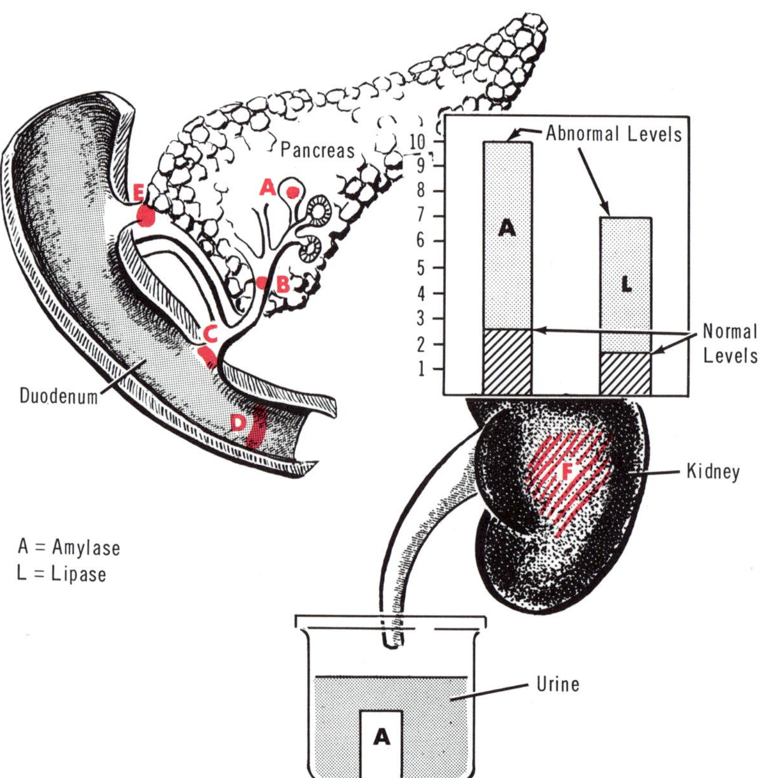

FIG. 13-1. Disorders of serum amylase and lipase. See text.

Renal Failure (F). The *rise* of *amylase* and *lipase* in this disorder is due to inadequate elimination in the urine.

Miscellaneous. Mumps and infective parotitis may lead to leakage of salivary amylase into the blood, with consequent rise. The lipase is normal in these conditions.

DISORDERS OF URINARY CATECHOLAMINES

The catecholamines epinephrine, norepinephrine, and dopamine are *produced* from tyrosine and phenylalanine in the brain, the sympathetic ganglia, postganglionic neurones, and the adrenal medulla. Of the catecholamine produced by the adrenal medulla, 75 to 80 per cent is epinephrine, and the remainder is norepinephrine. These are *secreted* into the circulation in response to activation of the splanchnic nerves by stress and other stimuli. Subsequently, 1 to 5 per cent is excreted into the urine, unchanged. Before secretion in the urine the rest undergoes *metabolic degradation* by methoxylation and oxidative deamination, with the formation of several derivatives, of which vanillyl mandelic acid (VMA) is the most abundant.

Pheochromocytoma. Whether in the adrenal medulla or extra-adrenal ganglionic tissue, these tumors secrete increased amounts of epinephrine and norepinephrine into the blood. As a result, *increased amounts* of *catecholamines* and their metabolic derivatives, such as *vanillyl mandelic acid,* appear in the urine. Twenty-four-hour urine specimens usually contain 20 to 40 gamma of catecholamines and less than 10 mg. of VMA. False positives may be produced by drugs such as methyldopa (Aldomet); foods such as coffee, tea, and bananas; and certain diseases (hemolytic anemias, Cushing's disease, lymphomas, etc.). A provocative test using tyramine is available. Plasma epinephrine and norepinephrine determinations are even more accurate and will eventually replace the above tests.

Further support for the diagnosis of a pheochromocytoma may be obtained by a Regitine test (in cases of consistent hypertension) or a histamine provocative test (in normotensive patients). The BMR and blood sugar (p. 72) are frequently elevated. Presacral air insufflation or arteriography may demonstrate a mass in the adrenal, but these patients should be explored if consistent elevations of urinary catecholamines are found. In cases of symptomatic hypertension, this diagnosis can be excluded only by repeatedly normal 24-hour urine catecholamines and vanillyl mandelic acid.

Neuroblastomas and Ganglioneuromas. These tumors usually also arise from the adrenal medulla so, as expected, often cause a significant elevation of urinary catecholamines and VMA. There is also an elevated urinary homovanillic acid (HVA), which helps to distinguish this condition from a pheochromocytoma.

DISORDERS OF COPPER METABOLISM

Copper is probably important in hemopoiesis, but its exact role here is not known.

Normal Metabolism

Intake. Approximately 2 mg. of copper is ingested daily in the average diet.

Absorption. Copper is absorbed in the upper part of the jejunum by both an active and a passive process, the exact nature of which is unknown.

Transport. Copper is transported by the blood, half of it in the plasma and the other half in the blood cell as erythrocuprein. Of plasma copper, 96 per cent is firmly bound to ceruloplasmin, an alpha-2 globulin. The rest is loosely bound to albumin. The normal adult has 65 to 165 mcg. of copper per 100 ml. of plasma.

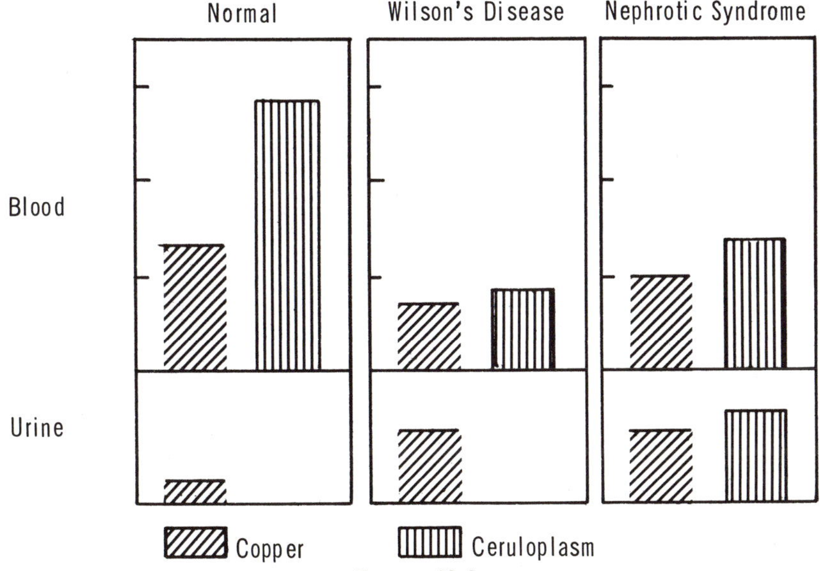

FIGURE 13-2

Storage. Approximately 125 mg. of copper is stored in the body. Most of this is in the liver, muscles, and bones.

Regulation. Both estrogens and androgens may increase the serum copper. Estrogen apparently does this by increasing the blood level of ceruloplasmin. This effect is similar to that of estrogen on the protein-bound iodine (p. 97).

Excretion. Copper is excreted by the intestinal tract, partly by way of the bile. Normally, imperceptible amounts are excreted in the urine.

Disorder

Wilson's Disease. In this disorder large amounts of copper accumulate in the liver, basal ganglia, cerebral cortex, kidney, and cornea. *Plasma copper* and *ceruloplasmin drop,* and large amounts of free *copper* are found in the plasma and *excreted* in the *urine* (Fig. 13-2). The exact cause of this disorder is not clear. It may be that the body cannot synthesize adequate ceruloplasmin. Plasma copper is then loosely bound to albumin and easily excreted in the urine or deposited in the tissues. There is also a high urine output of amino acids in this condition. Liver biopsy and slit-lamp examination of the cornea are also of assistance in diagnosis.

Low plasma ceruloplasmin and copper are found also in the *nephrotic syndrome,* in which ceruloplasmin is lost with other plasma proteins in the urine. Other causes of the low serum copper are kwashiorkor, sprue, and idiopathic hypocupremia of infancy.

DISORDERS OF URINE 5-HYDROXYINDOLEACETIC ACID

Urine 5-hydroxyindoleacetic acid (5-HIAA) is a product of the metabolic degradation of serotonin by monamine oxidase in the liver and lungs. Serotonin is *produced* from tryptophan in the Kulchitsky cells of the intestinal tract. It is secreted into the blood, where it serves as a powerful vasopressor substance. Serotonin is also produced in the nervous system, but this apparently accounts for only a small amount of circulating serotonin.

Two to 8 mg. of 5-hydroxyindoleacetic acid is excreted in the urine in 24 hours.

Malignant Carcinoid Tumors. These tumors arise from the Kulchitsky cells anywhere in the intestinal tract and most commonly in the ileum. Particularly after metastasis to the liver, they secrete large amounts of serotonin, which is converted to *5-hydroxyindoleacetic* acid in the liver. *Increased amounts* of 5-HIAA then appear in the urine. Further laboratory confirmation can be obtained by a serum serotonin. It is important to exclude intake of bananas and reserpine at least 24 hours before performing these tests, since these substances cause increased levels of 5-HIAA.

Bronchial adenomas may also be associated with increased secretion of serotonin.

Adult Celiac Disease. Urine 5-HIAA is increased in this disease, possibly because of an increase in the number of chromaffin cells in the intestinal wall. The levels are not nearly as high as those in the carcinoid syndrome.

DISORDERS OF SERUM IRON

Iron is important in the formation of hemoglobin and various cellular enzymes (cytochrome, catalase, etc.).

Normal Metabolism of Iron

Intake. Iron enters the body by way of the gastrointestinal tract. The average American ingests between 6 and 15 mg. of iron a day in such foods as eggs, liver, and spinach.

Absorption. Absorption takes place in the duodenum and upper jejunum by an active process, the exact mechanism of which is unknown. However, it is believed that the transfer through the mucosal cell is facilitated by an iron-amino acid complex. Granick believed this to be apoferritin, but this has not been confirmed by others.

Absorption of 2 mg. of ingested iron is usually sufficient to replace iron lost in menstruation, pregnancy, and excretion.

The growing child must absorb 1 to 1.5 mg. a day. Some pregnant women require as much as 3 mg. a day.

Certain factors influence iron absorption. The ferrous form of iron is more easily absorbed. The presence of hydrochloric acid assists iron absorption by reducing the ferric to the ferrous form of iron. Ascorbic acid increases iron absorption, whereas sodium phytate and phosphorus in various foods (e.g., cereals) inhibit it. Organically bound iron is more difficult to absorb. Erythropoietin (the humoral plasma factor that stimulates erythropoiesis) probably increases iron absorption. In pyridoxine deficiency the assimilation of iron continues in excess of body needs, an indication that this vitamin may have a direct effect on inhibiting iron absorption.

Transport. Iron is transported in the blood by a group of iron-containing beta globulins collectively called *transferrin.* The normal serum iron level is 75 to 175 mcg. per 100 ml. in the adult male. The serum iron-binding capacity (transferrin) is normally 150 to 300 mcg. per 100 ml. Iron is distributed to the bone marrow, liver, and other tissues.

Utilization. Iron is utilized to form the respiratory pigments hemoglobin and myoglobin, and several body enzymes (cytochrome, cytochrome oxidase, catalase, etc.). Only 7 per cent of the total body iron is not in the organic form.

Production. Iron is not produced by the body, but 20 to 25 mg. is released daily into the plasma during the degradation of hemoglobin. This iron is used over and over again by the body.

Storage. Twenty per cent (0.5 to 1.5 gm.) of total body iron is stored as ferritin and hemosiderin in the liver, spleen, and bone mar-

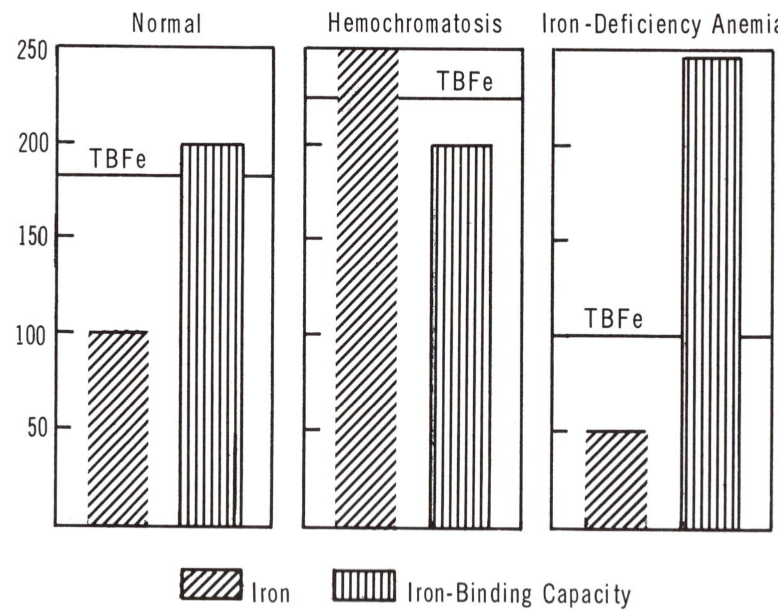

FIG. 13-3. Disorders of iron metabolism.

row. This can be readily mobilized for the synthesis of hemoglobin and other hemoproteins. Another 20 per cent of body iron is in the form of myoglobin, and 50 to 60 per cent is in the form of hemoglobin.

Excretion. Approximately 0.5 to 1 mg. of iron is lost daily in the feces, urine, and sweat, probably largely by desquamation of the cells from the skin and mucosal surfaces. Smaller quantities are lost in the bile and urine (as red cells). Women may be considered to "excrete" iron during menstruation. This amounts to between 16 and 32 mg. of iron each month.

Regulation. Both iron utilization and hemoglobin production are no doubt under hormonal control. Erythropoietin is believed to exert at least part of this control. A decreased oxygen supply to the intestinal mucosa may be responsible for the increased iron absorption in anemic states.

Disorders

(Fig. 13-3)

Hemochromatosis. Increased iron absorption in this disorder leads to *saturation* of *plasma transferrin* and an *elevated plasma iron* (A). Eventually iron spills over into the parenchymal tissue of the liver, pancreas, endocrine glands (testicles, etc.), and skin. Total body iron increases to 50 gm. The pancreatic involvement may lead to diabetes (p. 73). Thus a glucose tolerance test may assist the diagnosis. Liver function tests other than a BSP are often normal. A liver or skin biopsy is the most valuable diagnostic aid. If the tissue is stained for iron, iron deposits will be found in the parenchyma. Hemosiderin can also be demonstrated in the urine.

By contrast, in hemosiderosis iron is found in the reticuloendothelial tissue. Hemolytic anemias may give similar values for the serum iron and iron-binding capacity as hemochromatosis.

Iron-deficiency Anemia. In this disorder the *serum iron falls,* and iron stores are depleted because of a relative or absolute deficiency of iron intake to meet body requirements. Thus this condition may develop when body requirements increase, as in the growing child, the pregnant woman, or a gastrointestinal bleeder, or when the diet may be insufficient to meet the ordinary needs of the adult.

Iron-binding capacity often increases, perhaps in an attempt to compensate for the diminished serum iron. The characteristic hematologic features of iron-deficiency anemia develop. Staining of bone marrow for the presence of hemosiderin is an additional laboratory aid in diagnosis. Hemosiderin deposits are reduced in this disorder.

Serum iron levels are increased in other anemias but without diagnostic significance.

DISORDERS OF SERUM MAGNESIUM

Magnesium is extremely important in activating the phosphorylating enzymes of the body and promoting energy interchange.

Normal Metabolism

Intake. The average adult ingests 360 mg. of magnesium a day in practically all food stuffs.

Transport. Magnesium is transported in the blood, where it exists in a concentration of 1.5 to 2.5 mEq. per liter. Like calcium, approximately half of it is bound to protein, and the rest is free.

Storage. Magnesium is present throughout the body, chiefly intracellularly. The body contains 2,000 mg., but 50 to 75 per cent of this is in bone.

Excretion. The ionized portion of magnesium is filtered and partially reabsorbed in accordance with body needs. In depleted states urinary loss may fall to less than 1 mg./liter in 24 hrs.

Regulation. The hormonal influences on serum magnesium are many and diversified. Parathyroid hormone causes a distinct drop in magnesium excretion by the kidney. Growth hormone enhances the intestinal absorption of magnesium. The level of serum magnesium is high in Addison's disease. Thyroxine causes an elevation of the serum magnesium.

Disturbances in Disease States

Ulcerative Colitis. In this disease serum magnesium levels drop as a result of both diminished intestinal absorption of dietary magnesium and loss of intestinal secretions containing magnesium.

Diarrhea, whatever the cause, will produce the same picture.

Hypoparathyroidism. Diminished tubular reabsorption of magnesium in this disorder leads to a drop in serum magnesium.

Laennec's Cirrhosis. In this disorder there is a lack of absorption because dietary magnesium combines with ammonia in the intestines to produce an insoluble, nonabsorbable complex.*

DISORDERS OF MELANIN METABOLISM

The pigment melanin is formed by the oxidation of tyrosine in the melanocytes of the skin; this reaction is catalyzed by the enzyme tyrosinase (B in metabolic pathway 2 below). Tyrosine may come directly from the diet or be formed from parahydroxylation of the benzene ring, a reaction that is catalyzed by the enzyme phenylalanine hydroxylase (A in metabolic pathway 1 below). Catabolism of tyrosine and phenylalanine leads to the formation of homogentisic acid. The last is wholly degraded in the liver by homogentisic acid oxidase (C in metabolic pathway 4 below). Schematic outlines of these metabolic pathways follow:

Metabolic Pathway

1. phenylalanine $\xrightarrow{A}$ tyrosine
2. tyrosine $\xrightarrow{B}$ melanin
3. tyrosine $\longrightarrow$ homogentisic acid
4. homogentisic acid $\xrightarrow{C}$ degradation products

Phenylketonuria. In this disorder phenylalanine hydroxylase (A above) is inactive, so that phenylalanine is not converted to tyrosine. *Phenylalanine* accumulates in the body fluid, and some of it is *excreted* in the *urine.* A large amount of it is transaminated to *phenylpyruvic acid,* which is *excreted in the urine.* Phenylpyruvic acid is easily detected by a urine test that is being used as a screening procedure on newborn infants. False positives with this test (Phenistix) occur in ketonuria (as in diabetic acidosis) and salicylate poisoning and after ingestion of phenothiazines. A more reliable screening test is the Guthrie test for abnormal amounts of phenylalanine in the blood. This test involves comparing the growth of *Bacillus subtilis* bacteria on a culture medium deficient in phenylalanine with addition of normal blood and blood from a patient with phenylketonuria (PKU). Growth will be sustained best in the media with PKU blood.

Alkaptonuria. In this disorder homogentisic acid oxidase (C above) is deficient. Consequently, homogentisic acid is not degraded, and large amounts appear in the urine. The urine turns black on the addition of alkali or on standing. X-ray examination may show heavy calcification of the intervertebral discs.

Melanotic Sarcoma. Normally, melanocytes do not produce sufficient melanin to spill over into the blood and urine. However, in metastatic melanotic sarcoma large amounts of a colorless precursor of melanin (conjugated 5, 6-dihydroxyindole) appear in the urine and can be detected by the laboratory.

Albinism. In albinism there is a congenital deficiency of tyrosinase (B above), with consequent impaired melanin formation. This condition cannot as yet be detected by the laboratory.

* Duncan, G. G. (ed.): Diseases of Metabolism. ed. 5, p. 280. Philadelphia, W. B. Saunders, 1964.

DISORDERS OF PORPHYRIN METABOLISM

The porphyrins of the body are important in the formation of the hemoproteins (hemoglobin, myoglobin, cytochrome oxidase, etc.) that function as carriers of oxygen in the blood and tissues.

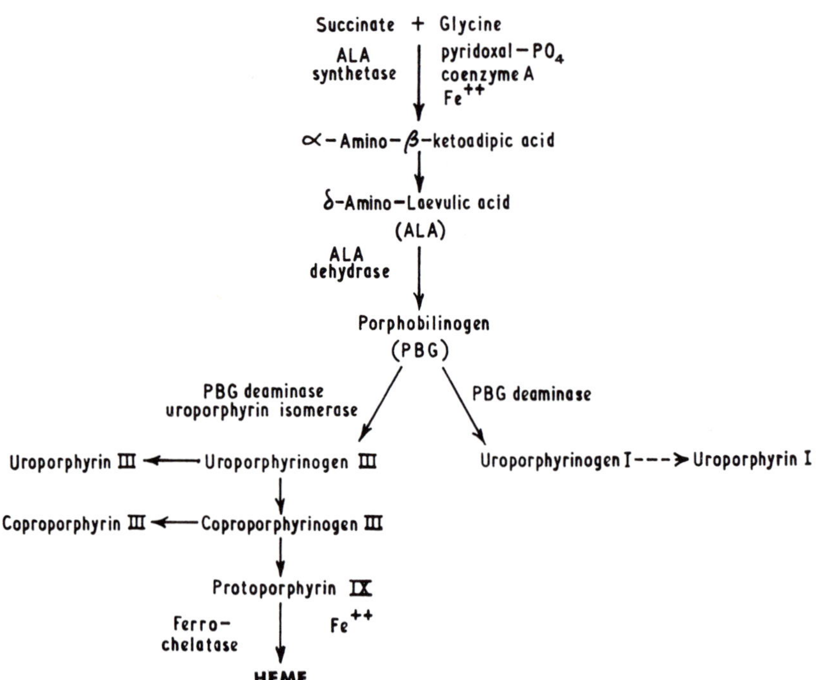

Fig. 13-4. The biosynthesis of heme. (Gray, C. H.: Miscellaneous disorders in metabolism: III. Porphyrias. *In* Thompson, R. H. G., and King, E. J. [eds.]: Biochemical Disorders in Human Disease. ed. 2, Chap. 22, p. 852, Fig. 5. New York, Academic Press, 1964)

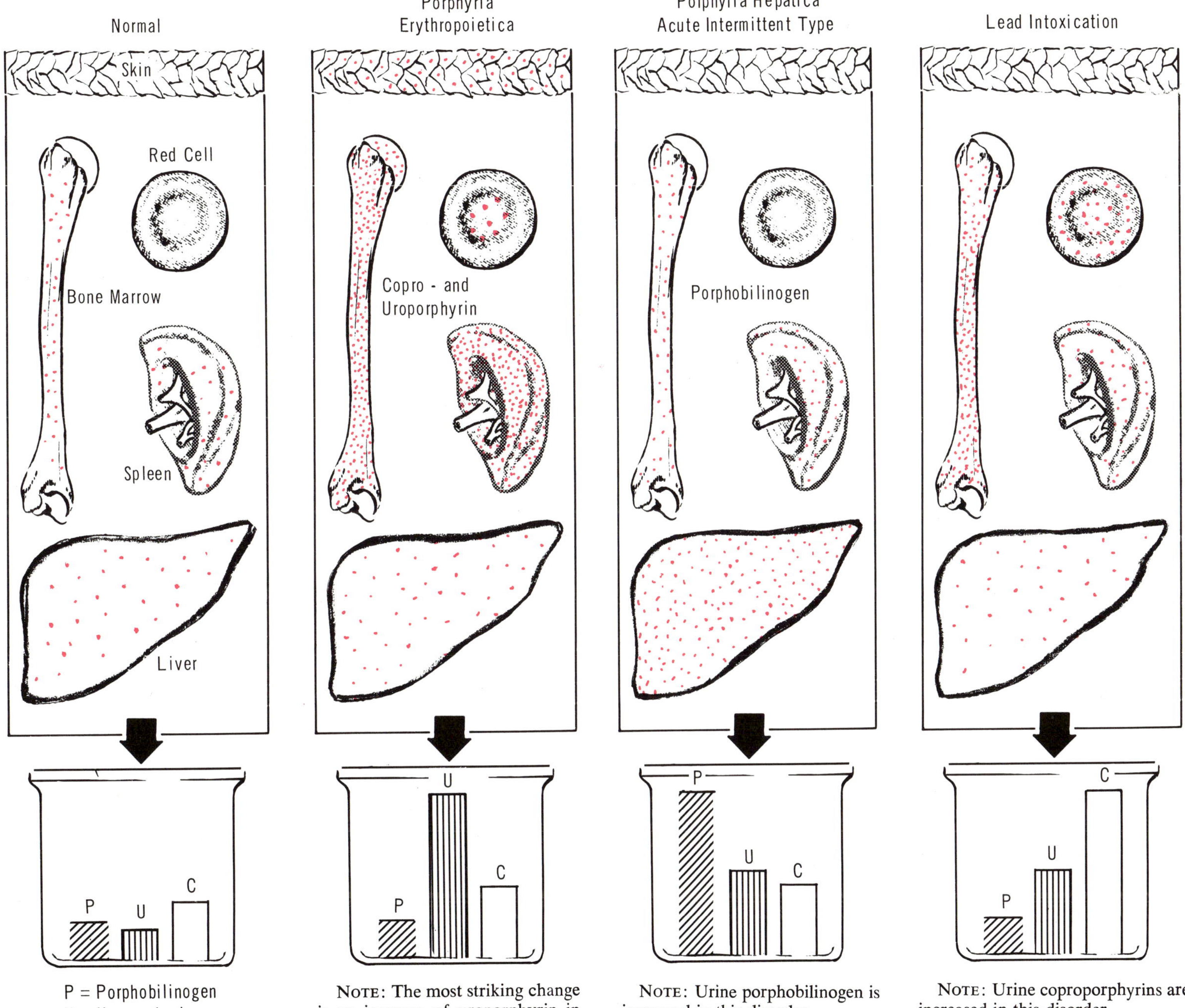
Normal
Porphyria Erythropoietica
Porphyria Hepatica Acute Intermittent Type
Lead Intoxication
Skin
Red Cell
Bone Marrow
Spleen
Liver
Copro - and Uroporphyrin
Porphobilinogen
P
U
C
P = Porphobilinogen
U = Uroporphyrin
C = Coproporphyrin
NOTE: The most striking change is an increase of uroporphyrin in the urine.
NOTE: Urine porphobilinogen is increased in this disorder.
NOTE: Urine coproporphyrins are increased in this disorder.

FIGURE 13-5

Production and Excretion

Production. Porphyrins are produced as intermediaries or by-products in the formation of hemoproteins from succinate and glycine (Fig. 13-4). In this synthesis small amounts of uroporphyrin, coproporphyrin, and porphobilinogen get into the blood and are excreted in the urine and feces. Most of the hemoproteins (catalases, peroxidases, cytochromes, etc.) may be synthesized in any cell in the body. However, hemoglobin is synthesized only in the hemopoietic organs.

Excretion. Porphyrins are excreted in the urine and feces. From 15 to 30 mcg. of uroporphyrin (mainly type I) is excreted daily in the urine and 20 to 60 mcg. in the feces. Between 300 and 1,400 mcg. of coproporphyrin (primarily type I) is also excreted in the feces each day. Equal amounts of porphobilinogen (approximately 4 mg./day) are excreted in the urine and feces.

Disorders

(Fig. 13-5)

Lead Poisoning. In this disorder there is a block in the synthesis of hemoglobin from succinate and glycine. The block may be in the formation of porphobilinogen from δ-*aminolevulinic acid,* for the latter is excreted in increased amounts in the urine (80 to 150 mg./day). The block may occur at other points in hemoglobin synthesis, since *coproporphyrin* (type III) is also excreted in large amounts in the urine and accumulates in both mature and immature red blood cells. A blood lead level establishes the diagnosis.

Coproporphyrin is also increased in aplastic anemias in which chemical toxicity is implicated, and in hemolytic anemias.

Hepatic Disease. In cirrhosis and other liver diseases there is an increase of urine coproporphyrin (200-800 mcg./day) of both the type I and the type III variety. The exact cause of this is unknown. Uroporphyrin may also be increased but not as frequently as the coproporphyrin.

Porphyria Erythropoietica. An inborn defect in the conversion of porphobilinogen to uroporphyrin, type III, in the course of hemoglobin synthesis occurs in this disorder, together with a marked overproduction of uroporphyrin, type I, in the bone marrow. Large amounts of uroporphyrin, type I, accumulate in the red cells, spleen, and skin and are excreted in the urine and feces. Urinary porphobilinogen is normal. The red cells hemolyze when exposed to light (as when they pass through the skin) because they may contain uroporphyrin, type I.

Porphyria Hepatica, Acute Intermittent Type. In this disorder there is a block in the conversion of porphobilinogen to uroporphyrins in the course of hemoprotein (cytochromes, peroxidases, etc.) formation in the liver, with an excessive production and excretion of porphobilinogen and δ-aminolevulinic acid in the urine. In addition, Watson has reported excessive production and excretion of uroporphyrins, types I and III, in this condition.

Porphobilinogen is also excreted in increased amounts in the urine in Hodgkin's disease, carcinomatosis, hepatic cirrhosis, and nervous system affections.

Porphobilinogen may be detected in the urine simply by adding Ehrlich's reagent to the urine and extracting with chloroform. In the presence of either porphobilinogen or urobilinogen, the urine turns red when mixed with Ehrlich's reagent. However, porphobilinogen is not extracted with chloroform, whereas urobilinogen is. Failure of butanol extraction is even more specific than chloroform. Further confirmation may be had by spectroscopic examination of porphobilinogen aldehyde. A strong absorption band is found at 552 to 556 mμ.

Porphyria Hepatica, Cutaneous Type. In this disorder coproporphyrin is excreted in large amounts in the feces and urine. Porphobilinogen excretion is usually normal.

THE DETECTION OF TOXIC SUBSTANCES IN THE BLOOD AND URINE

There are numerous drugs and poisons that are intentionally or accidentally ingested. Only the most common will be discussed here.

Arsenic. Hair, nails, and urine can be examined for arsenic content. Arsenic is no longer a popular means of homicide.

Barbiturates. In suspected barbiturate intoxication, both blood and urine levels may be determined. A blood level of more than 3 mg./100 ml. of blood is diagnostic, and 1–3 mg./100 ml. suspicious.

Bromides. Although Bromo Seltzer® is not as popular as it used to be, abuse of this analgesic is still seen. Blood-bromide levels should be determined, especially in patients with delirium, psychosis, or dementia of unknown cause. A bromide level of more than 150 mg./100 ml. is diagnostic. Blood levels should also be used to monitor therapy (epilepsy, etc.).

Carbon Monoxide. Poisoning from carbon monoxide may be determined by drawing blood for carboxyhemoglobin concentration. Above 5% saturation is abnormal. A quick qualitative method is to mix 1 ml. of blood with 200 ml. of distilled water. If there is over 20% saturation the resulting solution will be unusually pink.

Carbon Tetrachloride (and related compounds). Organic chlorine compounds can be tested for in the urine and body fat.

Digoxin. An accurate method of determining digitalis toxicity has long been sought. For years indirect methods such as the ECG and response of heart rate to intravenous potassium have been used. Now assay of blood for digoxin is available in most large community hospital laboratories. Normal levels are 1.2 to 3.0 ng./100 ml. 4–6 hours after ingestion. Assay for other digitalis preparations may be done also, but many clinicians are shifting their patients to digoxin because of the availability of this assay method.

Ethyl Alcohol. A blood–alcohol level is now more frequently asked for, especially by the state police. When the blood is obtained the needle, syringe and skin must not have been contaminated with alcohol. Sodium oxalate should be used as the anticoagulant. A blood level above 0.11% is abnormal, and above 0.18% is diagnostic of intoxication.

Lead. The best test for lead intoxication is the blood–lead level. More than 40 mcg. per 100 ml. is abnormal.

Marihuana. An in vitro test of a cigarette or particles of "tobacco" is available and should be resorted to when no other proof is evident.

Phenothiazines. A urine test for phenothiazines is easily performed. The urine is acidified with nitric acid and a few drops of tincture of ferric chloride are added. A violet color results if phenothiazines are present. A dipstick test with Phenistix (Ames Company) may also be used but is not as accurate.

Quinidine. Blood levels for quinidine can now be used to monitor therapy in cardiac patients.

Salicylates. Both blood and urine may be sent to the laboratory for salicylate levels. A serum salicylate level of more than 45 mg./100 ml. is considered toxic. Patients on aspirin for rheumatoid arthritis and allied diseases should have their blood–salicylate levels monitored from time to time. The urine test is simple, utilizing ferric chloride; but even simpler is the use of Phenistix.

14 Renal Function Tests

Determination of the blood levels of urea nitrogen and other waste products excreted by the kidney is a poor measure of renal function. They are not altered except in the late or severe stage of renal disease. When impairment of renal function is mild, more sensitive tests must be utilized. To understand the use of these tests it is necessary to understand how urine is formed.

URINE FORMATION

Normally, 1,200 ml. of blood, or 650 ml. of plasma, flows through the two kidneys each minute. In the first step of urine formation 19 per cent of the renal plasma flow, or 120 ml. per minute of plasma, is filtered through the glomeruli, most of its protein remaining behind in the glomerular capillaries. Thus most of the organic and the inorganic chemicals in the blood (glucose, amino acids, urea, uric acid, sodium, potassium, etc.) reach the tubular lumen in concentrations similar to those of the blood. The specific gravity of the glomerular filtrate is 1.010, the same as that of a protein-free filtrate of plasma. The tubules act on this filtrate by reabsorbing almost entirely substances that are useful to the body, such as glucose and amino acids, and large quantities of water. The greater part of the waste products, such as urea, phosphates, and sulfates, is allowed to remain in the urine, but moderate amounts of some of these are reabsorbed. Much of the sodium is reabsorbed in exchange for hydrogen and potassium ion under the influence of the aldosterone hormone of the adrenal cortex. Although the greater part of the water is reabsorbed by passive diffusion in the proximal tubules, some is reabsorbed in the distal and collecting tubules under the influence of the antidiuretic hormone (ADH) from the neurohypophysis. Finally, creatinine, potassium, penicillin, and other synthetic products are secreted into the urine by the tubules. Each day 180 l. of fluid containing 25,000 of mEq. of sodium and 25 gm. of urea is filtered through the glomeruli to form approximately 1 l. of urine containing 150 mEq. of sodium and 15 gm. of urea.

To summarize, urine is formed by the *filtering of plasma* through *the glomeruli* of the kidneys, and the tubules *selectively reabsorb* those substances useful to the body and leave behind or *secrete* into the urine those substances undesirable to the body. Laboratory tests have been developed to evaluate each of these processes of urine formation in health and disease.

LABORATORY TESTS

Glomerular Filtration

Suppose one is considering a substance that is excreted into the urine only by glomerular filtration. Then if the concentration of that substance appearing in the urine and the volume of urine excreted each minute is known, and the amount in each milliliter of blood passing through the kidney, it is possible to determine the amount of plasma that would have to pass through the glomeruli each minute to clear that amount of substance: this last is the glomerular filtration rate. The calculation is based on the old formula of volume times normality equals volume times normality. To rephrase this in another way, the urinary content of a substance that can be excreted only by glomerular filtration is directly proportional to the concentration of that substance in the plasma passing through the glomerular membrane (the glomerular filtrate).

It is easy to determine the *concentration of such a substance in the blood* (B). The amount of the substance in the urine can be determined by multiplying the *concentration* (U) by the *number* of milliliters of *urine excreted in a given period of time* (V). With these three figures at hand, it is possible to calculate the glomerular filtration rate (G.F.R.), or *renal clearance*, by the equation

$$\text{G.F.R.} = \frac{UV}{B}$$

Inulin is a substance that is excreted only by glomerular filtration. None is reabsorbed or secreted by kidney tubules. Thus the inulin clearance can be a useful test of glomerular filtration.

It is more practical, however, to use a substance such as urea, which obviates the introduction of a foreign substance into the body. There are two difficulties in using this substance. First, all the urea filtered by the glomeruli is not excreted in the urine. At least one third is reabsorbed passively in the proximal tubule. Thus, in the healthy subject only 75 ml. of the 120 ml. of plasma filtered through the glomeruli each minute can be completely cleared of its urea. Second, the amount of urea excreted depends on the volume of urine formed. If the volume of urine formed excedes 2 ml./min., the urea clearance bears a nearly constant relation to the filtration rate; when the volume formed is below this amount, the relation is not so constant.

Thus in performing this test it is important to force fluid so that urine formed exceeds 2 ml./min., giving the maximum urea clearance. Then the same formula may be used as that which was applied in determining the inulin clearance:

$$\text{Clearance} = \frac{UV}{B}$$

When the urine flow is below 2.0 ml./min., the formula must be modified as follows:

$$\text{Clearance} = \frac{U\sqrt{V}}{B}$$

This is called the *standard urea clearance*. But utilizing the square root does not always accurately correct for the lowered urine volume. The use of the above formulas is better illustrated by applying them to clinical problems.

Urea Clearance. In performing the urea clearance test the patient drinks 1,000 ml. of water in the morning, 1 hour later urine is collected for a 1-hour period, and in the middle of that period a specimen of blood for urea nitrogen determination is drawn. Suppose that the BUN (B in the formula) on a patient is 18 mg./100 ml., or .18 mg./ml., the urine volume during the 1-hour interval is 150 ml., or 2.5 cc./min. (V in the formula), exceeding maximum clearance, and the concentration of urea in the urine is 4 mg. per cc. (U in the formula). Then by using the formula for maximum clearance:

$$\text{Urea Clearance} = \frac{UV}{B} = \frac{4 \times 2.5}{.18} = 55.5 \text{ cc./min.}$$

This is substantially below the normal of 75 ml./min., an indication of renal disease even though the BUN is normal.

Suppose that the BUN is 20 mg./100 ml., or 0.20 mg./ml., the urine volume is 101 ml. in 1 hour, or 1.69 cc./min. (below the maximum clearance), and the concentration of urea in the urine is 3 mg./cc. Then by using the formula for standard clearance:

$$\text{Urea clearance} = \frac{U\sqrt{V}}{B} = \frac{3 \times 1.3}{.20} = 19.5 \text{ cc./min.}$$

This is considerably below the normal standard clearance of 55 ml./min., an indication of renal disease.

Endogenous Creatinine Clearance. Measuring the rate of endogenous creatinine excretion provides certain advantages over measuring urea clearance. The clearance of endogenous creatinine is very close to that of inulin in health. The blood level of creatinine, unlike that of urea, is very constant. Thus the clearance of creatinine can be measured over a 24-hour period. Finally, the clearance is unaffected by the volume of urine.

Urine is collected for a 24-hour period, and a single blood sample is taken at the end of the test. The creatinine clearance is then computed with the same formula used above:

$$\text{Clearance} = \frac{UV}{B}$$

The normal value is 150 to 180 l./24 hrs. per 1.73 sq m. of body surface.

Tubular Reabsorption

Defective tubular reabsorption may be suggested by finding glucose or amino acids in the urine or by a persistently alkaline urine. This function is best evaluated by the *concentration test.* The test depends on the ability of the distal tubule to reabsorb water in the presence of adequate amounts of antidiuretic hormone (ADH). If the tubules are able to reabsorb water, the urine will become concentrated and have a high specific gravity in states of water deprivation.

The Fishberg concentration test is one of the simplest of these procedures. The subject to be tested is given nothing by mouth after 6 P.M. on the night before the collection of test samples of urine. Dehydration results, inducing maximal endogenous ADH secretion. The following day specimens of urine are collected at 9, 10, and 11 A.M. The specific gravity is normally 1.025 or greater in one of these specimens.

In patients with *chronic nephritis* the damaged tubules are unable to reabsorb water. Thus the urine appearing in the collecting tubules from these nephrons has a specific gravity like that of the glomerular filtrate (1.010). Since in many cases many glomeruli have also been destroyed, the other glomeruli are required to excrete a greater load of solutes. This creates an osmotic diuresis and prevents the normal tubules from reabsorbing much water.

The urine specific gravity is invariably low in patients with *nephrogenic diabetes insipidus,* who fail to concentrate the urine because of an hereditary defect in the renal tubular reabsorption of water. These patients have adequate antidiuretic hormone secretion (p. 50).

Patients with *disease of the posterior pituitary* (diabetes insipidus) do not produce adequate ADH. Therefore they also do not reabsorb enough water in the distal tubules to concentrate the urine even in states of water deprivation. Specific gravities of 1.003 to 1.008 are common. Recently, to eliminate the water deprivation of the Fishberg test, a single 5-unit injection of pitressin tannate in oil is given in the late afternoon. Urine collections at 6 A.M., 9 A.M., and 12 A.M. are made the following day.

Tubular Secretion

This is evaluated by introducing a substance into the blood that is excreted almost entirely by tubular secretion. Such a substance is the dye phenosulfophthalein (PSP). After the patient drinks 600 to 800 ml. of water, he receives 1.0 ml. (6 mg.) of the dye intravenously and empties his bladder at 15, 30, 60, and 120 minutes afterward. The percentage of PSP in each urine specimen is measured. Normally, 25 to 50 per cent of the dye is excreted in the first 15 minutes, a total of 40 to 60 per cent in the first hour, and 80 to 85 per cent within the first 2 hours. An abnormal result indicates either *renal tubular disease* or diminished renal plasma flow, as might occur in *shock* and *heart failure.* If the latter conditions are excluded, then the abnormal results are probably due to renal disease.

This test may help to indicate where the renal disease is most prominent. For example, in acute glomerulonephritis the PSP may be normal when creatinine clearance is depressed, an indication that glomerular damage exceeds tubular damage. On the other hand, the PSP excretion may be reduced when creatinine clearance (or glomerular filtration) is normal, as in pyelonephritis, hydronephrosis, and tubular disease due to prolonged hypokalemia.

PRIMARY PURPOSE

Generally, renal function tests such as these cannot be used to establish the cause of renal disease. They are primarily utilized merely to detect renal damage when it is suspected clinically. This test can be of great value in evaluating the severity of hypertension. Renal function tests are also of value in following acute and chronic nephritis whatever the cause.

15 Radioactive Isotopes in Diagnosis

Radioactive isotopes have now achieved an important place in laboratory diagnosis. Since these tests are performed by specially trained personnel, the clinician needs to know very little about the technical aspects of the tests. It is important for him to know which tests are valuable for clinical use, their physiological basis, their limitations, and the indications for their use. Some of these tests have already been mentioned in other sections of this text.

GASTROINTESTINAL TRACT

Schilling Test. Vitamin B_{12} tagged with radioactive coballt (Co^{60}) is given orally to patients suspected of having pernicious anemia, and the urinary output of tagged B_{12} is measured. Because their gastric mucosa fails to elaborate intrinsic factor, patients with pernicious anemia are unable to absorb the tagged B_{12}. Consequently, they excrete less than 5 per cent of it in the urine. Patients with sprue or a severe malabsorption syndrome are also unable to absorb B_{12} even though their stomachs elaborate sufficient intrinsic factor. To differentiate the two disorders, the test is repeated, but this time the intrinsic factor is given along with the radioactive B_{12}. The urinary output of tagged B_{12} is returned to normal in pernicious anemia, whereas it remains low in malabsorption syndrome. The test may be modified by measuring the output of radioactive B_{12} in the feces or the liver uptake of this substance.

Cr^{51} Quantitation of Blood Loss Through the Gastrointestinal Tract. Very small amounts of gastrointestinal bleeding (5 ml. or less) may be detected by tagging a sample of the patient's blood with Cr^{51} and measuring the radioactivity in the stool. When there is strong clinical suspicion of gastrointestinal bleeding in the presence of repeatedly negative stools for occult blood, this test may settle the question.

Radioactive Triolein Uptake. A test meal of triolein tagged with I^{131} is given to patients suspected of having a malabsorption syndrome, and plasma, urine, and feces are scanned for radioactivity. Normally, less than 2 per cent of the tagged triolein is excreted in the feces in the subsequent 48 hours, and plasma levels of 12 per cent or higher are obtained in 6 hours. In malabsorption syndrome less is absorbed, so that the fecal level is higher, whereas the plasma level is lower (Fig. 15-1A). Patients with chronic pancreatitis may also have diminished absorption of radioactive triolein. The reason is that they lack the enzymes to digest triolein to oleic acid and glycerol. To differentiate the two conditions, oleic acid tagged with I^{131} is administered (Fig. 15-1B). This is easily absorbed in chronic pancreatitis, but it suffers the same fate as triolein in a malabsorption syndrome.

HEMOPOIETIC SYSTEM

Blood Volume. A specific amount of serum albumin labeled with a specific number of microcuries (20 or thereabout) of radioactive iodine is injected intravenously. After allowing time for sufficient mixing in the circulation (about 10 minutes), a blood sample is withdrawn and analyzed for radioactivity. The blood volume can be indirectly determined by dividing the number of radioactive units injected by the radioactivity per milliliter of blood after dilution. Red cells tagged with Cr^{51} may be used in a similar fashion, and this is a more accurate but more time-consuming procedure. It may be wise to use both methods at the same time to get best results. This procedure is of great value in differentiating hemorrhagic shock from other forms of peripheral circulatory failure. It is also useful in following cases of acute renal failure, in diagnosing early congestive heart failure, and in following gastrointestinal bleeders and intestinal obstruction.

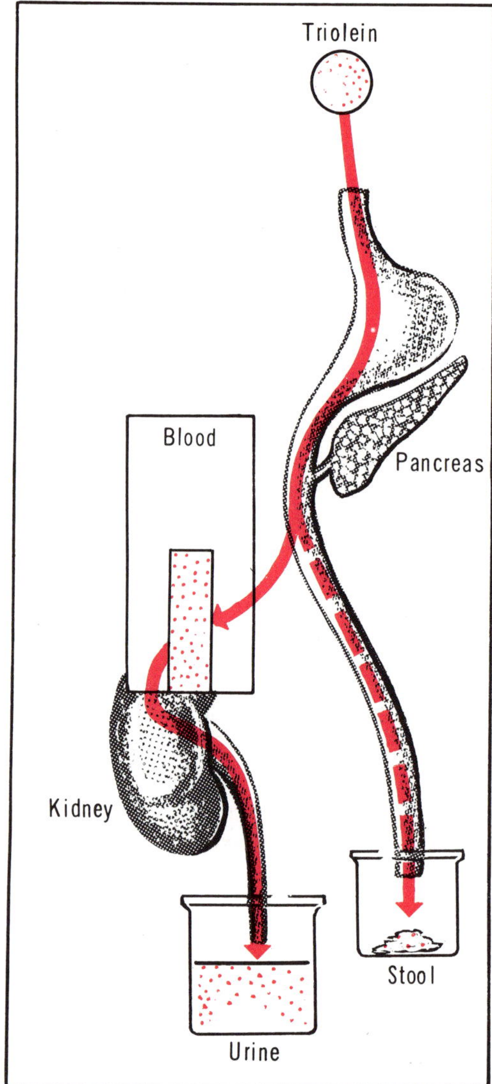

Normal

NOTE: Triolein is broken down to oleic acid and glycerol and absorbed.

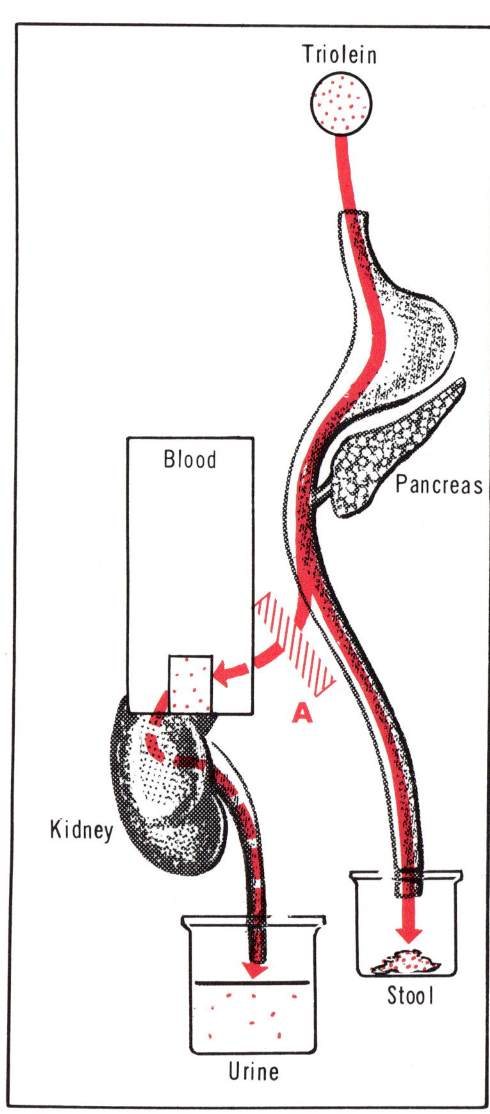

Malabsorption Syndrome

NOTE: A mucosal block (A) prevents the absorption of neutral fats.

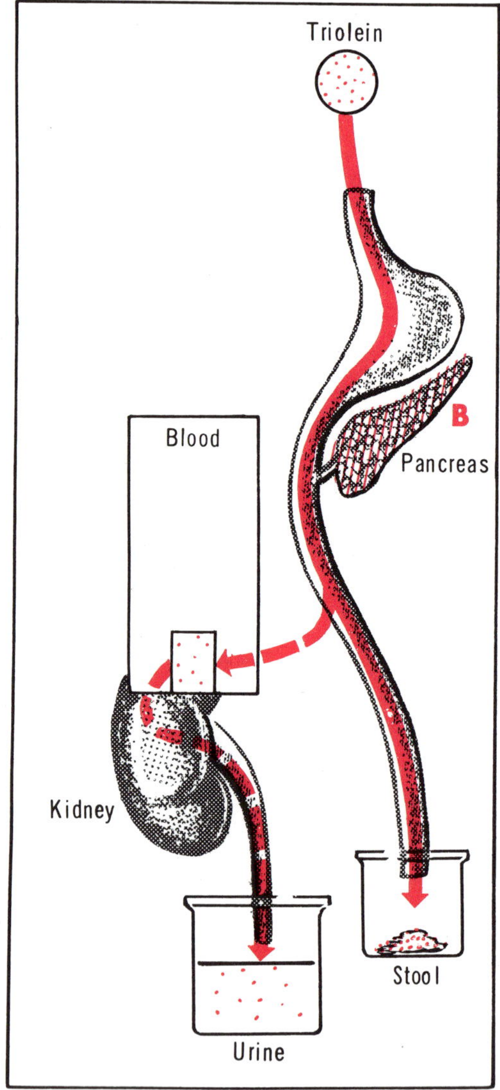

Pancreatitis

NOTE: Lack of lipolytic enzymes (B) prevents breakdown of triolein to fatty acids that may be absorbed.

FIG. 15-1A. Radioactive triolein uptake.

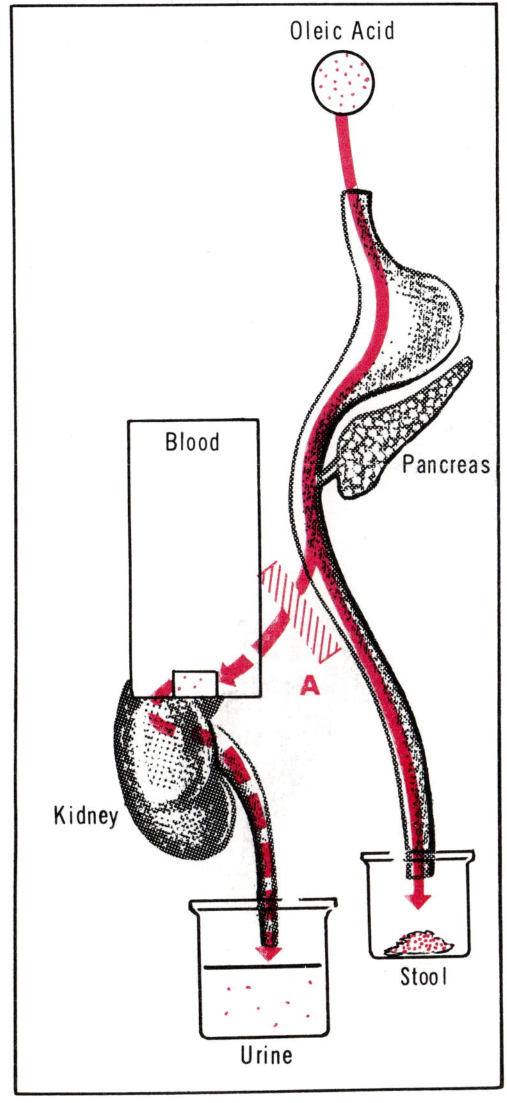

Malabsorption Syndrome
due to Celiac Disease

NOTE: Oleic acid cannot be absorbed because of the mucosal block (A).

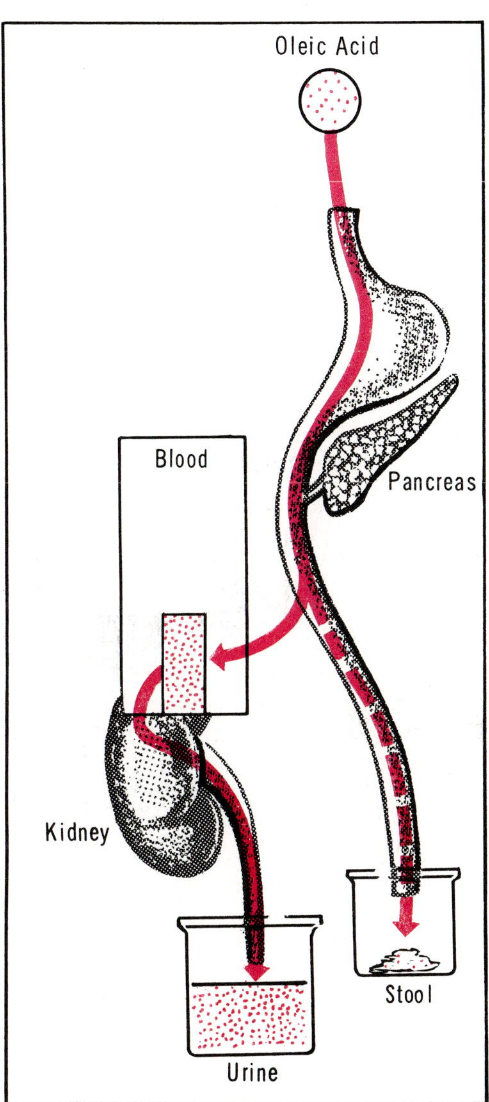

Malabsorption Syndrome
due to Pancreatitis

NOTE: Oleic acid is absorbed as there is no mucosal block.

FIG. 15-1B. Radioactive oleic acid uptake.

Red Cell Survival Time. A sample of blood is taken from a patient suspected of a hemolytic anemia, and the red cells are tagged with Cr^{51} and reinjected. Serial blood samples are assayed for radioactivity over a period of 2 weeks. An erythrocyte half-life below 26 days suggests hemolytic anemia. Once the diagnosis of hemolytic anemia is established, it is well to determine whether this is due to intrinsic abnormalities in the patient's red cells or to toxic or immunologic effects of the patient's plasma. This can be done by injecting a sample of tagged red cells from the patient into a normal but compatible recipient. If these red cells survive normally, it can be assumed that some factor in the patient's plasma is responsible for the hemolysis. If they still show a short survival time, the cells themselves probably have some intrinsic defect. To verify that a hemolytic factor is present in the patient's plasma, tagged red cells from a compatible normal donor may be injected into the patient. These cells should show a shortened survival under such circumstances.

ENDOCRINE SYSTEM

Radioactive I^{131} Uptake. Five to 25 μc of radioactive iodine (I^{131}) is administered orally, and the amount of radioactivity in the thyroid is measured in 6 and 24 hours (and in 2 hours when indicated). The normal gland traps between 15 and 45 per cent of the dose after 24 hours. In myxedema the 24-hour uptake rarely exceeds 15 per cent (Fig. 15-2). In pituitary myxedema the uptake will return to normal after an injection of thyrotropic hormone, but this will not be the case in primary myxedema. In hyperthyroidism, 24-hour uptakes of 50 to 70 per cent are the rule. Occasionally, the maximum uptake is reached earlier in this disorder, and so it is important to measure the uptake at an earlier time (2, 6, or 8 hours).

The urinary excretion of radioactive iodine has also been used in the diagnosis of dysfunction of the gland. A 24-hour urine test is required. Normally, 30 to 70 per cent of the dose is excreted in the 24 hours after administration. Less is excreted in hyperthyroidism and more in hypothyroidism. The test is less reliable than the uptake because dependable results are obtainable only if renal function is unimpaired (a fact that is not easy to ascertain).

The radioactive I^{131} uptake is affected by the ingestion of both organic and inorganic iodides, steroids, and other drugs. The pitfalls of this test have been reviewed in other textbooks.*

* See Quimby, E. H., Feitelberg, S., and Silver, S.: Radioactive Isotopes in Clinical Practice. Philadelphia, Lea & Febiger, 1958.

Radioactive T_3 Red Cell Uptake. This test is an in vitro test with the advantage that no radioactive material need be administered to the patient. Radioactive triiodothyronine (T_3) is mixed with the patient's blood, and the percentage that combines with the surface of the patient's red cells is measured. Normally, 25 to 35 per cent combines with the red cells. If the thyrobinding protein is saturated with thyroxine (T_4), as in hyperthyroidism, most of the radioactive T_3 will combine with the red cells, and the T_3 uptake will be above 40 per cent (Fig. 15-3). If the thyrobinding protein is bound to very little thyroxine, as in hypothyroidism, most of the radioactive T_3 will combine with the thyrobinding protein and very little with the red cells (less than 25%). This test is very useful in patients who have recently ingested iodides or had radiocontrast studies (with Hypaque, etc.), in which case the PBI would be inaccurate. Neither organic nor inorganic iodine distorts the test results. A resin sponge that will pick up the radioactive T_3 has now been substituted for the red cells.

T_4 by Isotope. This test is also called the Murphy-Pattee or T_4 by competitive binding. One milliliter of the patient's serum is mixed with 2 ml. of ethyl alcohol and allowed to stand. The alcohol extracts almost all of the thyroxine in the serum. The extract is then added to a standard solution of TBP-thyroxine I^{125}. While the solution stands, the patient's thyroxine competes with the radioactive thyroxine for binding sites on the TBP and displaces some of the radioactive thyroxine into a free state. A resin sponge is dropped into the solution to pick up the free thyroxine I^{125}. The resin is separated from the solution and the radioactivity measured by a Geiger counter. The amount of thyroxine I^{125} counted will be proportional to the level of thyroxine in the patient's serum.

Scintillation Scanning. By using a Geiger-Mueller tube or a similar device, the radioactive uptake of I^{131} is measured systematically over small sections of the thyroid at a time. In this way the clinician can determine whether the uptake is the same in each area of the gland or whether there are localized areas of increased or decreased uptake (Fig. 15-4). The uptake is uniform in all areas of the gland in the normal, hyperplasia, and myxedema. In benign adenomas small areas of increased uptake ("hot" nodules) or decreased uptake ("cold" nodules) may be noted. In carcinoma areas of decreased uptake ("cold" nodules) are the rule. A "hot" nodule is invariably benign. Only a small percentage of "cold" nodules are malignant. Scintillation scanning is also useful in detecting substernal thyroids, ectopic thyroid tissue, and metastatic deposits of thyroid carcinoma.

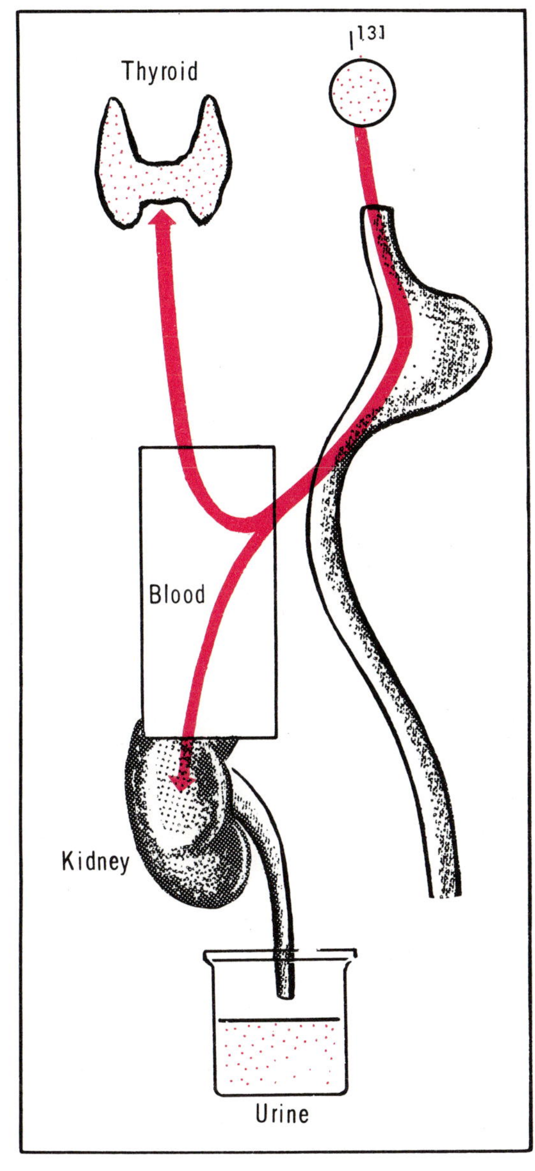

Normal

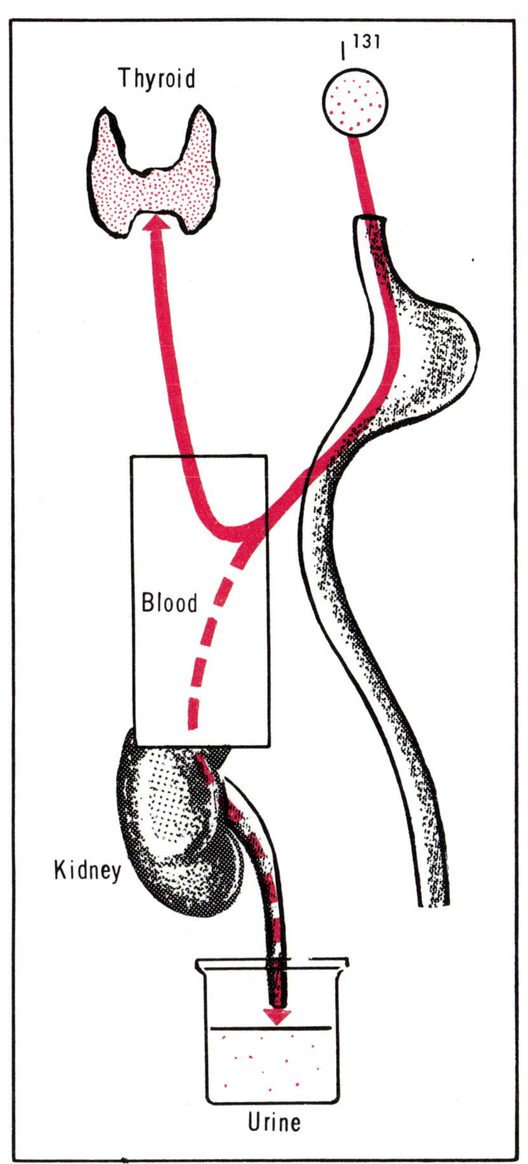

Hyperthyroidism
(Graves' Disease)

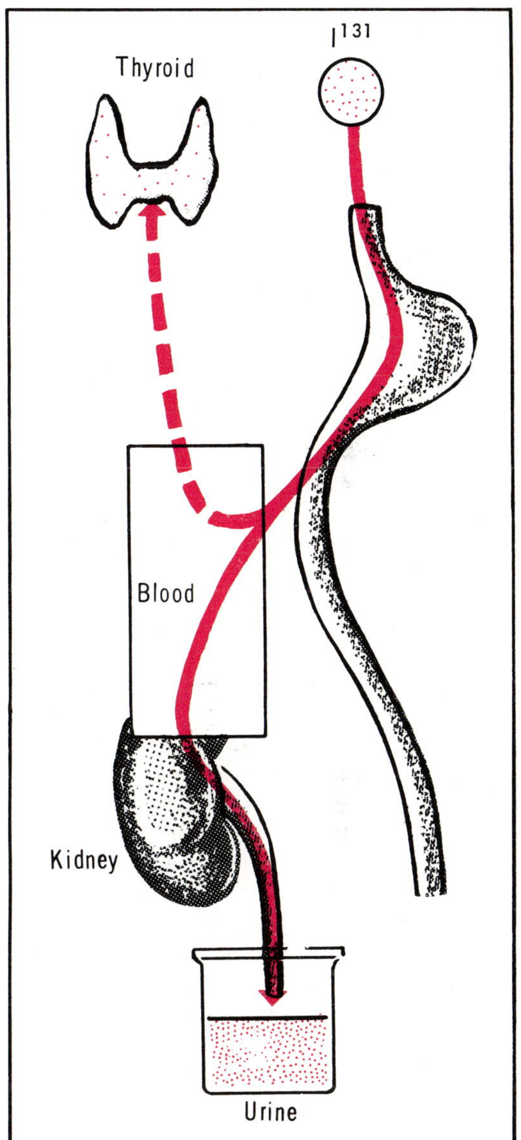

Hypothyroidism

FIG. 15-2. Radioactive I^{131} uptake.

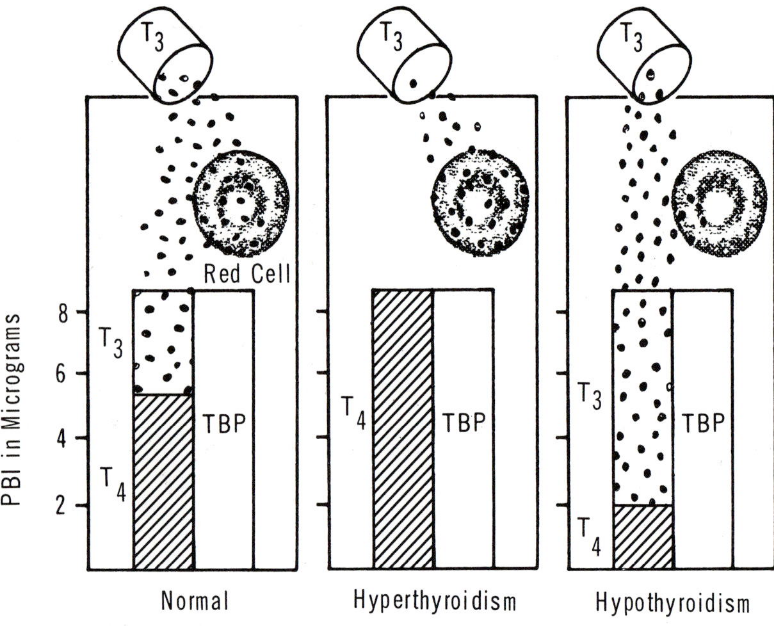

Note: Part of T_3 is bound to TBP and part to red cell.

Note: Most of T_3 is bound to red cell as TBP fully saturated.

Note: Most of T_3 is bound to TBP (which is bound to very little T_4).

T_3 = triiodothyronine
T_4 = thyroxine
TBP = thyrobinding protein

FIG. 15-3. Radioactive T_3 red cell uptake.

NERVOUS SYSTEM

Brain scanning with technetium-99m pertechnetate has become a widely used test for diagnosing space-occupying lesions of the brain. Tumors, abscesses, and hematomas can be picked up by this method. A negative scan does not rule out a brain tumor, as basilar tumors and posterior fossa tumors do not show well and the great majority of tumors under 2 cm. will be missed. Subdural hematomas usually cannot be picked up until they are 2 weeks old. Cerebral infarctions cause a positive brain scan, but this will usually disappear in 6 weeks. If infarction is suspected surgery can often be delayed until a repeat scan is done. Despite the above false negatives and false positives brain scanning is 85-90% accurate. It is harmless and can be done with little preparation of the patient and no discomfort. Figure 15-5 shows the anterior-posterior and lateral view of a brain scan positive for a parasagittal meningioma. Note that the tumor shows up as a "hot" nodule.

LIVER

Next to thyroid and brain scanning, liver scanning has become the most popular use of radioisotopes. Technetium–99m colloid and I^{131} rose bengal are used. There are involved little preparation and discomfort to the patient. The bone, liver, and spleen can be done together so an accurate picture of the size and function of the reticuloendothelial system can be obtained. Primary and metastatic tumors, cirrhosis, and fatty livers can be diagnosed. Figure 15-5 shows characteristic scans in these conditions. Note that tumors characteristically produce a "cold nodule" or decreased uptake. Liver scans will miss 10-15% of metastatic carcinomas and yield 10% false positives, probably due to cirrhosis.

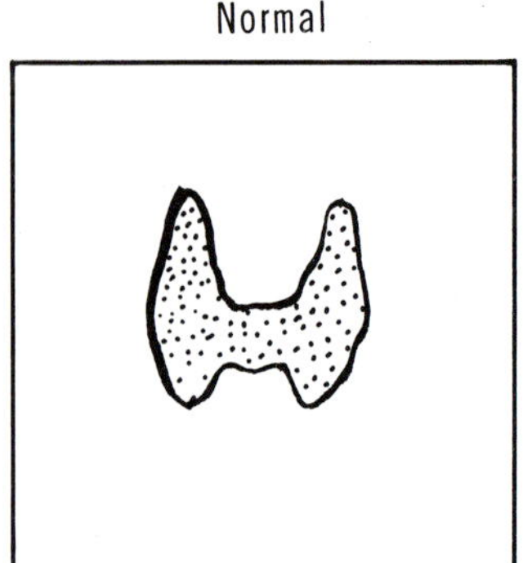

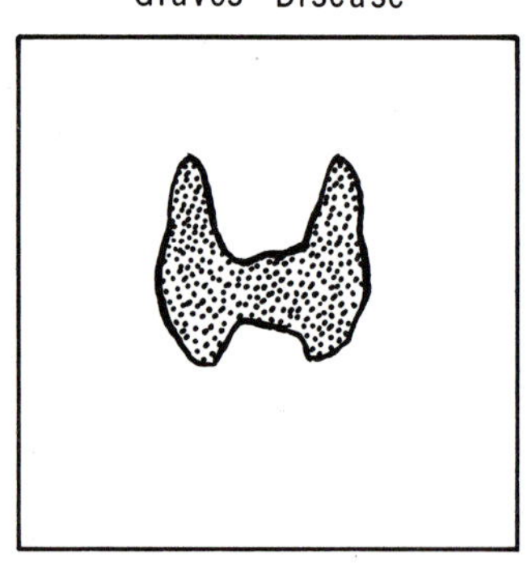

Hypothyroidism

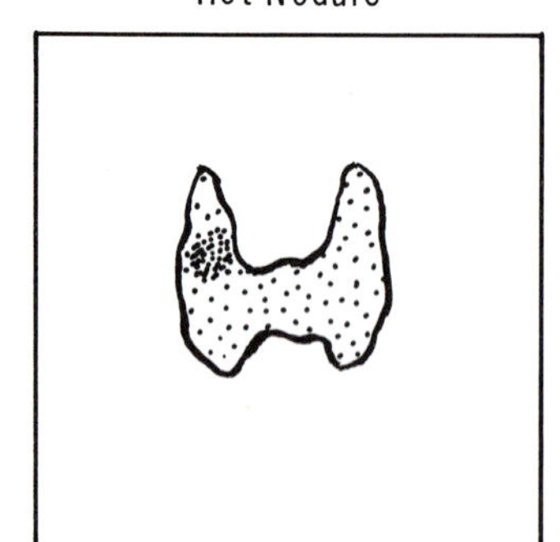

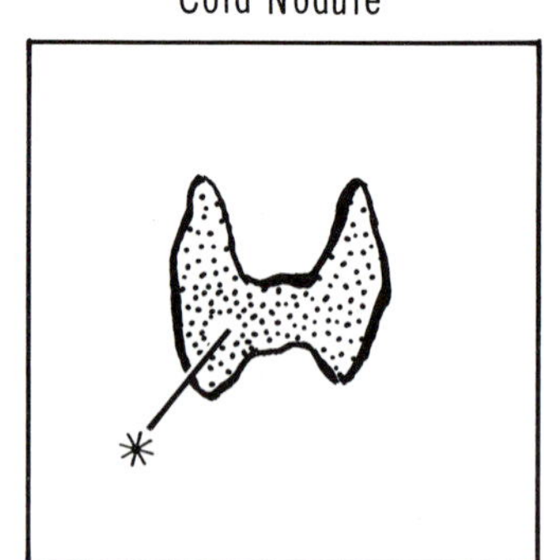

FIG. 15-4. Thyroid scans.

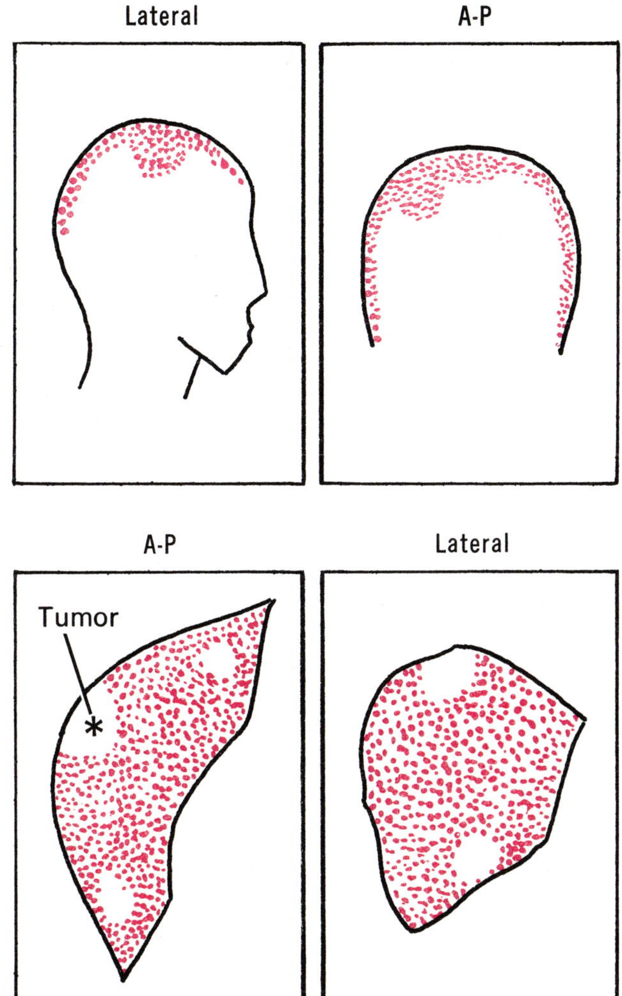

Fig. 15-5. (*Above*) Brain scan; (*below*) liver scan.

RESPIRATORY SYSTEM

Radioisotopes yield information about lung disease in two ways. They are useful in scanning for pulmonary emboli and bullae. They are used in estimating lung function. Unfortunately, scans are of little help in diagnosing early lung cancer. Technetium–99m macroaggregated albumin or I^{131} macroaggregated albumin is injected intravenously, and the material collects in the pulmonary capillaries, where it usually remains for 2 hours and then is washed away. Emboli and bullae show up as "cold nodules." Figure 15-6 demonstrates typical scans. Repeat scans are valuable in following the course.

By inhaling radioactive xenon a good test of ventilatory distribution is obtained. Normally the xenon is distributed to the alveoli symmetrically, but in emphysema and space-occupying lesions "cold nodules" will indicate areas of fibrosis or obstruction. Xenon can also be injected intravenously to demonstrate areas of decreased capillary perfusion (especially important in emphysema).

PANCREAS

Pancreatic scanning with selenomethionine is useful in diagnosing pancreatic carcinoma, pancreatitis, and other conditions. After a high-protein meal a normal pancreatic scan is effective in ruling out serious pancreatic disease.

BONE

With radioactive strontium-85 many cases of metastatic bone tumors can be diagnosed by bone scanning before the lesions are evident on x-ray. Unfortunately the strontium remains in the bone for some time, so the test is hazardous in patients without proven cancer. Recently fluorine-16 and technetium–99m polyphosphate have been introduced. These isotopes circumvent the hazards of strontium-85.

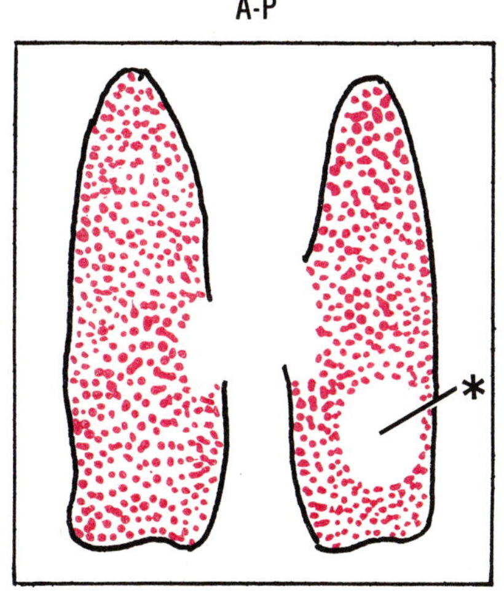

Fig. 15-6

16 Comparative Analysis of Body Fluids

The various alterations that may take place in body fluids other than the blood are remarkably similar. Furthermore, similar alterations are often caused by similar etiologies. For these reasons a comprehensive discussion of the urine, gastric juice, duodenal fluid, sputum, feces, vaginal discharge, and the cerebrospinal, pleural, peritoneal, and synovial fluids will be undertaken in this chapter.

OBTAINING THE SPECIMEN

Urine for routine analysis is easily obtained. If a culture is desired, a washed midstream specimen should be obtained. Catheterization carries the hazard of introducing infection into the bladder and should not be done routinely. Recently, the technique of suprapubic aspiration of urine from the urinary bladder has become popular for obtaining sterile specimens in women and infants. The patient should not have voided for 4 hours. After the area is cleansed a 10 cc. syringe with a #22 needle 1½ inches long is inserted in the midline just above the symphysis and directed slightly caudally. Urine is aspirated and the needle removed. Complications are rare. A 24-hour urine specimen will be necessary for certain tests (steroids, etc.).

Gastric juice is obtained by passing a Levin tube into the stomach by way of the nose, pharynx, and esophagus after applying an appropriate lubricant (Lubertine, glycerin). A fasting specimen is first obtained by sucking out the gastric contents. If this is inadequate, a test meal using histamine or Histalog (an analogue of histamine) is given. Histalog has the advantage of having few of the undesirable side-effects of histamine. A quantitative overnight specimen will be useful in certain disorders (Zollinger-Ellison syndrome, etc.).

Duodenal fluid is obtained by introducing a Levin or Rehfuss tube into the duodenum by way of the nose or mouth. Considerable patience and experience are needed, and fluoroscopy is helpful in ascertaining that the tube has reached the proper position. A double lumen gastroduodenal tube is required to assure that no gastric juice gets into the specimen when a specimen of pancreatic juice is desired. If a specimen of bile is sought, magnesium sulfate (33% solution) is given orally to relax the sphincter of Oddi. If pancreatic juice is sought, secretin (1 unit per kilogram of body weight) is given intravenously.

Sputum can at times be difficult to obtain. In fulminating bacterial infections of the respiratory tree no difficulty is encountered. However, when a specimen is required in chronic conditions (tuberculosis, etc.) it is a different story. The best time to obtain it is in the early morning at the time the patient arises. A French catheter may be passed to cause irritation and thus provoke a good cough, and some warm saline may be injected to make the cough productive. Nebulization with propylene glycol may aid in obtaining a good specimen for cytology. By injecting 10 cc. of normal saline through the crycothyroid membrane with a #22 needle ¾ inch long, an excellent specimen can be obtained. A 24-hour sputum, like a 24-hour urine, is preferred for detecting tubercle bacilli. If no sputum can be obtained, morning specimens of gastric juice can be taken for acid-fast smears and culture.

There is usually no difficulty in obtaining a specimen of **feces,** but in cases of constipation a specimen can be obtained by digital palpation. If parasites are suspected, the specimen should be examined while still warm. Several specimens and even a "cathartic stool" may be necessary to expose the parasite.

Vaginal or **cervical discharge** can be aspirated by a vaginal pipette with a suction bulb or picked up on a cotton swab and applied to the slide for examination. If cytology is to be done, special applicators are used to scrape the cervical os.

Cerebrospinal, pleural, peritoneal, and **synovial fluids** are obtained by paracentesis, that is, by inserting an appropriate needle into the cavity in question. Of course, sterilization of both patient and instruments is required as well as local anesthetics. In abdominal paracentesis the bladder should be emptied first. In thoracocentesis the needle is inserted along the upper border of the rib to avoid the intercostal vessels. Lumbar punctures are performed by inserting the needle in the lower lumbar spine to avoid the spinal cord. The fluid should be removed slowly to avoid herniation of the cerebellar tonsils.

VOLUME

Urine. The volume of urine is normally between 1,000 and 2,000 ml. a day. This represents about 0.5 per cent of the glomerular filtrate. The rest is absorbed by the renal tubules. For the most part, urine output depends on intake, glomerular filtrate rate, and tubular reabsorption.

Urine volume is increased by an increased intake of fluid, as in *hysterical diabetes insipidus,* and in the presence of increased solute load, as in *diabetes mellitus.* In *hyperthyroidism* the urine volume is increased by an increased rate of glomerular filtration. In *diabetes insipidus* and *chronic nephritis* it is increased because of decreased tubular absorption.

Urine volume is decreased when intake is diminished, as in *dehydration;* when there is abnormal loss of body fluids, as in *hemorrhagic shock, diarrhea,* or *vomiting;* and when glomerular filtration rate is diminished, as in *shock, congestive heart failure, nephritis,* and *toxic* and metabolic diseases of the *kidney.* In addition, it is decreased by obstructive lesions of the bladder and urethra, such as *prostatic hypertrophy, neurogenic bladder,* and *urethral strictures.* Rarely, bilateral ureteral obstruction is the cause.

Gastric Juice. The volume of gastric juice is normally 60 to 80 ml. per hour. The volume is increased in duodenal ulcer. Large volumes are obtained in the *Zollinger-Ellison syndrome* (noninsulin secreting islet cell adenomas of the pancreas). The volume is diminished in *gastric carcinomas, pernicious anemia,* and *gastric atrophy.*

Duodenal Fluid. This is significantly reduced after intravenous secretin in *chronic pancreatitis* and *carcinomas* of the *ampulla.*

Sputum. The volume of sputum is normally negligible. Increased volumes occur in infections of the respiratory tree, but the largest volumes are noted in pulmonary edema, *bronchiectasis,* and *lung abscess.*

Feces. Normally, 100 to 200 gm. of feces is excreted each day. The volume is, of course, increased in any condition that will cause *diarrhea* (enteritis, ulcerative colitis, etc.), but its measurement does not constitute a laboratory test. It is important to look for increased volume of feces in *malabsorption syndrome* and in *fibrocystic* disease of the *pancreas.*

Vaginal Discharge. This is normally minimal but may increase during ovulation and during bacterial and parasitic infections.

Cerebrospinal Fluid. The volume of cerebrospinal fluid is normally 60 to 120 ml. It is measured indirectly by determining the spinal fluid pressure. Normally, this is 75 to 200 mm. It is most often increased by *infections, neoplasms,* and *trauma* of the brain and meninges. *Vascular diseases* that lead to hemorrhage (berry aneurysms, A-V anomalies, etc.) also cause increased pressure. Conditions that cause increased venous pressure will elevate the spinal fluid pressure. *Congestive heart failure, pulmonary emphysema,* and *superior vena caval syndrome* are just a few. In this respect the spinal fluid is similar to pleural and peritoneal fluid.

Decreased pressure is associated with *subarachnoid block* above the level of the needle. This should be confirmed by performing a Queckenstedt test. If the jugular veins are compressed, the spinal fluid pressure normally rises from 150 mm. to 300 mm. In complete subarachnoid block a rise will not occur, and in partial block there will be a slow rise and/or a slow return to normal. A Valsalva maneuver or abdominal compression should be performed (which will cause a rise in pressure whether or not there is a block) to ascertain that the needle communicates freely with the subarachnoid space.

Pleural Fluid. This is normally negligible. Like spinal fluid, it is increased in *trauma, infections,* and *neoplasms* (but of the pleural cavity). It is similarly increased in *congestive heart failure* and disease associated with *hypoalbuminemia. Vascular disorders* (pulmonary infarct, etc.) are an infrequent cause of marked pleural effusion.

Peritoneal Fluid. This, too, is negligible under normal circumstances. It is increased by the same etiologic states that increase pleural fluid. In addition, certain *ovarian tumors,* a *ruptured ectopic pregnancy,* and *portal cirrhosis* may lead to increased peritoneal fluid. *Obstructions* of the *hepatic* or the *portal vein* are at times responsible. These would be analogous to the production of pleural fluid associated with a pulmonary infarct or congestive heart failure.

Synovial Fluid. As with pleural and peritoneal fluid, the volume is normally insignificant. It may be increased in *traumatic, neoplastic,* and *inflammatory conditions of the joint.* Most commonly, increases are due to osteoarthritis and rheumatoid arthritis.

pH

Determinations of the pH of urine, gastric juice, duodenal fluid, and vaginal discharge are important aids to clinical diagnosis.

Urine. Urine pH is normally 6 to 7.8. Changes in the urine pH are frequently a reflection of blood pH. For example, in *metabolic acidosis* the urine pH is more acid, and in *metabolic alkalosis* the urine pH is alkaline. When there is a defect in the tubular mechanism for conserving bicarbonate, however, the urine remains alkaline in the presence of acidosis. Thus in *chronic glomerulonephritis, de Toni-Fanconi syndrome, renal tubular acidosis,* and during *acetazolamide therapy* the urine may be persistently alkaline. In some cases of renal failure the ability to excrete a highly acid urine is preserved. Infecting organisms such as *Proteus,* which breaks down urea to form ammonia, and *Pseudomonas* produce an alkaline urine. On the other hand, *tubercle bacilli* are associated with a persistently acid urine.

Gastric Juice. Like urine, the pH of gastric juice is normally low but reaches much lower levels. It is consistently below 3.5. In *peptic ulcer* the concentration of hydrochloric acid as well as the volume secreted is usually high, especially in the *Zollinger-Ellison syndrome.* A 3–hour gastric analysis is useful in detecting this disorder. First a basal sample is collected for 1 hour. If this is over 10 mEq./hour the Z-E syndrome is suspected. Then Histalog (1.7 mg./kg.) is given subcutaneously and 4, ½–hour specimens are taken. HCl of over 45 mEq./hour is highly suspicious of the Z-E syndrome. This is called the MAO test (maximum acid output test). A 12–hour overnight gastric analysis will help diagnose this and other disorders (see Table 16-1).

Table 16-1. Overnight Gastric Analysis

Carcinoma of stomach	–	6.7 mEq.
Normal	–	10–30 mEq.
Duodenal ulcer	–	above 60 mEq.
Zollinger-Ellison syndrome	–	95–300 mEq.

To test the completeness of a gastric vagotomy, a gastric analysis with insulin (0.3 units/kg.) i.v. is performed. An increase of less than 20 mEq. of HCl per liter above the resting free HCl means the vagotomy was fairly complete. In *pernicious anemia, gastric atrophy,* and *gastric carcinoma,* achlorhydria is frequently found, and hypochlorhydria is usual. A good screening test for achlorhydria has been developed called the Diagnex Blue test. When ingested orally, an azure A-resin compound is broken up into azure A indicator and resin by the hydrogen ion of the gastric juice. The azure A can then be absorbed and excreted in the urine. If there is no free acid present, none will be broken down, absorbed, or excreted in the urine.

Duodenal Fluid. The pH here is normally alkaline. Its measurement is of no significance, but the measurement of the total bicarbonate after intravenous secretin is. In patients with good pancreatic function this should reach 90 mEq./liter in any 20-minute specimen. In chronic pancreatitis it will often be less.

Sputum. When there is doubt as to whether bloody expectoration is from the respiratory tract or the stomach, determining the pH with Nitrazine paper is useful. If the specimen is markedly acid, it comes from the stomach.

Vaginal Discharge. The normal pH of vaginal discharge is 3.5 to 4.5. It becomes more alkaline in *atrophic vaginitis* and infections of the vagina, notably *gonococcus.*

SPECIFIC GRAVITY

It is important to measure the specific gravity of specimens of urine as well as pleural and peritoneal fluids. Although this is not specifically determined on feces, feces that float in water are suggestive of *malabsorption syndrome.*

Urine. The specific gravity of urine indicates the degree of reabsorptive power of the kidney. The normal specific gravity of urine is 1.015 to 1.025. In *chronic nephritis* there is a gradual loss of concentrating or reabsorptive power of the kidney until the specific gravity reaches 1.010, the specific gravity of the glomerular filtrate (a "protein-free plasma filtrate"). Special concentration tests (Fishberg, etc.) are discussed on page 182. Recently the urine osmolality has been a useful alternative to the specific gravity. It is a measure of the number of osmotically active ions or particles in the urine (or any solution). Normally it is 800-1300 milliosmoles/liter after a 14–hour period of dehydration. Both tests have the same significance. The specific gravity is also reduced in *pituitary diabetes insipidus,* in which there is insufficient antidiuretic hormone to maintain distal tubular reabsorption of water, and in *renal diabetes insipidus,* in which there is renal tubular unresponsiveness to antidiuretic hormone. The specific gravity may also be diminished in *primary aldosteronism* (p. 51).

Diabetes mellitus (by increasing urine solute, i.e., glucose) and dehydration cause high urine specific gravities.

Pleural, Peritoneal, and Synovial Fluids. Determination of the specific gravity of these fluids helps to differentiate transudates from exudates. Transudates have a specific gravity of 1.006 to 1.018, whereas exudates because of a greater content of protein have a specific gravity of over 1.020. Transudates usually result from *congestive heart failure* or *hepatic* and *renal disorders* associated with *hypoproteinemia.* Exudates are, of course, caused by *infection, tumor cells,* or *bleeding.* Transudates in synovial fluid often result from *osteoarthritis.*

EXAMINATION FOR CLOTTING

Cerebrospinal Fluid. When clear spinal fluid forms a clot on standing, serious consideration should be given to the diagnosis of a *spinal cord tumor.* The turbulent spinal fluid of *tuberculous meningitis* forms a delicate weblike clot on standing. This has also been observed in *syphilitic meningitis, poliomyelitis,* and *aseptic meningitis.* The purulent fluid of *acute bacterial meningitis* almost invariably forms a coarse fibrin clot. The bloody fluid of *subarachnoid hemorrhage,* on the other hand, does not usually clot because defibrination has occurred within the subarachnoid space. This helps to differentiate it from a *traumatic tap,* in which a clot will form if there is much blood. The same can be said of bloody fluid obtained from the pleura, pericardium, or peritoneum. If it clots it is traumatic in origin. If it does not clot it signifies a disease state.

Synovial Fluid. Normal synovial fluid does not clot. When a clot forms, it almost invariably signifies an inflammatory joint.

The character of the *mucin* of the synovial fluid is important to ascertain in cases suspected of rheumatoid arthritis. This is a precipitate of hyaluronic acid. The synovial fluid is specially prepared by centrifugation, and acetic acid and distilled water are added to make a 1 per cent solution. Normal fluid forms a tight clump of ropy material (mucin) surrounded by clear fluid that is unchanged after standing for 24 hours. In *rheumatoid arthritis* either no coagulum is formed, or that which is formed may disappear shortly thereafter. Poor mucin is also found in *gouty, tuberculous,* and *gonococcal arthritis.*

APPEARANCE

Urine. Urine is normally amber. Red urine usually signifies hematuria or hemoglobinuria. This is more fully discussed under Blood (see below, this chapter). Red urine is also found in *congenital porphyria.* Urine that turns reddish brown on standing is found in acute *intermittent porphyria hepatica.* Pyridium (a urinary analgesic) turns urine orange-red. Urine that turns black on standing is characteristic of alkaptonuria. Green urine is found in *Pseudomonas infections,* and blue urine is noted after methylene blue administration. Brown smoky urine is associated with *glomerulonephritis.* Brown urine is also seen in *obstructive jaundice* (due to the presence of bilirubin).

Gastric Juice. This is normally clear but becomes red after fresh bleeding and black or coffee-ground in appearance if the blood has had a chance to undergo breakdown to heme before the specimen is taken.

Sputum. Normal sputum is clear with a slight turbidity. Like urine and gastric juice, it becomes red after *bleeding* anywhere in the respiratory tree. In *pneumococcal pneumonia* it is rusty, since the red cells have been broken down to heme. The sputum of *lung abscesses* is green or brown and foul-smelling. It often separates into layers. *Pseudomonas infections* of the respiratory tract give rise to green sputum.

Feces. Feces are normally brown. In *severe diarrhea* they become green because the pigment biliverdin has not had a chance to be converted to bile and urobilinogen. In *breast-fed infants* they are golden yellow due to the presence of unconverted bilirubin. A red stool usually signifies *bleeding* in the lower G.I. tract but may be seen after eating beets or carrots. A black stool is seen after *ingestion* of *iron but usually indicates upper gastrointestinal bleeding* (see under Blood, this chapter). Clay-colored stools are found in *obstructive jaundice,* in which bile pigments are absent from the stool.

Vaginal Discharge. This is normally colorless and slightly turbid. It becomes green in vaginal infections, particularly *gonorrhea,* and bloody during *menses* and *intermenstrual bleeding.* The discharge in *trichomoniasis* is thin, greenish, and foamy, whereas in *candidiasis* it is thin and watery with clumps of thick cheesy exudate. *Cervicitis* is associated with a white mucopurulent discharge.

Cerebrospinal Fluid. This is clear and colorless under normal circumstances. It becomes turbid and milky in *infections* and bloody in *cerebral hemorrhage.* Yellow spinal fluid may signify *previous bleeding* with lysis of the red cells, *jaundice,* or *tumor.*

Pleural and Peritoneal Fluids. Many color changes in these fluids have the same significance as those in the spinal fluid although pleural and peritoneal fluids are normally slightly yellow. Greenish purulent fluid is often seen in infections, particularly *Pseudomonas.* Bloody fluid will be more fully discussed below. Greenish peritoneal fluid may indicate a *biliary fistula.*

Synovial Fluid. This is normally clear and amber. It becomes milky in infections and turbulent and red following trauma.

BLOOD

Bleeding

This presence of blood may be determined by gross or microscopic examination or by using the benzidine or the guaiac test for occult blood. A very sensitive test of *gastrointestinal bleeding* is the radioactive chromium-tagged red cell excretion test (p. 183). The patient's red cells are tagged with radioactive chromium, reinjected into the patient, and stools are examined for radioactivity. In the presence of even minimal bleeding (5-10 ml.) the stools may contain significant radioactivity.

Determining the site of bleeding in any of the body fluids usually involves the use of selected x-ray pictures, radiocontrast studies, and endoscopy, as well as other special diagnostic procedures such as biopsy. For example, the site of gastrointestinal bleeding is determined by an upper gastrointestinal series or barium enema, gastroscopy or sigmoidoscopy. Mesenteric arteriography should also be performed. When these tests are unsuccessful, a *fluorescein string test** may be used. In studying hematuria an intravenous or retrograde pyelogram and cystoscopy are often helpful in diagnosis. A subarachnoid hemorrhage is best evaluated with arteriography.

Before considering bleeding pathological, the clinician must be sure that it is not due to trauma in obtaining the specimen (see page 190). Catheterization of the urinary tract; intubation of the gastrointestinal tract, or insertion of a needle into the subarachnoid space, the pleural or the peritoneal cavity—all of these procedures may cause bleeding. Bloody urine is often due to menstruation in females, so a washed midstream specimen must be obtained under these circumstances.

* Traphagen, D. W., and Karlan, M.: Fluorescein string test for localization of upper gastrointestinal hemorrhage. Surgery, 44:644-645, 1958.

Pathological bleeding, regardless of where it occurs, is usually due to one of five causes: trauma, inflammation, neoplasm, vascular diseases, or a coagulation disorder. The last of these is frequently forgotten. When other diagnostic procedures fail to locate a cause for the bleeding, a bleeding time, a coagulation time, a partial thromboplastin time, and a prothrombin time should be ordered to evaluate the clotting mechanism. It is of interest to compare the relative incidence of bleeding from each of these causes in the various body fluids.

Urine. Grossly bloody urine is frequent in *urethrotrigonitis,* but the most common causes are *neoplasm* and *renal calculi.* Microscopic hematuria regularly occurs in *glomerulonephritis* and often in *renal tuberculosis.* Vascular disorders such as *embolic glomerulitis* and *renal vein thrombosis* are less common causes. *Pyelonephritis* may be associated with microscopic hematuria, but *cystitis* is a more frequent cause.

It is helpful to know in what stage of micturition the urine is bloody. For this purpose a two-glass test is employed. If the initial urine is bloody, the urethra is probably the source of the bleeding, whereas if the terminal urine is bloody, the prostate or the trigone is probably responsible. When both specimens are bloody, the kidney or the bladder is the most likely source.

Gastric Juice. Bloody gastric juice commonly occurs in *esophageal varices, peptic ulcers, gastritis,* and *hiatal hernias* with *esophagitis. Mallory-Weiss syndrome* and *carcinoma* of the stomach are less common causes. In all patients with a history of hematemesis a Levine tube should be inserted and gastric washings for blood performed as part of the "physical" examination. If positive, esophagoscopy and gastroduodenoscopy should be done immediately rather than wait for x-ray studies. Coffee-ground vomitus has the same significance as bright red blood.

Sputum. Bloody sputum, like bloody urine, is frequently caused by *carcinoma* and *tuberculosis. Bronchiectasis* is another common cause. Vascular disorders such as *pulmonary infarction* and *congestive heart failure* also cause bloody sputum. Grossly bloody sputum is seen in *viral influenza* and *Klebsiella pneumoniae. Calculi* (broncholiths) are rare causes of bleeding in contrast to the calculi in the urinary tract.

Feces. Bloody stools usually result from bleeding in the lower gastrointestinal tract unless upper gastrointestinal bleeding is associated with diarrhea. Upper gastrointestinal bleeding usually produces black stools, because the blood is digested to some unknown pigment. Occult blood is detected best by the guaiac test. This is less sensitive than the Hematest but yields fewer false positives, and the patient need not be on a meat–free diet.

The commonest causes of upper gastrointestinal bleeding have already been mentioned (see Gastric Juice, above). In contrast with upper G.I. bleeding, lower gastrointestinal bleeding is most commonly due to *neoplasms.* Inflammatory conditions such as *bacilliary* and *amebic dysentery* and *ulcerative colitis* are important causes. Bleeding from *diverticulitis* is encountered frequently in the aged. Vascular disorders, such as a *mesenteric artery thrombosis,* are less common causes of bloody stools, in contrast with the frequent association of bloody spinal fluid with cerebrovascular disease. In children with a clinical picture of *intestinal obstruction, intussusception* should be remembered. Rectal bleeding is most commonly associated with *anal fissures, hemorrhoids,* and *rectal carcinomas.*

Vaginal Discharge. This is normally bloody for 3 to 5 days every 21 to 35 days. An average of 50 ml. is lost during this time, but it may be as much as 150 ml. Normal menstrual blood fails to clot. Bloody vaginal discharge is said to be pathological if it occurs between periods (when it is called metorrhagia), or if menstrual bleeding is excessive or prolonged and contains clots. Abnormal bleeding is most commonly *dysfunctional* (hormonal) or due to complications of *pregnancy.* It is often due to *neoplasms,* such as carcinomas of the cervix or endometrium and uterine fibromata, and after the menopause it should be considered as such until proven otherwise. *Coagulation defects* and *thrombocytopenia* should not be overlooked. In many cases no cause can be found. *Retained placental parts* are also at times responsible.

Cerebrospinal Fluid. In distinct contrast to other bloody fluids, bloody spinal fluid is most commonly caused by vascular disorders. These include ruptured *congenital* or *mycotic aneurysms, arteriovenous anomalies,* and *cerebral arteriosclerosis* and *hypertension. Trauma* of the brain and meninges is another frequent cause. Infection of the central nervous system rarely causes bleeding. Nor do intracranial tumors with the exception of the *glioblastomas.*

Pleural and Peritoneal Fluids. Bloody pleural or peritoneal fluid is very suggestive of a *neoplasm* in the absence of a history of trauma. *Pulmonary infarct* may be associated with a bloody pleural effusion. A red cell count of greater than 100,000/cu. mm. is almost certain evidence of this or neoplasm. A *ruptured ectopic pregnancy* or a *ruptured uterus* secondary to abruptio placenta are common causes of bloody peritoneal fluid in females of childbearing age. *Coagulation disorders* must be considered as in other body fluids.

Synovial Fluid. Bloody synovial fluid usually signifies previous *trauma,* but *hemophilia* and other coagulation disorders should be considered.

Cell Study

White Blood Cells. Under normal circumstances significant numbers of white cells are found in most body fluids except the spinal fluid. From 1 to 2 million are found in a 24–hour urine. The synovial fluid normally contains 50 to 200 white cells/cu. mm., most of which are neutrophils. Pleural and peritoneal fluids contain up to 5,000 cells/cu. mm. Although not normally suggested by examination of the feces, numerous white cells are present microscopically. Spinal fluid, on the other hand, contains less than 5 WBC's/cu. mm. Gastric and duodenal contents are not ordinarily examined for white cells. In the absence of bleeding, inflammation is usually responsible for the increased number of white cells in the body fluids, but the differential count will vary with the type of inflammation.

Inflammation and Infection

Urine. *Inflammation* anywhere in the urinary tract will produce gross or microscopic pyuria. The reader is reminded, however, that bacterial infection may occur without pyuria. If the suspicion of infection is high, the urine should be cultured even in the absence of pyuria. *Glomerulonephritis* will also produce significant pyuria, but the presence of increased red cells and granular casts will distinguish this from *pyelonephritis.* The differential white count of the urine is of little significance. However, large leukocytes with brownian movement of their cytoplasmic granules (so-called "granular motility cells" or "glitter cells") are believed to indicate *active pyelonephritis* as opposed to infection elsewhere in the urinary tract. These granules exhibit special staining characteristics with the Sternheimer-Malbin supravital stain.*

Sputum. Purulent sputum indicates infection of the respiratory tract. The differential count on a stained smear is of great diagnostic significance. In *acute bacterial infections* neutrophils predominate,

* Sternheimer, R., and Malbin, B.: Clinical recognition of pyelonephritis, with a new stain for urinary sediments. Am. J. Med., *11*:312-323, 1951.

whereas in chronic bacterial infections (tuberculosis, etc.), the *mycoses,* and *viral pneumonias,* mononuclear cells dominate the picture. As expected, the latter cells are also found in significant numbers in healing bacterial pneumonia. Mononuclear cells containing heme granules are found in *chronic congestive heart failure.* Mononuclear cells containing fat-staining vacuoles (with Sudan III, etc.) are seen in *lipoid pneumonia.* Eosinophilia of the sputum is very helpful in the diagnosis of *bronchial asthma* and other allergic conditions of the respiratory tree. These are best brought out by Giemsa stain, but Wright's stain may also be used.

Feces. Pus in the stool usually indicates inflammation of the lower colon and rectum, including *diverticulitis, ulcerative colitis,* and *amebic* or *bacillary dysentery.* The pus in these disorders is often associated with blood.

The presence of pus is unusual in the watery stools of patients with *irritable colon,* a helpful diagnostic point.

Vaginal Discharge. The discharge of *acute vaginitis* invariably contains pus cells. Pus cells are also seen in *endometritis* and occasionally in salpingitis. They are not found in significant numbers in the discharge of *cervical* and *endometrial carcinoma.*

Cerebrospinal, Pleural, Peritoneal, and Synovial Fluids. Alterations in the white cell count and differential in spinal, pleural, peritoneal, and synovial fluids have relatively the same significance. A neutrophilic leukocytosis indicates *acute bacterial infection* (meningitis, pleuritis, peritonitis, septic arthritis). However, the etiology of the infection differs from one fluid to another. *Acute bacterial meningitis* is usually due to the pneumococcus, influenza bacillus, or meningococcus. *Acute pleuritis* is most commonly due to the pneumococcus. On the other hand, *acute peritonitis* may be due to gonococcus, pneumococcus, or the *E. coli* bacillus following a ruptured viscus. *Acute septic arthritis* is most commonly gonococcal or streptococcal in origin. *Viral meningitis* or encephalitis (poliomyelitis, etc.) may produce neutrophilia in the early stages. More commonly, however, lymphocytes predominate the count. No matter which compartment *tuberculosis* involves, it is associated with a predominance of mononuclear cells. Syphilitic meningitis also produces a predominance of these cells. *Neoplasms* of the brain and spinal cord occasionally are responsible for slight elevations of the spinal fluid white count. *Cryptococcal organisms* often resemble mononuclear cells, and therefore an India ink stain should be done if there is any doubt.

CASTS

Casts are found in *sputum* and *urine.* Bronchial casts may be fibrinous, hemorrhagic, or mucous in character. They are found in *bronchitis, resolving pneumonia, tuberculosis,* and *cardiovascular diseases.* Curschmann spirals are yellowish-white masses of delicate fibrils and mucus found in *bronchial asthma.* Both the number and character of casts in the *urine* are important in diagnosis. Casts originate from the renal tubules. Occasional hyaline casts (1–2 per high-power field, 0–5,000 in a 24–hour specimen) are seen in normal urine. Large numbers appear after exercise. Red cell casts almost invariably signify injury to the glomerulus. This is most commonly the result of *glomerulonephritis,* but *embolic glomerulitis* from a subacute bacterial endocarditis or mural thrombus of the heart may be responsible, or various *collagenous diseases.* Casts containing heme pigment may result from *acute tubular necrosis* secondary to intravascular hemolysis. White cell casts invariably indicate *pyelonephritis* (acute or chronic). Epithelial cell casts characteristically appear after *acute tubular necrosis* of toxic or metabolic origin. Waxy and granular casts are probably epithelial cell casts that have degenerated. Thus they have the same significance as epithelial cell casts. "Fatty" casts, so-called because they contain lipid droplets, are seen in the *nephrotic syndrome.*

Elastic or Muscle Fibers. Such fibers may be seen in both sputum and feces. In the sputum they are formed from destruction of alveoli, bronchi, or blood vessels and indicate chronic infection, as in *bronchiectasis, abscess,* or pulmonary tuberculosis. In the feces they are undigested meat and indicate defective digestion, as in *chronic pancreatitis* and *fibrocystic disease* of the pancreas.

Farber Test. This is an excellent test for intestinal obstruction of the newborn. A specimen of the meconium is examined for amniotic squames (lanugo skin cells and hairs and vernix). These are normally swallowed but will not appear in the stool if there is intestinal obstruction.

CRYSTALS

Urine. Crystals of uric acid, calcium phosphate, calcium oxalate, cystine, and sulfonamide might lend support in diagnosing the various types of *renal calculi.*

Duodenal Fluid. Cholesterol and calcium bilirubinate crystals found in duodenal fluid are very suggestive of biliary calculi, even in the presence of a normal cholecystogram.

Sputum. Charcot-Leyden crystals, colorless pointed hexagons derived from disintegrated eosinophils, are found in the sputum of patients with *bronchial asthma.*

Synovial Fluid. The finding of urate crystals in synovial fluid is diagnostic of *gout.* Calcium pyrophosphate crystals are found in the joints of nongouty subjects with acute arthritis (pseudogout).

BIOCHEMICAL ALTERATIONS

Fat. The presence of lipid droplets in the urine is very suggestive of the *nephrotic syndrome.* They are best visualized with polarized light. Increased fat content in the stool (steatorrhea) suggests *malabsorption syndrome.* This may be due to *celiac disease, chronic pancreatitis, fibrocystic disease* of the pancreas, or biliary obstruction. Fat in the pleural or peritoneal fluid signifies obstruction and rupture of the lymphatics, with loss of chyle into these cavities. This is commonly due to *neoplasms* or *tuberculosis.* The fluid may appear to be milky.

Protein. Increased protein is a significant diagnostic finding in all body fluids except sputum, vaginal discharge, feces, gastric and duodenal juices.

Less than 0.1 gm. of protein is excreted in the *urine* in 24 hours. *Spinal fluid* also contains insignificant amounts normally (15–45 mg./100 ml.). On the other hand, the small amount of *pleural, peritoneal,* and *synovial* fluids present under normal circumstances contains 0.2 to 0.4 gm./100 ml.

Urine. Normally, less than 0.1 gm. of protein is excreted in the urine in 24 hours, and none is noted by qualitative tests on random specimens. These insignificant amounts are due to incomplete tubular reabsorption of the small amounts of protein in the glomerular filtrate (30 mg./100 ml.).

Protein appears in the urine in increased amounts in *inflammatory, toxic, metabolic,* and *vascular diseases* of the kidney and in association with hematuria. In most cases the protein is nearly all albumin. When it occurs in the absence of hematuria, it is most frequently due to increased permeability of the glomerulus. *Infections* confined to the lower urinary tract do not usually cause a significant increase in urine protein. Therefore proteinuria in the presence of pyuria should make the clinician suspect *kidney infection* (pyelonephritis, etc.). *The most significant renal cause of proteinuria is glomerulonephritis.* In the acute stage it is usually associated with significant hematuria (frequently microscopic). In the nephrotic stage (subacute stage) it may occur without hematuria and in massive amounts. *Collagenous diseases* also cause proteinuria, frequently with increased red cells and casts. *Chronic granulomatous conditions* (tuberculosis, sarcoidosis, syphilis, etc.) are rarely responsible.

Toxic conditions are frequently associated with proteinuria in *renal tubular necrosis* secondary to mercury, carbon tetrachloride, and other poisonings. More commonly, in women *preeclampsia* is responsible.

Diabetes mellitus in the form of Kimmelstiel-Wilson's disease is a common *metabolic condition* associated with proteinuria. *Gout* and *amyloidosis* should be mentioned.

Vascular diseases are also frequently associated with proteinuria. *Essential hypertension* associated with nephrosclerosis and *congestive heart failure* are the most prominent of these. The showers of emboli from *subacute bacterial endocarditis* may also be responsible, but this is usually associated with microscopic hematuria. In *multiple myeloma* a peculiar type of globulin is responsible for the proteinuria. It is called Bence-Jones protein. It precipitates after being heated to 45° to 70° and then redissolves at 100° C.

Benign orthostatic albuminuria should be ruled out before undertaking extensive diagnostic studies to expose other causes.

Stool. Large amounts of protein (10 to 50 per cent of the total plasma pool) may be lost in the stool in protein loosing enteropathy. The protein is difficult to detect as it is either digested or "eaten" by bacteria. However, a radioactive PVP test (I^{131} polyvinyl pyrrolidone test) will be useful. The radioactive substance is injected intravenously, and the stools are checked for radioactivity for the next 4 days. Patients with protein loosing enteropathy excrete up to 33% of the PVP in the stools.

Duodenal Fluid. The mucoproteins of the duodenal fluid of normal people will dissolve in distilled water, but the mucoproteins of cases of cystic fibrosis will not. This is the basis for an excellent diagnostic test. The various sweat tests should also be given.

Pleural and Peritoneal Fluids. The protein content of these body fluids is most significantly increased (above 3 gm./100 ml.) in *neoplasms* and *tuberculosis. Empyema, pulmonary infarcts,* and *lupus erythematosus* also cause high protein content in the pleural fluid. On the other hand, *congestive heart failure* and *portal cirrhosis* are associated with smaller increments of protein (less than 3 gm./100 ml.) in pleural and peritoneal fluids, respectively. Protein electrophoresis on these body fluids may be done to differentiate further the various disorders.

Spinal Fluid. As in the other body fluids, increased protein is invariably associated with hemorrhage. Just as *pyelonephritis* and *empyema* are associated with marked elevations of protein in their respective fluids, so *bacterial meningitis* is associated with a high spinal fluid protein. In the absence of cells, and elevated spinal fluid protein is very suggestive of a *neoplasm* of the central nervous system. A high protein without increased cells is also seen in *Guillian-Barré's syndrome,* occasionally in *central nervous system lues,* and in certain metabolic diseases, notably *diabetes mellitus* and *hypothyroidism.* As in urine, the presence of abnormal proteins is significant in spinal fluid. In *multiple sclerosis* there is an increase in the gamma-globulin fraction of spinal fluid protein. This is determined by protein electrophoresis after concentrating the fluid by dialysis. Abnormal spinal fluid proteins are also found in *central nervous system lues.* These are best demonstrated by the *colloidal gold test.* The test is performed by adding a colloidal solution of gold to serial dilutions (10 in all) of spinal fluid. Various changes in color appear according to the proportion of albumin to globulin in the fluid. Normally, there should be no change in color in the various dilutions. In *general paresis* and *multiple sclerosis* the color changes are most notable in the first 3 tubes (first-zone reaction). In *tabes dorsalis* the color changes usually occur in the middle 3 tubes (mid-zone reaction), although many other conditions produce the same reaction. The presence of central nervous system lues is more definitely established by serologic tests (p. 290).

Glucose

Change in the *urine* and *spinal fluid* glucose concentration is an important diagnostic aid, but this is an unimportant determination in the diagnosis of disorders of other body fluids.

Ordinarily, only minute quantities of glucose occur in the urine, while the *spinal fluid* sugar contains only 20 mg./100 ml. less than the concentration in the blood (normal value of spinal fluid glucose is 50–75 mg./100 ml.). Increased glucose has the same significance in both fluids, namely, *primary* or *symptomatic diabetes mellitus.* Symptomatic diabetes occurs in Cushing's syndrome, acromegaly, thyrotoxicosis, and pheochromocytomas. These are discussed more fully in Chapter 5, Disorders of Blood Glucose (pp. 58-75). Glycosuria is also associated with *acute central nervous system disorders* (meningitis, cerebrovascular accidents, etc.). The dipstick papers, Tes-Tape (Eli Lilly & Co.) and Clinistix (Ames Co., Inc.), are specific for glucose, but Benedict's solution or Clinitest tablets (Ames Co., Inc.) will give positive results with other reducing substances such as fructose, lactose, homogentisic acid, etc. (See Chap. 5, Disorders of Blood Glucose.) Various disaccharides (lactose, etc.) appear in the stool in deficiency of their respective enzymes (lactase, etc.). The lactic acid may be high in the stool in lactase deficiency. This disorder is best diagnosed by an oral lactose tolerance test.

Decreased glucose is of significance only in disorders of the spinal fluid. *Bacterial meningitis* is associated with a significant drop, but the most marked drop occurs in *tuberculous meningitis.* The spinal fluid glucose determination is of significance only if a blood sugar is drawn concomitantly for comparison, since drops in cerebrospinal fluid sugar regularly occur in *hypoglycemia* from whatever cause.

Amino Acids

Amino acids appear in the urine in a wide variety of inborn errors of metabolism in addition to diseases with renal tubular defects, already mentioned (Fanconi syndrome, etc.). In *phenylketonuria* moderate amounts of phenylalanine appear in the urine as well as phenylpyruvic acid. In *maple syrup urine disease* leucine, isoleucine, and valine are found in the urine. *Hartnup disease* is characterized by the presence of all the common amino acids except proline, hydroxyproline, methionine, and arginine. In addition, urinary indican and indoleacetic acid are increased in this disease. *Cystinuria* is associated with the urinary excretion of cystine, lysine, arginine, and ornithine. The cystine may crystallize to form renal calculi. Two other rare conditions associated with amino aciduria are *β-aminoisobutyric aciduria* and *argininosuccinic aciduria.* Undoubtedly more will be found.

Miscellaneous Biochemical Alterations

Urine. The urine ketones are important in diabetes mellitus (p. 75) and starvation (p. 105). Other chemicals that should be searched for in special clinical instances are discussed elsewhere in this book: bilirubin (p. 13), urobilinogen (p. 14), phenylpyruvic acid (p. 176), homogentisic acid (p. 176), melanin (p. 176), porphyrins (p. 178), catecholamines (p. 172), steroids (p. 76), and amylase (p. 171).

Stool. Examination of the stool for *trypsin* is important when chronic pancreatitis is suspected. In this condition trypsin will be diminished or absent. Stool urobilinogen and stercobilin are important tests in the evaluation of the jaundiced patient (p. 14).

Gastric Juice. Certain mucoproteins occur in gastric carcinoma.

Duodenal Fluids. *Bile* will not be present in duodenal juice in complete biliary obstruction.

Peritoneal Fluid. Peritoneal fluid may contain *bilirubin* in the presence of a biliary-peritoneal fistula. It may contain *amylase* in large quantities in acute pancreatitis.

Cerebrospinal Fluid. Spinal fluid *chloride* may be low in acute meningitis and tuberculous meningitis but is usually associated with a low blood chloride, and therefore the significance of this finding is open to question. Spinal fluid *bilirubin* is elevated in jaundice. It may also be elevated in cerebro-vascular diseases associated with minimal hemorrhage or a hemorrhage that has preceded the lumbar puncture a few days, during which the red cells have lysed. Spinal fluid LDH and transaminases are useful in the diagnosis of neoplastic and vascular diseases of the brain.

CYTOLOGY

Papanicolaou smears of the sputum, cervical and vaginal discharge, and pleural and peritoneal fluids are extremely valuable in detecting occult carcinomas. Excellent sputum specimens can be obtained by brushing the bronchial mucosa at bronchoscopy. Smears are not of much use in diagnosing neoplasms of the central nervous system with the exception of ependymomas. Cytologic examination of the gastric juice and urine requires considerable experience but is becoming more widespread as interested pathologists gain greater experience. Table 16-2 lists the method of reporting cytological smears according to Papanicolaou (1954).

Table 16-2. Cytology Reports

Class I:	Absence of atypical or abnormal cells.
Class II:	Atypical cytologic picture but no evidence of malignancy.
Class III:	Cytologic picture suggestive, but not diagnostic, of malignancy.
Class IV:	Cytologic picture strongly suggestive of malignancy.
Class V:	Cytologic picture diagnostic of malignancy.

17 The Autoanalyzer

The SMA® 12/60 analyzer is one of the most remarkable advances in medicine in the past decade. Now every hospitalized patient and numerous outpatients can be screened for more than a hundred diseases with one sample of blood at a very low cost. The newer machines can perform 60 or more tests an hour. Significant unsuspected diseases have been found in at least 4% of hospitalized patients screened. Abnormal profiles giving the clinician excellent leads to the diagnosis of vague symptoms have been found in 20-30% of all patients screened.

APPARATUS AND TEST METHOD

Laboratory procedure has generally been omitted from this book. Because it is such a widely used and new instrument, however, the use of the autoanalyzer should be discussed.

A simplified diagram of the autoanalyzer is shown in Figure 17-1. The autoanalyzer consists of 6 basic components: the sampler, the proportioning pump and manifold, the dialyzer, the heating bath, the colorimeter, and the recorder. These 6 components are interconnected by plastic tubing which transfers the patient's serum and reagents from one component to the other under the force of the proportioning pump. The patient's serum is placed in the small cups of the sampler (A). Samples of known standard solutions are also placed at various intervals in the sampler cups. Reagents to be used in the analysis are placed in the *reagent bottle* (or bottles) (B). Under the force of the *proportioning pump* (C) serum is aspirated from the sampler into one tube and reagent (or reagents) from the reagent bottles into one or more other tubes. The serum and reagents pass through the proportioning pump and on to the *dialyzer* (D). In the dialyzer a proportion of the patient's serum or standard solution is filtered through a fine membrane and picked up by the reagent tub-

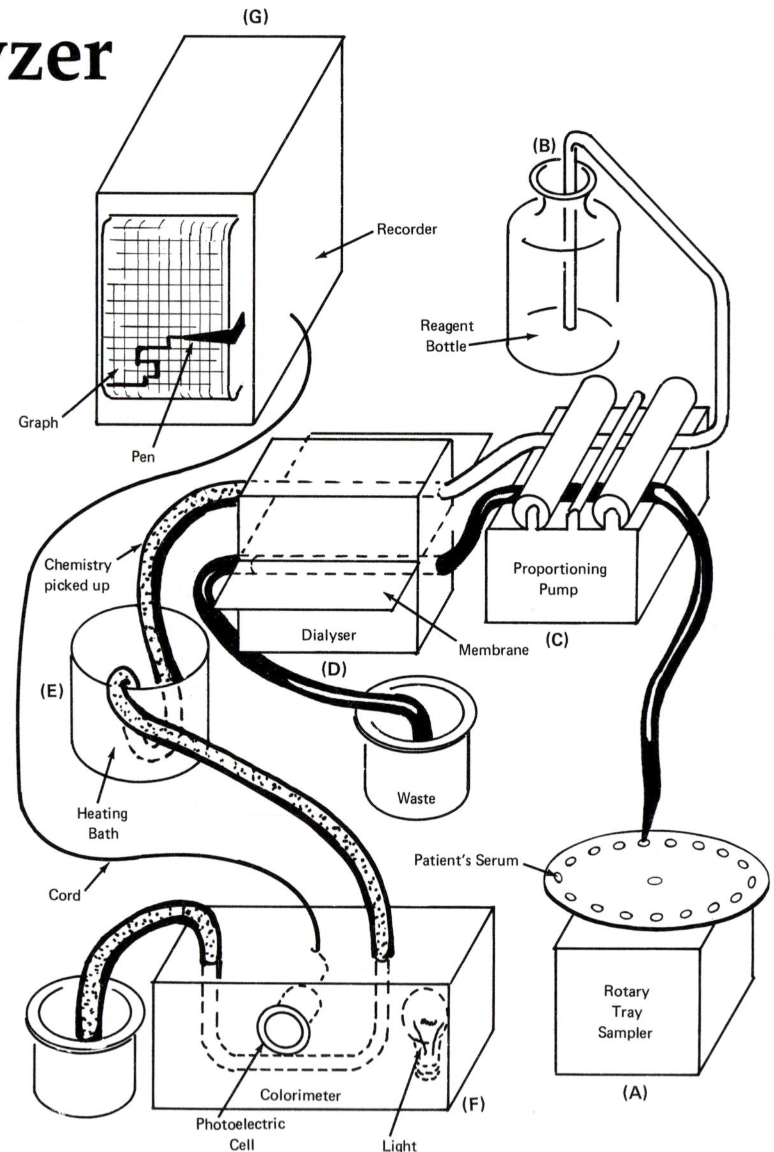

FIG. 17-1. The autoanalyzer.

ing, where a chemical reaction eventually occurs. While not all the chemical to be tested (glucose, urea, etc.) passes from the patient's serum into the reagent tubing, the proportion picked up from the serum and known standard solution will be the same, so the actual amount in the serum can be extrapolated. The "reagent" tube containing the reagents and the chemical being tested passes these on to the *heating bath* (E) where they can be brought to the temperature necessary to cause a chemical reaction, if one has not already occurred. The substance resulting from the reaction, which by now has developed a characteristic color, is passed on to the *colorimeter* (F) which measures the percentage of light (of a certain wave length) transmitted through the chemical solution. The concentration of the chemical being tested for (in the patient's serum or the standard solution) can be determined by the degree to which the colored light is transmitted or absorbed by the solution of combined dialyzed patient's serum and reagent (or reagents).

The colorimeter makes its measurements by means of a photoelectric cell and transmits them to the recorder (G) where the result is recorded on a graph and can be compared with the results from the standards and also from other patients. Therefore this type of analysis is extremely accurate. Many controls can be run in little time; and if there is a trend toward higher or lower values due to contaminants or other factors, it will be quickly spotted.

The procedure described above is for a single–channel system designed to determine 1 blood chemistry (i.e., glucose) on 20 to 60 patients an hour. The SMA-12, a multichannel system which divides a patient's serum sample into 12 portions, is distributed into 12 flow patterns (sets of tubing) so that analyses for 12 blood chemistries can be made simultaneously. This is possible because of time–delayed coils in the system and because of a colorimeter that has different light filters that can rotate into position, depending on the chemical susbtance to be measured.

Interpreting the SMA-12/60 Profiles

In Figure 17-2 is the serum-chemistry graph with which most physicians are familiar. The 12 chemistries (albumin, calcium, etc.) are listed on the horizontal axis; and the range of their concentration in milligrams, grams, or units is shown numerically on the vertical axis. The range of normal values for each chemistry is shaded in gray. The pen of the recorder traces (usually in red) the actual concentration value in the unknown sample of serum or standard

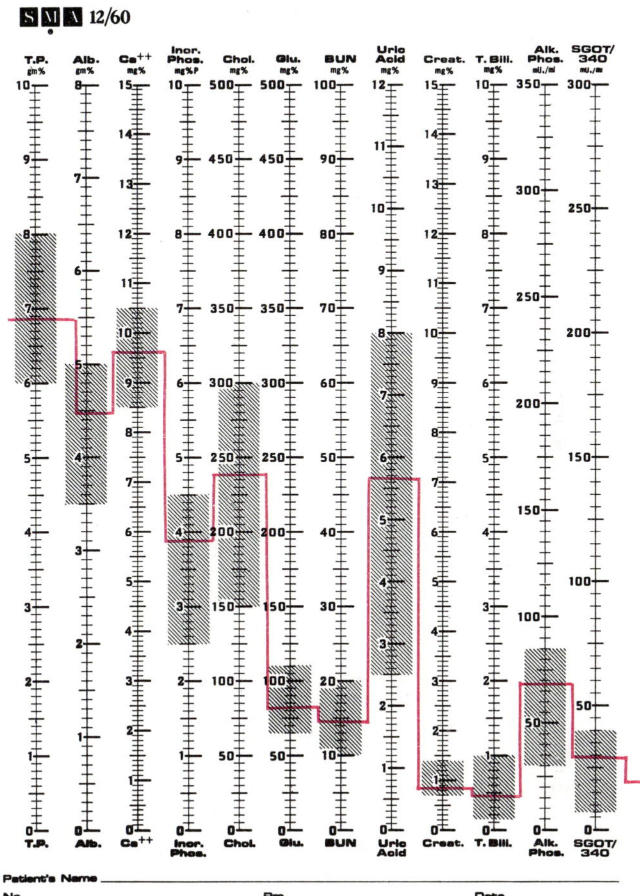

FIG. 17-2A. Normal.

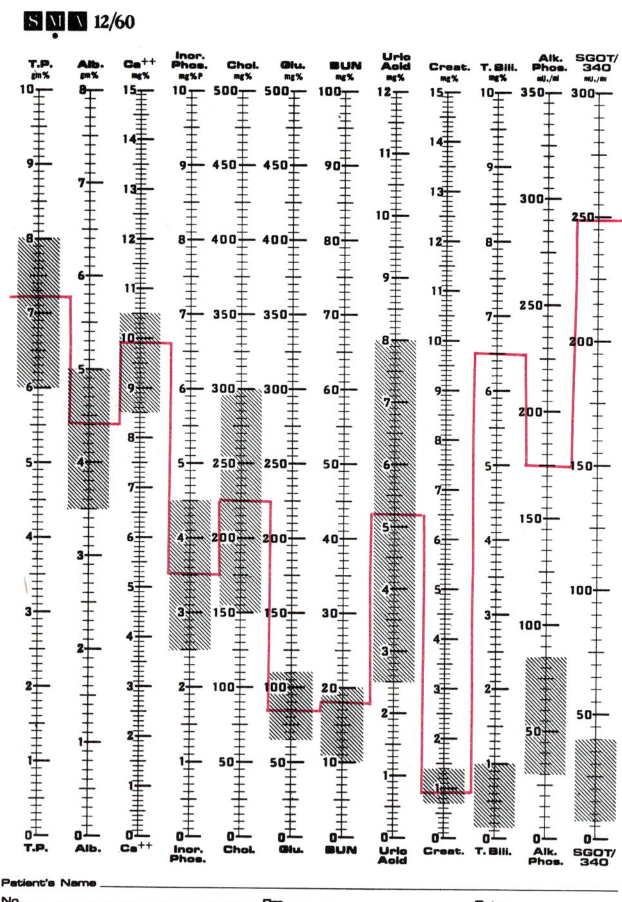

FIG. 17-2B. Viral hepatitis.

solution. This type of representation allows the clinician to determine at a glance which values are abnormal. A normal profile is shown in Figure 17-2A. After years of using the SMA-12 certain profiles (actually combinations of abnormal values for one or more blood chemistries) have emerged as typical of a certain disease. These are shown in the following pages.

Autoanalyzer Profiles

Viral Hepatitis. The combination of hepatocellular damage and intrahepatic cholestasis in this disorder causes a marked elevation of the *bilirubin,* and *SGOT* and a mild elevation of the *alkaline phosphatase.* The *total protein* is also elevated, as there is hypergammaglobulinemia. In contrast to cirrhosis, the albumin does not usually drop. A liver biopsy is important for the diagnosis. (See Fig. 17-2B.)

Severe Laennec's Cirrhosis of the Liver. The SMA-12 pattern in this disorder is best typified by a low *albumin* and *total protein,* a low *BUN,* and moderate elevations of the *SGOT.* The *bilirubin* and *alkaline phosphatase* may or may not be elevated. The prothrombin time is usually elevated and fails to respond to parenteral vitamin K. A liver biopsy is axiomatic in the diagnosis. (See Fig. 17-2C.)

Carcinoma of the Head of the Pancreas. When this tumor obstructs the common bile duct, the SMA-12 shows an elevated *total bilirubin* (mostly direct), *alkaline phosphatase,* and *cholesterol.* The SGOT may be elevated in some cases. The alkaline phosphatase is heat stable in contrast to alkaline phosphatase originating from bone, which is heat labile. Diagnosis is established by exploratory laparotomy, but a positive CEA (carcinoembryonic antigen) is also helpful. *Fasting blood sugar* may also be *elevated* (page 73). (See Fig. 17-2D.)

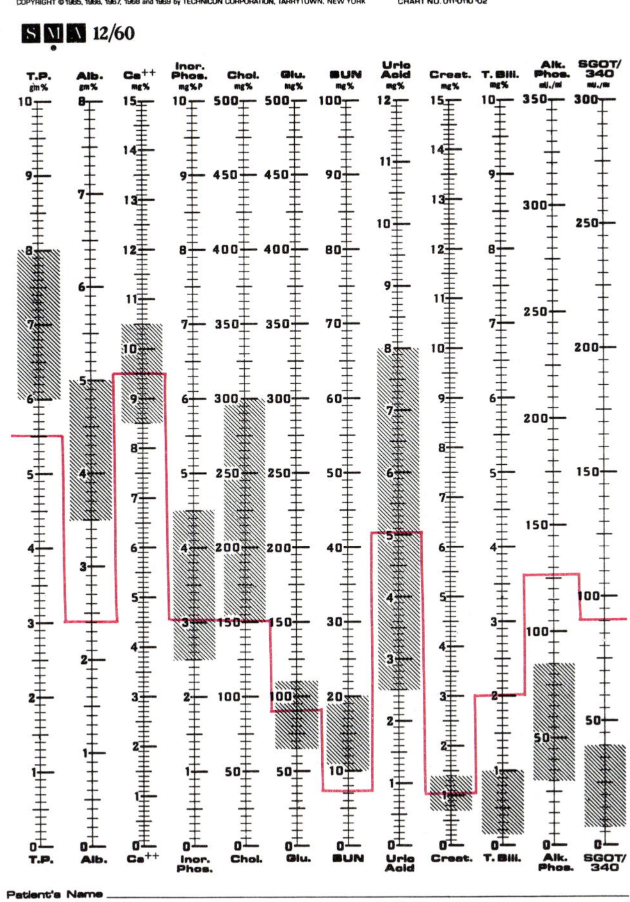

FIG. 17-2C. Laennec's cirrhosis.

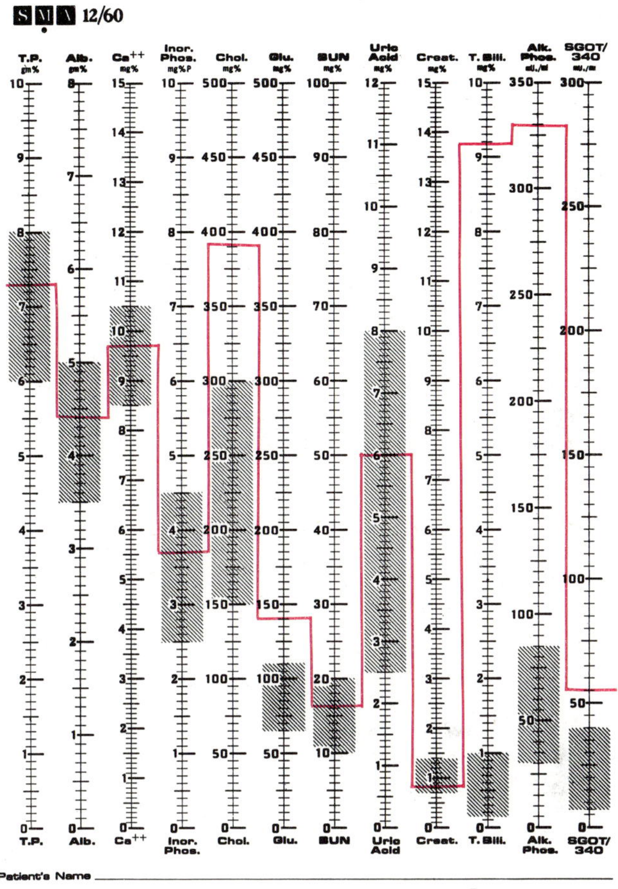

FIG. 17-2D. Carcinoma of the head of the pancreas.

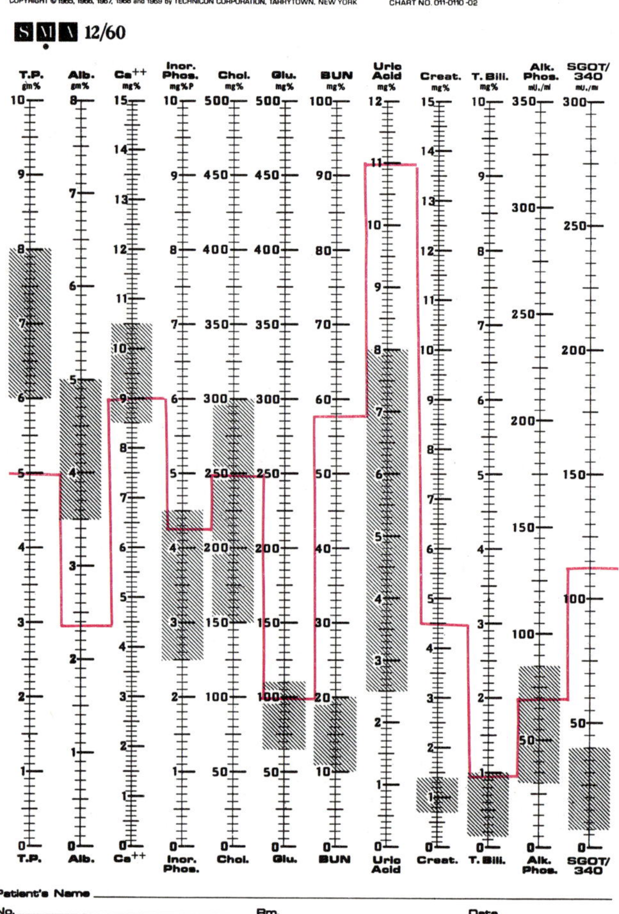

FIG. 17-2E. Acute eclampsia.

Acute Eclampsia. Renal involvement in this disorder causes an *elevated BUN, uric acid,* and *creatinine,* and a *drop* in *albumin* and *total protein.* Liver–cell necrosis is evidenced by the *elevated SGOT.* This pattern plus the urinalysis may be diagnostic. (See Fig. 17-2E.)

Metastatic Carcinoma of the Liver. The typical pattern of metastatic carcinoma of the liver is an isolated elevation of the alkaline phosphatase on the SMA-12 profile. This isolated *alkaline phosphatase* rise may also be seen in bone metastases but there is usually an elevation of the serum calcium with bone metastasis (page 29). The two may be differentiated by heating the serum, as liver alkaline phosphatase is heat stable while bone alkaline phosphatase is heat labile. A liver scan and liver biopsy assist in the diagnosis. (See Fig. 17-2F.)

Multiple Myeloma. The proliferating plasma cells invade the bone, which breaks down and releases *calcium* into the blood. The blood-calcium is elevated, but surprisingly the alkaline phosphatase is normal. The *uric acid* is elevated due to tumor proliferation (as in many myelo-proliferative diseases), and the *total protein* is markedly elevated by hypergammaglobulinemia. (See Fig. 17-2G.)

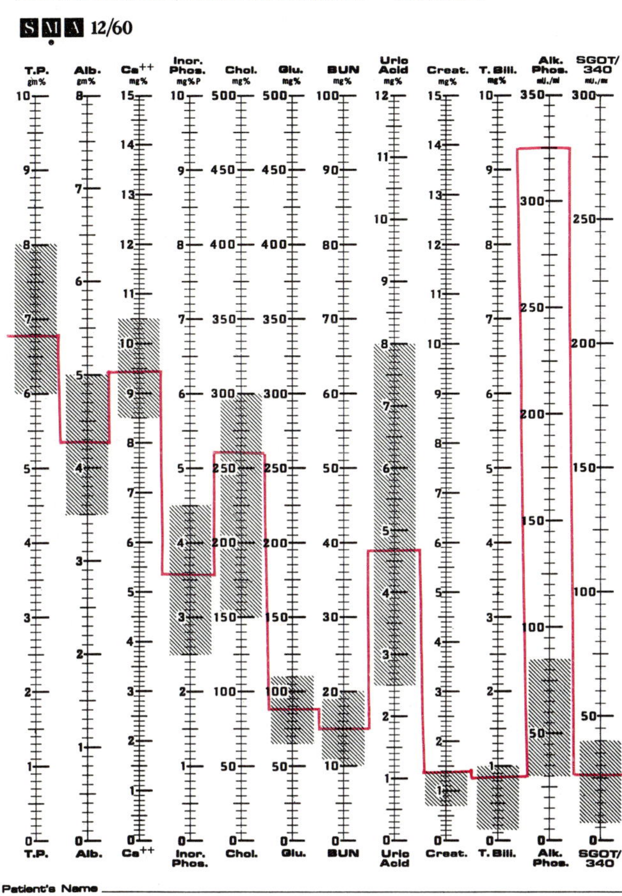

FIG. 17-2F. Metastatic carcinoma of the liver.

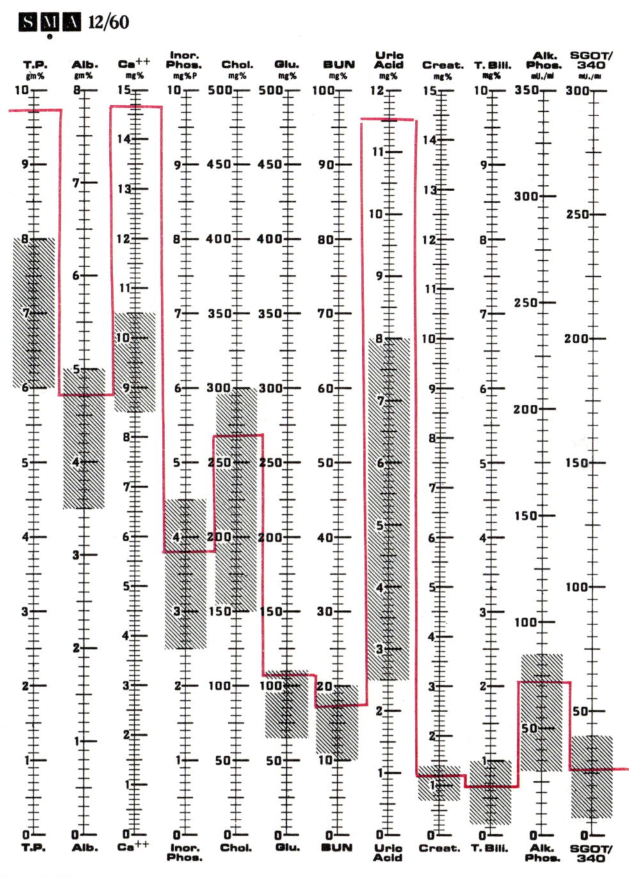

FIG. 17-2G. Multiple myeloma.

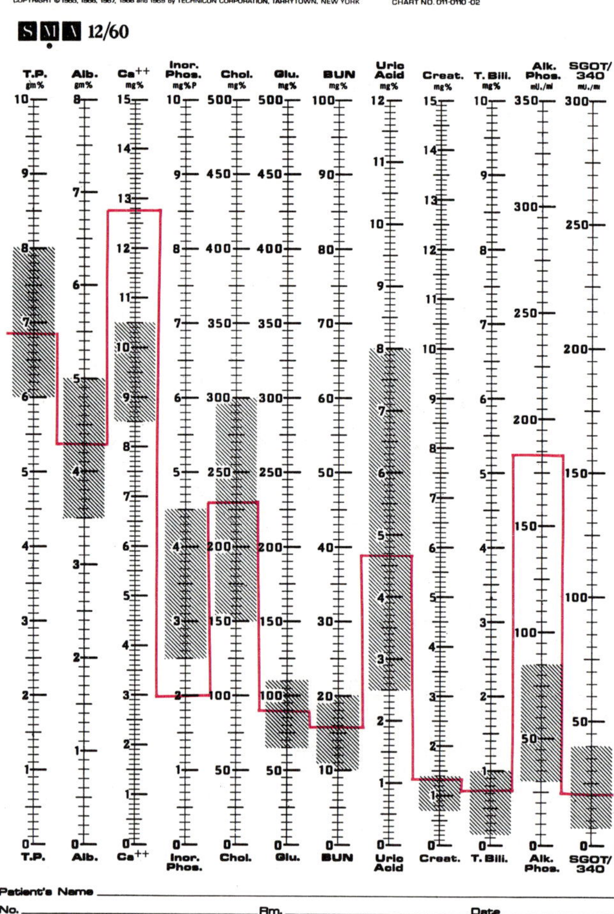

FIG. 17-2H. Primary hyperparathyroidism.

Primary Hyperparathyroidism. This profile is typical of a parathyroid adenoma discussed on page 32. The *calcium* and *alkaline phosphatase* are *elevated,* while the inorganic phosphorus is *decreased.* This pattern is almost diagnostic. (See Fig. 17-2H.)

Severe Malabsorption Syndrome. In this disorder there is poor absorption of calcium, fat, protein, sugar, and many other substances. Thus the *serum calcium* is low, precipitating a secondary hyperparathyroidism with an elevated *alkaline phosphatase* and often a *low phosphorus.* Serum *total protein, albumin,* and *cholesterol* are *reduced.* The glucose is not usually low because of gluconeogenesis. (See Fig. 17-2I.)

Myxedema. The asymptomatic elevation of *cholesterol,* uric acid, and *SGOT,* in the absence of other abnormal liver function tests, is rather typical and should prompt a thyroid survey. The L.D.H. is often elevated also. (See Fig. 17-2J.)

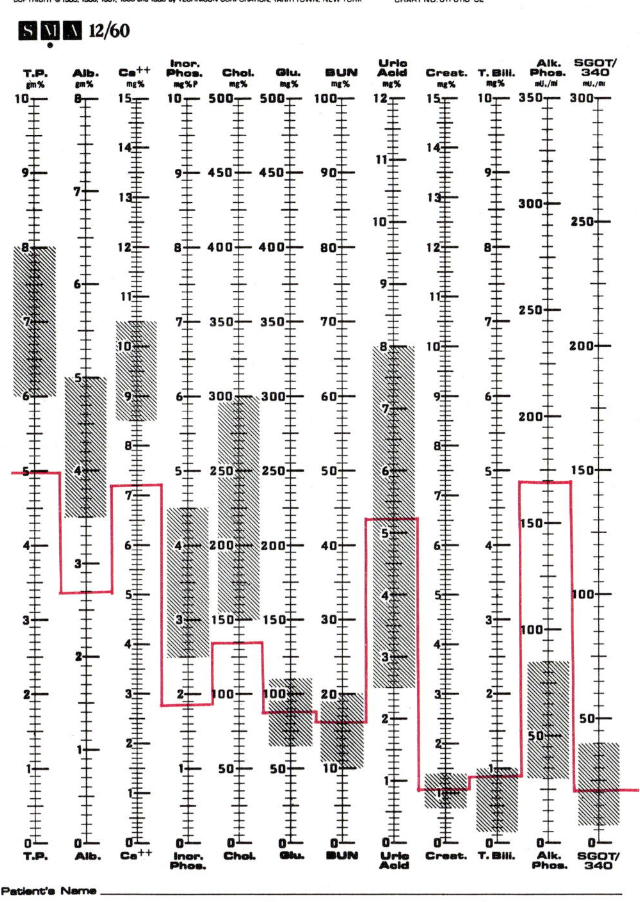

FIG. 17-2I. Severe malabsorption syndrome.

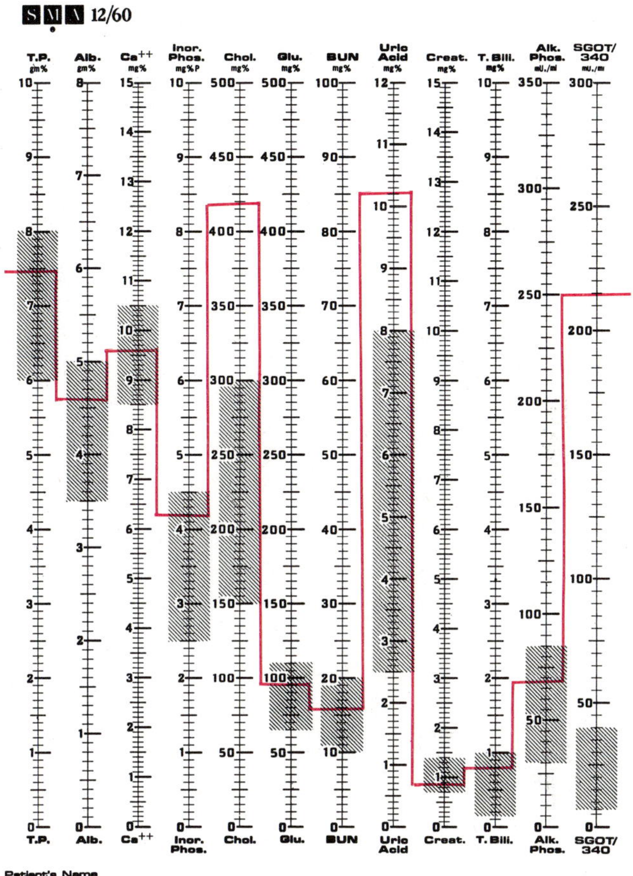

FIG. 17-2J. Myxedema.

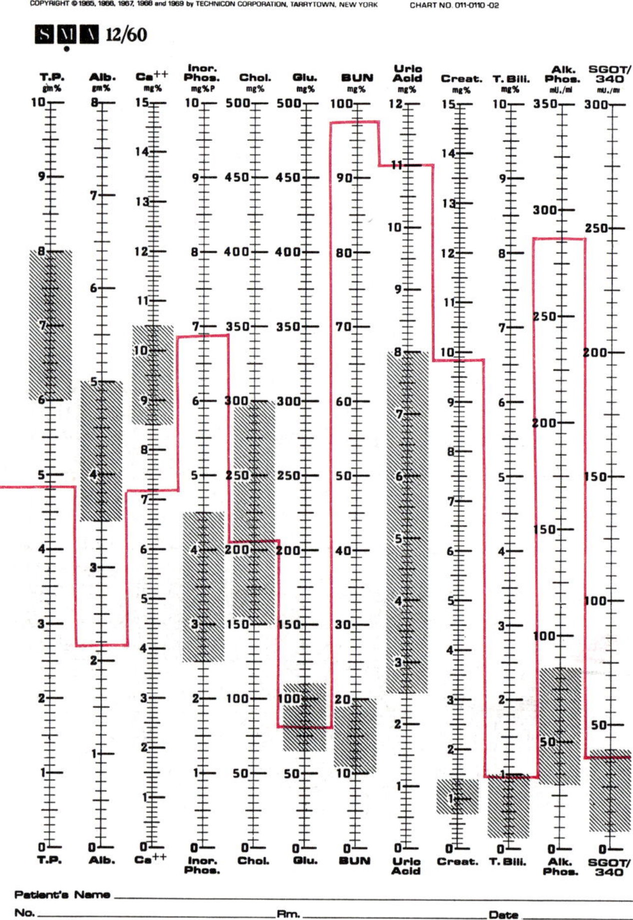

FIG. 17-2K. Chronic glomerulonephritis.

Chronic Glomerulonephritis. Severe renal disease causes a low *calcium* with a high *inorganic phosphorus* and *alkaline phosphatase* and a high *BUN, uric acid,* and *creatinine*. Serum *total protein* and *albumin* are decreased by the persistent albuminuria. The only normal values are the glucose, bilirubin, and SGOT. (See Fig. 17-2K.)

Nephrotic Syndrome. The profile in this disorder is signified by the very *high cholesterol* with a very low *total protein* and *albumin* in the presence of moderate elevations of the BUN. No other condition gives this picture. (See Fig. 17-2L.)

Metastatic Carcinoma of Bone. When tumors metastasize to the bone, there is breakdown of bone and *calcium* is released, which *increases* in the blood and urine. Osteoblasts may proliferate in an attempt to lay down more bone, and the *alkaline phosphatase increases*. (See Fig. 17-2M.)

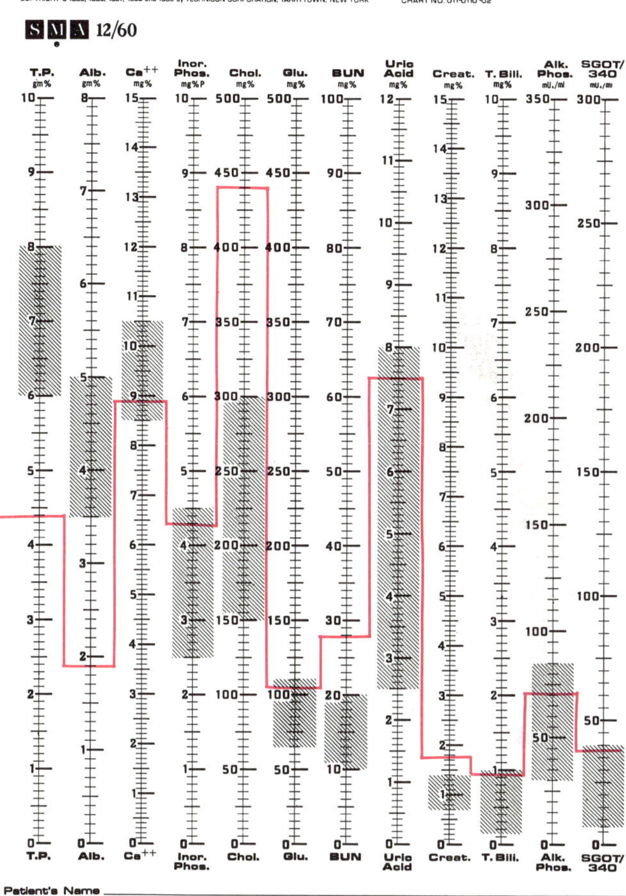

Fig. 17-2L. Nephrotic syndrome.

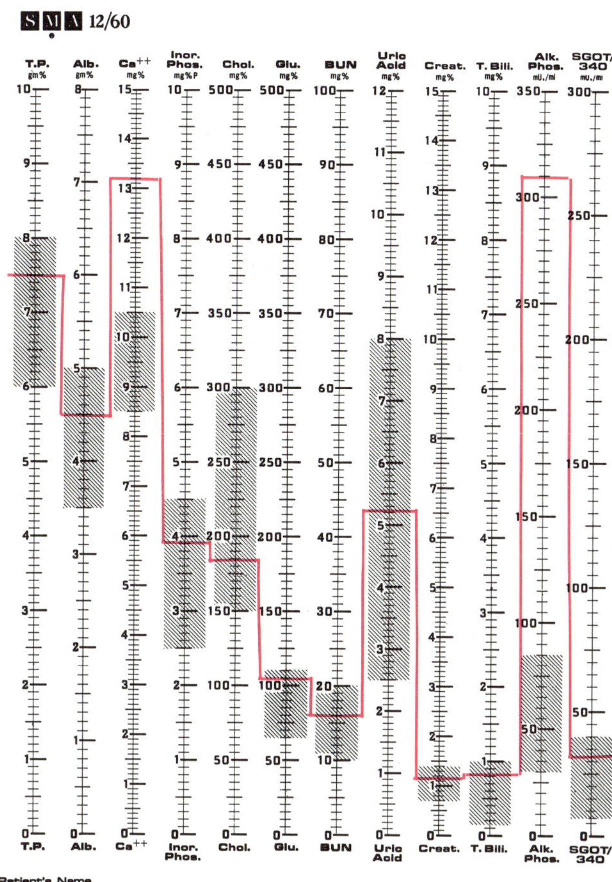

Fig. 17-2M. Metastatic carcinoma of bone.

18 Disorders of the Erythrocytes

NORMAL METABOLISM

Production. In the normal adult, red cells are formed in the bone marrow by a process called erythropoiesis. In diseased states, however, they may be formed in the spleen and other organs of the reticuloendothelial system. Red cell production depends on an adequate intake of protein, carbohydrate, fat, minerals, and vitamins. The most important of the last two groups are iron, folic acid, and vitamin B_{12}. Pyridoxine and ascorbic acid also seem to be essential. Including these in the diet does not assure their utilization. They must be absorbed. Absorption of iron is favored by hydrochloric acid and ascorbic acid. It may depend on the formation of an iron-amino-acid compound in the intestinal wall.

Absorption of vitamin B_{12} requires the intrinsic factor, secreted by the fundus and the body of the stomach. Both folic acid and vitamin B_{12} depend on a normally functioning intestinal mucosa for their absorption. Ascorbic acid facilitates the transformation of folic acid to its active form, citrovorum factor (folinic acid). Iron, folic acid, and vitamin B_{12} are all stored in the liver. Thus an individual can maintain a normal red cell count without their daily inclusion in the diet.

The red cells of the peripheral blood are the product of a progressive maturation and cell division of stem cells called megaloblasts in the bone marrow. Through a steady reduction in size and changes in the character of the nucleus and cytoplasm, the myeloblast becomes a pronormoblast, a basophilic normoblast, a polychromatophilic normoblast, an orthochromic normoblast, and a reticulocyte, in that order, before being released into the peripheral blood. Since the interpretation of bone marrow smears is relegated to the specialist, a description of the morphologic characteristics of most of these primitive cells is omitted.

The reader should be acquainted with the appearance of the orthochromic normoblast and the reticulocyte because both of these appear in the peripheral blood in many anemias, and a few reticulocytes (0.5 to 1.5%) are present normally. An orthochromic normoblast contains orange-red cytoplasm, a small, shrunken, dark-staining nucleus, and is about the same size as the mature erythrocyte. The reticulocyte resembles a mature erythrocyte on staining with Wright's stain except for a purplish hue, but on staining with brilliant cresyl blue, fine granular basophilic filaments appear.

Transport. Erythrocytes are transported in the intravascular space by the force of the heart and somatic muscle "pumps." When the vascular wall is injured, they may enter the extracellular space of the body cavity or be brought to the exterior through the skin, the gastrointestinal, respiratory, or urinary tract. The primary function of the erythrocyte is to carry oxygen to and carbon dioxide from the cells.

In studying anemias it is very important to know the morphologic characteristics of the mature red cell. They are round, red-staining, and nonnucleated with a central thin portion. They measure from 7.2 to 7.9 microns. There are between 4.5 and 5.5 million of these cells per cubic millimeter of blood in the normal adult male. The accuracy of this test has been increased by the Coulter Counter.

Destruction. The normal red cell survives an average of 120 days. Thus, about 0.8 per cent of the total red cells in the circulation are destroyed each day. Whether most of the red cells disintegrate spontaneously in the blood stream or are broken down by the spleen and reticuloendothelial system is not clear. It is certain that the spleen and reticuloendothelial system pick up the debris and degradate the hemoglobin to bilirubin (see Chap. 2, Disorders of Serum Bilirubin, Normal Metabolism, p. 13).

Regulation. It is not clear what physiologic mechanism is responsible for maintaining the normal balance between red cell production and destruction. A factor that stimulates erythrocyte production, erythropoietin, has been isolated, but its precise chemical structure and site of action are unknown. It is considered to be produced by the kidney and possibly some other organs. A reduced blood oxygen saturation has long been known to stimulate red cell production, but here again the mechanism is unknown. Hydrocortisone is believed to stimulate the bone marrow, but whether this effect is significant in the regulation of the production of erythrocytes in the normal individual is conjecture. It is understandable that thyroid hormone would have some influence on bone marrow as it does on other body cells, namely, to stimulate their metabolism; but the possibility of a direct effect of thyroxine on erythropoiesis is not proven. The possibility that a splenic hormone depresses the bone marrow has been considered but is not conclusively established experimentally.

The destruction of red cells is determined by their morphology and the activity of the reticuloendothelial system, but the influence of regulatory mechanisms such as hormones is unknown.

Storage. Red cells are stored in the spleen and may be released under stressful conditions in response to epinephrine.

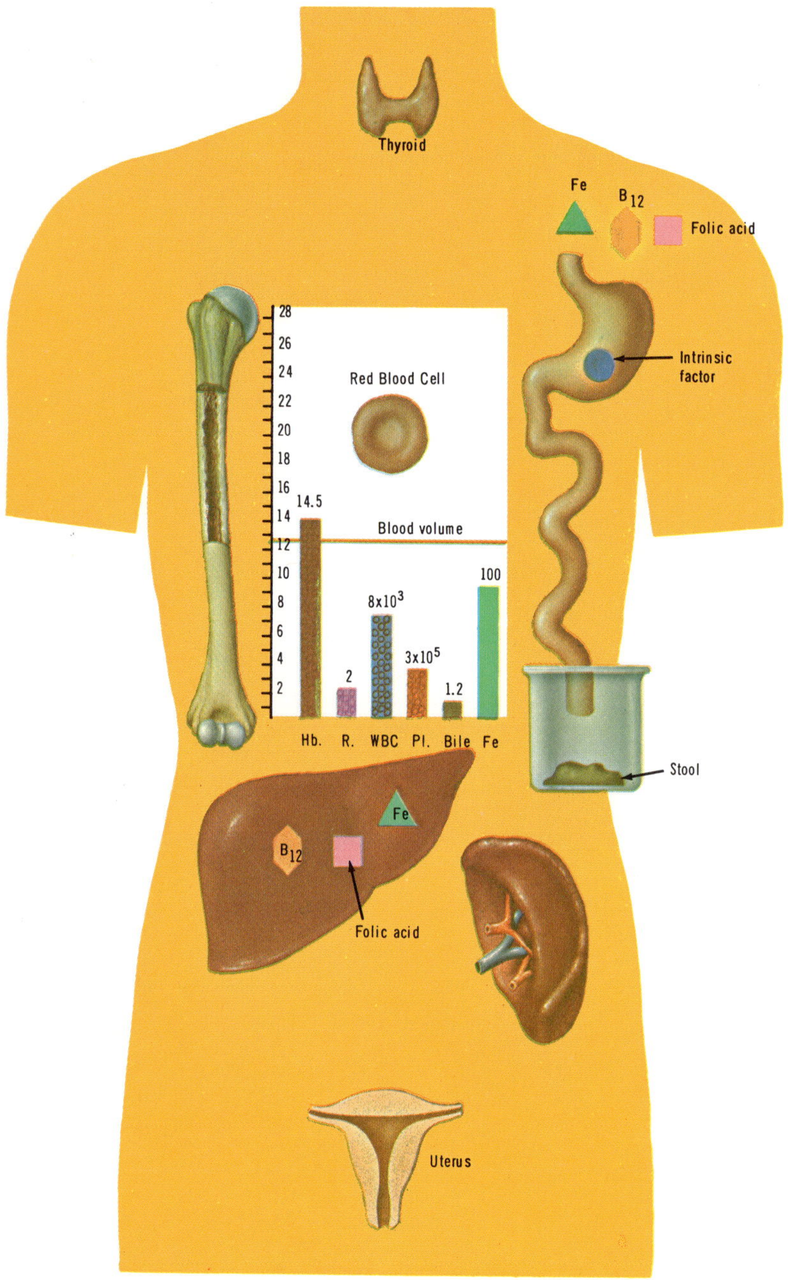

THE APPROACH TO THE DIAGNOSIS

Disorders of the erythrocytes are grouped into the anemias, in which there is a reduction in circulating red cells, and polycythemia, in which there is an increase in circulating red cells. Anemias may be due to three basic mechanisms: decreased red cell production, increased red cell destruction, and blood loss. It is well to approach the problem with these mechanisms in mind.

The nine tests included in the profiles of red cell disorders will be an excellent start in deciding whether an anemia exists, and which of the above three mechanisms is responsible. (1) The **hemoglobin** and **hematocrit** will establish the presence and severity of the anemia. (2) A **blood smear** will establish the morphologic type of anemia (normocytic, macrocytic, microcytic, etc.) and often be diagnostic, as in sickle cell anemia and hereditary spherocytosis. This is a very important test and too often neglected. Blood obtained by a finger puncture is best for blood smears, because oxalate anticoagulant produces W.B.C. and R.B.C. artifacts. The red cell indices (mean corpuscular hemoglobin, mean corpuscular volume, and mean corpuscular hemoglobin concentration) may be ordered, but inaccuracy of the red cell count limits the value of all but the MCHC. An increased (3) **reticulocyte count** and (4) **indirect bilirubin** will indicate an anemia of increased red cell destruction. The (5) **stool** for **occult blood** often exposes an anemia of blood loss. (6) The **white blood cell count** and (7) **platelet** will be of value in diagnosing an anemia of decreased red cell production, in which case the white blood cells and platelets are usually decreased. The (8) **serum iron** may establish a nutritional basis for an anemia of decreased red cell production. (9) A **gastric analysis** will show no free acid in pernicious anemia. The use of more specific tests is noted in each disorder. While the clinician does not need to know how to read a *bone marrow,* he should know the indications for its use. A bone marrow should probably be done in all cases suspected of megaloblastic anemia, aplastic anemia, agranulocytosis leukemia, multiple myeloma, thrombocytopenia, metastatic neoplasm of the marrow, and Hodgkin's disease. It may also be indicated in selected cases of chronic anemia or iron deficiency anemia. *Therapeutic trials* with iron or B_{12} are still useful.

Abbreviations Used in Plates:

Hb = Hemoglobin in gm. per 100 ml. of blood
R = Reticulocyte count as per cent of normal erythrocytes
WBC = White blood cell count per cu. mm. of blood
Pl = Platelet count per cu. mm. of blood
Bile = Serum bilirubin in mg. per 100 ml. of blood
Fe = Micrograms per 100 ml. of blood

HYPOCHROMIC ANEMIA OF INFANCY

Infants fed almost entirely on milk formulas do not have an adequate dietary intake of iron (A). *Serum iron levels diminish,* and liver and bone marrow stores are depleted (B). With the constant increase in the growing infant's blood volume, there is a corresponding demand for increased red cell mass. Without adequate iron supplies to meet this demand, a *drop* in *hemoglobin* and *hematocrit* occurs. The red cells have a decreased hemoglobin content and are thus small (microcytic) and pale (hypochromic) in the center (C). This accounts for a mean corpuscular hemoglobin concentration of less than 30 per cent and a mean corpuscular volume of less than 80 cu. microns. The red cells also vary in size and shape. Production of platelets and leukocytes is not usually affected because they do not rely on iron for their normal development. The bone marrow is hyperplastic, and there is a decrease in stainable iron. Little or no iron in the bone marrow may be the first laboratory proof of iron deficiency.

Premature infants are even more prone to this type of anemia, as they have a lower amount of total hemoglobin in their blood at birth.

Dietary deficiency of iron is rare in adults. However, an iron deficiency anemia may occur in achlorhydria, whether due to gastric atrophy or gastrectomy, and in malabsorption syndrome. It is not unusual in pregnancy, in which the demand for iron is greater. Although hypochromic anemia almost invariably means iron deficiency, the reader must remember that it also may be seen in thalassemia. A microcytic, hypochromic anemia also occurs in acquired or congenital sideroblastic anemia. Unlike iron deficiency anemia there is an increase in total body iron and the anemia may respond to pyridoxine.*

Summary of Laboratory Findings:

Hemoglobin and hematocrit: Decreased

Reticulocyte count: Normal

Cell morphology: Microcytosis, hypochromia, and anisocytosis

White cell count: Normal

Platelet count: Normal

Serum bilirubin: Normal

Serum iron: Decreased

*Hines, J. D., Grasso, J. A.: The sideroblastic anemias. Semin. Hematol., 7:86, 1970.

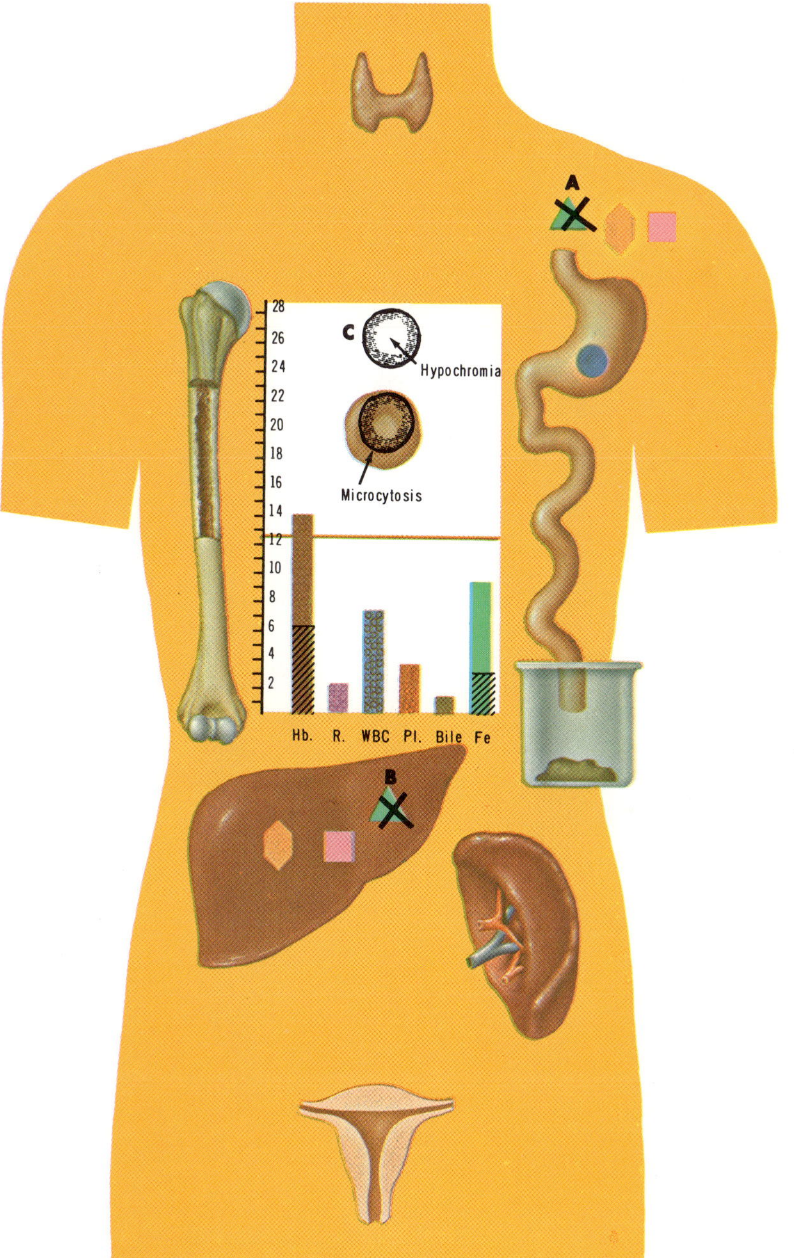

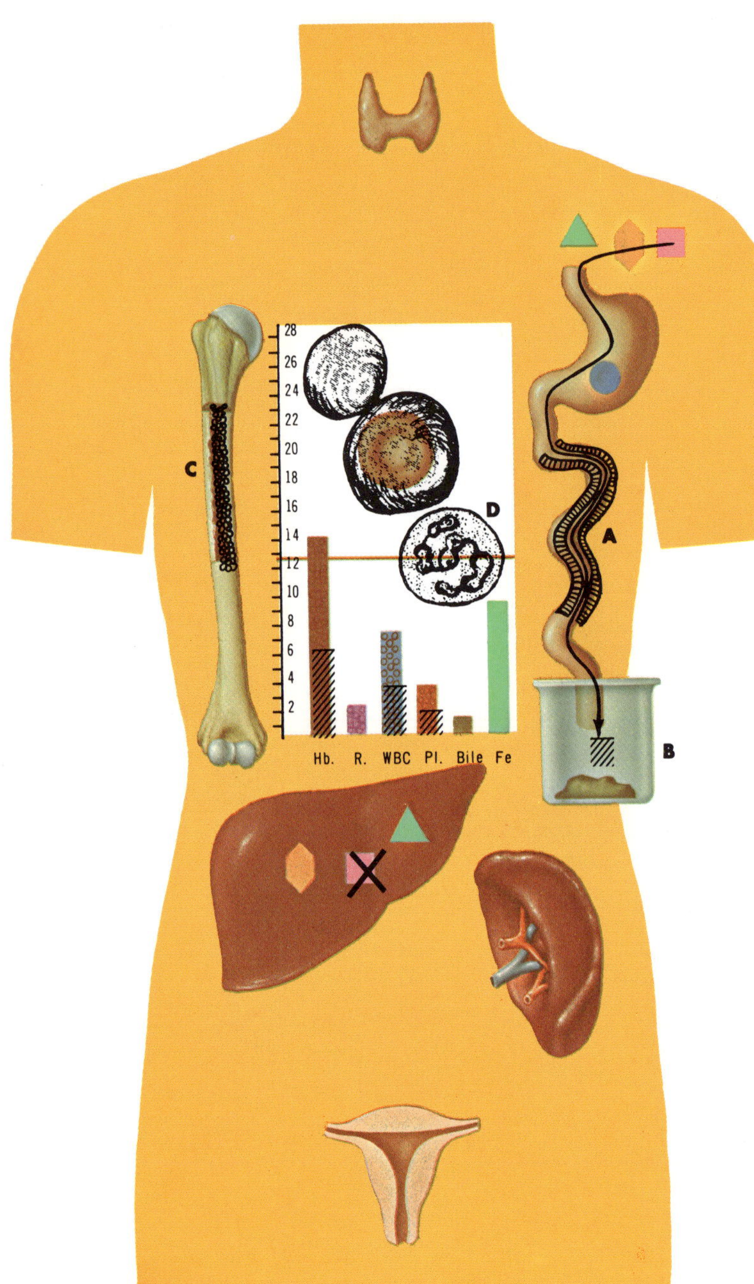

IDIOPATHIC STEATORRHEA

In this disorder the diseased intestinal wall is unable to absorb folic acid (A) and occasionally B_{12} or iron. These substances pass into the stool (B). When folic acid absorption is blocked, the liver and body stores of this substance are depleted over a period of months. Megaloblasts accumulate in the bone marrow due to the arrested maturation and give the marrow a richly cellular appearance (C). The red cells of the peripheral blood are commonly hyperchromic and macrocytic. There are hypersegmented neutrophils (D) as in pernicious anemia. Since folic acid is just as important for the maturation of the granulocytes and megakaryocytes, *leukopenia* and *thrombocytopenia* are present as well.

Because poor absorption of iron may occur also in this disorder, a microcytic, hypochromic anemia is occasionally seen. And sometimes the anemia is normochromic and normocytic.

Folic acid deficiency leading to the above picture may occur likewise in malnutrition, in which a reduced supply does not meet the normal demand, and in pregnancy, in which an increased demand taxes the normal supply. Anticonvulsant drugs such as diphenylhydantoin may also cause this picture.

Although the diagnosis of a malabsorption syndrome will be supported by such ancillary diagnostic procedures as the stool fat and trypsin, the D-xylose uptake, the serum carotene, and radioactive triolein-I^{131} uptake, the diagnosis of folic acid deficiency must rest on the therapeutic response to this substance. Urinary formiminoglutamic acid is increased in this disorder, but its determination is not within the diagnostic armamentarium of the average clinical laboratory. Performance of the test after a histidine load has made the test more accurate.

Summary of Laboratory Findings:

Hemoglobin and hematocrit: Decreased

Reticulocyte count: Normal

Cell morphology: Hyperchromia and macrocytosis, anisocytosis and poikilocytosis, hypersegmented neutrophils

White cell count: Decreased

Platelet count: Decreased

Serum bilirubin: Increased occasionally

Serum iron: Normal, increased, or decreased

PERNICIOUS ANEMIA

In pernicious anemia the atrophied cells of the gastric mucosa are unable to produce the intrinsic factor of Castle (A). Despite adequate B_{12} intake, it is not absorbed and passes into the stool (B). Liver stores of B_{12} are eventually depleted (C). B_{12} synthesis of deoxyribonucleic acid (DNA) is disturbed, and maturation of the myeloblasts is arrested. The bone marrow becomes hypercellular (D). The marrow cells may not appear megaloblastic if there has been a recent blood transfusion (even as little as 12 hours previously). Fewer mature cells are released into the circulation, with a corresponding *drop* in the *hemoglobin* and *hematocrit.* The cells that are released are large (macrocytic) and laden with hemoglobin. Some are nucleated and of various sizes and shapes (anisocytosis and poikilocytosis, respectively). They fail to survive as long as normal red cells. Thus the *total serum bilirubin* may be *elevated* in this disorder.

The disordered DNA synthesis affects the maturation of the granulocytes and megakaryocytes as well. Consequently, there are *leukopenia* and *thrombocytopenia.* However, in early cases there may be only anemia. The leukocytes are multilobulated (E). Iron utilization diminishes because of the decreased red cell synthesis and diminished incorporation of iron into the developing red cells. Thus the *serum iron rises.*

More definitive diagnosis of this disorder may be made by a gastric analysis and a Schilling test. There is a histamine-resistant achlorhydria. The Schilling test reveals very little tagged vitamin B_{12} in the urine, indicating a lack of its absorption. When intrinsic factor is administered with the tagged vitamin B_{12} orally, the urine level of tagged vitamin B_{12} returns to normal (p. 183). A radioimmunoassay of serum B_{12} can now be done and should be diagnostic.

B_{12} deficiency may also occur in idiopathic sprue due to poor absorption, in dietary deficiency due to lack of intake, and in *Diphyllobothrium latum* infection because the worm ingests dietary B_{12}. Gastrectomy is yet another cause.

Summary of Laboratory Findings:

Hemoglobin and hematocrit: Decreased

Reticulocyte count: Normal

Cell morphology: Hyperchromia and macrocytosis, anisocytosis and poikilocytosis

White cell count: Decreased

Platelet count: Decreased

Serum bilirubin: Increased

Serum iron: Normal or increased

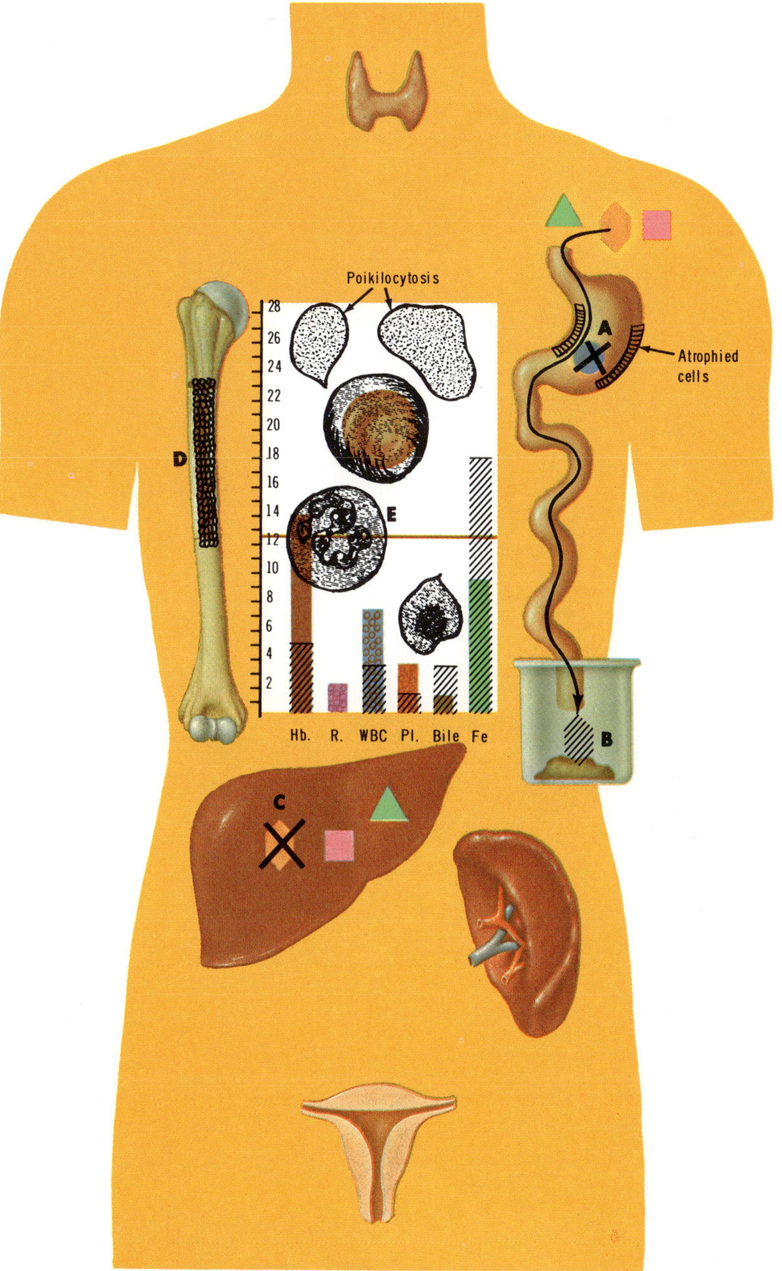

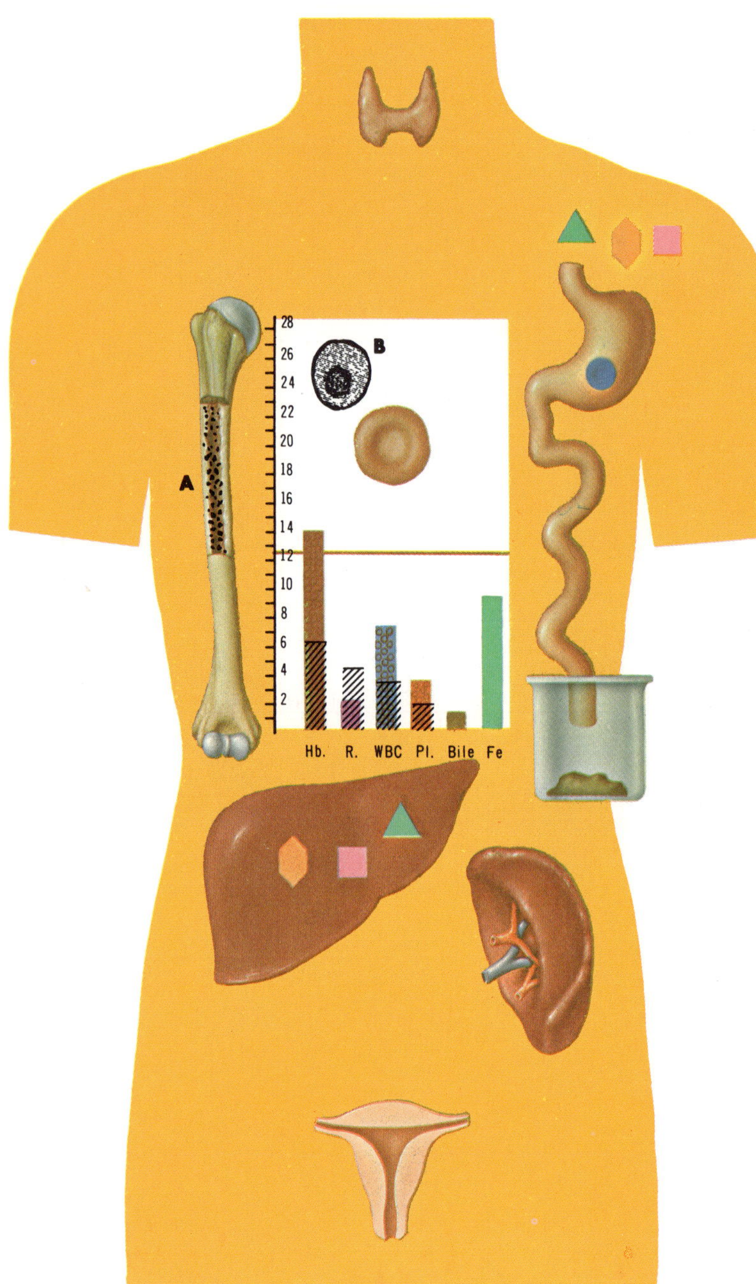

MYELOPHTHISIC ANEMIA

In this disorder the bone marrow is overrun by metastatic carcinoma, multiple myeloma, lymphomas, primary xanthomatoses, and other tissue (A). For this reason these conditions have been termed space-occupying lesions of the bone marrow. The total volume of bone marrow is depleted, and *anemia* of varying degree ensues. What marrow is left probably produces at an increased rate to compensate for the blood loss. Consequently, as many as 50 per cent of the red cells in the peripheral blood may be nucleated (B). *Reticulocyte count* is usually *elevated*. Myeloproliferation and platelet proliferation are affected as well, and so often there are *leukopenia* and *thrombocytopenia*. A bone marrow examination will frequently determine the diagnosis, but a systematic search for malignancy is most important.

Differentiating this condition from myelofibrosis may be difficult. A surgical biopsy of the marrow may reveal diffuse sclerosis and hypoplasia in the latter disorder. Splenomegaly and primitive leukocytes in the peripheral blood are more common in myelofibrosis, whereas the presence of numerous normoblasts in the peripheral blood is more common in myelophthisis.

Summary of Laboratory Findings:

Hemoglobin and hematocrit: Decreased

Reticulocyte count: Increased or normal

Cell morphology: Normal cellular morphology aside from nucleated red cells and occasional myelocytes

White cell count: Decreased

Platelet count: Decreased

Serum bilirubin: Normal

Serum iron: Normal

IDIOPATHIC APLASTIC ANEMIA

In this condition the bone marrow for unknown reasons becomes aplastic and is replaced by fat (A). Red cell production comes almost to a halt. Thus there is *pancytopenia* in the blood. The *reticulocyte count* is *normal* for obvious reasons, and unless there is extramedullary erythropoiesis, there are no nucleated red cells in the peripheral blood. The red cells are usually normal in size and configuration. However, up to one third of patients may have a predominance of macrocytes. *Plasma iron* is often *increased.* a bone marrow examination is essential in establishing this diagnosis. A bone marrow biopsy is more useful than a smear in estimating cellularity.

Idiopathic aplastic anemia is to be differentiated from aplastic anemia secondary to various chemical and physical agents. Among these are ionizing radiation, mustards, urethane, Myleran, benzene, 6-mercaptopurine, Mesantoin, and chloramphenicol. It must also be differentiated from simple chronic anemias. (See p. 235.)

Summary of Laboratory Findings:

Hemoglobin and hematocrit: Decreased
Reticulocyte count: Normal or decreased
Cell morphology: Normal
White cell count: Decreased
Platelet count: Decreased
Serum bilirubin: Normal
Serum iron: Normal or increased

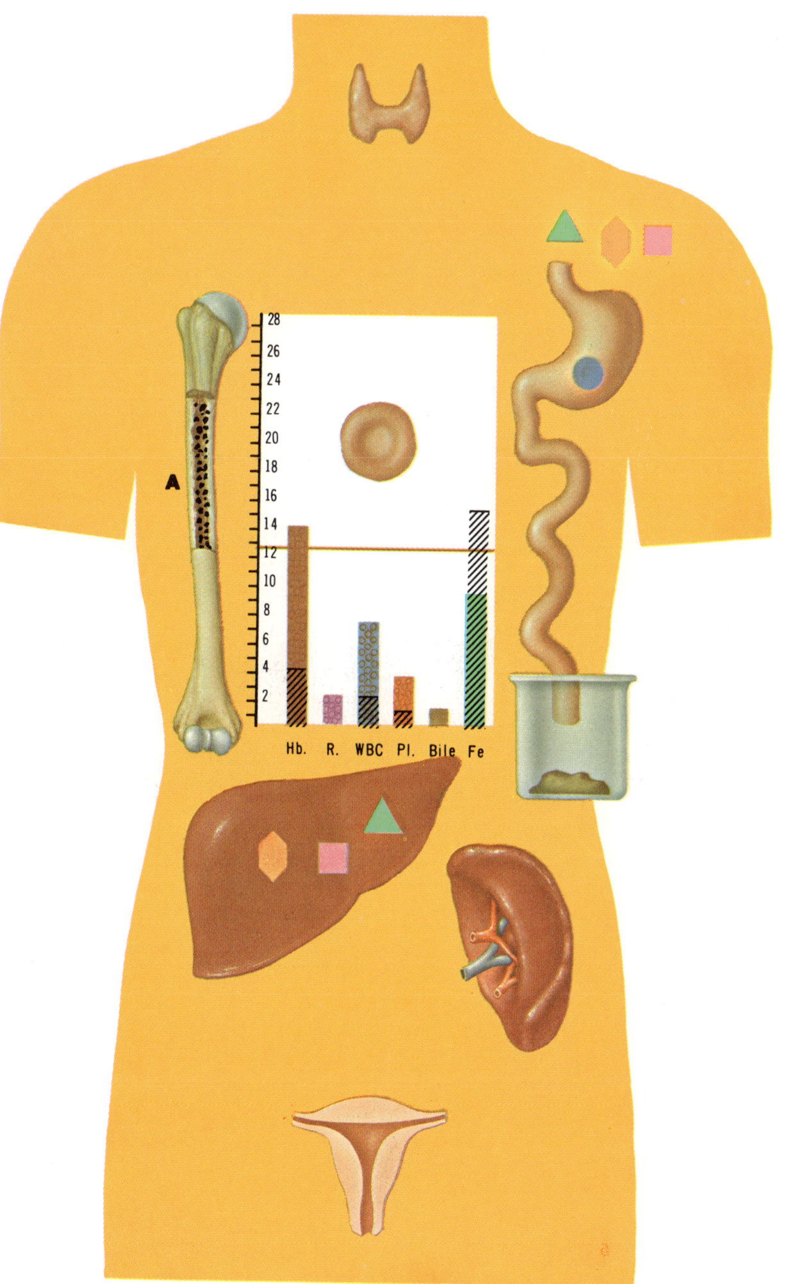

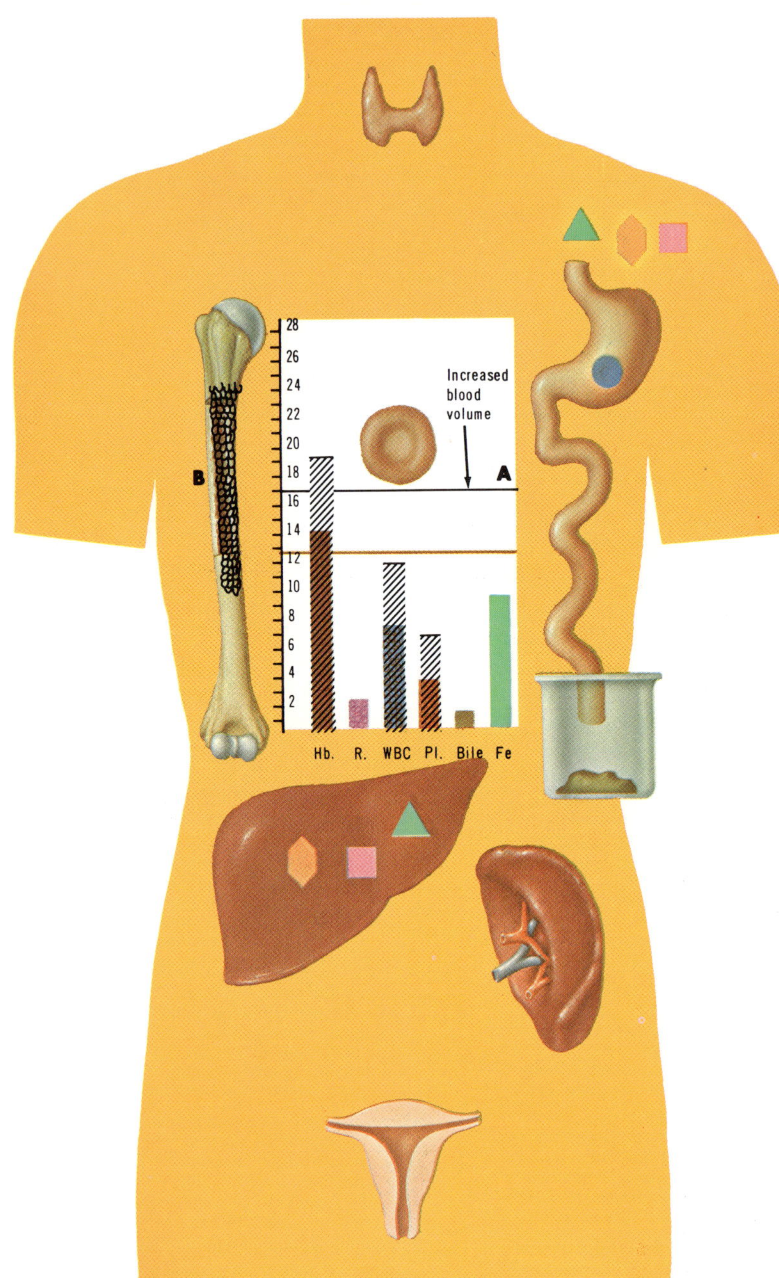

POLYCYTHEMIA VERA

For unknown reasons there is an absolute increase in total red cell mass in this condition. Thus the blood volume (A), *hemoglobin,* and *hematocrit* are all *increased.* The red cells are "packed in like sardines" in some cases. They are normal in appearance, and there is no reticulocytosis. Usually, *leukocytosis* is present, with a "shift to the left" (immature neutrophils). Commonly, the *increase* in blood *platelets* is five- to tenfold. Thus all the cellular elements of the blood are augmented in number. Serum bilirubin is not usually elevated even though increased blood destruction is probable in most cases. As one might expect, the bone marrow is hyperplastic (B), but the myeloid-erythroid ratio is not altered.

Measuring the blood volume will help to differentiate this condition from relative polycythemia, in which the blood volume does not increase. If the uric acid is elevated, the polycythemia is probably not secondary to some other condition. Polycythemias secondary to pulmonary or cardiovascular disease may be excluded by a normal arterial blood oxygen saturation test, since the blood volume is often increased in these conditions. Polycythemia secondary to Cushing's disease and unilateral renal disease must be excluded by performing urine tests for steroids and an intravenous pyelogram, respectively.

Summary of Laboratory Findings:

Hemoglobin and hematocrit: Increased
Reticulocyte count: Normal
Cell morphology: Normal
White cell count: Increased
Platelet count: Increased
Serum bilirubin: Normal
Serum iron: Normal
Blood volume: Increased

BLEEDING PEPTIC ULCER, ACUTE STAGE

Acute bleeding, whether internal or external, does not result in an immediate drop in hemoglobin unless more than 1,000 ml. is lost. The full extent of the resulting *anemia* may not be evident until 24 to 48 hours later. There are *leukocytosis* and an *increase* in *platelets*, however, possibly due to the stress reaction. In massive bleeding from a peptic ulcer, there will often be melena (A) and hematemesis (B). No change in the reticulocyte count will be noted at first. The diagnosis is usually established by a G.I. series or gastroscopy. It should be pointed out that the finding of even 3 or 4 stools negative for occult blood does not exclude a peptic ulcer or G.I. cancer, as these may bleed intermittently.

The same picture will be found in massive bleeding from whatever cause. This includes trauma, childbirth, gastritis, hiatal hernia, and retroperitoneal or peritoneal hemmorrhage from a ruptured or an ectopic gestation.

Summary of Laboratory Findings:

Hemoglobin and hematocrit: Normal or decreased
Reticulocyte count: Normal
Cell morphology: Normal
White cell count: Increased
Platelet count: Increased
Serum bilirubin: Normal
Serum iron: Normal
Blood volume: Decreased

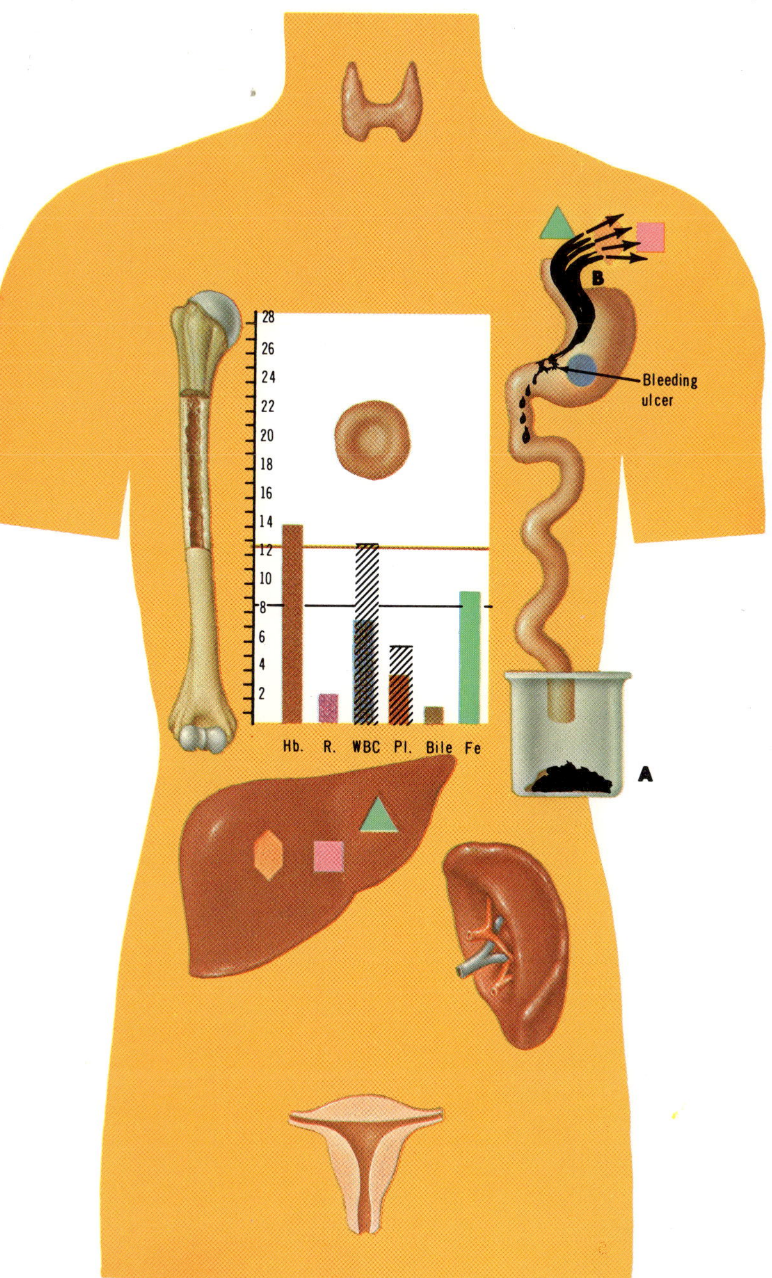

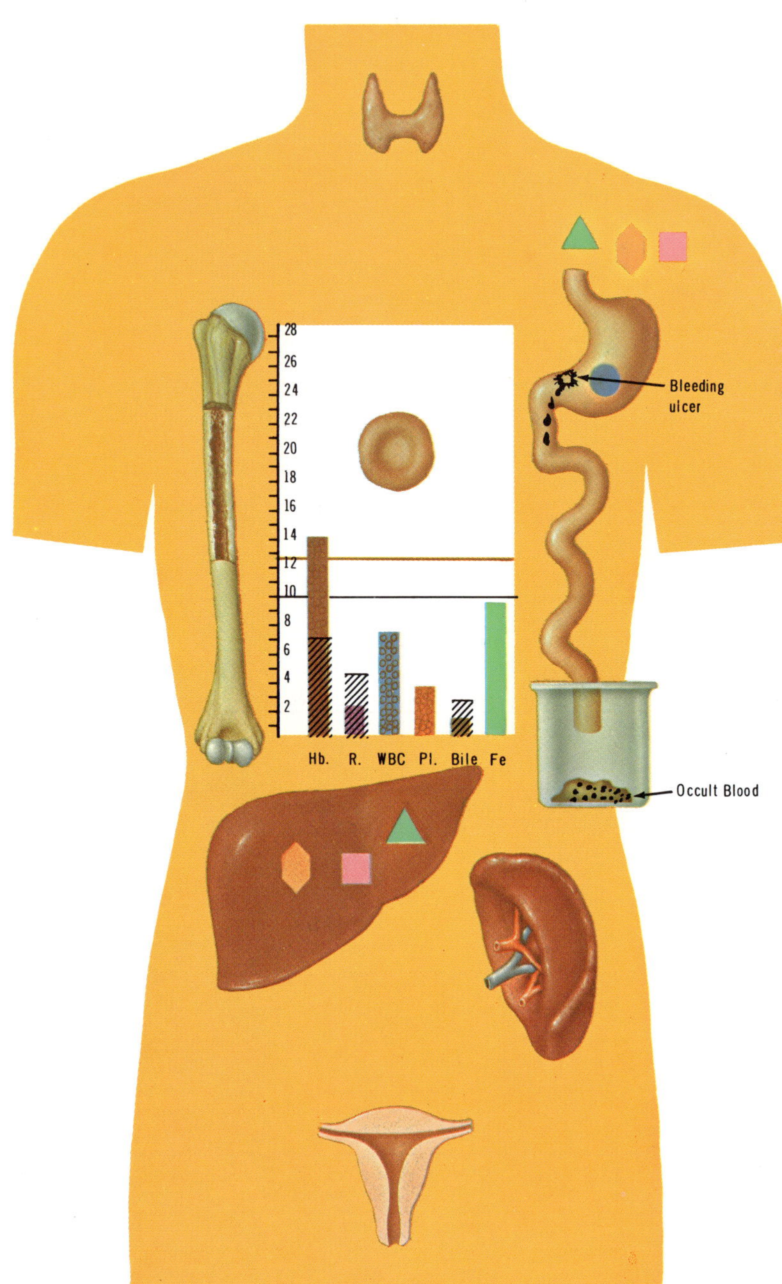

BLEEDING PEPTIC ULCER, SUBACUTE STAGE

After the first 24 hours hemodilution occurs in this disorder, and a definite *drop* in *hemoglobin* and *hematocrit* will be observed. The *reticulocyte count* rises as the bone marrow begins to compensate for the blood loss. Reabsorption of hemoglobin and its metabolites from the gastro-intestinal tract may lead to a rise in indirect bilirubin. The white count and platelets usually return to normal at this time.

Summary of Laboratory Findings:

Hemoglobin and hematocrit: Decreased

Reticulocyte count: Increased

Cell morphology: Red cell morphology normal except for polychromasia

White cell count: Normal

Platelet count: Normal

Serum bilirubin: Normal or increased

Serum iron: Normal or decreased

Blood volume: Decreased

CHRONIC MENORRHAGIA

Excessive menstrual bleeding (A), whether due to fibroids, endometrial carcinoma, or an endocrine disorder, will lead to the loss of as much as 200 ml. of blood during each period. Women who have a good diet may compensate for this loss of hemoglobin and iron. Those who have an inadequate intake of iron cannot (B). The blood picture is identical with that seen in hypochromic anemia of infancy (p. 213).

Metrorrhagia from gynecological conditions and chronic blood loss from gastrointestinal disorders will produce similar changes in the peripheral blood. "The appearance of iron deficiency anemia in an adult man or a postmenopausal woman means blood loss until proved otherwise."* It is much less common for hematuria, recurrent epistaxis, or hemoptysis to produce this picture.

Summary of Laboratory Findings:

Hemoglobin and hematocrit: Decreased

Reticulocyte count: Normal

Cell morphology: Hypochromia, microcytosis, and anisocytosis

White cell count: Normal

Platelet count: Normal

Serum bilirubin: Normal

Serum iron: Decreased

* Beeson, P. B., and McDermott, W. (eds.): Cecil-Loeb Textbook of Medicine. ed. 11, p. 1110. Philadelphia, W. B. Saunders, 1963.

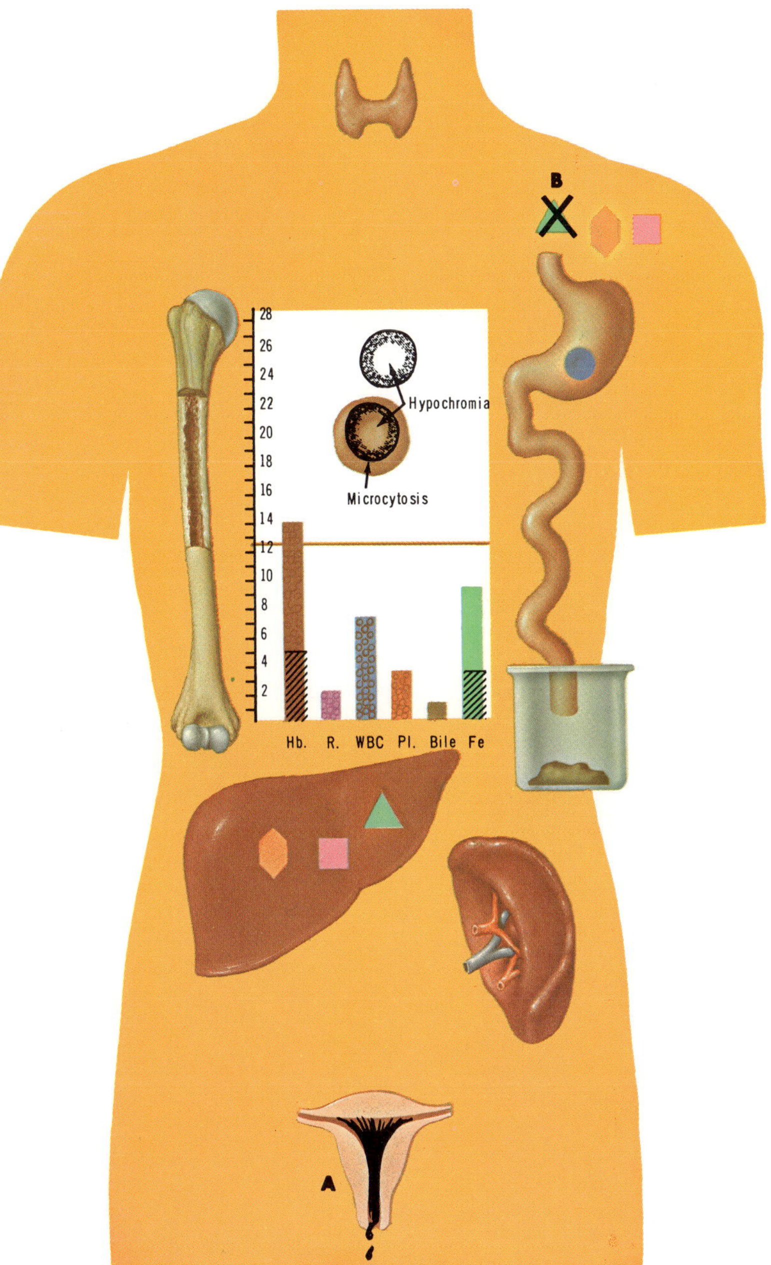

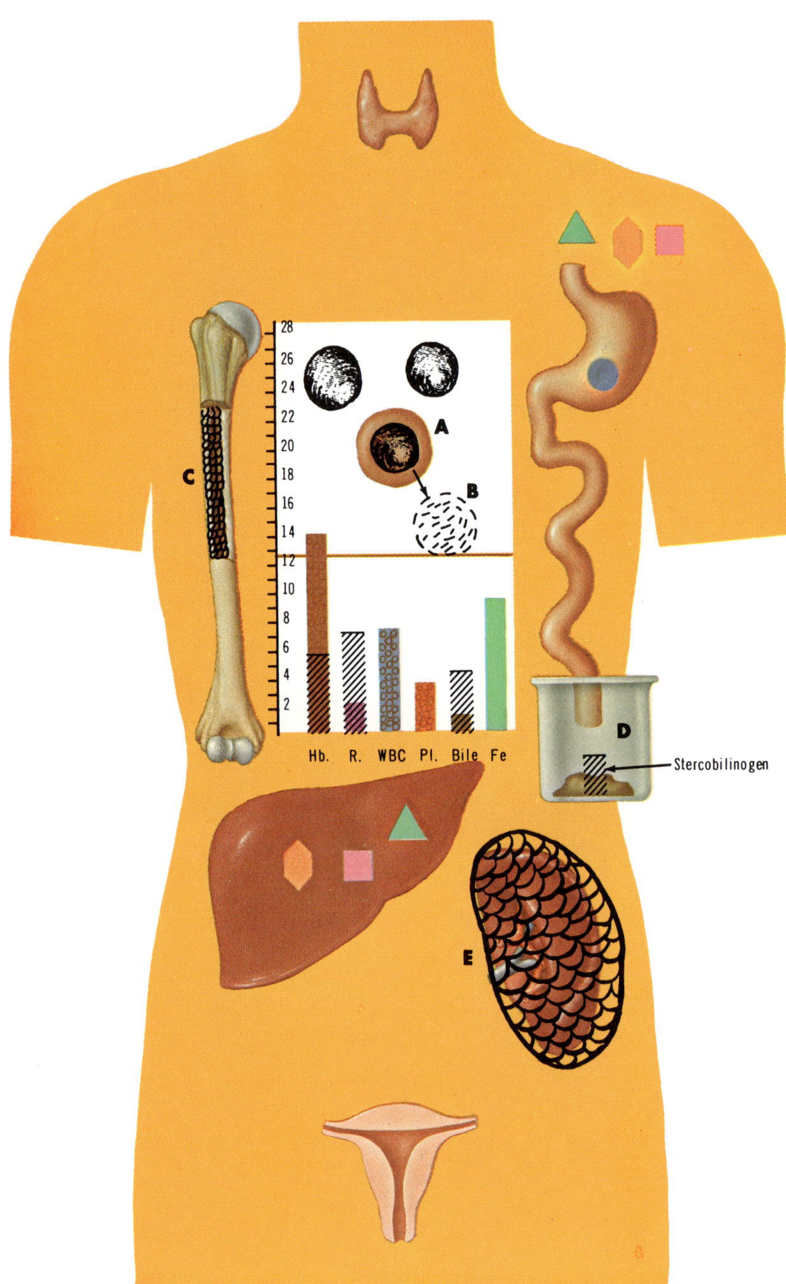

HEREDITARY SPHEROCYTOSIS

This condition is characterized by defective red cells that are small and spherical with no central pallor (A). They have diminished resistance to hypotonic saline. The mean corpuscular volume is usually low. The blood smear will often be diagnostic. During a crisis the fragile red cells hemolyze (B), and there is a rapid *drop* in *hemoglobin* and *hematocrit* attended by a *rise* in *reticulocytes*. Compensatory hyperplasia in the bone marrow (C) follows. The hemoglobin released by hemolysis is converted to *indirect bilirubin*, and this *rises* in the blood. Serum haptoglobins are decreased because of binding with the liberated hemoglobin. The increased breakdown of hemoglobin may also be reflected by an increase in stool stercobilinogen (D). The spleen enlarges (E) because of its increased work load in removing red cell debris.

A red blood cell fragility test with hypotonic saline should be performed. A Coombs' test as well as the determination of the chromium-tagged red cell survival will help to differentiate this condition from the acquired form of hemolytic anemia. The survival of chromium-tagged red cells from normal subjects injected into the patient is, of course, normal, as there are no antibodies. A bone marrow examination is unnecessary to establish the diagnosis.

Summary of Laboratory Findings:

Hemoglobin and hematocrit: Decreased

Reticulocyte count: Increased

Cell morphology: Microcytosis, spherical cells

White cell count: Normal or increased

Platelet count: Normal or increased

Serum bilirubin: Increased

Serum iron: Normal or increased

SICKLE CELL ANEMIA

The red cells in this hereditary disorder contain an abnormal hemoglobin that causes these cells to become sickle-shaped (A) under decreased oxygen tension. Such cells have a decreased survival time. During a crisis the *hemoglobin* and *hematocrit drop* precipitously as the cells hemolyze at a rapid rate. The hemoglobin released is converted to *bilirubin,* and the serum level of this pigment rises. If hemolysis is rapid the serum haptoglobins drop. The stools also contain increased stercobilinogen (B) as a reflection of the higher serum level of bilirubin. The bone marrow tries to compensate by hyperplasia, increasing the number of nucleated red blood cells, but frequently there is hypoplasia ("aplastic crisis"). The *reticulocyte count increases,* and normoblasts (C) appear in the peripheral blood. There are *leukocytosis* and an *increase* in *platelets.*

Wright's stain will often show a few sickle cells as well as normoblasts and target cells. If not, a preparation made under reduced oxygen tension either by using 2 per cent sodium metabisulfite or by sealing it under a cover slip will be diagnostic. These cells also show increased resistance to hypotonic saline solutions. Occasionally, sickle cell trait will produce the same picture and can be differentiated by hemoglobin electrophoresis. This reveals that 20-45% of the hemoglobin is sickle type (HbS) and the rest is normal adult type (HbA). Hemoglobin electrophoresis also may reveal sickle-cell hemoglobin C disease (HbC) and hemoglobin C trait disease (HbC and HbA combined).

Summary of Laboratory Findings:

Hemoglobin and hematocrit: Decreased
Reticulocyte count: Increased
Cell morphology: Sickle cells and target cells
White cell count: Normal or increased
Platelet count: Normal or increased
Serum bilirubin: Increased
Serum iron: Normal or increased

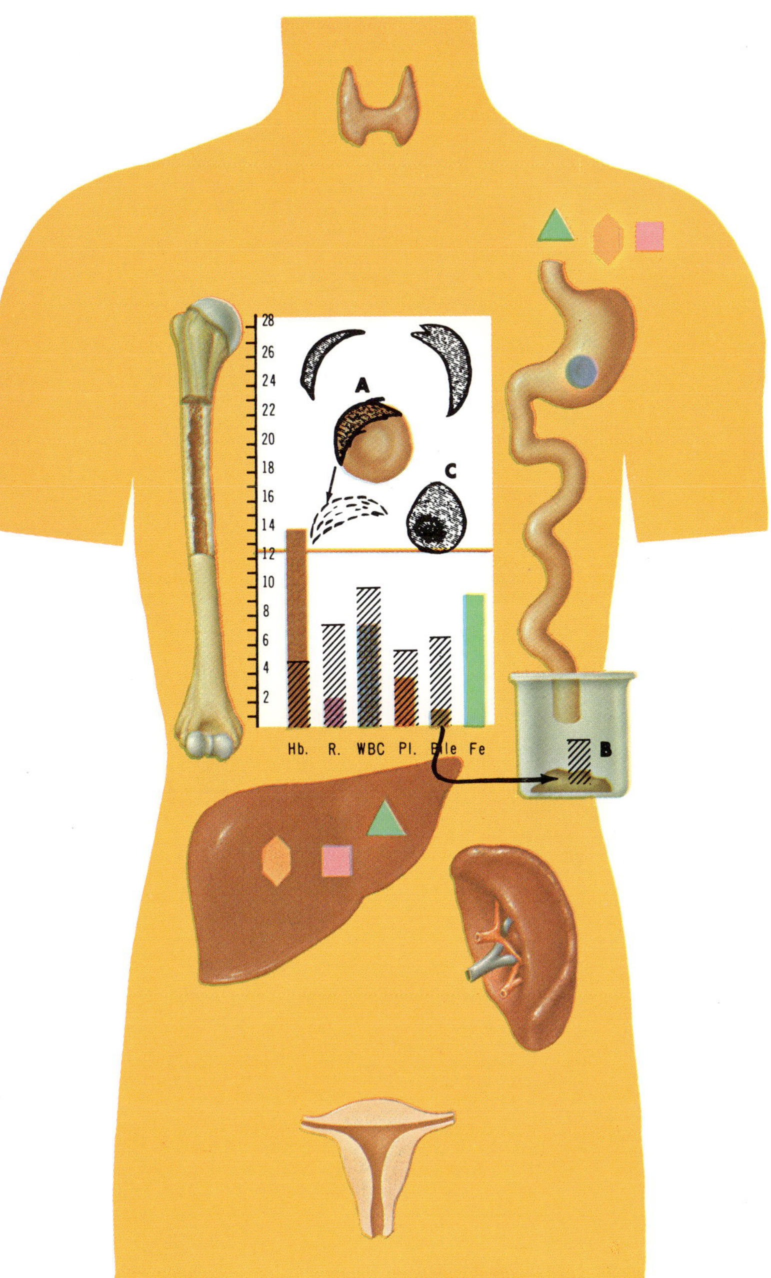

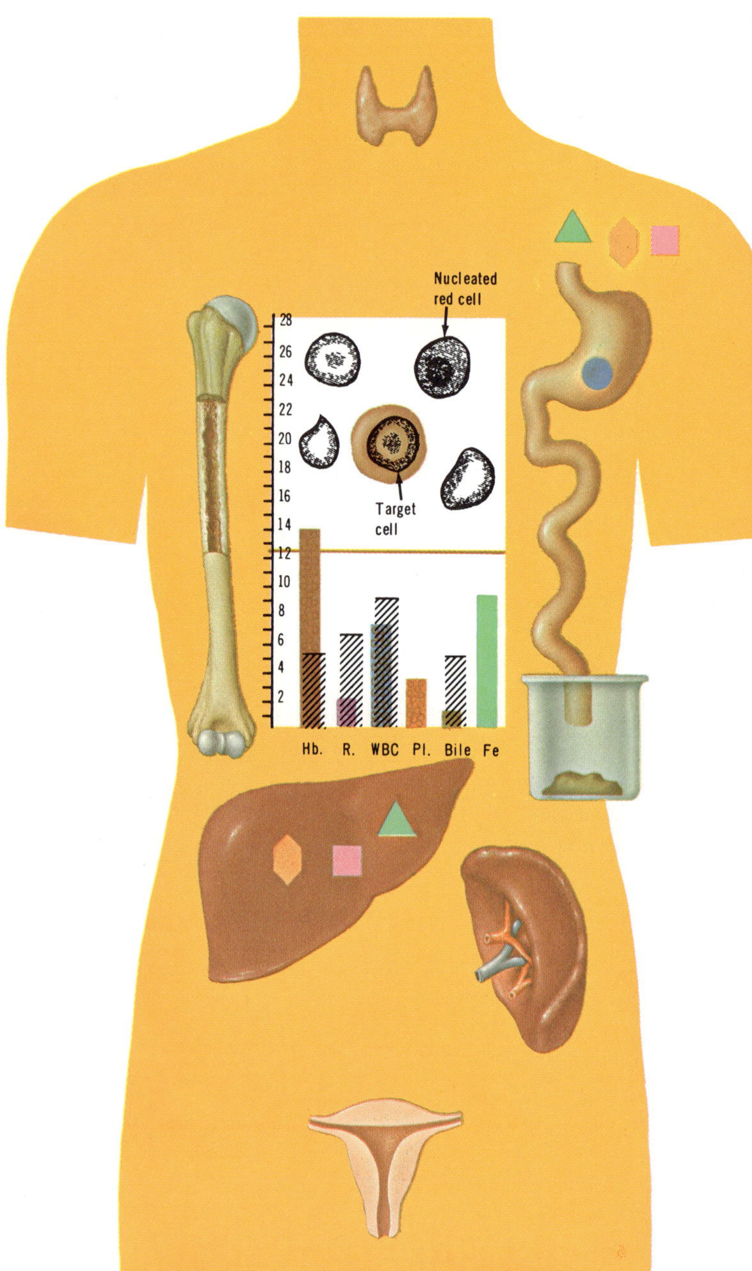

THALASSEMIA MAJOR

In this hereditary disorder there is a defect in total hemoglobin synthesis that may manifest in many ways (fetal, etc.).* On hemoglobin electrophoresis with alkali denaturation, the majority of patients have over 50 per cent HbF (fetal). The cells are small and hypochromic and have a decreased survival time. A marked *reduction* in *hemoglobin* and *hematocrit* from hemolysis occurs, indicated by a *rise* in *serum bilirubin*. The bone marrow tries to compensate for the hemolysis by hyperplasia, and an increase of nucleated red cells is noted. Some of these reach the peripheral blood, and the *reticulocyte count* is *increased*. Leukocytosis is common, but the platelet count is usually not altered. Roentgenograms of the skull and long bones may show characteristic changes that lend support to the diagnosis.

The distorted red cells have a characteristic appearance in the blood smear. They are hypochromic and microcytic and vary in size and shape (anisocytosis and poikilocytosis). What little pigment they have may be concentrated in the center (''target cells''). The fragility of these cells in hypotonic saline is usually decreased, a characteristic that helps to differentiate this anemia from hereditary spherocytosis.

Various forms of thalassemia Hb-C and thalassemia minor (HbA_2) may present a similar picture but can be differentiated by hemoglobin or starch block electrophoresis. In thalassemia Hb-S disease the sickle cell preparation will be positive.

Summary of Laboratory Findings:

Hemoglobin and hematocrit: Decreased

Reticulocyte count: Increased

Cell morphology: Hypochromia, microcytosis, target cells, and nucleated red cells

White cell count: Increased

Platelet count: Normal

Serum bilirubin: Increased

Serum iron: Normal or increased

* Beeson and McDermott, *op. cit.*, p. 1103.

ACQUIRED HEMOLYTIC ANEMIA

The alterations in the blood in this form of hemolytic anemia, as readily noted, are almost identical with those in the hereditary forms of hemolytic anemia. The principal difference is that on blood smear the bulk of the *red blood cells* are *normal* in appearance. Of course, there are often *normoblasts* (A) in the peripheral blood, especially in the acute stages. The basis for the hemolysis is an autoantibody (B) that agglutinates the red cells. These will be detected by the performance of Coombs' test.

Such antibodies may be found in *malignant lymphomas, chronic lymphocytic leukemia, lupus erythematosus, infectious mononucleosis,* and *viral infections* as well as in an idiopathic state. These cells exhibit increased mechanical fragility, whereas osmotic fragility may be normal.

Transfusion reactions and erythroblastosis are also associated with antibodies and produce the same changes in blood.

Hemolytic anemias due to infectious agents, such as *malaria, Oroya fever,* and *septicemia,* and physical agents, such as *phenacetin, nitrobenzene, primaquine,* and *lead,* will present a picture similar to that of acquired hemolytic anemia. History and a negative Coombs' test will usually differentiate them. Looking for intracellular parasites in malaria, Heinz bodies in primaquine sensitivity, and basophilic stippling in lead intoxication will be of further assistance in diagnosis. Paroxysmal (cold) hemoglobinemia also produces an acquired hemolytic anemia, but a positive serologic test for syphilis and the Donath-Landsteiner test, in which there is hemolysis following chilling of the blood, make the diagnosis clear.

Summary of Laboratory Findings:

Hemoglobin and hematocrit: Decreased
Reticulocyte count: Increased
Cell morphology: Normal except for nucleated red cells
White cell count: Increased during crisis
Platelet count: Normal
Serum bilirubin: Increased
Serum iron: Normal or increased

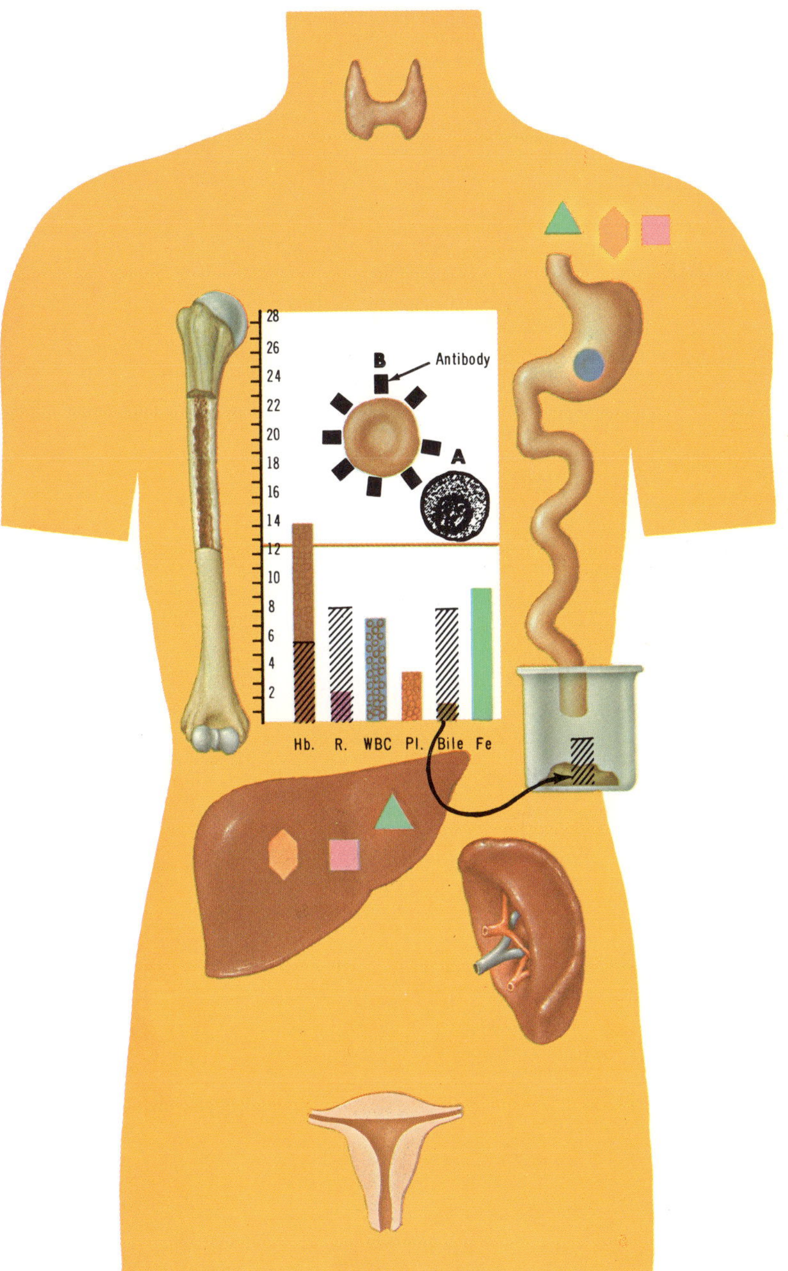

HEMOLYTIC TRANSFUSION REACTIONS

In this disorder either isoagglutinins present in the recipient's blood agglutinate the donor's red cells (most common), or isoagglutinins in the donor's blood agglutinate the recipient's red cells. Usually, an ABO or Rh incompatibility is responsible, but Kell, Duffy, and other factors may occasionally be involved. Intravascular or extravascular hemolysis (A) results with a consequent *drop* in *hemoglobin* and *hematocrit* (see plate on p. 229). At the same time there are *reticulocytosis* and *increased serum bilirubin* (indirect type). Red cell morphology is usually undisturbed. The *white count* may be *increased*. Serum haptoglobins decrease. Free hemoglobin is often present in the plasma and urine. The blood urea nitrogen will rise if there is hemoglobinuric nephrosis. A more definitive diagnosis is made by retyping and crossmatching the donor's blood and the recipient's blood in both pre- and post-transfusion samples. Coombs' test may be positive.

Common Types of ABO and Rh Incompatibility

These are illustrated in Tables 18-1 and 18-2.

ABO Incompatibilities. Anti-A antibodies occur in type B blood; anti-B antibodies occur in type A blood; both types of antibodies occur in type O blood. Type AB blood has neither anti-A nor anti-B antibodies. The principle to remember is that an individual will not produce antibodies against his own antigens.

It follows from the above that a transfusion reaction might result from agglutination of donor red cells when:

1. Type A blood is given to a type B recipient.
2. Type B blood is given to a type A recipient.
3. Type AB blood is given to recipients with either A, B, or O blood.

Type O blood may be given to any type of recipient without agglutination of donor cells. This has given rise to the concept of the "universal donor" (to be explained subsequently, p. 229).

Likewise, it follows that a transfusion reaction might result from agglutination of recipient red cells when:

1. Type B blood is given to type A recipients.
2. Type A blood is given to type B recipients.
3. Type A, B, or O blood is given to type AB recipients.

Any type of blood may be given to type O recipients without agglutination of recipient's red cells. Most important, no agglutination will occur if both donor and recipient have the same type of blood. One exception to this is donors with A_2 blood type because they have antibodies to A_1 blood. When their blood is given to A_1 recipients a transfusion reaction may occur.

Agglutination of recipient's red cells by the donor's blood is infrequent because the donor's blood is diluted by the recipient. However, if the donor's blood contains high titers of antibody, there may not be sufficient dilution.

Rh Incompatibilities.. In the Rh system natural antibodies do not occur, but Rh antibodies (called iso-immune antibodies) may be produced in response to transfusions and pregnancy. Thus the blood of Rh_0-negative (D-negative) persons who have been subjected to these circumstances may have Rh_0 antibodies. Rh_0-positive (D-positive) blood does not contain Rh_0 antibodies. It follows that donor's blood of type Rh_0-negative may agglutinate Rh_0-positive blood cells of a recipient. Likewise, red cells of a donor with type Rh_0-positive blood may be agglutinated by type Rh_0-negative blood of a recipient. There are six additional important types of Rh antibodies. These are anti-rh′ (anti-C), anti-rh″ (anti-E), anti-hr′ (anti-c), anti-hr″ (anti-e), anti-C^w and anti-D^u. These antibodies may be produced by any individual who does not have the corresponding antigen (C, E, c, e, etc.) when he is transfused with blood containing that antigen. Sensitization of this type is infrequent. Thus transfusion reactions of this type are just as infrequent.

Prevention of Transfusion Reactions

Prevention of transfusion reaction depends on careful selection of the donor. First, the donor's blood and the patient's blood should be of the same type. Second, the donor's blood and the blood of the patient must be compatible when crossmatched. The following is a brief outline of one accepted procedure of typing and crossmatching.

Typing. Standard serums containing anti-A and anti-B antibodies are separately mixed with red cells of the untyped blood (whether it be donor or recipient). Type A red cells will be agglutinated by anti-A serum, type B red cells will be agglutinated by anti-B serum, and type AB red cells will be agglutinated by both. Type O cells will not be agglutinated by either. This is only half the job. The serum of the unknown blood must be mixed separately with standard suspensions of type A and B erythrocytes to eliminate most sources of error.

Table 18-1. Agglutination of Donor Cells (Major Reaction)

Recipient / Donor	Type A	Type B	Type AB	Type O
Type A	None	Reaction (A) Anti-A	None	Reaction (A) Anti-A
Type B	Reaction (B) Anti-B	None	None	Reaction (B) Anti-B
Type AB	Reaction (AB) Anti-B	Reaction (AB) Anti-A	None	Reaction (AB) Anti-A Anti-B
Type O	None	None	None	None

O = Red cell
▭ = Antibody

Recipient / Donor	Rh_o-Positive	Rh_o-Negative
Rh_o-Positive	None	Reaction (Rh_o) Anti-Rh_o
Rh_o-Negative	None	None

Table 18-2. Agglutination of Recipient Red Cells (Minor Reaction)

Recipient / Donor	Type A	Type B	Type AB	Type O
Type A	None	Reaction 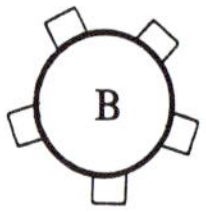 B Anti-B	Reaction 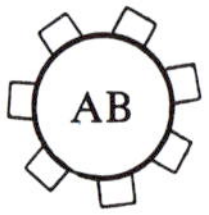 AB Anti-B	None
Type B	Reaction 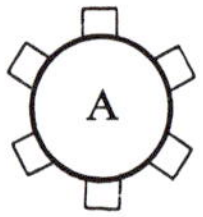 A Anti-A	None	Reaction 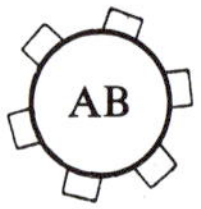 AB Anti-A	None
Type AB	None	None	None	None
Type O	Reaction 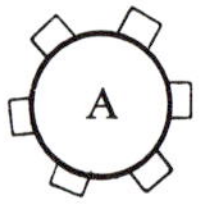 A Anti-A	Reaction 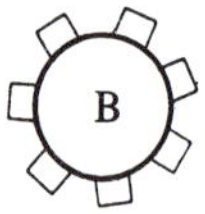 B Anti-B	Reaction 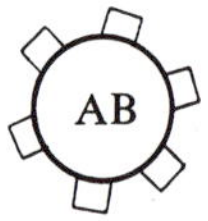 AB Anti-A Anti-B	None

O = Red cell
▭ = Antibody

Recipient / Donor	Rh$_o$-Positive	Rh$_o$-Negative
Rh$_o$-Positive	None	None
Rh$_o$-Negative	Reaction 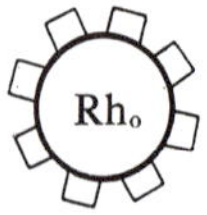 Rh$_o$ Anti-Rh$_o$	None

In like manner red cells resuspended from a clot of the unknown blood are tested separately with a standard serum containing Rh antibodies (Rh_0). If the blood is Rh-positive, the red cells will agglutinate immediately or at least after incubation and centrifugation. Those that fail to agglutinate are classified as Rh-negative. Rh-negative donors should be further tested for D^u and "C" antigens.* By using anti-D (Rh_0) serum known to contain these D variants, an indirect Coombs' test is performed. In general, routine testing of Rh_0 (D) antigen is sufficient, but occasionally a screening must be made for the other Rh antigens.

Crossmatching. First, the donor's cells are mixed with the serum of the recipient (major crossmatch). If there is any clumping, the two bloods are incompatible. Next the donor's serum is mixed with the recipient's cells (minor crossmatch). Again there should be no clumping if they are to be considered compatible.

Type O red cells will not be agglutinated by the serum of recipients with type O, A, B, or AB blood because anti-O isoagglutinins do not exist. This is the reason that type O donors have been labeled "universal donors." However, type O donors' blood contains anti-A and anti-B antibodies. In high titers these agglutinins will not be sufficiently diluted by the transfusion to prevent agglutination in recipients with type A, B, or AB blood. Therefore, except in emergencies, type O blood should not be given to type A, B, or AB recipients.

Summary of Laboratory Findings:

Hemoglobin and hematocrit: Decreased
Reticulocyte count: Increased
Cell morphology: Normal
White cell count: Increased
Platelet count: Normal or increased
Serum bilirubin: Increased
Serum iron: Normal

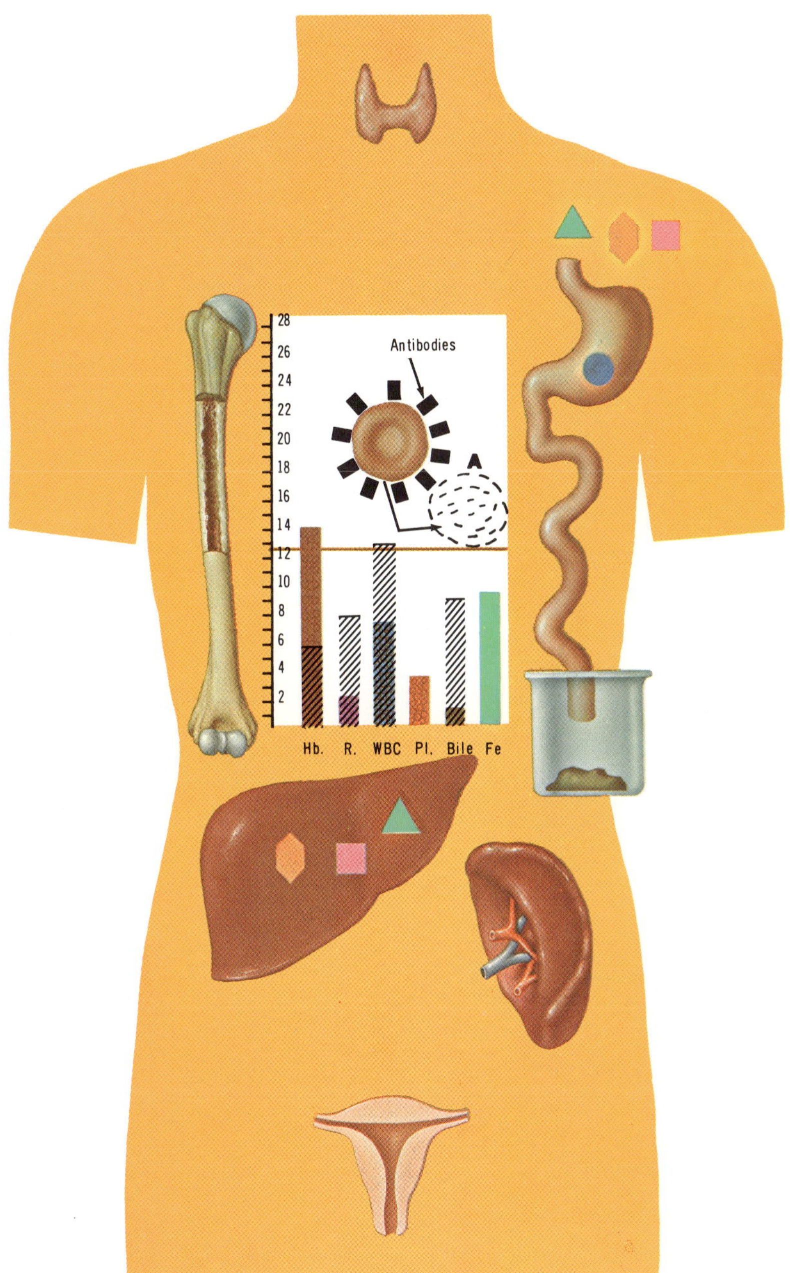

* Subcommittee on Transfusion Problems, Division of Medical Sciences, National Academy of Sciences-National Research Council (Strumia, M. M., *et al.*, eds.): General Principles of Blood Transfusion. Philadelphia, J. B. Lippincott, 1963.

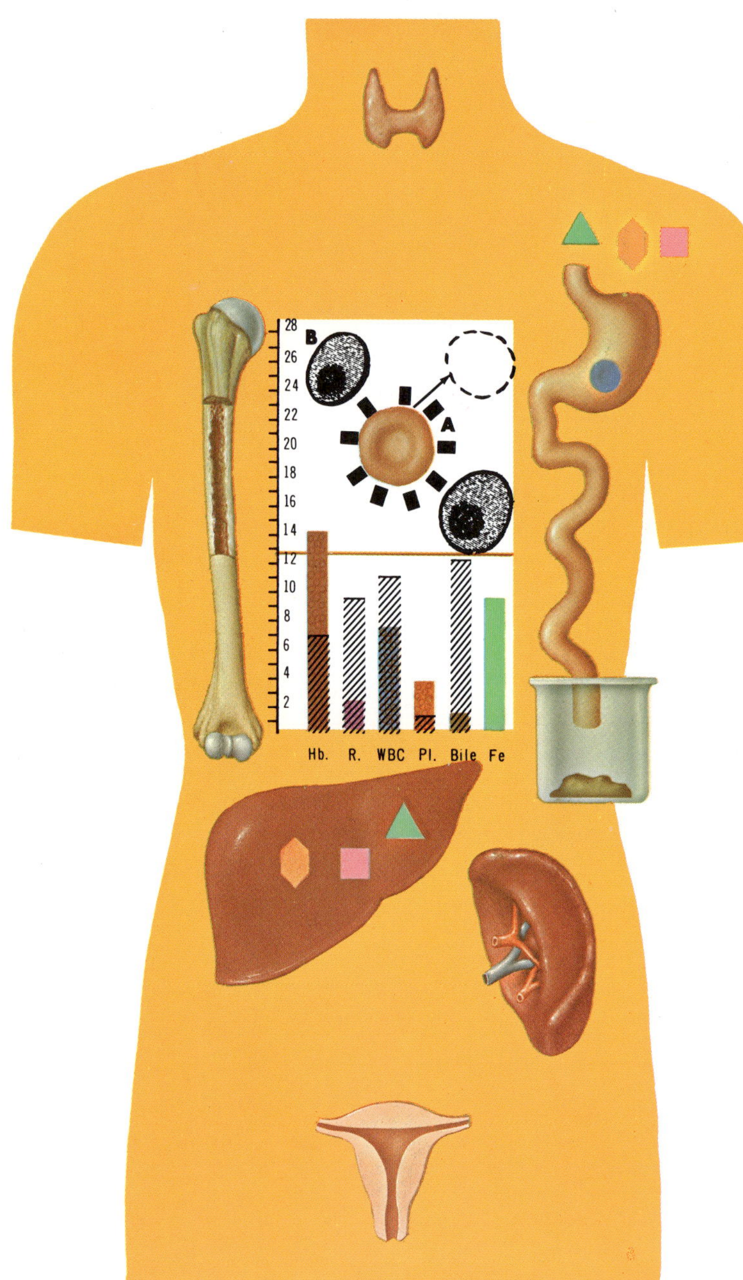

ERYTHROBLASTOSIS FETALIS

This disorder is essentially the consequence of a "transfusion reaction" between mother and fetus. If blood cells (or their components) of an Rh-positive fetus (the donor) cross the placenta into the circulation of an Rh-negative mother (the recipient), she forms Rh-antibodies. Once these antibodies (A) reach a sufficient titer in the mother's blood, they, too, cross the placenta into the fetal circulation, where they cause hemolysis. The *hemoglobin* and *hematocrit* of the fetus *drop*. A *rise* of *bilirubin* (the indirect type) occurs. This can be detected while the fetus is in utero by amniocentesis. Thus delivery can be planned early. There is *reticulocytosis,* and massive numbers of *nucleated red cells* (B) (10,000 to 100,000/cu. mm.) appear in the peripheral blood. (Normal newborn infants have 200 to 2,000 nucleated erythrocytes/cu. mm.).

In addition, there is *leukocytosis,* whereas the *platelets* often *diminish*. A direct Coombs' test (adding rabbit antihuman globulin to red cells suspected of being sensitized) on the infant is positive. An indirect Coombs' test (adding suspect serum to fresh Rh-positive red cells and then to rabbit antiglobulin) on the mother is positive.

It is unlikely that the above reaction will occur unless the mother has been sensitized by a previous transfusion or pregnancy. Erythroblastosis fetalis may occur also in babies of Rh-positive mothers. In these cases the incompatibility may be based on one of the other Rh antigens (C, E, c, e). For example, the infant's red cells may contain C-antigen, whereas the mother's do not. The mother may therefore form anti-C antibodies to the infant's blood cells. In sufficient titers these antibodies can cross the placenta to hemolyze the infant's red cells.

As in transfusion reactions, the reaction between mother and fetus may be based on an ABO incompatibility ("icterus praecox"). For example, a mother with group B blood may carry a fetus with group A blood. If her titer of anti-A antibodies is high enough, these antibodies will cross the placenta and agglutinate and hemolyze the infant's red cells. She may have a naturally high titer of anti-A antibodies or a high titer may develop in the same way as in Rh incompatibilities (transfusions, etc.).

Summary of Laboratory Findings:

Hemoglobin and hematocrit: Decreased
Reticulocyte count: Increased
Cell morphology: Nucleated red cells
White cell count: Increased
Platelet count: Normal or decreased
Serum bilirubin: Increased
Serum iron: Normal

ACUTE MYELOBLASTIC LEUKEMIA

The mechanism of anemia in this condition is obscure. Although it was previously thought to have a myelophthisic etiology, recent evidence reveals that decreased erythropoiesis or increased red cell destruction occurring alone or together are probably responsible (Wintrobe*). Nevertheless, the blood picture is best understood if one imagines it to be due to myelophthisis (A). There are *normocytic anemia* and *thrombocytopenia* in the face of *leukocytosis*. The count of leukocytes is rarely higher than 35,000, and in approximately 25 per cent of the cases it is normal or below normal. The importance of using Wright's stain in diagnosing anemia is well emphasized here. The finding of a large percentage of blast cells (B) makes the diagnosis unmistakable. Despite the frequent occurrence of increased red cell destruction, a rise in serum bilirubin is not usually detected. The reticulocyte count is often increased, and normoblasts (C) are found in the peripheral blood. Examination of the bone marrow is superfluous in the diagnosis of all but the aleukemic variety of leukemia.

Acute lymphoblastic anemia will give a picture very similar to the above, but the chronic leukemias usually show a much more marked leukocytosis, and the vast majority of the cells are more mature (see p. 241). Chronic lymphocytic leukemia is associated with a hemolytic anemia (p. 242).

Summary of Laboratory Findings:

Hemoglobin and hematocrit: Decreased

Reticulocyte count: Increased

Cell morphology: Myeloblasts

White cell count: Increased

Platelet count: Decreased

Serum bilirubin: Normal

Serum iron: Normal or increased

* Wintrobe, M. M.: Clinical Hematology. ed. 5. Philadelphia, Lea & Febiger, 1961.

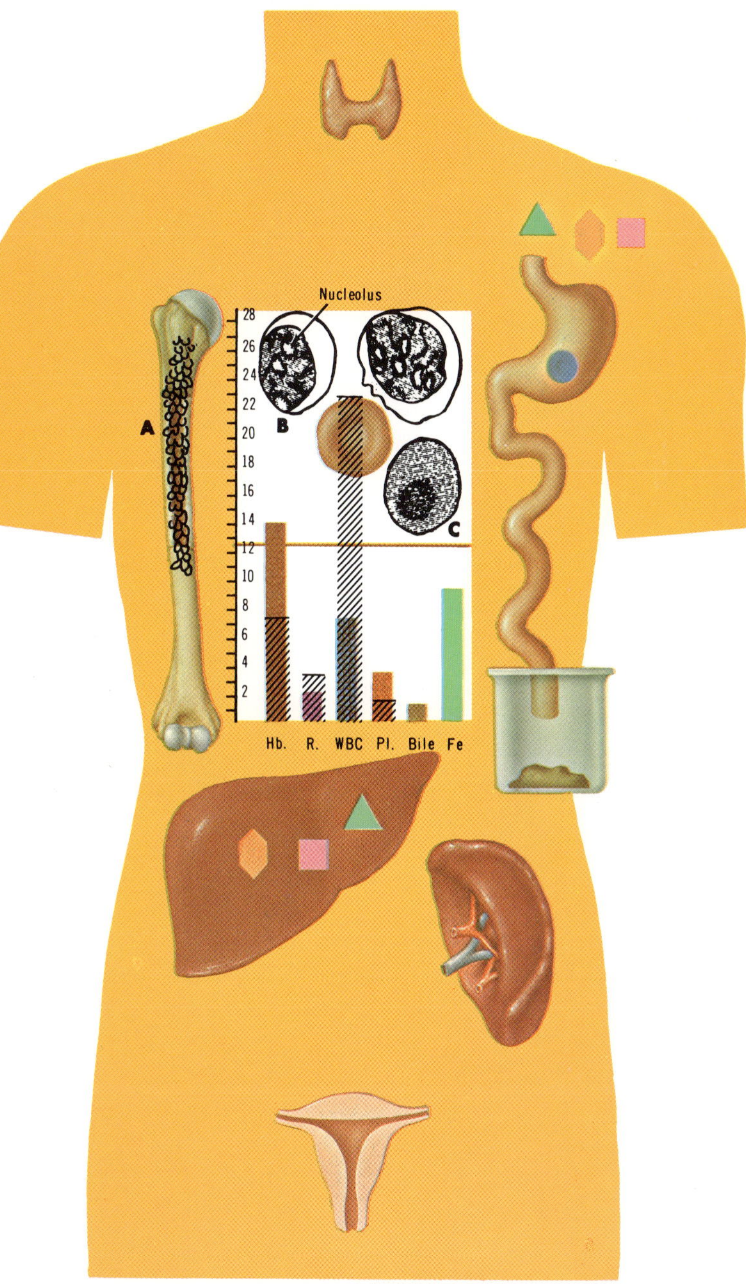

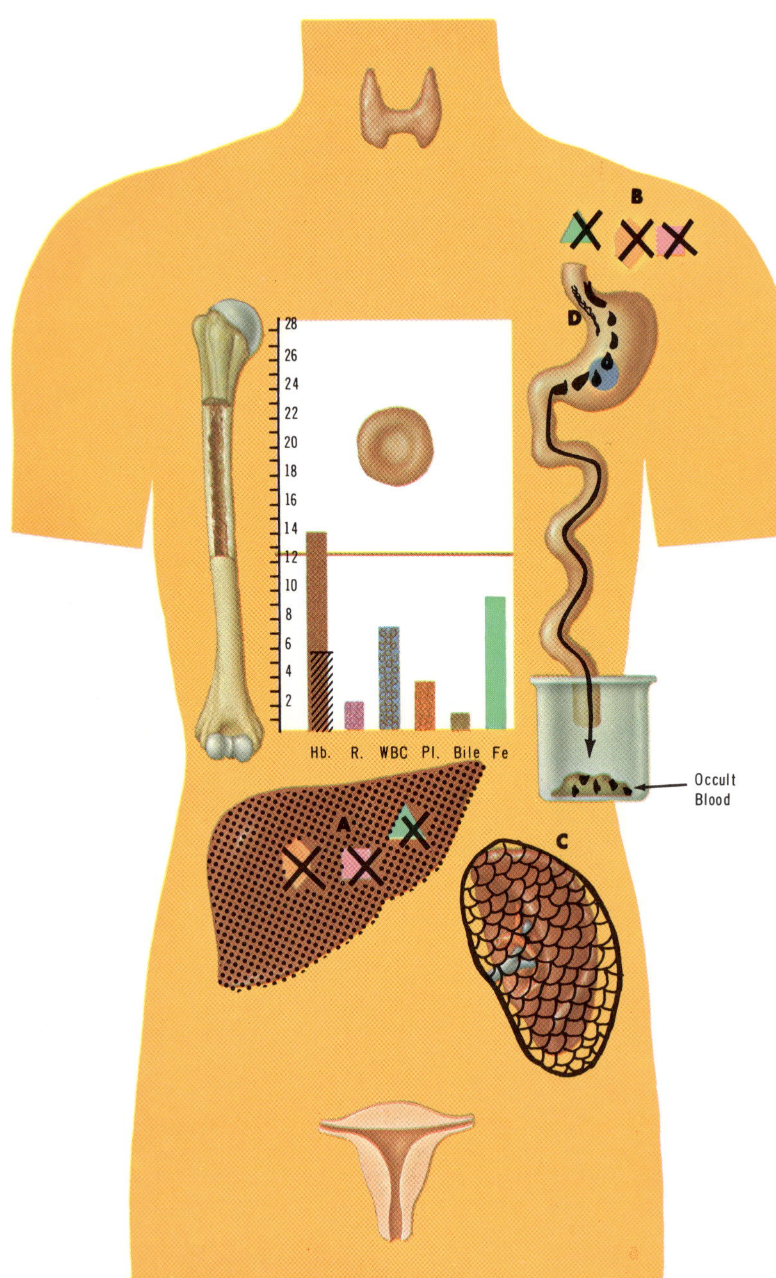

CIRRHOSIS OF THE LIVER

The anemia of cirrhosis may be due to any one of the three basic mechanisms of anemia. The storage of important nutritional elements such as B_{12}, iron, and folic acid may be impaired (A). The intake of these substances may be limited (B) because of the poor dietary habits of these individuals. *Red cell production may be decreased* for these reasons. On the other hand, *red cell survival* as determined by Cr^{51}-tagged red cells may be *diminished*. Whether this is primarily due to the production of defective cells or increased cell destruction by an enlarged spleen (C) or a hyperactive reticuloendothelial system is undetermined. Finally, anemia may result from *blood loss* through ruptured esophageal varices (D). The deficiency of clotting factors such as prothrombin predisposes to this.

From the above discussion it is easily understood why the anemia may be macrocytic, normocytic, or microcytic. There may be target cells in the peripheral smear. The *platelet* and *leukocyte* count are usually *unaltered*. Unless red cell destruction is proceeding at a rapid rate, the *reticulocyte count* and *serum bilirubin* are *normal* (on the assumption that hepatocellular damage is not severe enough to cause jaundice). The *serum iron* is *unaltered* unless poor diet is a factor in the pathogenesis. The history along with a battery of liver function tests and possibly a liver biopsy will establish the diagnosis in most cases.

Summary of Laboratory Findings:

Hemoglobin and hematocrit: Decreased
Reticulocyte count: Normal
Cell morphology: Varied
White cell count: Normal or decreased
Platelet count: Normal
Serum bilirubin: Normal or increased
Serum iron: Normal or decreased

CHRONIC CONGESTIVE SPLENOMEGALY (BANTI'S SYNDROME)

In this disorder portal hypertension leads to progressive splenic enlargement (A) and its consequences. Increased destruction of the formed elements of the blood or possibly bone marrow inhibition by a splenic humoral factor results in *anemia, leukopenia,* and *thrombocytopenia,* either alone or in combination. *Reticulocytes* are *increased.* The anemia is characteristically normocytic. A bone marrow examination is a valuable adjunct in diagnosis and usually reveals normal or increased cellularity with a variable myeloid-erythroid ratio. Chromium-tagged red cell survival is decreased. Subcutaneous injection of epinephrine will produce a rise in circulating red cells, white cells, or platelets. After chromium tagging of the patient's red blood cells and injecting them back into the blood, a spleen scan will reveal a large stasis compartment.

Chronic congestive splenomegaly may occur in any condition that produces portal hypertension. Among the commonest causes are cirrhosis of the liver, schistosomiasis, portal vein thrombosis or obstruction from an extrinsic tumor (pancreatic, etc.). Hypersplenism may develop in congenital hemolytic anemias, such as hereditary spherocytosis, or in acquired conditions, such as Gaucher's disease, Hodgkin's disease, and chronic granulocytic leukemia.

Summary of Laboratory Findings:

Hemoglobin and hematocrit: Decreased
Reticulocyte count: Increased
Cell morphology: Normal
White cell count: Decreased
Platelet count: Decreased
Serum bilirubin: Normal or increased
Serum iron: Normal or increased

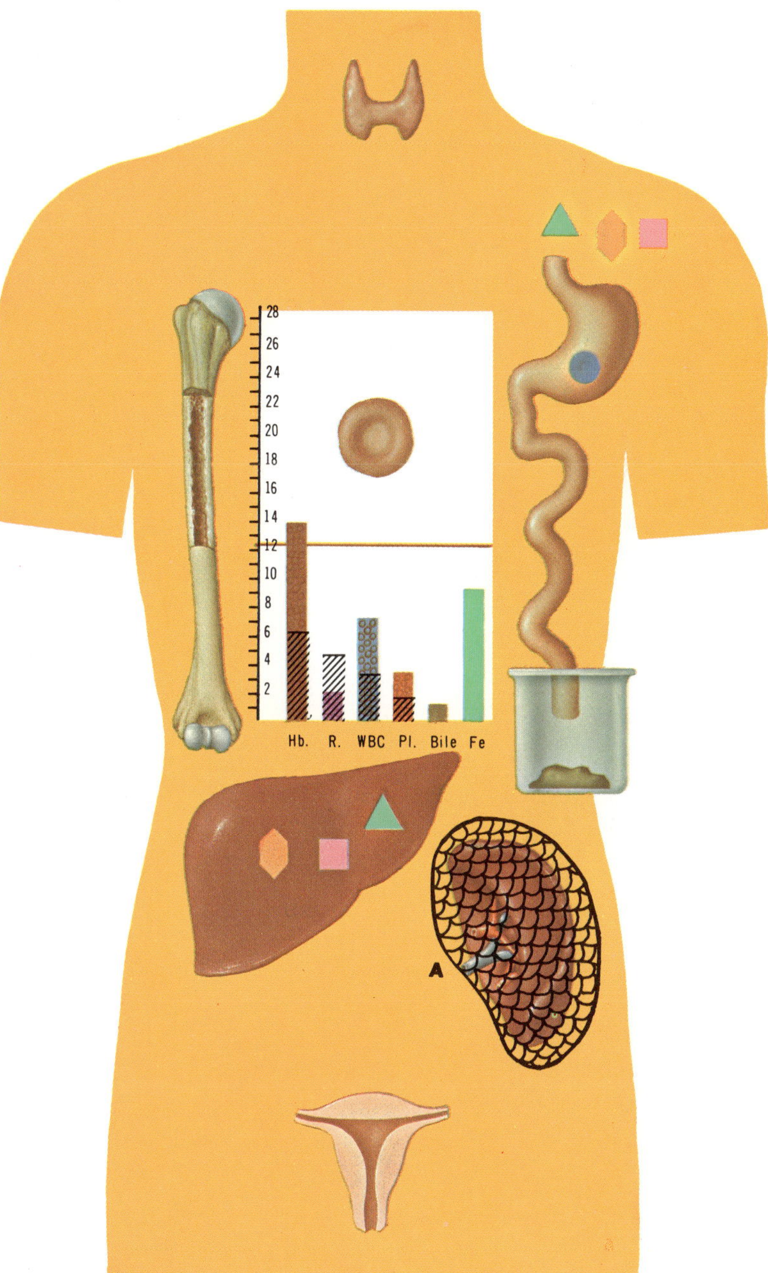

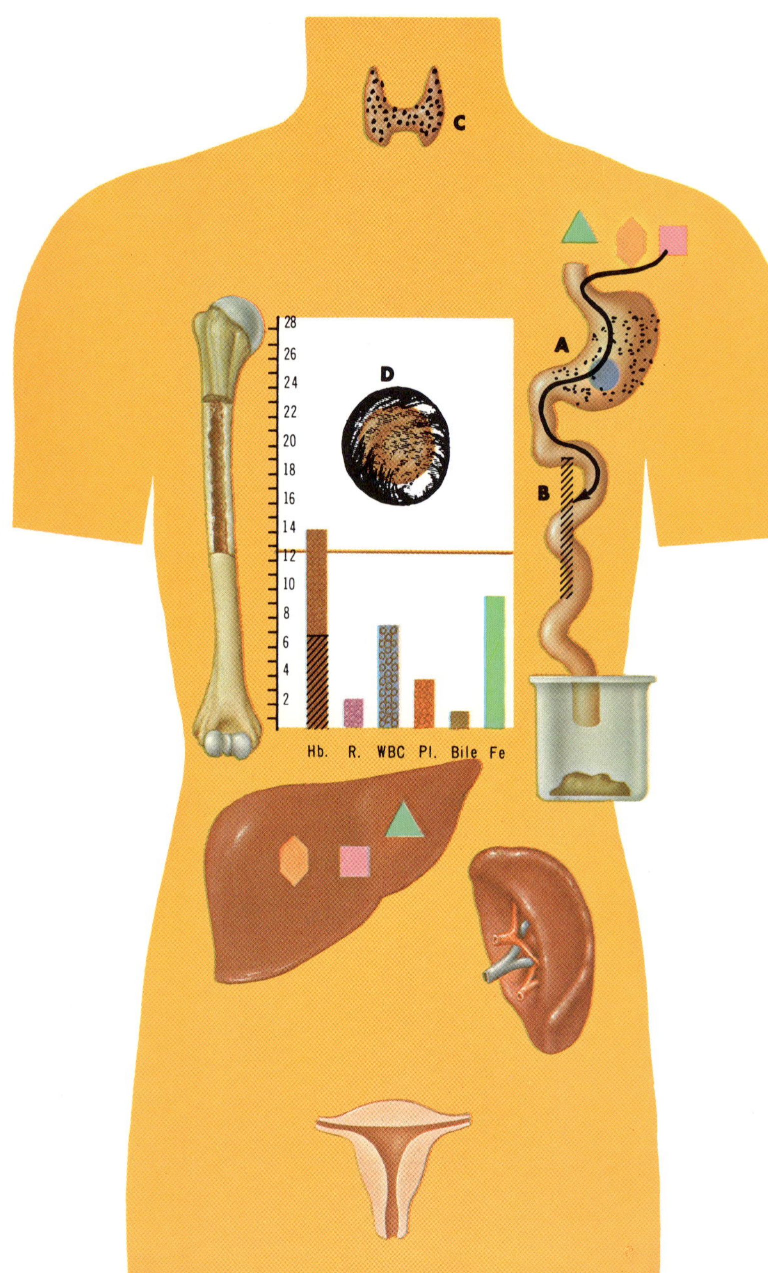

HYPOTHYROIDISM

This is another condition in which the anemia may be due to multiple factors. In over 50 per cent of these cases there is achlorhydria (A). Poor B_{12} and iron absorption may result from this or from a true defect in intestinal absorption (B). Over and above this there is apparently a true anemia of hypothyroidism (C) that responds to the administration of exogenous desiccated thyroid alone. In this condition there is macrocytosis (D) with little anisocytosis and no poikilocytosis. *White cell* and *platelet counts* are usually *unaffected,* and there is a *normal reticulocyte count.* Unless there is associated achlorhydria or poor intestinal absorption of iron, the *serum iron* is *normal.* The bone marrow may be normal or hypoplastic. A protein-bound iodine (PBI) (see p. 89) and a radioactive iodine uptake will establish the diagnosis in most cases. A therapeutic test may be performed with desiccated thyroid.

Summary of Laboratory Findings:

Hemoglobin and hematocrit: Decreased
Reticulocyte count: Normal
Cell morphology: Macrocytosis
White cell count: Normal
Platelet count: Normal
Serum bilirubin: Normal
Serum iron: Normal

SIMPLE CHRONIC ANEMIA

Chronic inflammatory conditions, neoplasms, renal disease, and endocrine disorders are associated with refractory anemias that are probably due to impaired erythropoiesis as well as shortened red cell survival. Possibly because the bone marrow fails to compensate adequately for the increased blood destruction, there is *no reticulocytosis*. Nevertheless, the appearance of the bone marrow is usually normal in contrast with that in *aplastic anemia*. Despite the shortened red cell survival the *serum bilirubin* characteristically *does not rise*. The *red cells* are *normocytic* and *normochromic*, and the anemia is rarely severe. The leukocyte count depends on the etiology, but the platelets are usually normal. *Serum iron* and *iron-binding capacity* are often *reduced*.

Serum iron, gastric analysis, and bone marrow examination should be performed to exclude such disorders as iron deficiency anemia, pernicious anemia, and aplastic anemia, respectively.

Summary of Laboratory Findings:

Hemoglobin and hematocrit: Decreased
Reticulocyte count: Normal
Cell morphology: Normal
White cell count: Variable
Platelet count: Normal
Serum bilirubin: Normal
Serum iron: Decreased

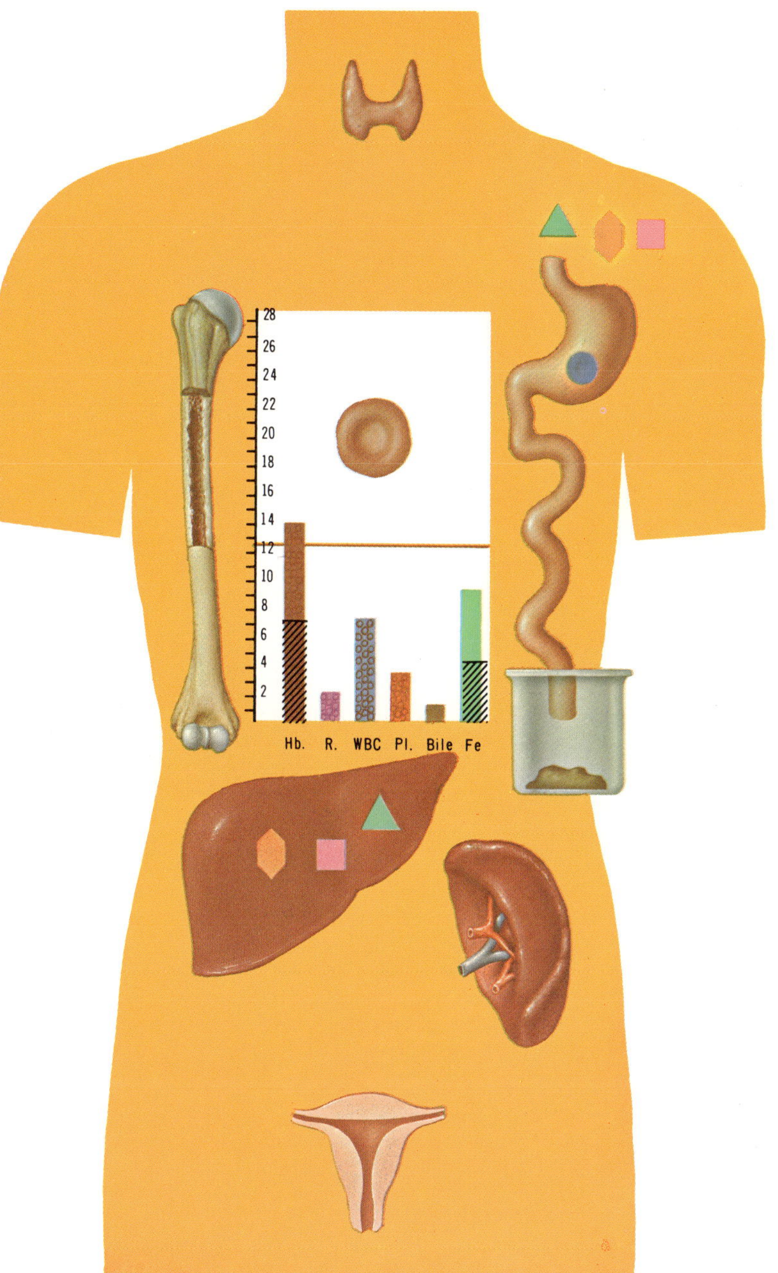

19 Disorders of the Leukocytes

NORMAL METABOLISM

Production. *Granulocytes* and *monocytes* are produced in the bone marrow by the progressive maturation and cell division of myeloblasts and monoblasts, respectively. Although the *lymphocytes* are produced primarily in the lymph nodes, the spleen, and lymphoid tissue throughout the body, they are also produced in the bone marrow. The bone marrow is one of the largest lymphocyte-containing tissues in the body, for lymphocytes make up approximately 15 per cent of the differential count on marrow aspirations. Lymphocytes originate from the maturation of the lymphoblast. *Plasma cells* are thought to originate from either the lymphocytes or primitive connective tissue cells. They are not normally found in the peripheral blood. Leukopoiesis probably depends on vitamin B_{12} and folic acid.

Since immature as well as mature cells of each series appear in the peripheral blood in disease states, it seems appropriate to comment on the structure and function of the most common of these at this point.

Myeloblast. This is a large cell with a large round nucleus containing 2 to 5 nucleoli and scanty blue nongranular cytoplasm that is occasionally foamy or reticular.

Myelocyte. The major difference between the myeloblast and the myelocyte is that granules are present in the cytoplasm of the myelocyte; the more granules, the more mature is the cell. In more mature cells the granules become neutrophilic, eosinophilic, or basophilic, depending on which type of cell they will ultimately produce. Nucleoli are usually absent.

Metamyelocyte. In these cells the nucleus is characteristically indented, and in their more mature stage it is divided into two lobes. The more mature forms are usually described as "band" cell (immature neutrophils) and increase in the blood in acute bacterial infections. The number of cytoplasmic granules increases, and they are neutrophilic, eosinophilic, or basophilic.

Neutrophil. The nucleus of this cell is a deep purplish-blue and divided into three or more lobes connected by thin strands of chromatin. The cytoplasm is pink and contains numerous pink-violet granules. The primary function of these cells is phagocytosis of both bacteria and cell debris.

Eosinophil. This cell is similar to that of the neutrophil except that the nucleus rarely contains more than two lobes, and the cytoplasmic granules are bright yellowish-red in color. Its function is not known.

Basophil. This cell is also similar to that of the neutrophil, but the granules are purplish or bluish-black, and the nucleus stains very light. Their function also is not clear, but they contain heparin and histamine.

Lymphoblast. This is a large cell containing a nucleus with coarse chromatin concentrated in the periphery, one to two nucleoli, and basophilic cytoplasm that rarely contains granules.

Lymphocyte. This is a small mononuclear cell about the size of an erythrocyte, with a large dense nucleus and scanty blue cytoplasm without specific granules. These cells contribute somewhat to antibody formation and may be phagocytic. Larger lymphocytes with paler nuclei and more cytoplasm are frequently found and are considered to be young forms.

Monoblast. This is a large cell containing a round or oval nucleus with abundant, stippled, finely reticulated purple chromatin and 1 to 2 nucleoli. The cytoplasm is basophilic and rarely contains granules.

Monocyte. This cell is much larger than that of the lymphocyte and contains more cytoplasm. The nucleus is indented or folded over and palestaining. There are no nucleoli. In a well-prepared stain, lilac granules are easily seen in the cytoplasm.

Plasmoblast. This cell contains a round or oval eccentric nucleus with reticulated chromatin and two to four nucleoli. The cytoplasm is less abundant than that in the plasmocyte but is basophilic.

Plasmocyte. This cell contains a round or oval, eccentrically placed nucleus that has coarse clumped chromatin but no nucleoli. The presence of a perinuclear halo and abundant blue-staining cytoplasm helps to distinguish it from the plasmoblast.

Transport. Granulocytes, monocytes, and lymphocytes are all transported in the blood and lymphatics. It is not certain how these cells get into the blood, but as the neutrophils are ameboid, they probably enter the circulation by ameboid movement. In the same way they leave the circulation when they are attracted by a focus of inflammation. In the circulation the granulocytes marginate to the periphery of the blood vessel, and this may facilitate their exodus. Once the neutrophils leave the circulation, they probably never return. The lymphocytes, however, may reenter the circulation.

Storage. White cells may be considered to be stored in the spleen, bone marrow, and lymph nodes. Large numbers of neutrophils are trapped and then released again by the lung.

Destruction. Some *neutrophils* are destroyed in the circulation; others, in the lung. They may be destroyed also in the spleen, liver, and other tissues. Their average life-span is 9 to 13 days. The fragments of disintegration are picked up by the reticuloendothelial system. *Lymphocytes* may be destroyed by the reticuloendothelial system. They have a lifespan of 100 to 200 days. The fate of eosinophils, basophils, and monocytes is not known.

Excretion. *Neutrophils* are "excreted" in the sputum and gastrointestinal tract, and a small number appear in the urine. *Lymphocytes* are lost in great numbers in the gastrointestinal tract.

Regulation. Many physiologic conditions (excitement, exercise, etc.) may alter the leukocyte count. Adrenal cortical hormones may increase the number of circulating neutrophils. It has not been proven that thyroid hormone causes lymphocytosis even though lymphocytosis is occasionally seen in Graves' disease. A splenic hormone that inhibits myelopoiesis has been postulated.

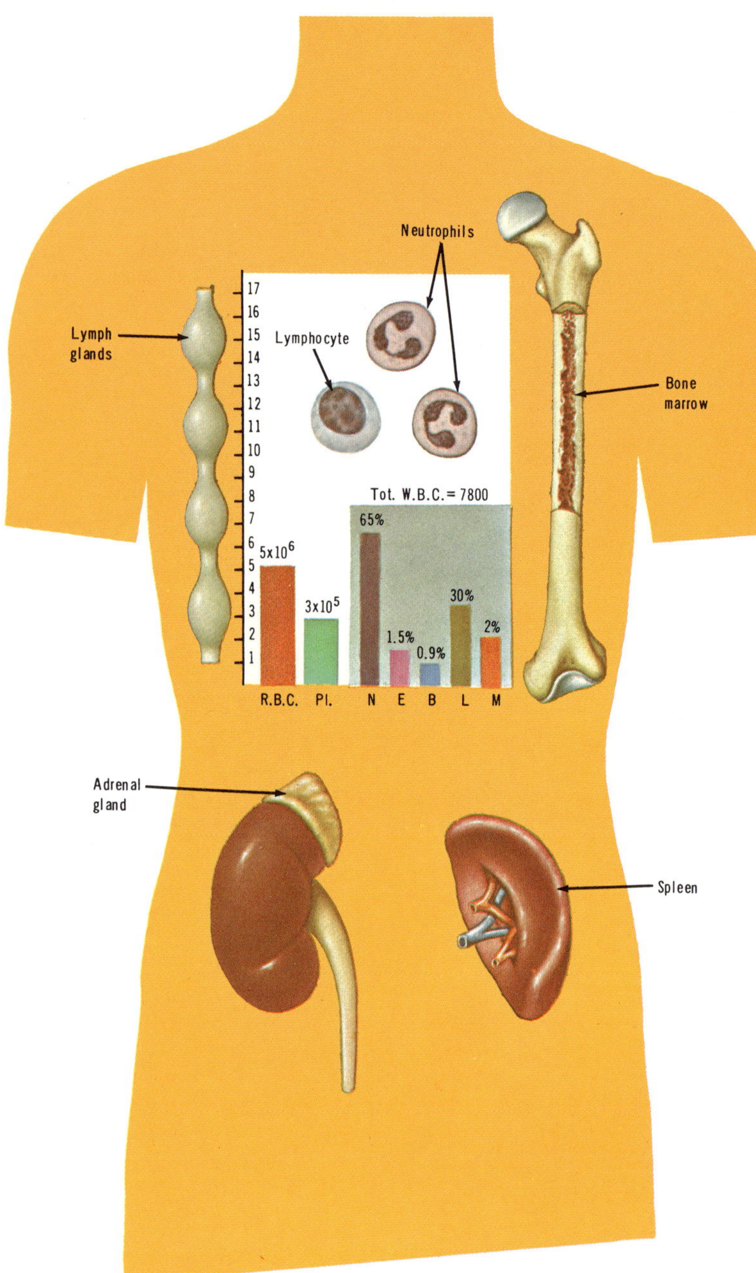

THE PRIMARY APPROACH TO THE DIAGNOSIS

A *total white count* and *differential* and a *peripheral smear* for cell morphology are the routine for beginning a study of leukocytic disorders. It is well to repeat these regardless of whether the clinical diagnosis is or is not supported by the first result. Eosinophilia can be better substantiated by a total eosinophil count. A *hemoglobin,* a *hematocrit,* and a *platelet count* are routinely ordered because disorders of the leukocytes are often associated with changes of the erythrocyte and platelet counts. A *bone marrow* is essential for the diagnosis of leukemia, multiple myeloma, and myeloid metaplasia.

These studies are illustrated. Tests for further investigation are discussed in each disorder.

Abbreviations Used in Plates:

Tot. W.B.C. = Total white blood cell count per cu. mm. of blood

R.B.C. = Red blood cell count per cu. mm. of blood

Pl = Platelet count per cu. mm. of blood

N = Neutrophils as per cent of total W.B.C.

E = Eosinophils as per cent of total W.B.C.

B = Basophils as per cent of total W.B.C.

L = Lymphocytes as per cent of total W.B.C.

M = Monocytes as per cent of total W.B.C.

THE WHITE COUNT OF INFANTS AND CHILDREN

The white count of infants and children may increase to 20,000 to 30,000 cells/cu. mm. during the first day of life. Throughout childhood and adolescence the range of normal is higher than that of adults. It ranges up to 15,500 cells/cu. mm. in infants and 13,000 cells/cu. mm. in adolescents. Children generally manifest a lymphocytosis of 40 to 50 per cent.

Summary of Laboratory Findings:

Red cell count: Variable

Platelet count: Normal or increased

Total white cell count: Increased

Differential: Lymphocytosis

Cell morphology: Normal

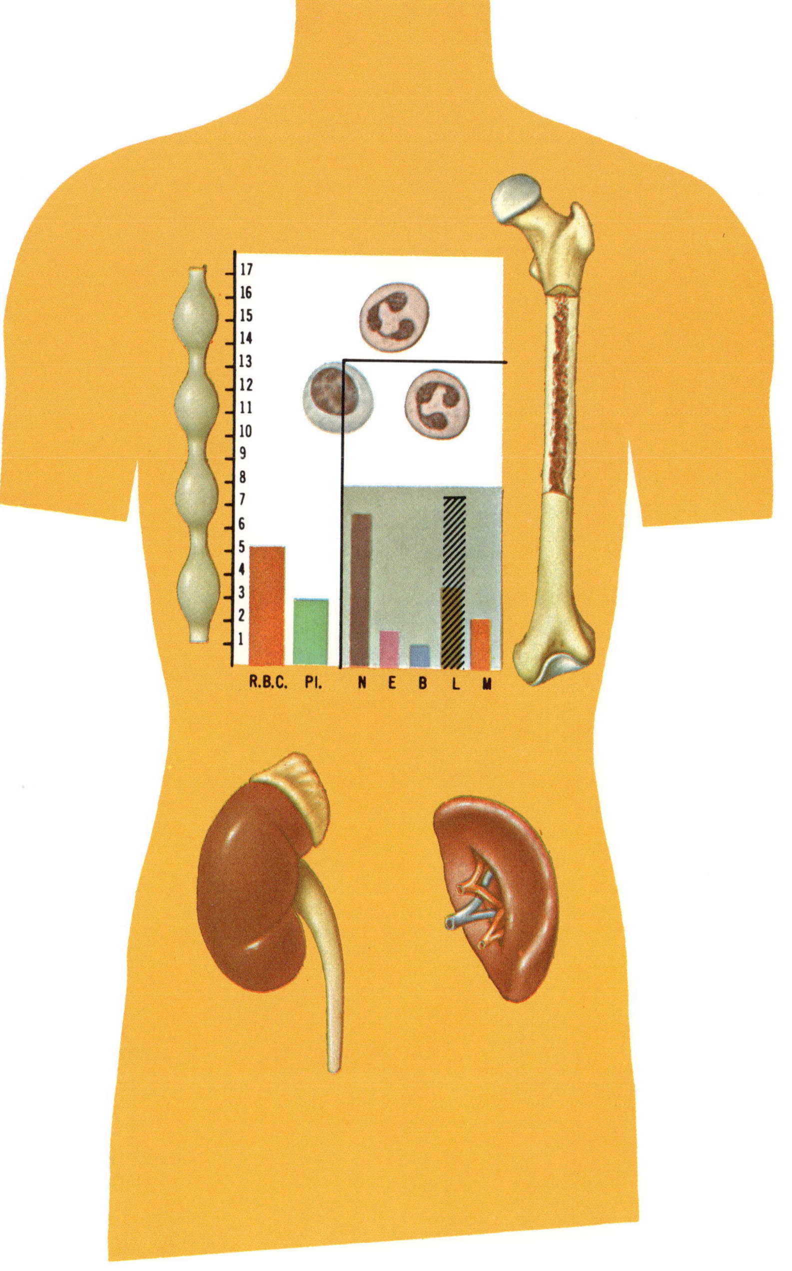

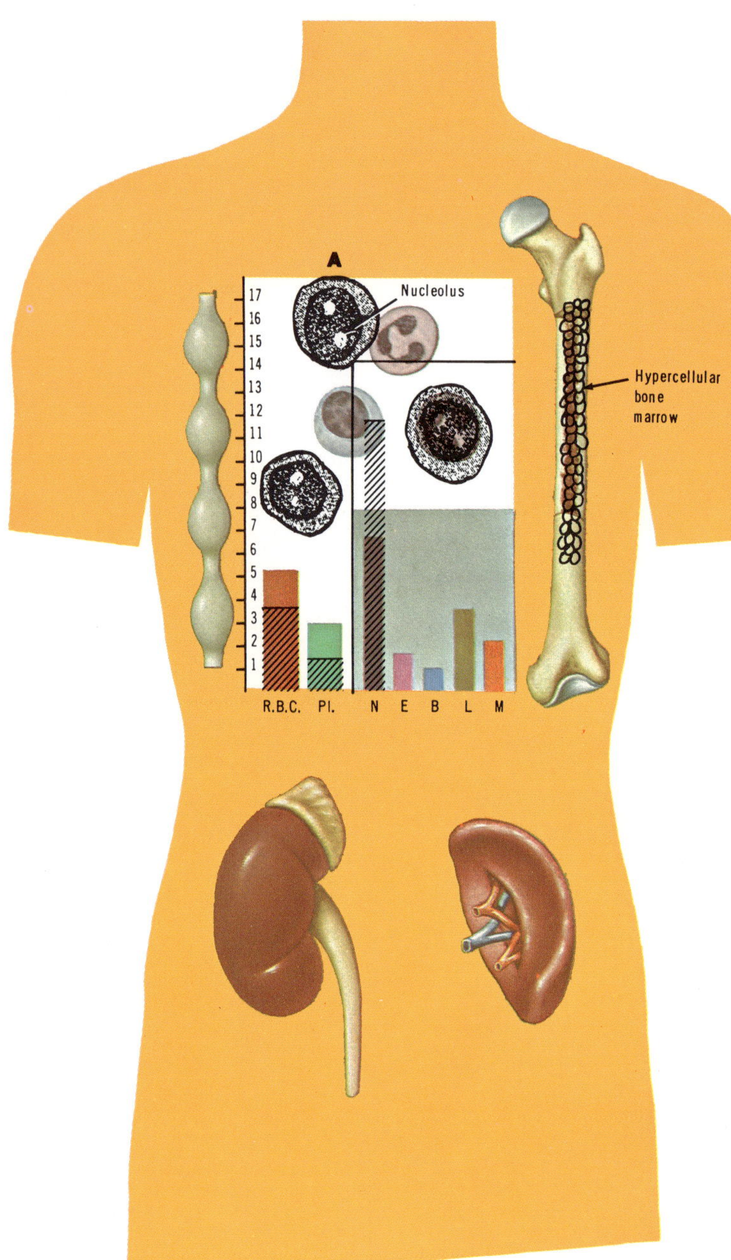

ACUTE LEUKEMIA

A neoplastic process, acute leukemia is characterized by a rapid proliferation of white blood cells of the granulocytic, lymphocytic, or monocytic series. In a few cases there is proliferation of the stem cells. *Immature cells,* particularly the blast forms (A) (myeloblast, lymphoblast, and monoblast), enter the peripheral blood, and the white cell count increases, usually between 30,000 and 50,000 cells per cubic millimeter. It is important to note that this is not invariably the case, and approximately 25 per cent of these patients have normal counts or leukopenia (aleukemic leukemia). In these cases bone marrow aspiration is often essential to the diagnosis. The marrow is characterized by a solid mass of immature cells with very few mature granulocytes, nucleated red blood cells, or megakaryocytes.

The number of granulocytes in the peripheral blood is reduced. The majority of cases are associated with normocytic, normochromic *anemia thrombocytopenia.*

Differentiation of the types of acute leukemia is in the scope of the experienced hematologist. A few distinguishing features deserve mention here. Both myeloblasts and lymphoblasts contain distinct nucleoli in contrast to the monoblasts. Unlike the myeloblasts, the lymphoblasts contain coarse chromatin arranged about the rim of the nucleus, suggesting a nuclear membrane. Lymphoblasts do not contain Auer bodies (rodlike cytoplasmic inclusions) or cytoplasmic granules (brought out by the peroxidase stain), which are regularly found in myeloblasts and monoblasts.

Summary of Laboratory Findings:

Red cell count: Decreased

Platelet count: Decreased

Total white cell count: Increased

Differential: Immature blast cells

Cell morphology: Huge nuclei with prominent nucleoli in blast cells

CHRONIC MYELOGENOUS LEUKEMIA

In this neoplastic disease of the hemopoietic system, increased proliferation of granulocytes *elevates* the *white count* to levels usually far exceeding those of acute leukemia. White counts of 200,000 to 500,000 cells/cu. mm. are frequent. There are many immature forms (*myelocytes* and *band cells*, etc.) in the peripheral blood, but myeloblasts are rarely found. The basophils and eosinophils are usually increased in number. A number of patients have slight to moderate normocytic *anemia*. The *platelet count* may be strikingly *high*. Isolated cases may have a normal or low white count, and thrombocytopenia often develops at some stage of the disease. Terminally there may be a picture of acute leukemia.

The bone marrow is hypercellular (A), and the myeloid/erythroid ratio is greatly increased. Mature and immature megakaryocytes are found in increased numbers here. The spleen may be huge, but the lymph nodes are not usually enlarged.

A decreased alkaline phosphatase in the granulocytic cells, plus an increased serum vitamin B_{12}, helps to differentiate this condition from leukemoid states and myeloid metaplasia (p. 256). The uric acid is also increased (p. 166). An abnormality in chromosome number 21 (Denver classification) called the Philadelphia chromosome is found in most cases.

Summary of Laboratory Findings:

Red cell count: Decreased

Platelet count: Increased or normal

Total white cell count: Markedly increased

Differential: Predominantly granulocytes, including neutrophils and eosinophils

Cell morphology: Myelocytes and band cells frequent

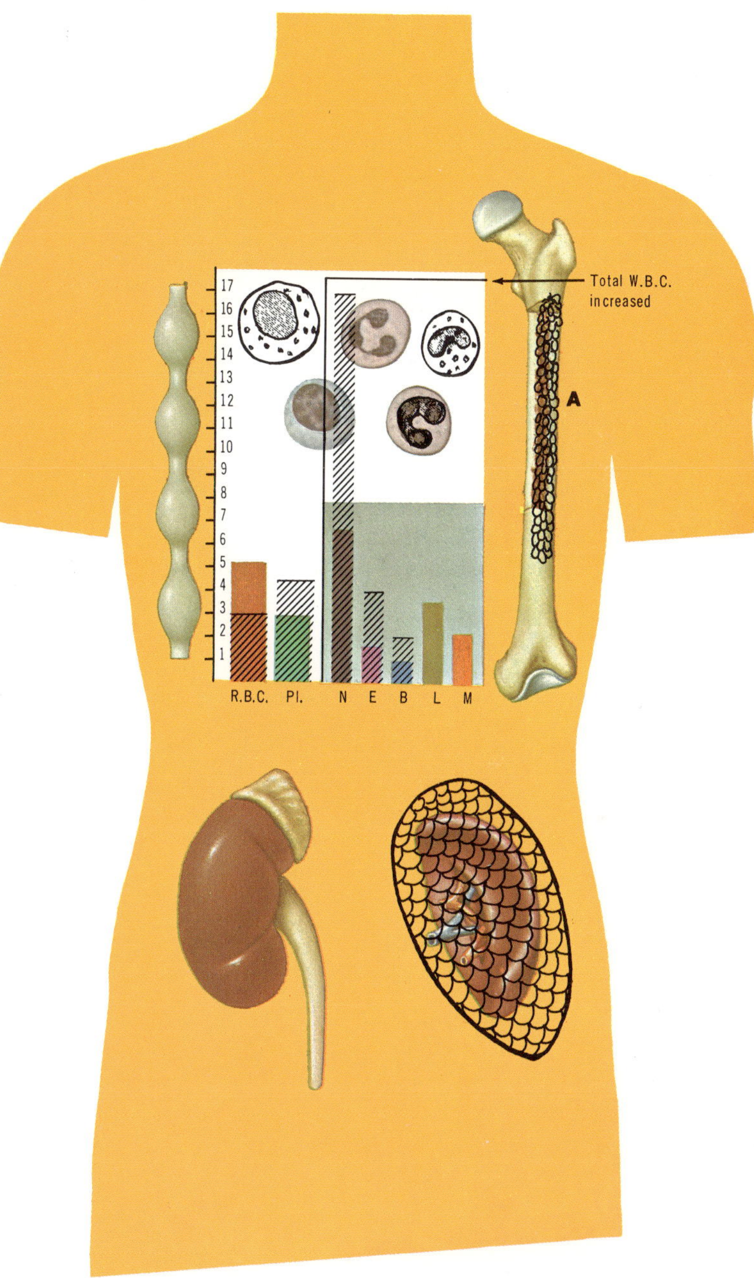

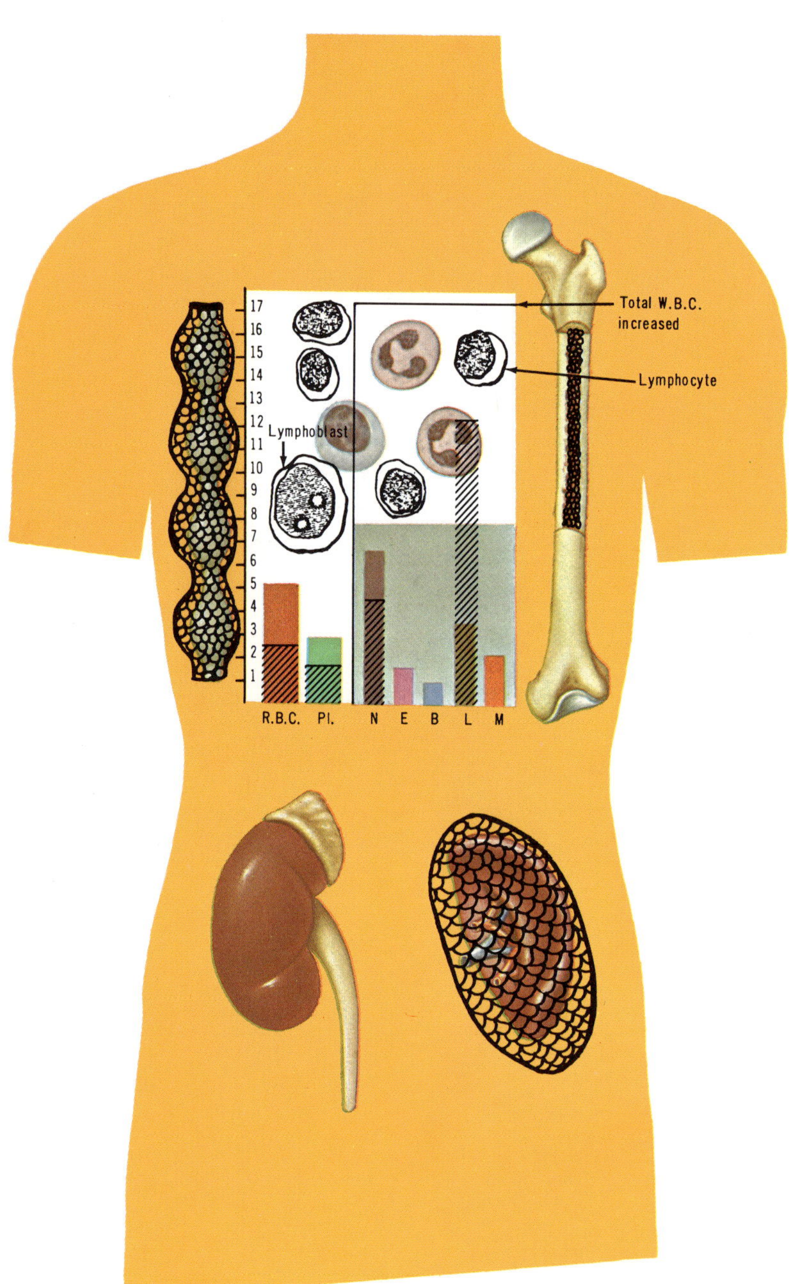

CHRONIC LYMPHOCYTIC LEUKEMIA

Like chronic myelogenous leukemia, this neoplastic disorder is characterized by a very *high white count.* In more than 50 per cent of the cases it exceeds 50,000 cells/cu. mm., and counts of 200,000 cells/cu. mm. are frequent. Only a small portion of patients have counts below 10,000 cells/cu. mm. Most of these cells are *small lynphocytes,* but occasionally the larger variety appear. In many cases a persistent *anemia* that seems to have an autoimmune basis is usual. In contrast to CGL (chronic myelogenous leukemia), an increased *platelet count* is unusual; more often it is *reduced.*

Lymphocytes make up 30 to 80 per cent of the bone marrow. This characteristic will differentiate this condition from infectious lymphocytosis and other disorders. Hypogammaglobulinemia is often found in the later stages of the disease. Both the spleen and lymph nodes are enlarged by the lymphocytic proliferation and infiltration. A lymph node biopsy may be useful where malignant lymphoma is suspected on clinical grounds.

Summary of Laboratory Findings:

Red cell count: Decreased

Platelet count: Decreased

Total white cell count: Marked increase

Differential: Lymphocytosis

Cell morphology: Lymphoblasts and immature lymphocytes infrequent

MULTIPLE MYELOMA

In this disorder there is abnormal *proliferation* of *plasma cells* in the *bone marrow* (A) and other organs. The *leukocyte count* is usually *normal.* A mild to severe *reduction* in *erythrocytes* is the rule. This is usually normocytic, but occasionally macrocytes are found. The most striking finding on the blood smear is rouleau formation (B), but plasma cells may be found. A large number of plasma cells are found on bone marrow examination. These are oval cells with abundant foamy basophilic cytoplasm and eccentric nuclei, often containing giant nucleoli. Serum electrophoresis (p. 153) and roentgenograms of the skull and long bones will confirm the diagnosis and differentiate this disorder from plasmocytosis of other causes (chronic infections, sarcoidosis, rheumatoid arthritis carcinomatosis, etc.).

Summary of Laboratory Findings:

Red cell count: Decreased

Platelet count: Normal

Total white cell count: Normal

Differential: Normal

Cell morphology: Rare plasma cells; frequent rouleau phenomena

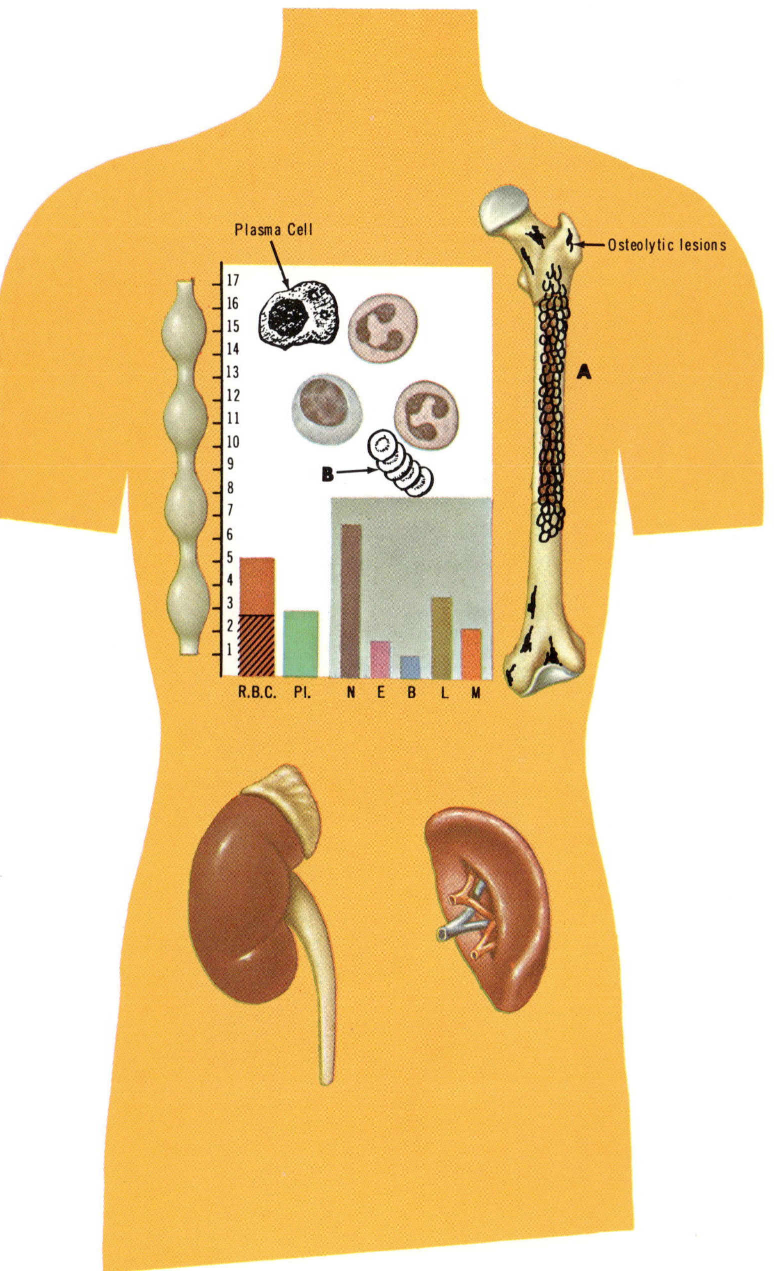

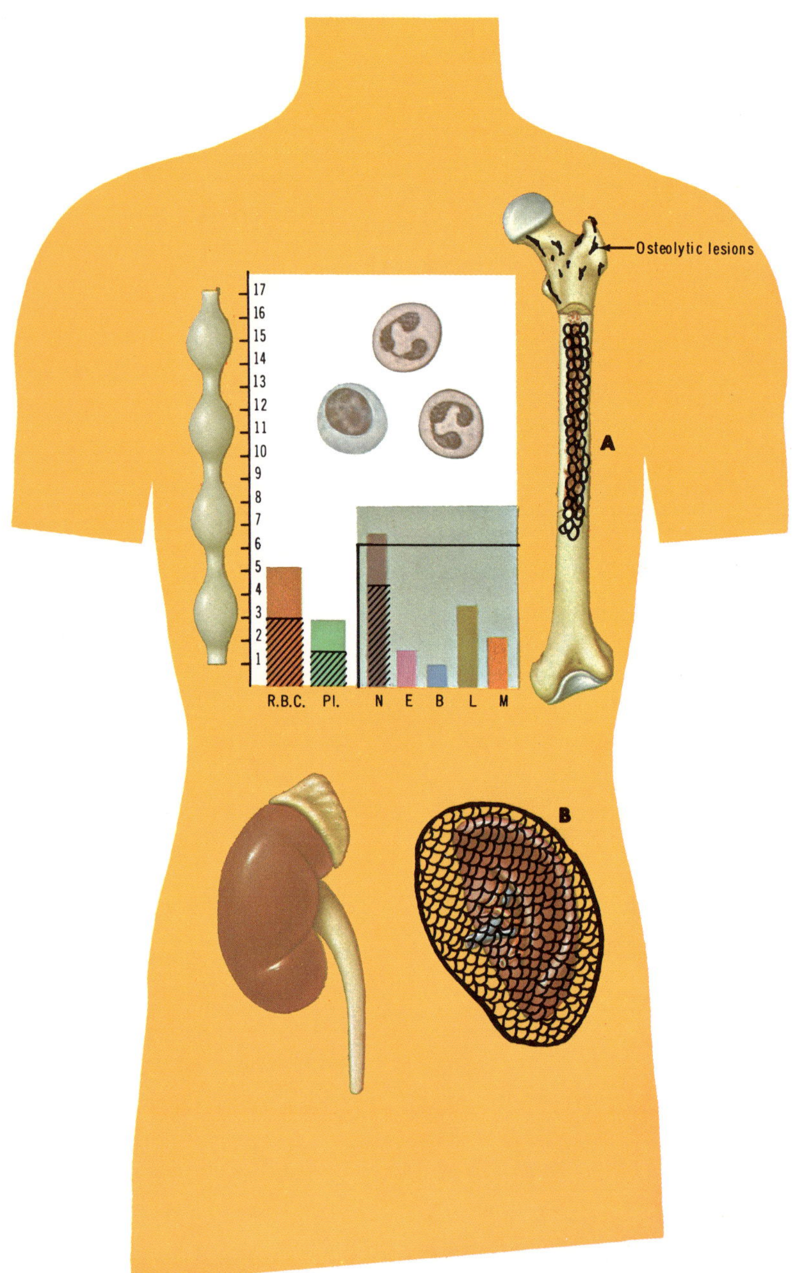

GAUCHER'S DISEASE

This disease is characterized by the presence of kerasin-containing reticulum cells and histiocytes in the *bone marrow* (A) and the entire *reticuloendothelial system* (spleen [B], etc.). In three fourths of the patients there are *normocytic anemia, leukopenia,* and *thrombocytopenia.* If hypersplenism develops, the blood manifestation of this is noted (p. 233). The diagnosis is usually readily established on clinical grounds, but a bone marrow aspiration is of great value in disputed cases. Blood lipids (p. 110) are consistently normal. The serum acid phosphatase is often elevated in this disorder (p. 6). X-rays of the bones reveal osteolytic lesions and "Erlenmeyer flask" deformity of the distal femur.

Summary of Laboratory Findings:

Red cell count: Decreased

Platelet count: Decreased

Total white cell count: Normal or decreased

Differential: Normal

Cell morphology: Normal

HODGKIN'S DISEASE

No hematologic abnormality is characteristic of Hodgkin's disease, but half the cases show a *decreased erythrocyte count* without changes in cellular architecture. This may be due to a hemolytic process, but a block in the utilization of iron has also been postulated. The white cell and platelet counts vary considerably. Twenty per cent of the cases manifest *eosinophilia.*

The bone marrow is often hyperplastic and may contain Sternberg-Reed cells. The diagnosis is more easily established by finding these cells in a biopsy of the associated *enlarged lymph nodes* (A). The spleen is also frequently enlarged.

In contrast to Hodgkin's disease, lymphosarcoma is frequently associated with a hemolytic anemia, lymphocytosis, and thrombocytopenia.

Summary of Laboratory Findings:

Red cell count: Decreased

Platelet count: Variable

Total white cell count: Variable

Differential: Predominance of eosinophils

Cell morphology: Normal

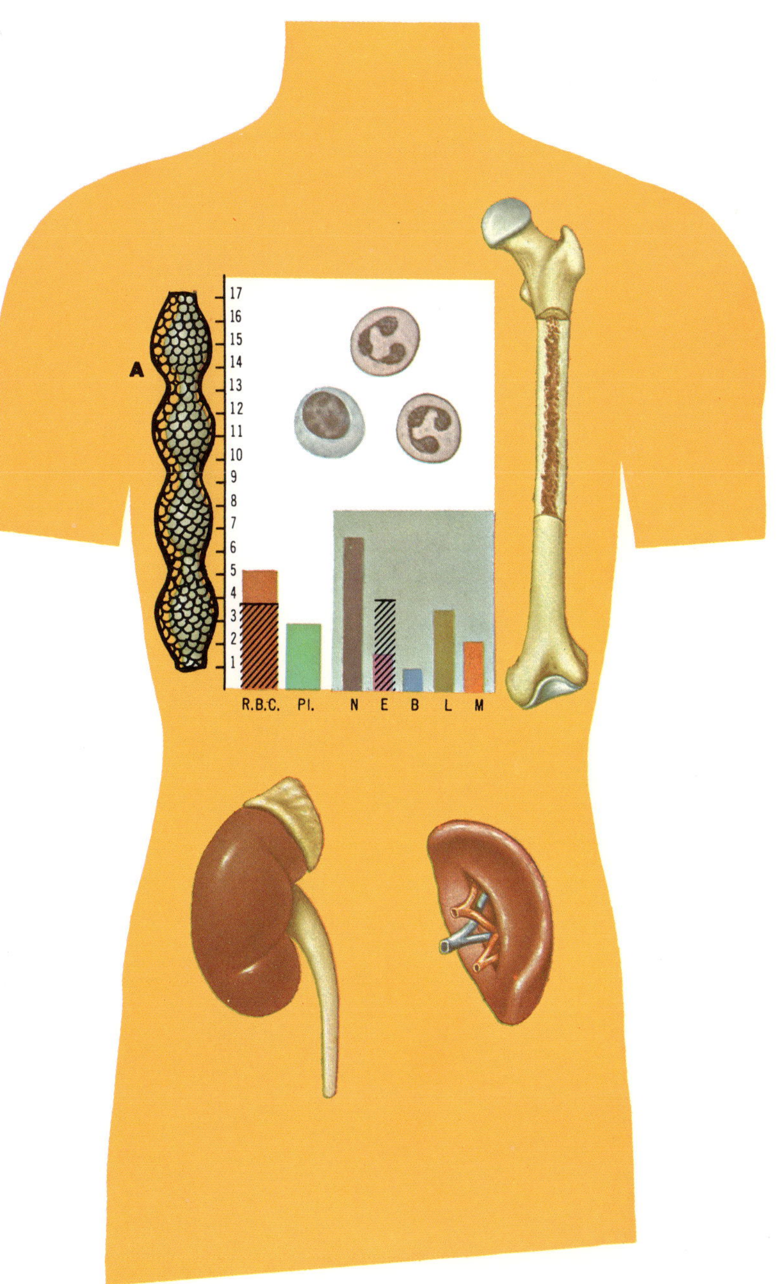

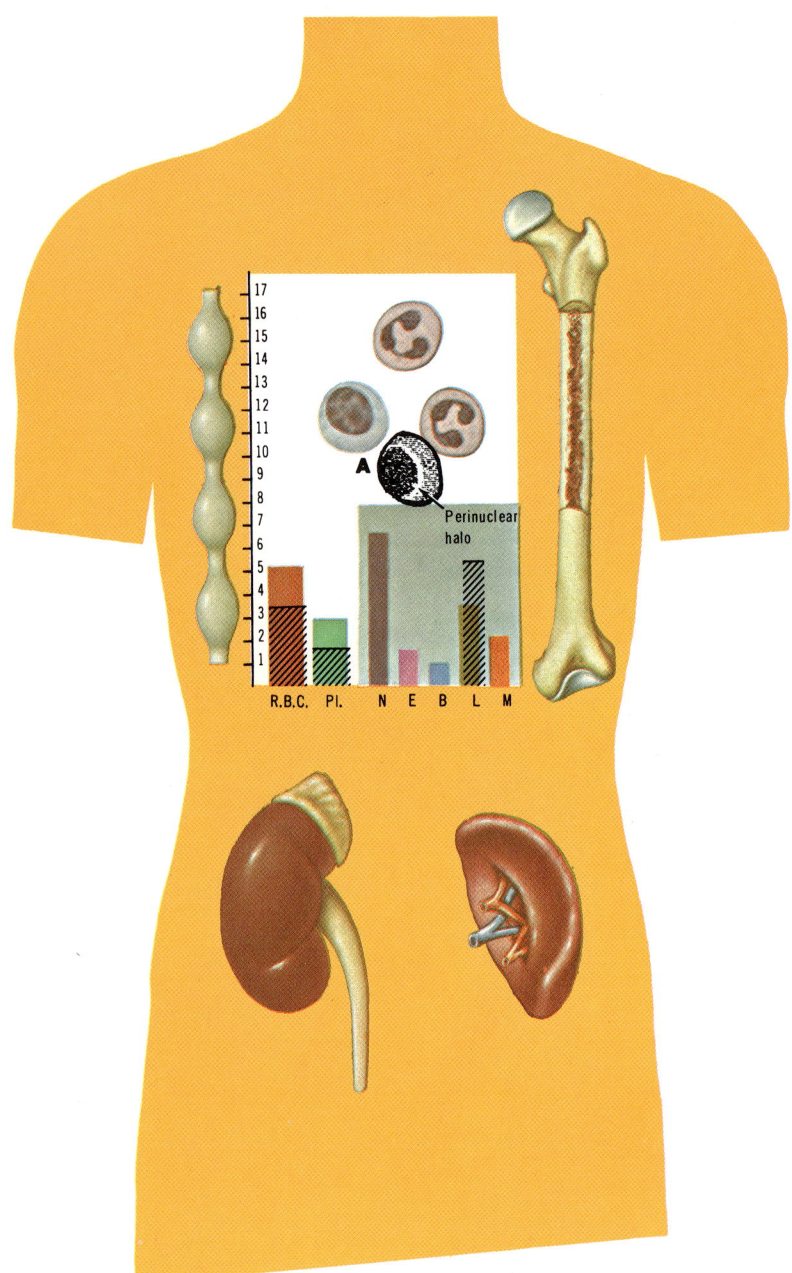

WALDENSTRÖM'S MACROGLOBULINEMIA

Although the most striking clinical feature of this disorder is bleeding diathesis, only 40 per cent of these patients have *thrombocytopenia,* and fibrinogenopenia is not a common manifestation. There are, however, normocytic *anemia* and *atypical lymphocytosis.* The lymphocytes (A) have eccentric nuclei with a clear perinuclear zone in the cytoplasm. Ultracentrifugation demonstrates the presence of macroglobulins, but serum electrophoresis, immunoelectrophoresis, and a Sia water test are also useful diagnostic aids. Punched-out lesions in the bone are rare in this disorder and help to distinguish it from multiple myeloma.

Summary of Laboratory Findings:

Red cell count: Decreased

Platelet count: Normal or decreased

Total white cell count: Normal

Differential: Lymphocytosis

Cell morphology: Atypical lymphocytes

ADDISON'S DISEASE

Lack of glucocorticoid production (A) in this disorder leads to *lymphocytosis* and *eosinophilia*. In addition, there is normocytic, normochromic *anemia*. The diagnosis is established by urinary 17-hydroxycorticoid and 17-ketosteroid determinations (p. 90). A Thorn test, in which parenterally administered epinephrine or ACTH fails to reduce the eosinophil count, supports the diagnosis.

Summary of Laboratory Findings:

Red cell count: Decreased
Platelet count: Normal
Total white cell count: Normal
Differential: Lymphocytosis and eosinophilia
Cell morphology: Normal

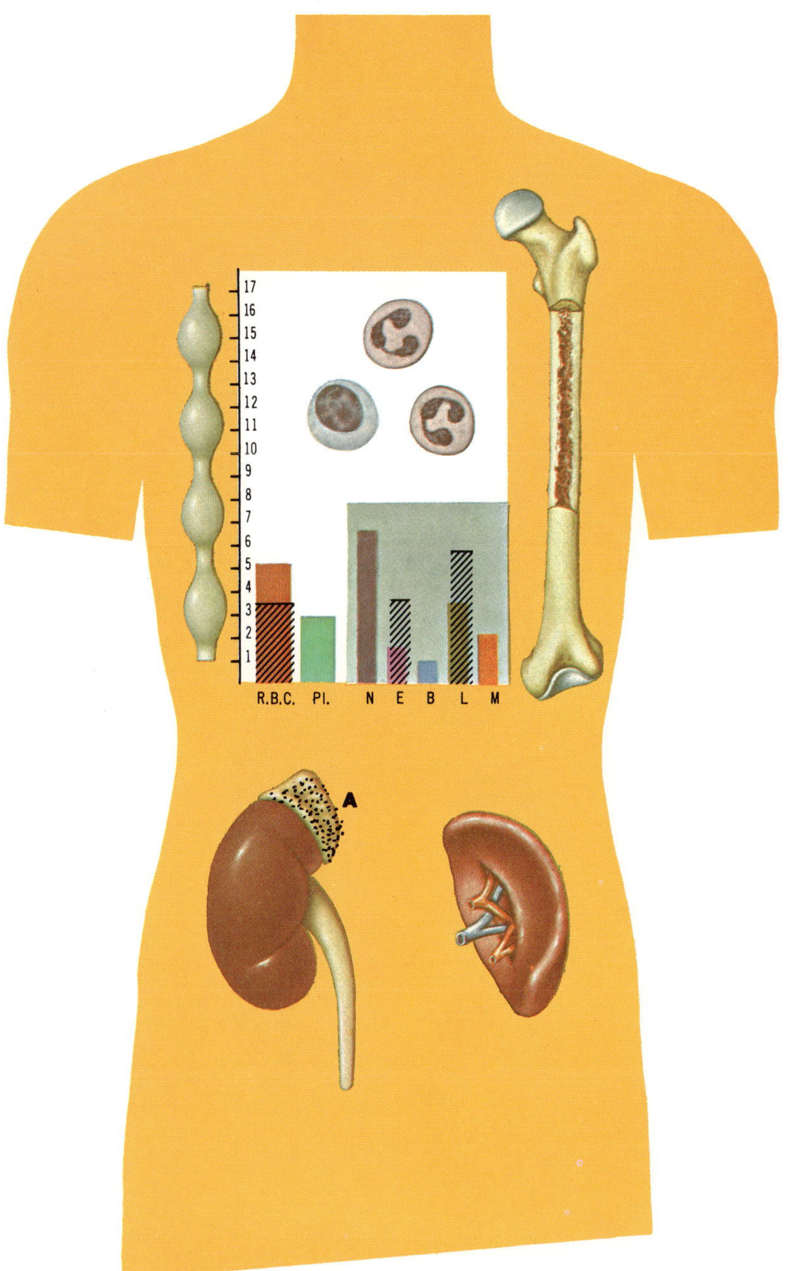

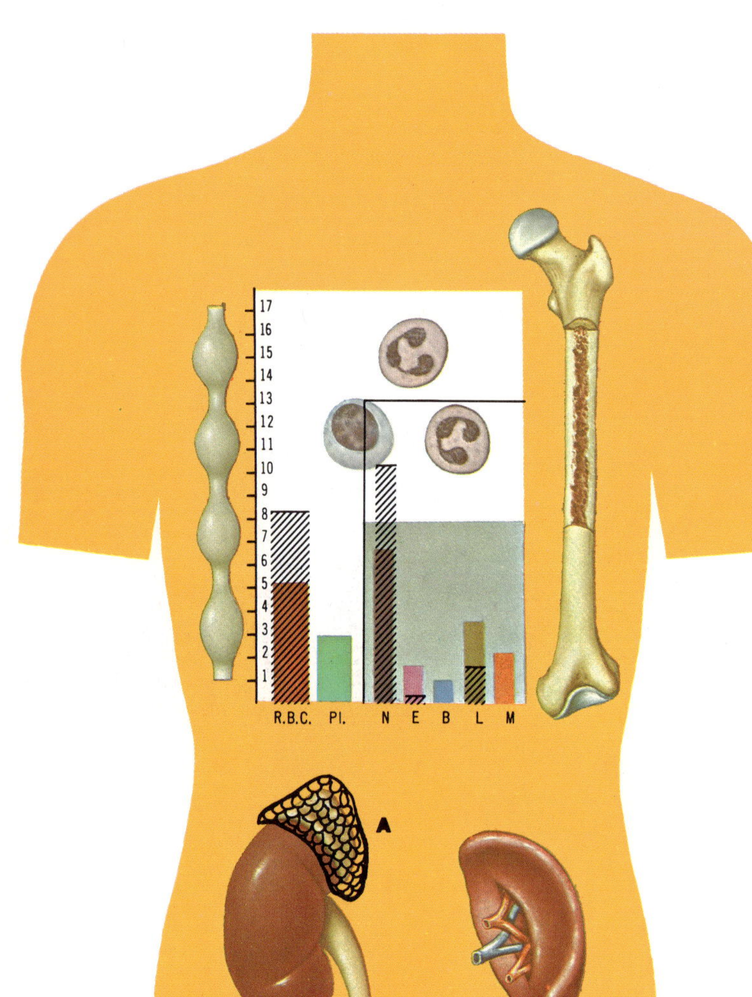

CUSHING'S SYNDROME

For unknown reasons the increased output of glucocorticoids (A) in this syndrome causes *lymphopenia, eosinopenia,* and *neutrophilia.* The total white count is increased or normal. *Polycythemia* is often present. Definitive diagnosis requires the determination of urinary 17-hydroxycorticoids and 17-ketosteroids (p. 92).

Summary of Laboratory Findings:

Red cell count: Increased

Platelet count: Normal

Total white cell count: Increased

Differential: Neutrophilia, lymphopenia, eosinopenia

Cell morphology: Normal

LUPUS ERYTHEMATOSUS

Probably because of the presence of circulating autoantibodies to red cells, platelets, and white cells, there are hemolytic *anemia, thrombocytopenia,* and *leukopenia* in this disorder. The reduction of the total white count is most often due to *lymphopenia,* but eosinophils also may be reduced in number. Definitive diagnosis is established by finding the characteristic L.E. cell on the blood smear (A). These cells are large neutrophilic granulocytes that contain a large, purple-red, globular inclusion body (the hematoxylin body) compressing the nucleus against the cell membrane. The inclusion body is the product of autoantibody destruction of the nucleus of other leukocytes. The L.E. cell is not routinely found on blood smears. The reason may be that the L.E. cell plasma factor cannot enter the intact cell membrane. Various techniques have been devised to produce cell damage. This may be accomplished by rotating with glass beads, permitting a coating of them to dry on a slide, or concentrating them under a clot. Smears of blood subjected to these techniques will often show L.E. cells in this disorder. An antinuclear antibody test (ANA) has now become widely used because it is positive in 95% of the cases if all antigens (DNA, RNA, etc.) are tested for with all methods (immunofluorescence, radioimmunoassay, etc.). There are false positives in rheumatoid arthritis and other collagen diseases. Serum complement is also reduced in this disorder.

Summary of Laboratory Findings:

Red count: Decreased
Platelet count: Decreased
Total white cell count: Decreased
Differential: Lymphopenia
Cell morphology: L.E. cells

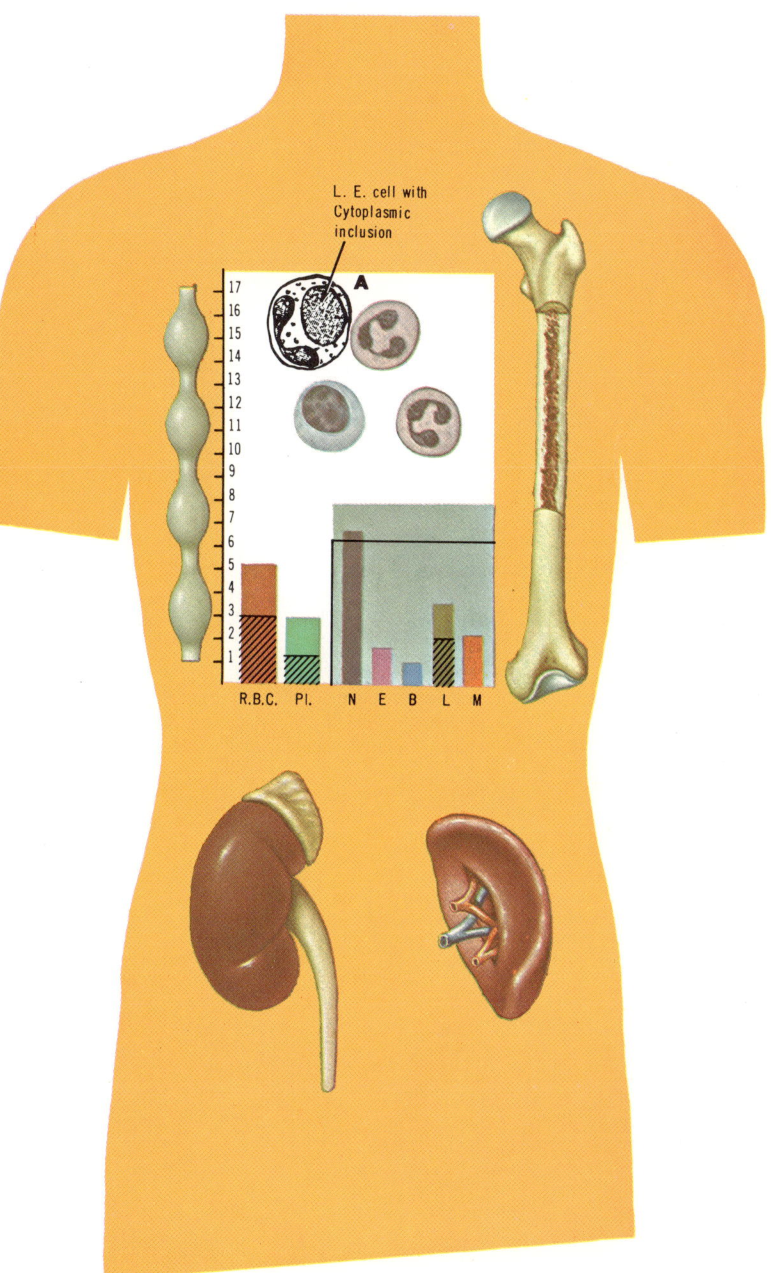

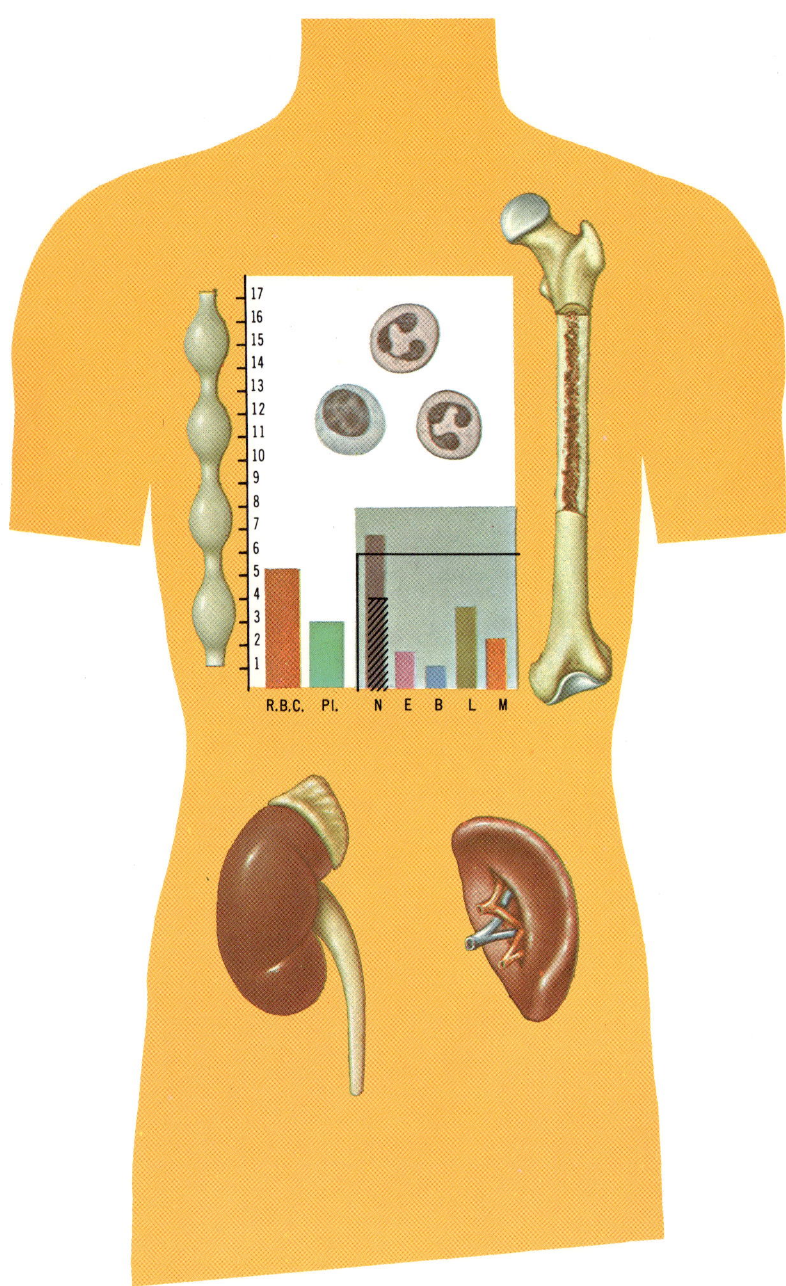

ACUTE VIRAL INFECTIONS

Typically, viral infections do not stimulate leukopoiesis and frequently inhibit it. Thus the white count is normal or *leukopenic,* usually due to a *decrease* in *neutrophils*. Occasionally there is an absolute lymphocytosis. Viral influenza, infectious hepatitis, and measles are just a few examples. Some bacterial infections (typhoid, brucellosis, etc.) and protozoal infestations (malaria, etc.) may produce a similar picture.

Summary of Laboratory Findings:

Red cell count: Normal

Platelet count: Normal

Total white cell count: Decreased

Differential: Neutropenia

Cell morphology: Normal

ACUTE BACTERIAL INFECTIONS

Acute bacterial infections generally stimulate the production of *neutrophils with resulting leukocytosis.* At the same time there is destruction of neutrophils at the site of inflammation. If destruction exceeds production, a normal white count or leukopenia is observed. The presence of increased numbers of *immature forms* (band cells, metamyelocytes) is frequent. The pyogenic cocci, such as pneumococcus, are the most common cause of infectious neutrophilia, but gram-negative bacilli and a few viruses (poliomyelitis, rabies, etc.) may also be responsible.

Summary of Laboratory Findings:

Red cell count: Normal
Platelet count: Normal
Total white cell count: Increased
Differential: Neutrophilia
Cell morphology: Juvenile forms and metamyelocytes

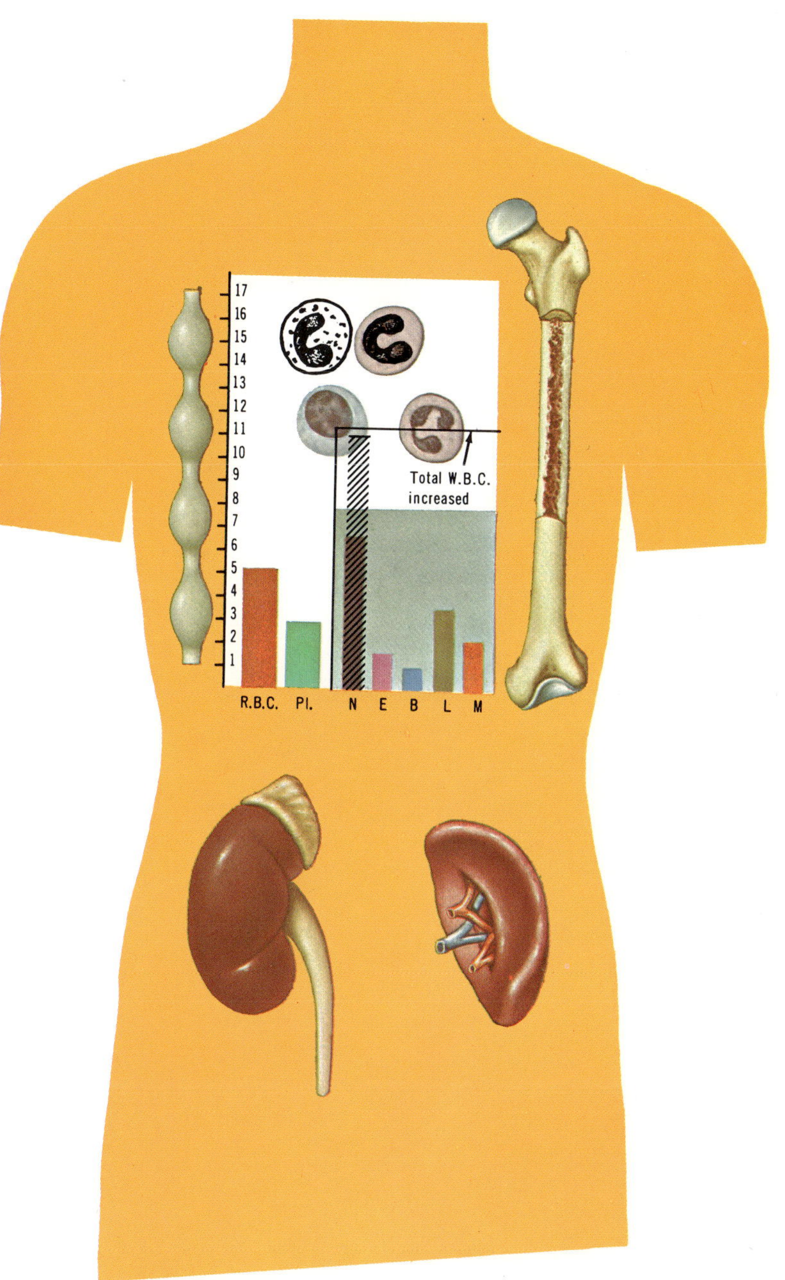

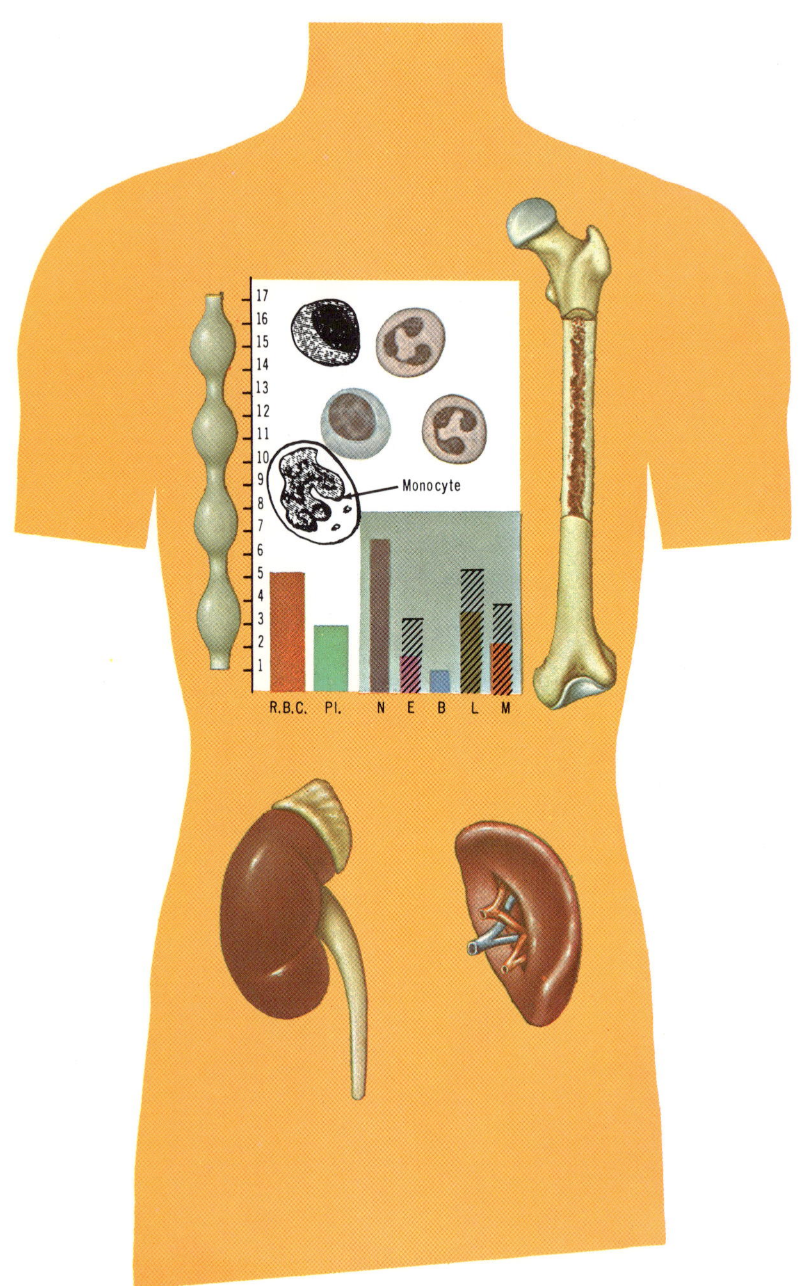

CHRONIC BACTERIAL INFECTIONS

Typically, after the acute stage of infection in chronic bacterial infections, the total *white count* and *neutrophil count drop* to near normal, and the number of *monocytes increases.* When recovery begins, there may be *lymphocytosis* and *eosinophilia.*

Summary of Laboratory Findings:

Red cell count: Normal or decreased

Platelet count: Normal

Total white cell count: Normal or increased

Differential: Lymphocytes and monocytes increased, and often with eosinophilia

INFECTIOUS MONONUCLEOSIS

Sometimes during the first week of this disorder there is an increase in lymphocytic production with a corresponding *leukocytosis*. About 10 to 90 per cent of the *lymphocytes* are considered *atypical*, because they are large, contain an oval kidney-shaped or lobulated nucleus with coarse chromatin strands, and have a vacuolated or foamy nongranular cytoplasm. The most important confirmatory test is the heterophile agglutination test, which is usually positive in a titer above 1:112. These agglutinins, unlike those of normal individuals or patients with serum sickness, are absorbed by ox red cells but not by guinea pig kidney. This is the basis for a differential test in those cases in which the total titer shows a borderline elevation. The cellular origin for these agglutinins is not known. It is now believed that this condition is caused by a virus named Barr-Epstein, the same virus associated with Burkitt's lymphoma.

Infections such as pertussis, infectious lymphocytosis, and tuberculosis may produce lymphocytosis, but as a rule the cells are not atypical.

Summary of Laboratory Findings:

Red cell count: Normal
Platelet count: Normal
Total white cell count: Increased
Differential: Lymphocytosis
Cell morphology: Atypical lymphocytes

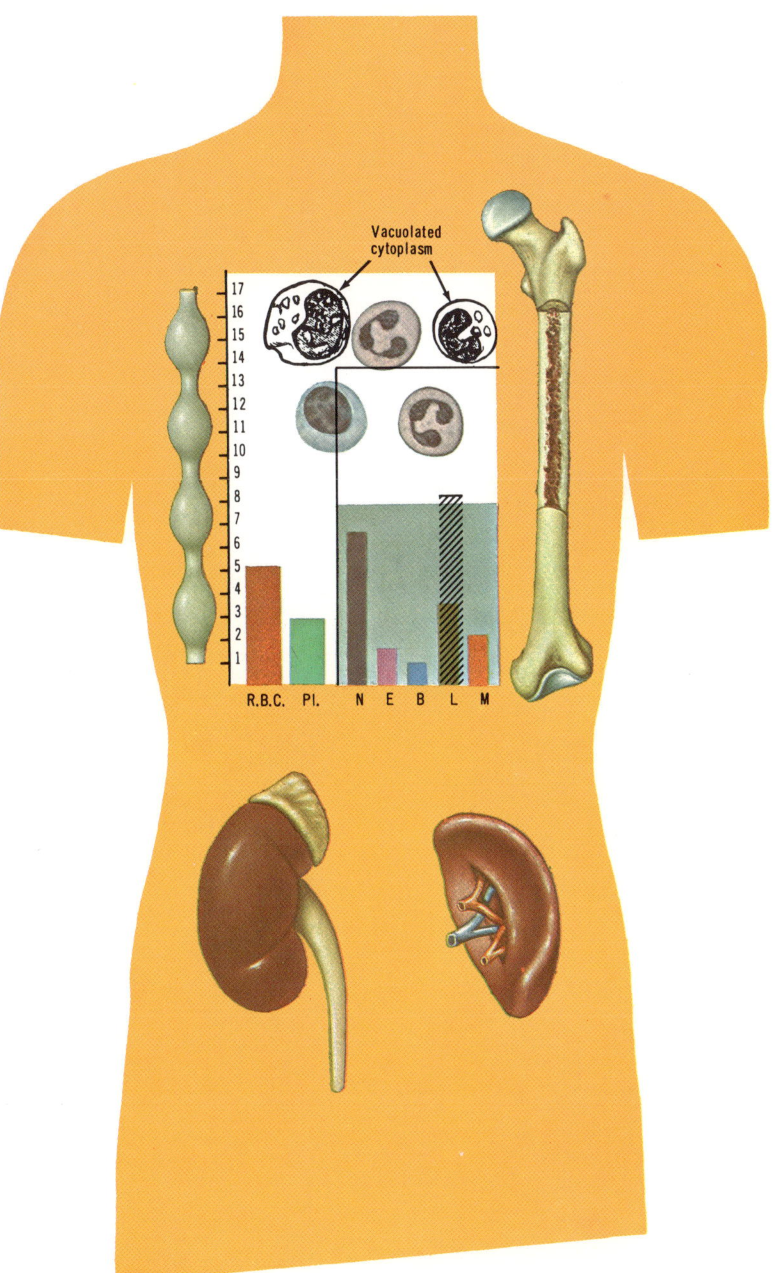

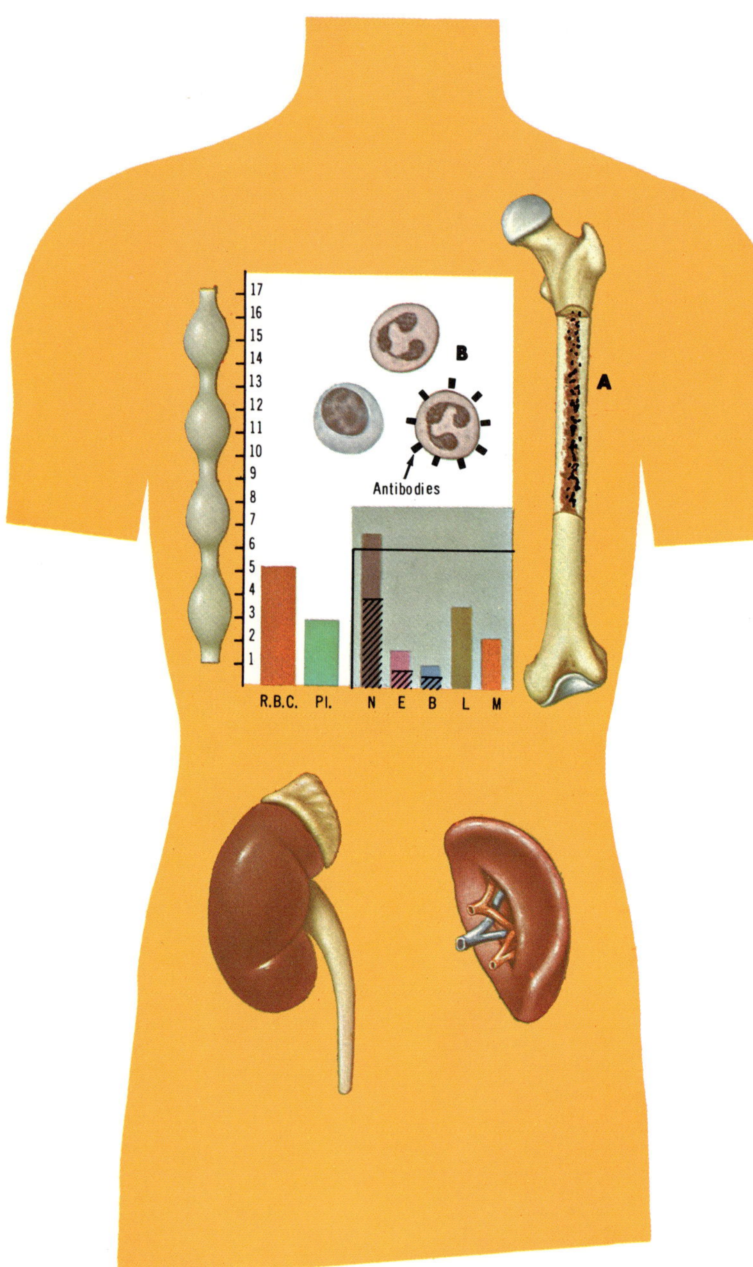

AGRANULOCYTOSIS

In this disorder all *granulocytes decrease* in number, sometimes to zero. There is a corresponding *decrease* in the *total white count,* and the lymphocytosis is relative. Platelets and red cells may decrease also. Immature red cells are rarely seen in the peripheral blood until the recovery phase. This disorder may result from toxic suppression of the bone marrow (A) (as in chlorpromazine-induced agranulocytosis) or an immunologic reaction (B) (as in aminopyrine-induced agranulocytosis*). The agranulocytosis of bone marrow invasion and aplastic anemia usually are associated with pancytopenia. Chloromycetin and other drugs produce a similar picture.

Summary of Laboratory Findings:

Red cell count: Normal or decreased

Platelet count: Normal or decreased

Total white cell count: Decreased

Differential: Neutropenia

Cell morphology: Toxic granulations in the neutrophils

* Moeschlin, S., Meyer, H., Israels, L. G., and Tarr-Gloor, E.: Experimental agranulocytosis. Its production through leukocyte agglutination by antileukocytic serum. Acta Haemat., *11*:73, 1954.

TRICHINOSIS

For unknown reasons there is an *increased* production of *eosinophils* in this disorder, often to 40 to 60 per cent of the *total white count,* which is also *increased.* Skin tests and immunologic tests are available, but a muscle biopsy is most helpful in establishing the diagnosis.

Other parasitic infestations such as the tapeworm, hookworm, and amebiasis produce the same picture.

Summary of Laboratory Findings:

Red cell count: Normal
Platelet count: Normal
Total white cell count: Increased
Differential: Eosinophilia
Cell morphology: Normal

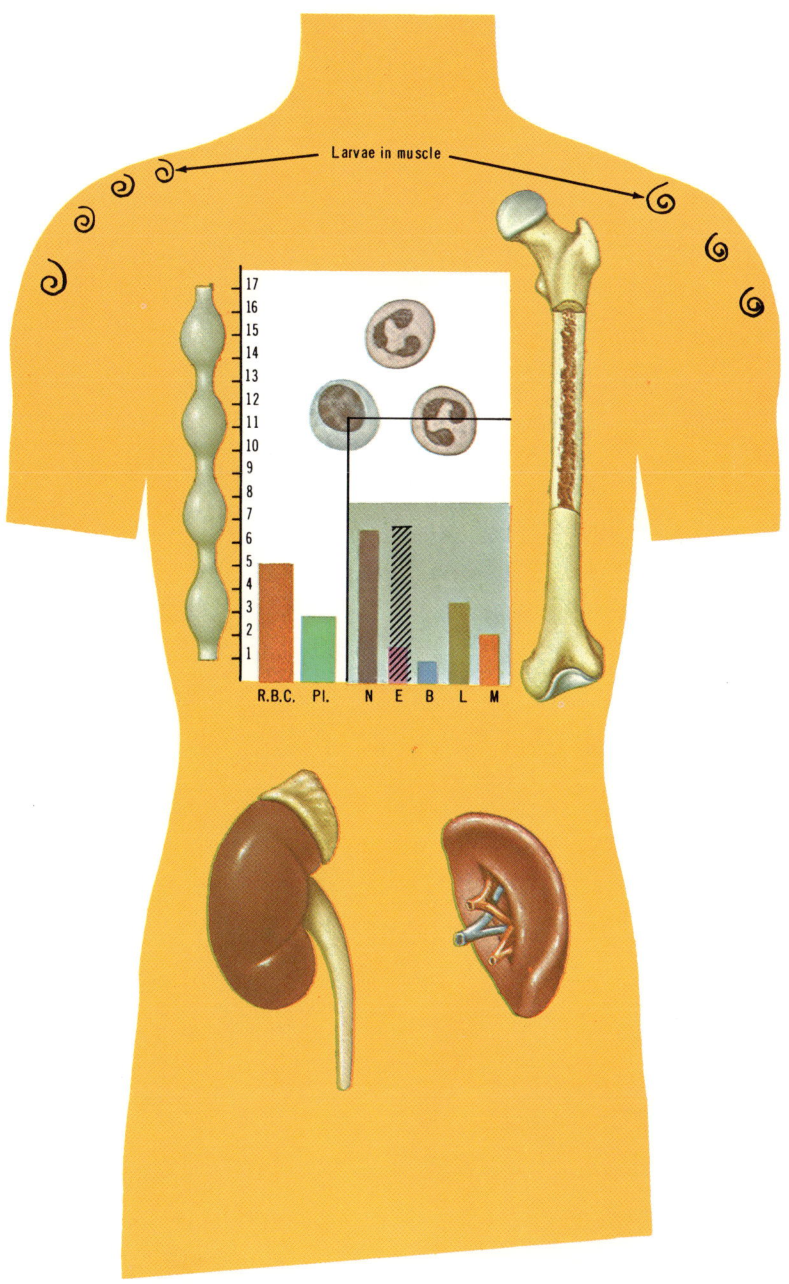

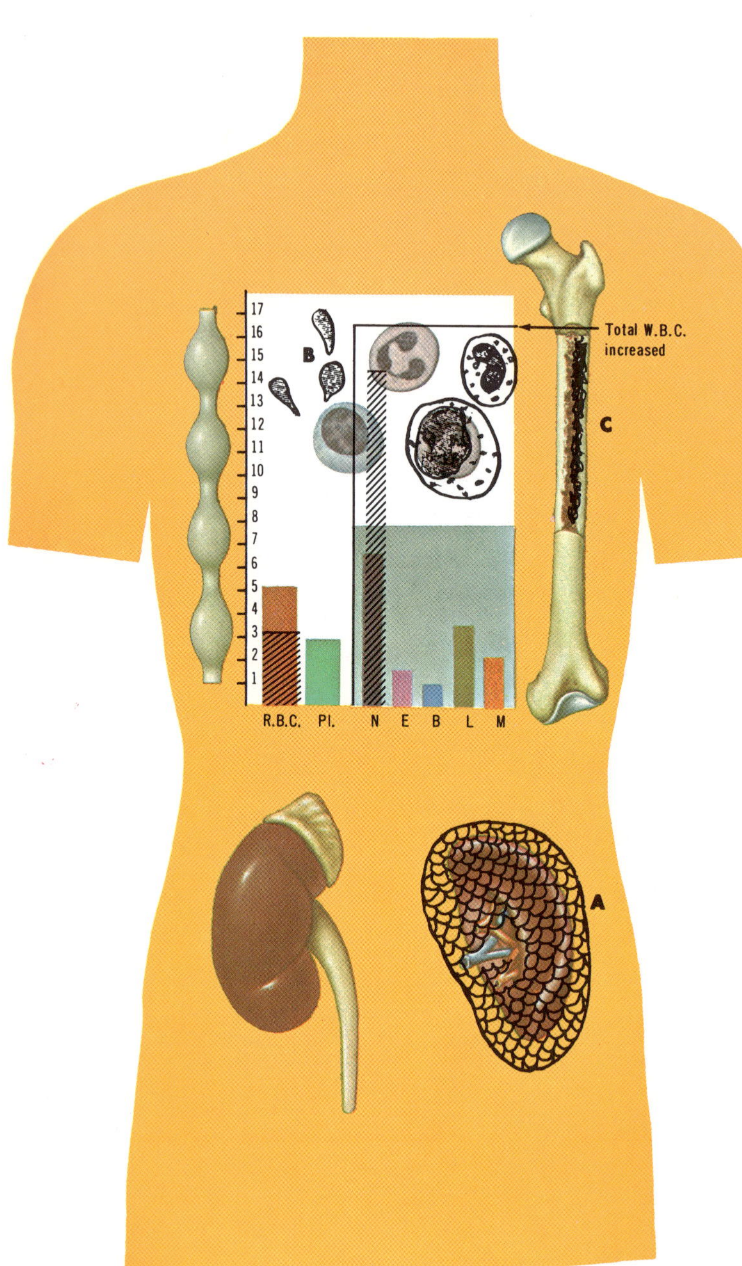

AGNOGENIC MYELOID METAPLASIA

In this myeloproliferative disorder there is hematopoiesis in the spleen (A), liver, and other reticuloendothelial tissues. *Immature granulocytes* enter the peripheral blood, and the *white blood count rises* to between 30,000 and 50,000 cells/cu. mm. in 50 per cent of the cases. Usually 2 per cent or less of these are myeloblasts in contrast to acute leukemia. A normocytic, normochromic *anemia* is a regular occurrence, and the red cells assume bizarre shapes (B) (teardrops, etc.), an unusual finding in chronic granulocytic leukemia. The *platelet count* is variable but often *increased*.

There may at times be great difficulty in differentiating this condition from chronic myelogenous leukemia. In agnogenic myeloid metaplasia bone marrow is hypocellular or acellular (C), and is often replaced by fibrous tissue, a useful diagnostic feature. There is a normal alkaline phosphatase level in the granulocytic cells in contrast to CGL (p. 241). Roentgenograms of the long bones often reveal increased bone density and trabeculation. A spleen biopsy will be helpful in doubtful cases.

Summary of Laboratory Findings:

Red cell count: Decreased

Platelet count: Variable

Total white cell count: Increased

Differential: Neutrophilia

Cell morphology: Immature granulocytes

20 Disorders of Hemostasis

NORMAL MECHANISMS OF HEMOSTASIS

In the not-so-distant past a discussion of hemostasis has been extremely confusing because of the lack of agreement on terminology. Now a standard nomenclature for the plasma coagulation factors has been established (Table 20-1).

In the normal individual there are three lines of resistance to bleeding: *extravascular resistance,* including the skin, subcutaneous tissue, and muscle; *vascular resistance;* and *intravascular resistance,* comprising the platelets and coagulation factors of the blood.

Extravascular Resistance

Because too little emphasis is placed on this subject in most textbooks, the reader may be surprised to learn that alterations in the skin and extravascular tissues are a common cause of bleeding. Senile purpura is just one example.

Tissue integrity depends on many factors that will not be elaborated here. Heredity and nutrition are most important. The ability to resist bleeding depends on the distensibility, denseness, and elasticity of the tissues. This will vary from one tissue to the next. Bone, of course, will be most resistant, whereas the mucous membranes of hollow organs, such as the gastrointestinal tract, will be least resistant. Tissues contain a thromboplastic substance that is released by injury and thereby assists in the coagulation of extravasated blood. The concentration of this substance varies from organ to organ, and this variation may explain in part the differences in bleeding tendency found in different parts of the body.

Vascular Resistance

Vascular resistance is another insufficiently stressed defense against bleeding. Disorders of the vascular wall account for the greatest incidence of pathologic bleeding. Vascular factors concerned with hemostasis are vessel size, elasticity, strength, tone, and contractility.

Although the arteries are best able to resist bleeding, once they are ruptured, they must oppose extravasating blood under high pressure. Thus they are often less successful in controlling bleeding than the capillaries. Vascular resistance depends on good nutrition, particularly vitamin C (for formation of capillary intracellular cement).

Intravascular Resistance

Platelets. At least ten platelet factors or activities have been postulated to play a role in hemostasis. They probably play a part in vasoconstriction, but whether this is due to the release of serotonin is not clear.* More important, they function by agglutinating at the site of a broken vessel, thus impeding the flow of blood temporarily. Of no less significance are the platelet clotting factors. Platelet thromboplastin activity, plasma factor V-like activity, and antiheparin activity are just a few. Finally, platelets possess clot retraction activity, which has been developed as an important test of their quantity and quality.

* Chambers, R., and Zxeifack, B. W.: Vasomotion in the hemodynamics of the blood capillary circulation. Ann. N. Y. Acad. Sci., *49*: 549, 1948.

Table 20-1. Plasma Coagulation Factors*

International Nomenclature	Terminology Frequently Used in Literature
	PRO-COAGULANTS
Factor I	Fibrinogen
Factor II	Prothrombin
Factor III	Thromboplastin, Thrombokinase, Prothrombinase
Factor IV	Calcium
Factor V	Labile Factor, Proaccelerin, Plasma Accelerator Globulin (AC-G) Plasma Prothrombin Conversion Accelerator, Plasmatic Co-factor of Thromboplastin
Factor VI	not used
Factor VII	Serum Prothrombin Conversion Accelerator (SPCA), Proconvertin, Stable Factor, Cothromboplastin, Autoprothrombin I
Factor VIII	Antihemophilic Factor (AHF) Antihemophilic Factor A (AHFA) Antihemophilic Globulin (AHG) Platelet Co-factor I, Thromboplastinogen
Factor IX	Plasma Thromboplastin Component (PTC), Christmas Factor, Antihemophilic Factor B (AHFB), Platelet Co-factor II, Autoprothrombin II
Factor X	Stuart Factor,† Prower Factor†
Factor XI	Plasma Thromboplastin Antecedent (PTA), Antihemophilic Factor C (AHFC)
Factor XII	Hageman Factor, Antihemophilic Factor D (AHFD), Glass Factor, Contact Factor
	INHIBITORS
	Anti-thromboplastin, Antithrombin, ? Heparin, Heparin Co-factor

* MacBryde, C. M. (ed.): Signs and Symptoms. ed. 4, p. 544, Table 24. Philadelphia, J. B. Lippincott, 1964.

† Factors VII and X were first clearly differentiated in 1957. Prior to that time the terms listed for Factor VII actually could refer to either Factor VII or X or both.

It is now generally agreed that platelets are cellular structures produced by the megakaryocytes for the most part in the bone marrow. Folic acid and vitamin B_{12} may be involved in their synthesis. They are colorless, usually spherical, moderately refractile bodies, measuring 2 to 4 microns in diameter. They take a basophilic stain with Wright's preparation. Approximately 100,000 platelets are formed per cubic millimeter per day.† These have a life-span of approximately 9 to 11 days. Little is known about the *regulation* of platelet production. A plasma factor referred to as thrombopoietin, which promotes megakaryocytic maturation, has been described.‡ The spleen may produce a humoral factor that depresses platelet production.

The mode of *destruction* of platelets is also uncertain. They may be removed by the spleen or simply utilized in intravascular coagulation. A decrease in the number of circulating platelets may result from decreased production, increased destruction, or increased utilization of platelets.

Coagulation. As a group, disorders of blood coagulation are the most infrequent cause of pathologic bleeding, and yet more attention is given to them in teaching than to the other causes of bleeding. Reference should again be made to Table 19-1 for the standard nomenclature of the factors involved in coagulation. Although there is not yet full agreement on the exact role of each of these factors in coagulation, there is enough agreement to provide a clinically useful outline of the events occurring in this unusual process.

Stages. For the convenience of this discussion, the process of coagulation will be divided into three stages. In Stage I, coagulation factors from platelets plus Factors V (Ac-globulin), VIII (AHG), IX (PTC), X, XI (PTA), and XII combine in the presence of calcium to form thromboplastin (Factor III). The exact role of each of the above factors in forming thromboplastin is disputed.

In Stage II, thromboplastin (Factor III), in the presence of Factors V, VII, and X and calcium ions, activates prothrombin (Factor II) to form thrombin. Finally, in Stage III, thrombin activates fibrinogen (Factor I) to form fibrin.

† Tocantins, L. M.: The mammalian blood platelet in health and disease. Medicine, *17*:175, 1938.

‡ Schulman, I., Pierce, M., Lukens, A., and Currimbhoy, Z.: Studies on thrombopoiesis. I. A factor in normal human plasma required for platelet production; chronic thrombocytopenia due to its deficiency. Blood, *16*:943, 1960.

Synthesis. The metabolism of most of the above factors is not well understood. However, the synthesis of prothrombin, Factors V, VII, IX, and X, and fibrinogen are better understood and deserve further consideration.

Prothrombin. True prothrombin is an alpha-1 globulin of the plasma with a molecular weight of about 62,700. It is formed in the liver, where its *production* depends on an adequate *intake* and *absorption* of vitamin K. Vitamin K, which is abundant in eggs and green leafy vegetables, is produced by the normal intestinal flora, so that a deficiency of the vitamin is unusual in the otherwise healthy adult. Bile aids in the absorption of vitamin K. Factors VII, IX, and X are also formed in the liver and depend on vitamin K for their synthesis. Although Factor V is probably synthesized by the liver, its dietary precursors are not known.

Fibrinogen. Fibrinogen is a protein with a molecular weight of about 450,000. It is probably formed in the liver, as its plasma level is severely reduced in acute yellow atrophy and hepatectomy.

Destruction. The mechanism of destruction of the many coagulation factors is not clear, but it may be a function of the reticuloendothelial system, particularly the liver.* In addition, circulating blood contains anticoagulants, such as antithromboplastin, antithrombin, and profibrinolysin, which may be important in inactivating coagulation factors under normal conditions as well as during coagulation. A very effective inhibitor of fibrinolysins is epsilon-amino-caproic acid (EACA), which is also useful in certain clinical disorders.

THE APPROACH TO THE DIAGNOSIS

Since only a few of the many coagulation factors have been isolated, the clinician is forced for the most part to rely on indirect tests. The seven tests illustrated in the profiles provide a firm basis to begin any study of pathologic bleeding. Because the clinician should be acquainted with the use of each of these, a description of each test follows.

Platelet Count. There are numerous methods for performing this test, and a discussion of each is not profitable for a manual of this scope. Normal values are from 140,000 to 340,000 per cu. mm.† The error may be as high as 10-20%. It is just as well to estimate the count from a peripheral smear. One platelet per h.p.f. equals 10,000/cu. mm. By definition the platelets are reduced in all thrombocytopenic states. In addition, they are elevated in certain disease states (polycythemia vera, etc.). Clot retraction should probably be performed every time a platelet count is ordered, because it will confirm thrombocytopenia or abnormal platelet function.

Tourniquet Test. After placing a sphygmomanometer cuff around the patient's arm and inflating it to a pressure of 70 to 90 mm. of mercury for 10 minutes, a count is made of the number of petechiae on the forearm within a circle having a diameter of 2 to 3 cm. Normally, there are less than 10.

Bleeding Time. This is a recording of the time needed for a small puncture wound of the skin to stop bleeding. The normal range in most laboratories is 3 to 10 minutes. The test is of most value in detecting vascular and platelet abnormalities or deficiencies.

Partial Thromboplastin Time. This test is performed just like a prothrombin time except an "incomplete" thromboplastin reagent (which lacks all thromboplastin factors except those in platelets) plus calcium is added to the patient's plasma. This test is of most value in detecting deficiencies of Stage I clotting factors.

Prothrombin Consumption Test.. In this test the prothrombin remaining in serum after the coagulation of whole blood is measured by the same method as that for the prothrombin time (see next paragraph). Normal values are 25 seconds or more, as most of the prothrombin has been utilized in the clot. This test is most useful in diagnosing Stage I clotting defects. A patient with a defect in Stage I will not convert as much prothrombin to thrombin in coagulation, and thus a great deal of prothrombin may be left in the serum.

Prothrombin Time. This test measures the time needed for citrated or oxalated plasma to clot after tissue thromboplastin and calcium chloride have been added. Normally, clotting takes place in approximately 11 to 14 seconds (but depends on the control). An abnormal result is not pathognomonic of prothrombin deficiency, as any one of the factors necessary for Stage II and Stage III of the clotting process may be involved. These include Factors V, VII, and X as well as prothrombin and fibrinogen. If a patient is not deficient in fibrinogen (as indicated by the thrombin time), then a Stage II defect is probable.

Thrombin Time. This test measures the time needed for oxalated

* Spaet, T. H., *et al.*: Reticuloendothelial clearance of blood thromboplastin by rats. Blood, *17*:196, 1961.

† Wintrobe, M. M.: Clinical Hematology. ed. 5, p. 269. Philadelphia, Lea & Febiger, 1961.

plasma to clot when thrombin is added. Normally, a clot is formed instantly. If not, a Stage III defect (fibrinogen deficiency) is undoubtedly present.

Protamine Sulfate Test. When low concentrations of this are added to the patient's plasma, fibrin monomers are released from the "split products" produced by secondary fibrinolysins (produced by activation of the natural fibrinolysin system) and allowed to polymerize (clot). The test is positive in fibrinogenopenia due to disseminated intravascular coagulation (DIC) as in obstetrical complications (page 268). It is negative in diseases associated with primary fibrinolysins (usually exogenous or produced by neoplasms).

These tests will usually indicate which of the lines of resistance or stage of coagulation is affected. Table 20-2 outlines the alterations of these tests in the various categories of disordered hemostasis.

Table 20-2. Alterations in Test Responses Indicative of Disordered Hemostasis*

	Platelet Count	Bleeding Time	Tourniquet Test	Partial Thromboplastin	Prothrombin Consumption	Prothrombin Time	Thrombin Time
Vascular and extravascular resistance		Prolonged	Positive				
Platelet deficiency	Decreased	Prolonged	Positive		Decreased		
Stage I deficiency				Prolonged	Decreased		
Stage II deficiency				May be prolonged		Prolonged	
Stage III deficiency				May be prolonged		Prolonged	Prolonged

* A blank signifies normal.

Abbreviations Used in Plates:

Plat. = Platelet count in hundred thousands per cu. mm. of blood
B. T. = Bleeding time in minutes
P. T. T. = Partial Thromboplastin time in seconds
P. C. T. = Prothrombin consumption time in seconds
P. T. = Prothrombin time in seconds
Pro. = Prothrombin
T. T. = Thrombin time in seconds
Vit. K = Vitamin K
Ht. = Hematocrit

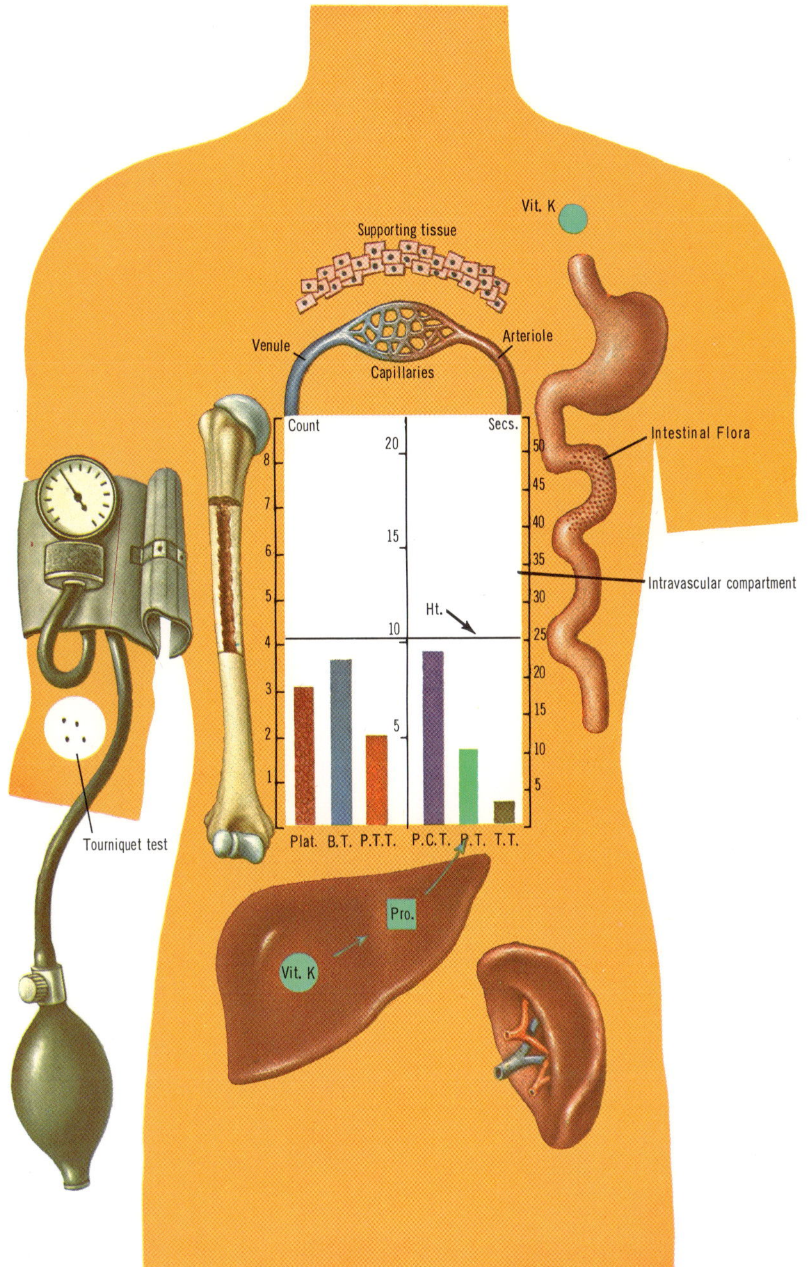

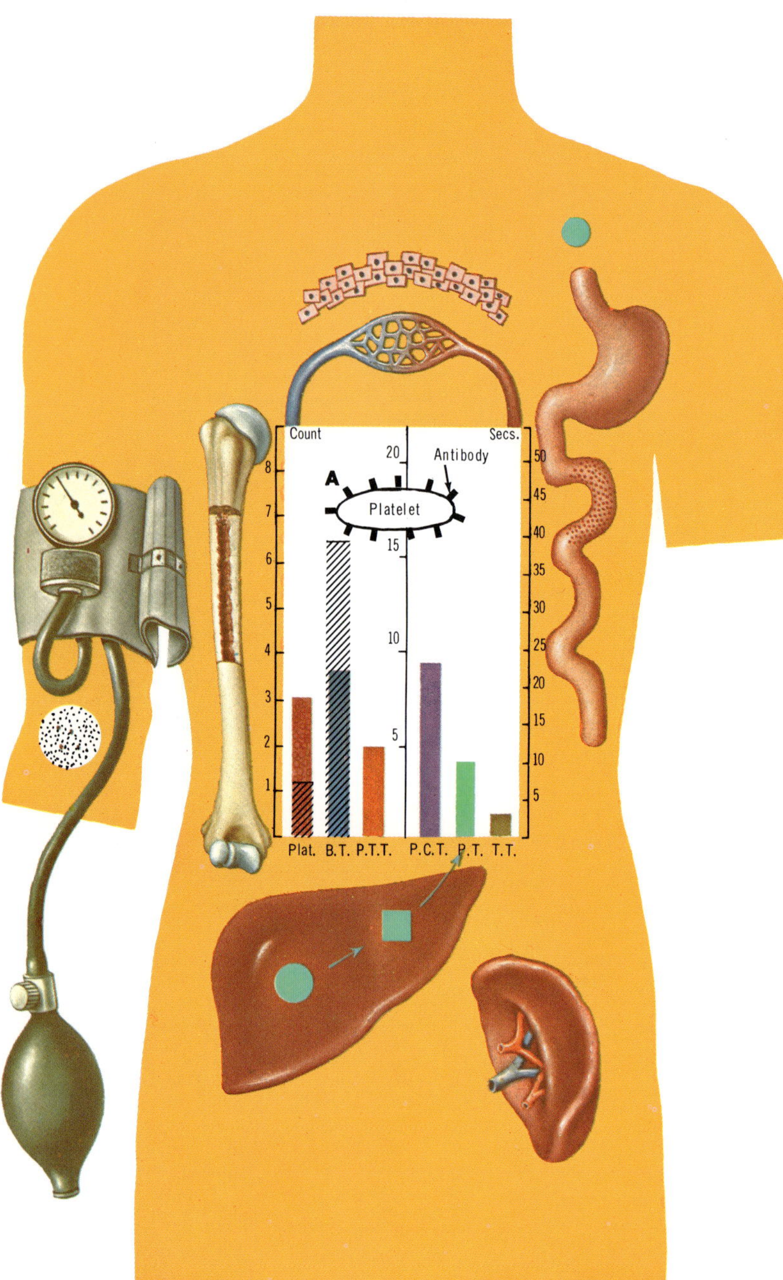

IDIOPATHIC THROMBOCYTOPENIC PURPURA

In most of these cases there is increased platelet destruction due either to an autoimmune thrombocytopenic factor (A) or to some other mechanism. The *platelet count diminishes,* leading to an *increase* of *bleeding time* and *capillary fragility*. The megakaryocytes of the bone marrow are normal or increased in number. Clot retraction is defective. In those cases with a circulating thrombocytopenic factor, the platelet survival time is short.

Thrombocytopenia due to increased platelet destruction may also be seen in drug sensitivity (sulfonamides, chlorothiazide compounds, etc.), in infections (measles, mumps, streptococcus, typhus, etc.), in collagen diseases, and in lymphoproliferative diseases.

There is also a group of disorders in which thrombocytopenia results from decreased production of platelets. Many of these conditions have already been illustrated in Chapters 18 and 19 (aplastic anemia, etc.). Coagulation studies are usually identical to the above. However, a bone marrow examination will show decreased megakaryocytes and often indicate the etiology.

Summary of Laboratory Findings:

Platelet count: Decreased
Bleeding time: Increased
Capillary fragility: Increased
Partial thromboplastin time: Normal
Prothrombin consumption: Normal
Prothrombin time: Normal
Thrombin time: Normal

HEREDITARY HEMORRHAGIC THROMBASTHENIA (GLANZMANN'S DISEASE)

In this condition there is a normal number of platelets in the peripheral blood, but the platelets fail to function normally because of a qualitative defect. Thus *bleeding time* and *capillary fragility* are usually *increased,* and clot retraction is defective. Gross* believes the defect is due to diminished platelet content of two enzymes important to glycolysis.

Familial and acquired forms of thrombocytopathic purpura exist in which the qualitative defect in the platelet is a deficient release of platelet Factor III during coagulation. In these disorders prothrombin consumption is abnormal. Platelet dysfunction is also seen in uremia and chronic liver disease.

Summary of Laboratory Findings:

Platelet count: Normal

Bleeding time: Increased

Capillary fragility: Increased

Partial thromboplastin time: Normal

Prothrombin consumption: Normal

Prothrombin time: Normal

Thrombin time: Normal

* Gross, R.: Metabolic aspects of normal and pathological platelets. *In* Henry Ford Hospital: Blood Platelets. p. 407. Boston, Little, Brown & Co., 1961.

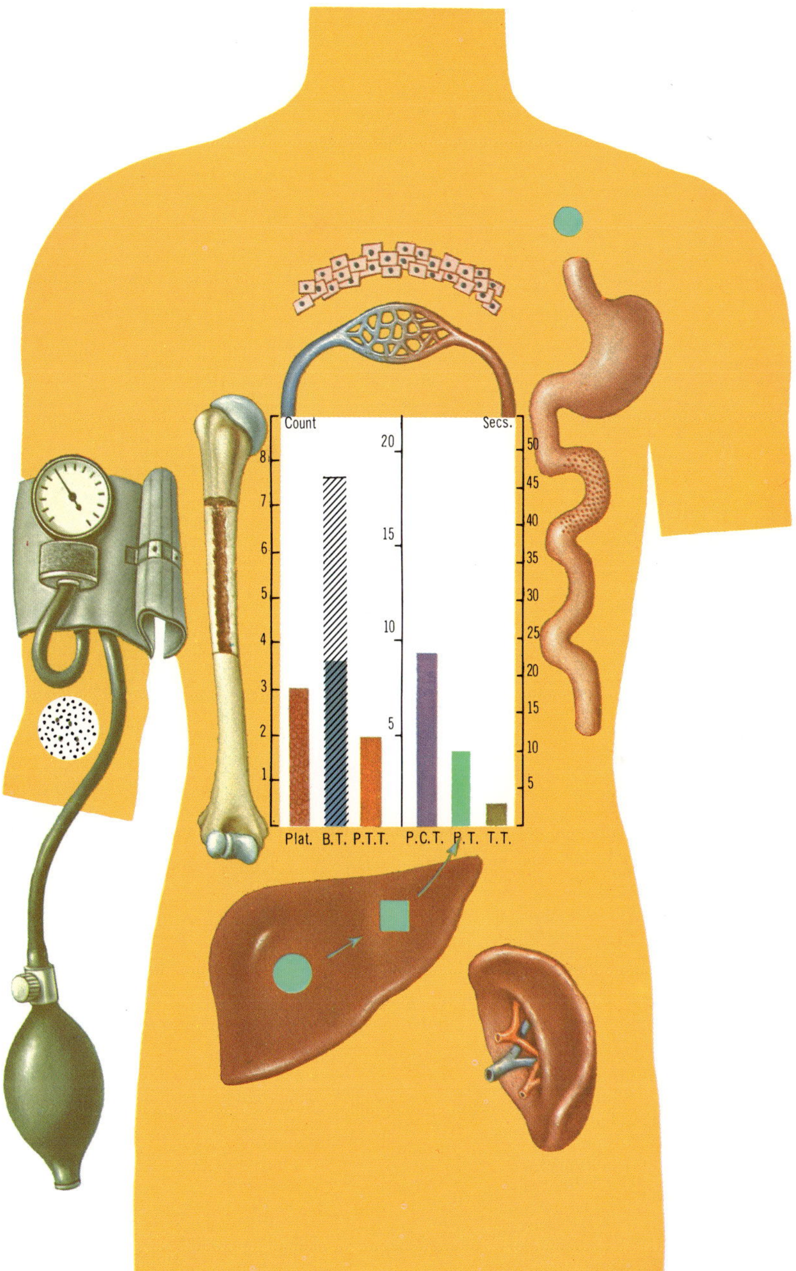

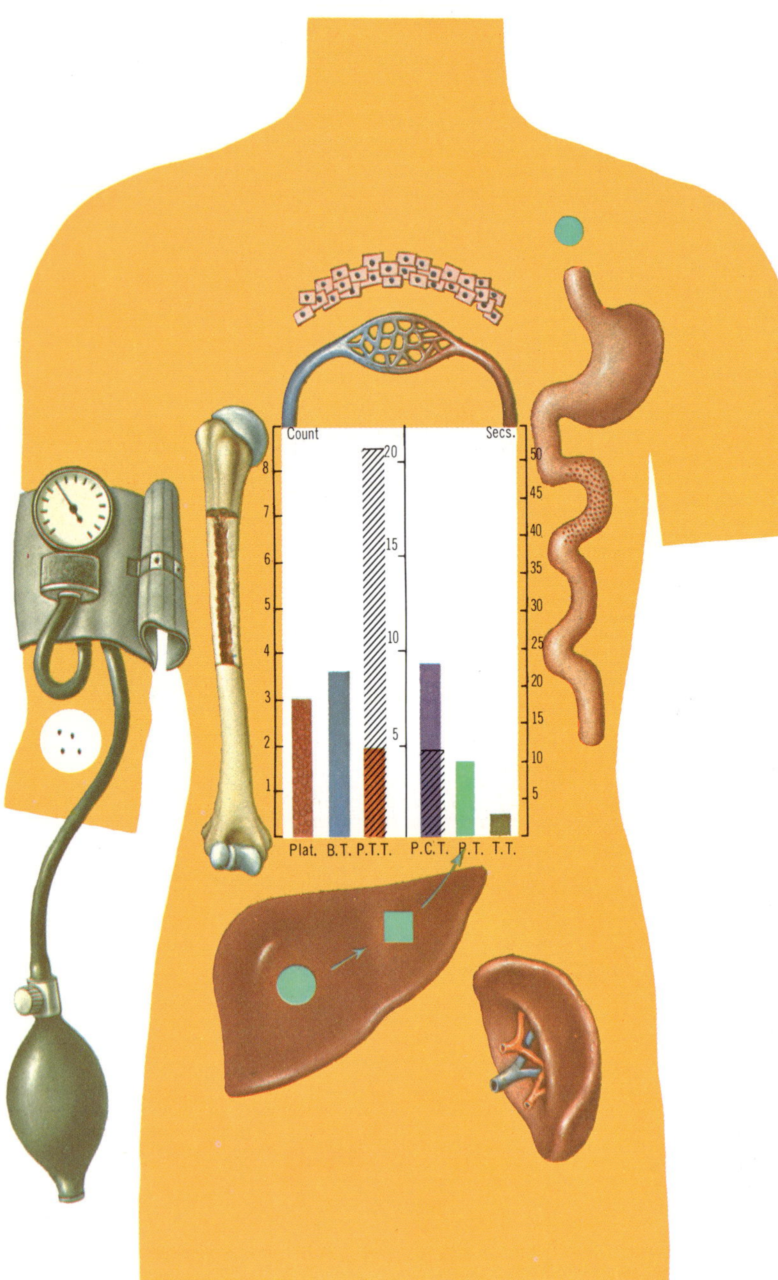

HEMOPHILIA A (CLASSICAL HEMOPHILIA)

In this sex-linked hereditary disorder there is a deficiency of Factor VIII (antihemophilic globulin), an essential precursor of thromboplastin. As a result, the partial thromboplastin *time* is classically *prolonged,* and the *prothrombin consumption is decreased.* Prothrombin time, thrombin time, and platelet count are normal. Bleeding time is rarely prolonged. The coagulation time is not a very sensitive test of Factor VIII deficiency and may be normal even in the presence of severe bleeding. A thromboplastin regeneration test is more sensitive and will also yield abnormal results. The newer partial thromboplastin time (PTT) is also abnormal. Deficiency of Factors IX (PTC), X, and XI (PTA) produce the same picture.

Factor VIII deficiency may be differentiated from the other hemophiliac syndromes by the fact that the results of the coagulation time, prothrombin consumption test, and thromboplastin generation test may be returned to normal by both normal plasma and adsorbed ($BaSO_4$-treated) plasma but not by normal or adsorbed serum.

In Factor IX deficiency these test results will become normal if normal plasma and serum are *added* but not with the addition of adsorbed ($BaSO_4$-treated) plasma or adsorbed serum. By contrast, Factor XI deficiency will be corrected by both normal and adsorbed plasma and serum.

Summary of Laboratory Findings:

Platelet count: Normal
Bleeding time: Normal
Capillary fragility: Normal
Partial thromboplastin time: Increased
Prothrombin consumption: Decreased
Prothrombin time: Normal
Thrombin time: Normal

DICUMAROL THERAPY

In the presence of Dicumarol the liver fails to synthesize prothrombin (A) and Factors VII, IX, and X from vitamin K. Thus *prothrombin time* is *prolonged.* However, clotting time does not increase until the deficiencies of Factors IX and X are great. Before this time the partial thromboplastin time and thromboplastin generation tests will become abnormal.

Salicylates produce the same picture by a similar mechanism.

Summary of Laboratory Findings:

Platelet count: Normal
Bleeding time: Normal
Capillary fragility: Normal
Partial thromboplastin time: Normal or increased
Prothrombin consumption: Normal
Prothrombin time: Increased
Thrombin time: Normal

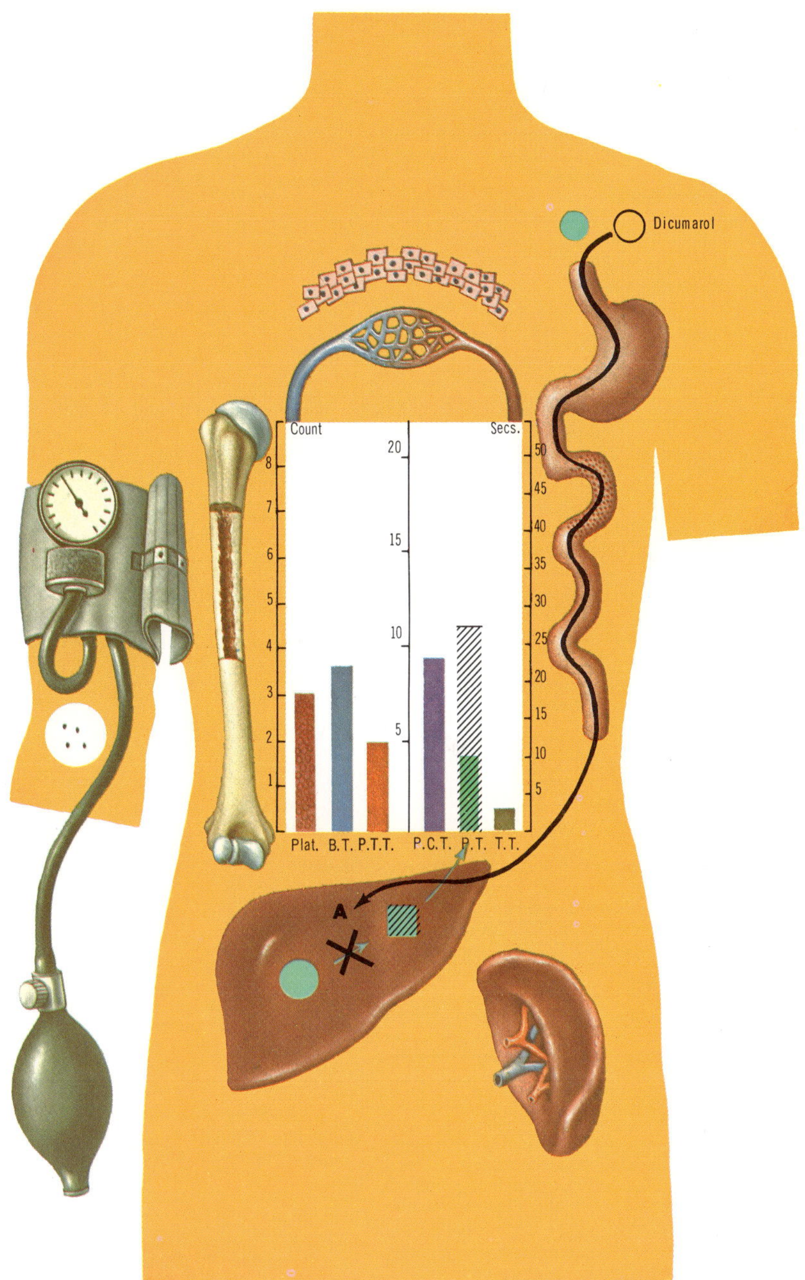

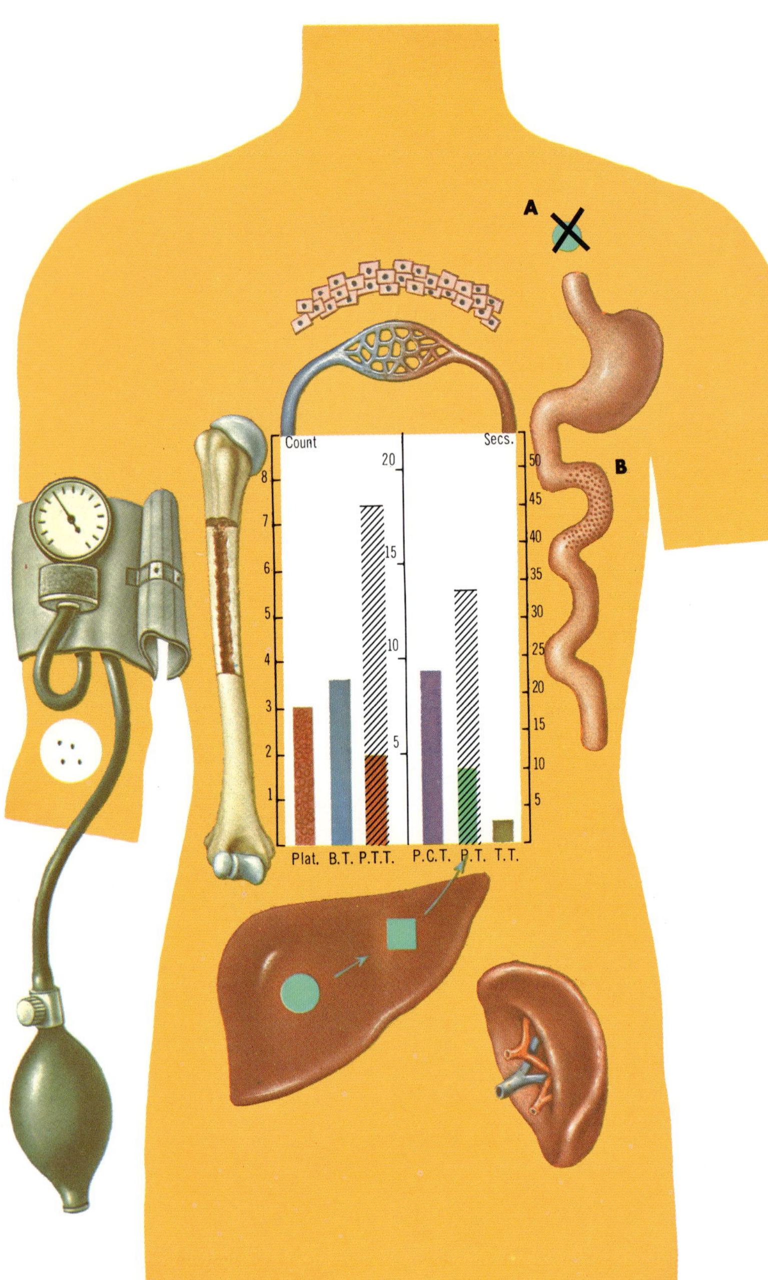

HEMORRHAGIC DISEASE OF THE NEWBORN

The newborn infant, already deficient in prothrombin, Factors VII, IX, and X, which depend on vitamin K for their synthesis, is very sensitive to further deficiency of vitamin K. If it is not supplied by the diet (A) or by the establishment of normal intestinal flora (B), he may bleed between the second and the sixth days of life. The *prothrombin time* and the partial thromboplastin *time* are usually *increased,* whereas the remainder of the tests are normal. Dietary deficiency of vitamin K is unusual in an adult.

However, prolonged use of oral or parenteral antibiotics, which destroy the intestinal flora, may occasionally cause an identical picture to the above.

Summary of Laboratory Findings:

Platelet count: Normal
Bleeding time: Normal
Capillary fragility: Normal
Partial thromboplastin time: Increased
Prothrombin consumption: Normal or decreased
Prothrombin time: Increased
Thrombin time: Normal

OBSTRUCTIVE JAUNDICE

Obstruction of the bile duct prevents bile from reaching the intestine. Since vitamin K absorption depends on bile, vitamin K absorption is blocked (A). Consequently, liver synthesis of prothrombin (B), Factors VII, IX, and X decreases. The *prothrombin time* is *increased*, and the *clotting time* and partial thromboplastin time are often *prolonged*. Increased oral intake of vitamin K will not improve the situation. In contrast, intravenous vitamin K will usually relieve the hypoprothrombinemia. Other liver function tests, intravenous cholangiography, and exploratory laparotomy make possible a more definitive diagnosis.

Poor absorption of vitamin K, resulting in the same picture, may occur in malabsorption syndrome.

Summary of Laboratory Findings:

Platelet count: Normal

Bleeding time: Normal

Capillary fragility: Normal

Partial thromboplastin time: Increased

Prothrombin consumption: Normal or decreased

Prothrombin time: Increased

Thrombin time: Normal

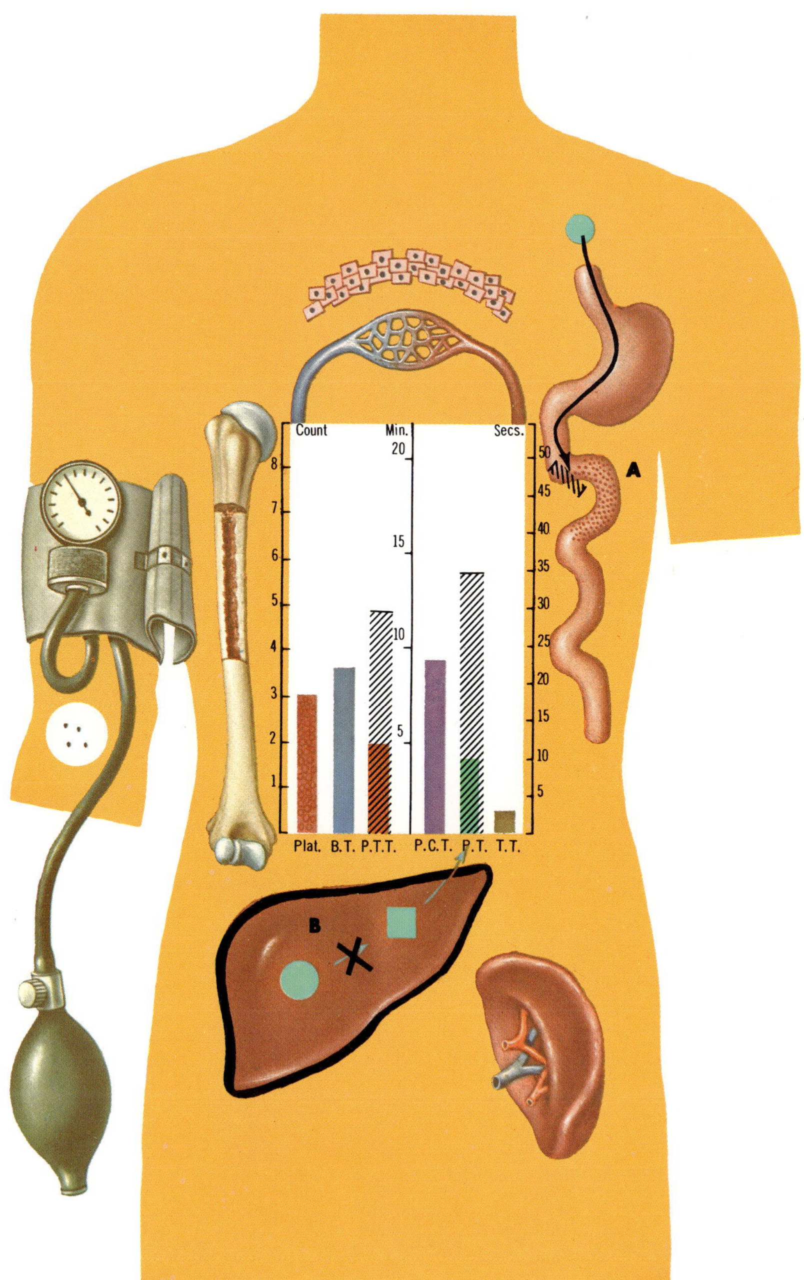

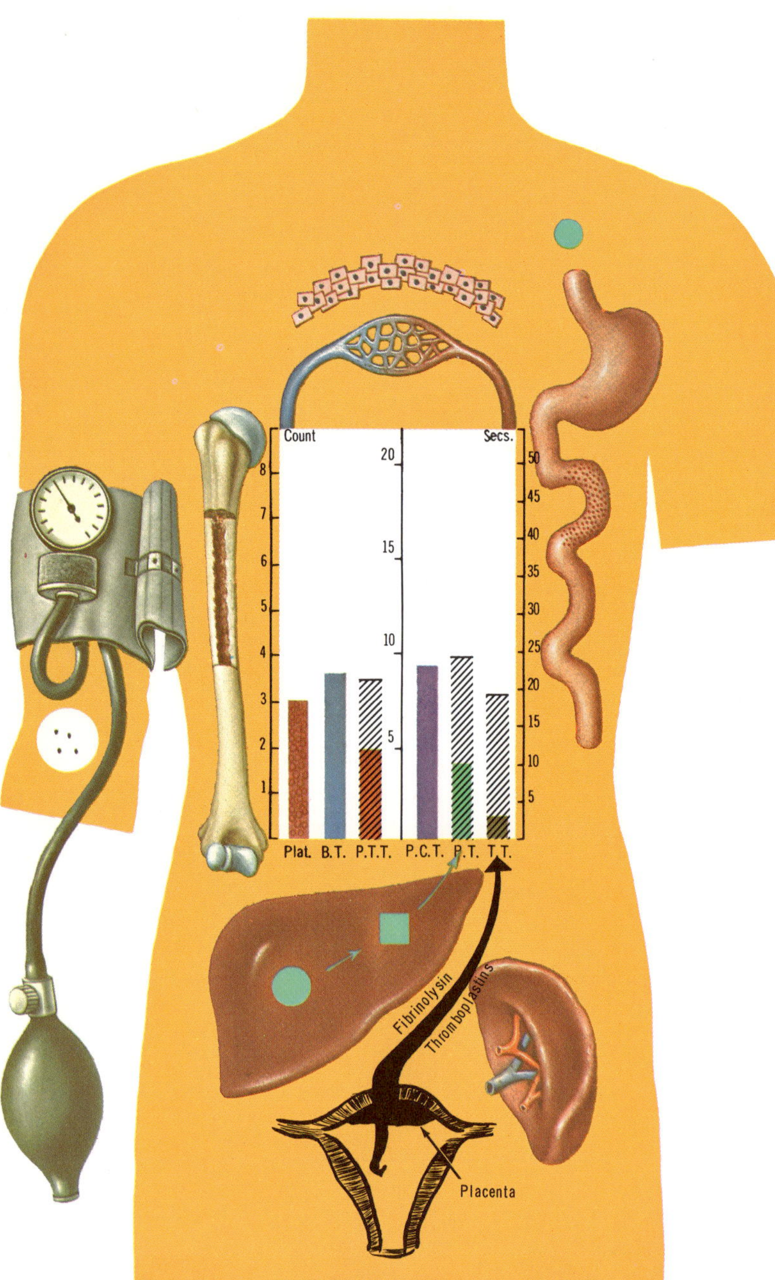

ABRUPTIO PLACENTAE

In this obstetrical complication, thromboplastic substances released from the placenta cause intravascular coagulation, consuming fibrinogen, and activate the fibrinolysin system.* The *thrombin time* (qualitative fibrinogen test) is *prolonged,* an indication of a *low level of blood fibrinogen.* The partial thromboplastin *time* and *prothrombin time* are also *prolonged.* In addition, deficiencies in Factors V and VIII and in platelets have been reported in this condition. The protamine sulfate test is positive, indicating the presence of secondary fibrinolysins in the blood.

Fibrinogenopenia may also occur in severe liver disease, due to reduced production, following transurethral prostatectomy, and in congenital afibrinogenemia. Circulating fibrinolysins, as seen in leukemia and disseminated carcinomas, probably account for more cases of fibrinogenopenia than either of the above.

Summary of Laboratory Findings:

Platelet count: Normal
Bleeding time: Normal
Capillary fragility: Normal
Partial thromboplastin time: Increased
Prothrombin consumption: Normal
Prothrombin time: Increased
Thrombin time: Markedly increased

* Schneider, C. L.: "Fibrin embolism" (disseminated intravascular coagulation) with defibrination as one of the end results during placenta abruptio. Surg. Gynec. Obstet., *92*:27, 1951.

VASCULAR HEMOPHILIA (VON WILLEBRAND'S DISEASE)

In this disorder the *bleeding time is prolonged,* possibly due to defective platelets. *Capillary fragility is increased* in half the cases. Although a deficiency of Factor VIII has been found in a number of these cases, the partial thromboplastin time usually is not prolonged, and prothrombin consumption is normal.* In addition, many investigators have found *abnormal capillaries* (A) in this disease.

Summary of Laboratory Findings:

Platelet count: Normal

Bleeding time: Increased

Capillary fragility: Increased

Partial thromboplastin time: Normal or increased

Prothrombin consumption: Normal or decreased

Prothrombin time: Normal

Thrombin time: Normal

* Biggs, R. P., and Macfarlane, R. G.: Human Blood Coagulation and Its Disorders. ed. 3. Oxford, Blackwell Scientific Publications, 1962.

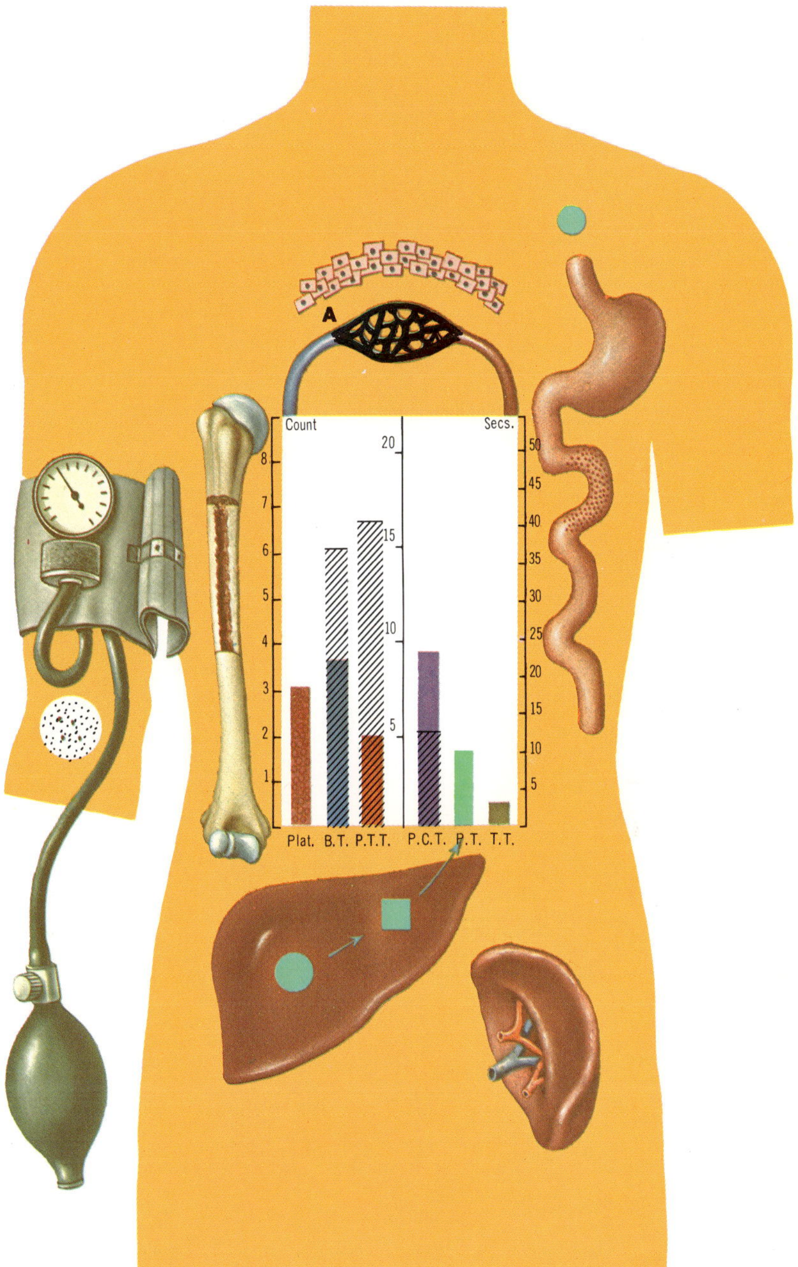

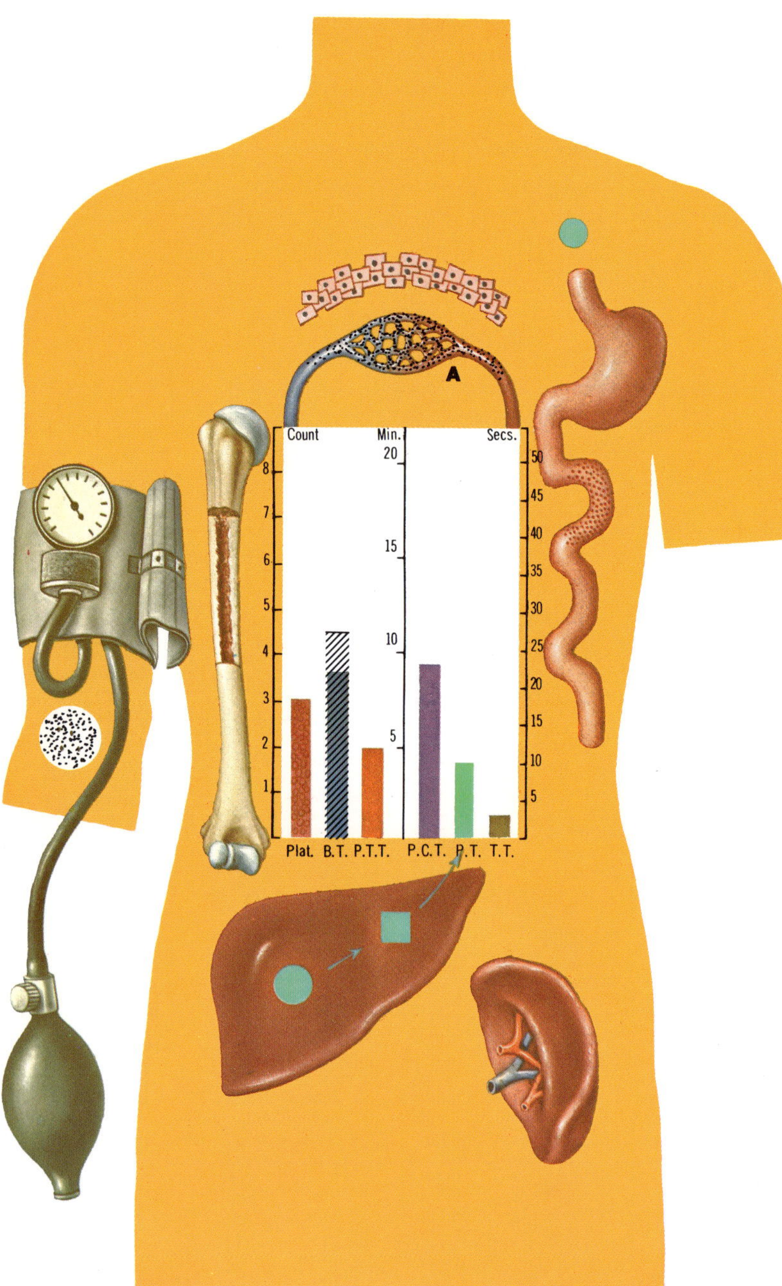

ANAPHYLACTOID PURPURA (HENOCH-SCHÖNLEIN PURPURA)

In this condition inflammation of the walls of the arterioles and capillaries (A), presumably on an immunologic basis, makes them rupture and bleed. As a rule all *tests of hemostasis are normal* except during exacerbation, when *capillary fragility* and *bleeding time* are *increased.*

Other vascular anomalies characteristic of the above are Schamberg's disease and Majocchi's disease.

Summary of Laboratory Findings:

Platelet count: Normal

Bleeding time: Normal or increased

Capillary fragility: Normal or increased

Partial thromboplastin time: Normal

Prothrombin consumption: Normal

Thrombin time: Normal

HEREDITARY HEMORRHAGIC TELANGIECTASIA

In this disorder the muscle and connective tissue of the small vessels (arterioles, capillaries, and venules) fail to develop properly (A). The vessels become dilated and rupture and bleed easily. The lesions are scattered throughout the body but occur particularly on the skin of the palms, fingernails, ears, and face and in the mucous membranes of the nose, tongue, respiratory tract, and gastrointestinal tract.

All the tests of hemostasis are normal.

Summary of Laboratory Findings:

Platelet count: Normal

Bleeding time: Normal

Capillary fragility: Normal except where lesions occur

Partial thromboplastin time: Normal

Prothrombin consumption: Normal

Prothrombin time: Normal

Thrombin time: Normal

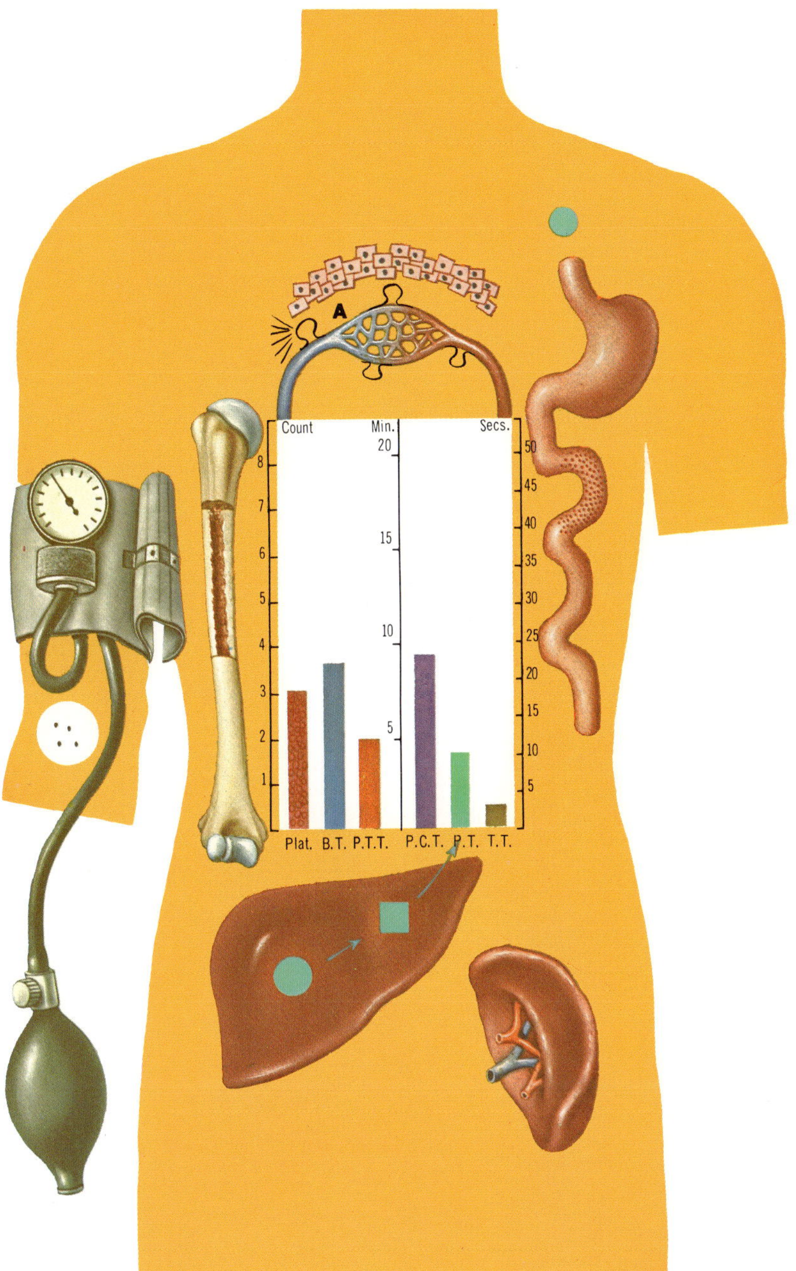

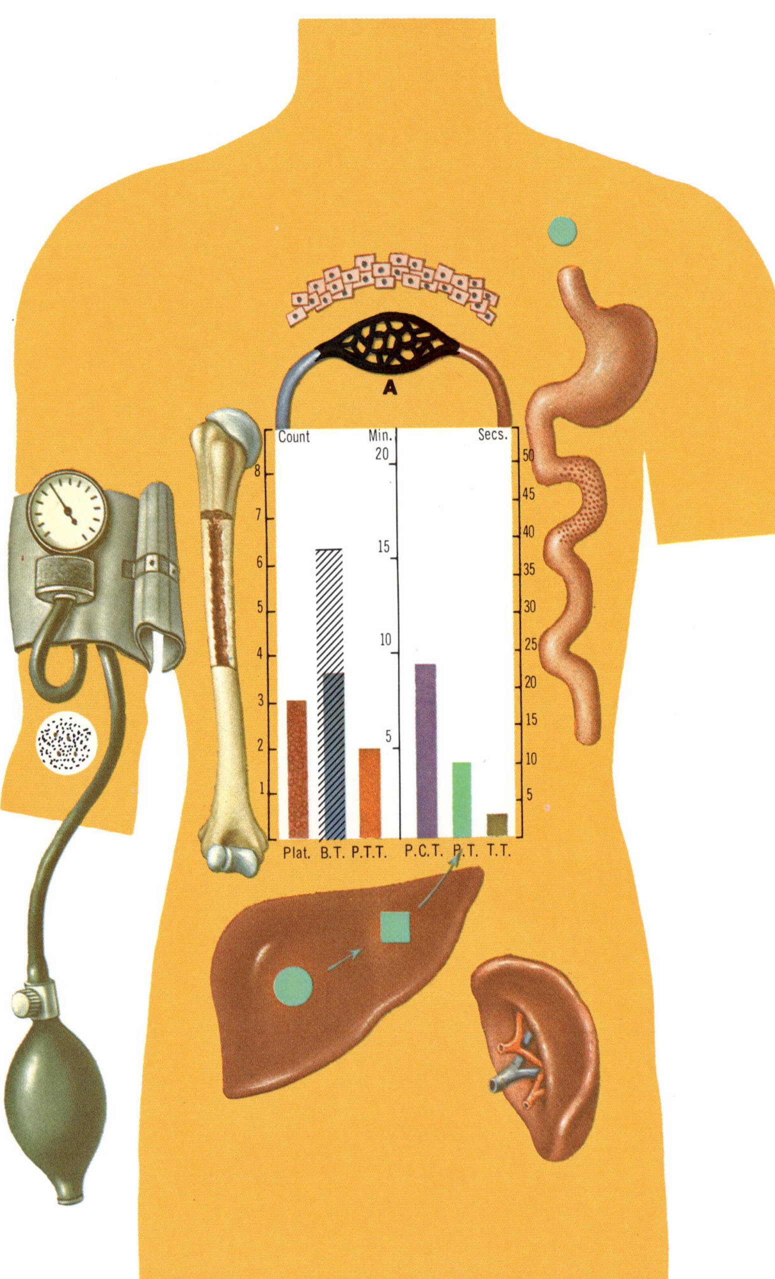

SCURVY

Lack of vitamin C leads to defective formation of the endothelial intercellular collagenous cement substance (A), and *increased capillary fragility* and *bleeding time* result. In some cases a thrombocytopenia occurs. All *other tests* of *hemostasis are* usually *normal.*

Summary of Laboratory Findings:

Platelet count: Normal
Bleeding time: Increased
Capillary fragility: Increased
Partial thromboplastin time: Normal
Prothrombin consumption: Normal
Prothrombin time: Normal
Thrombin time: Normal

HEPARIN THERAPY

Heparin in the presence of a cofactor (lipoprotein) in plasma delays the thrombin-fibrinogen reaction and inhibits the formation of thrombin from prothrombin.* Heparin also probably prevents the formation of plasma thromboplastic activity. These effects are reflected in a *decreased prothrombin consumption* and an *increased partial thromboplastin time, prothrombin time,* and *thrombin time.* Increased circulating heparin is also found in systemic mast cell disease. It is now more useful to follow heparin therapy with the P.T.T. instead of the clotting time.

Summary of Laboratory Findings:

Platelet count: Normal
Bleeding time: Normal
Capillary fragility: Normal
Partial thromboplastin time: Increased
Prothrombin consumption: Decreased
Prothrombin time: Increased
Thrombin time: Increased

* Biggs, R. P., and Macfarlane, R. G.: *Op. cit.*

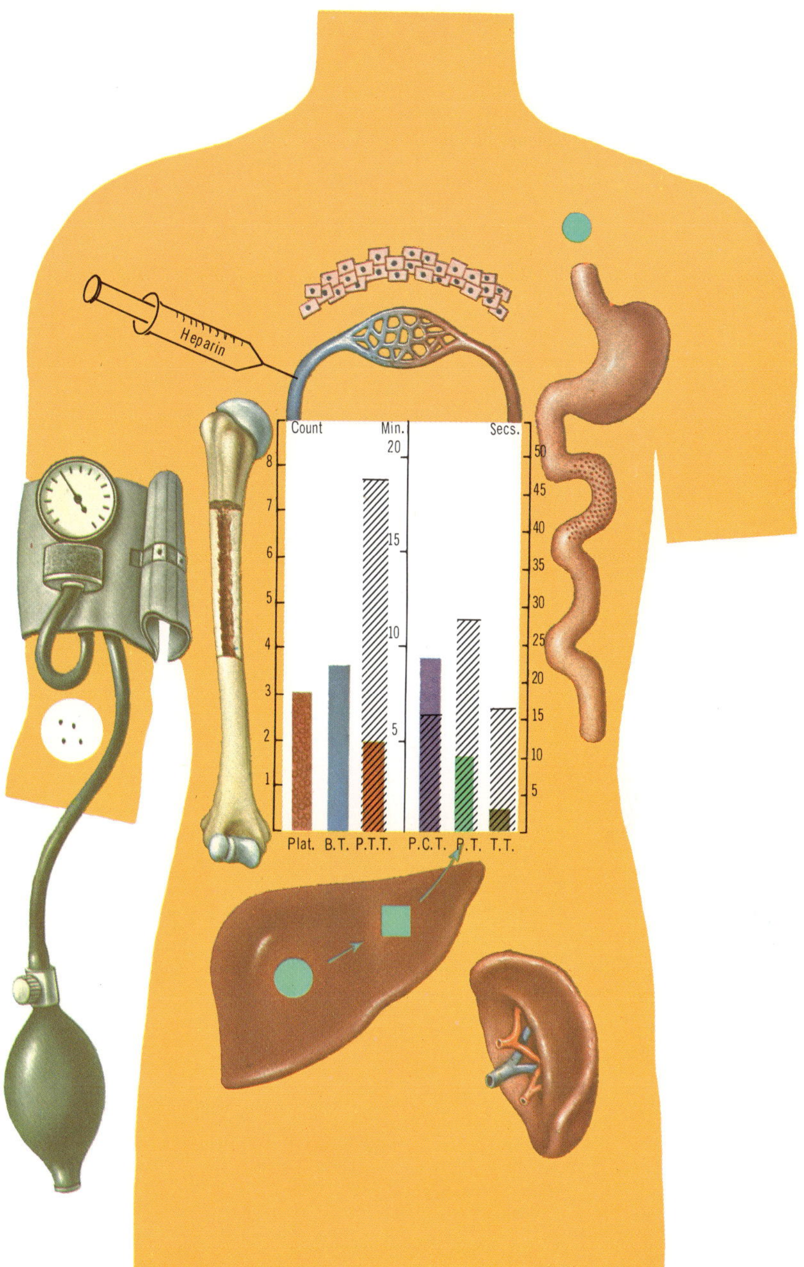

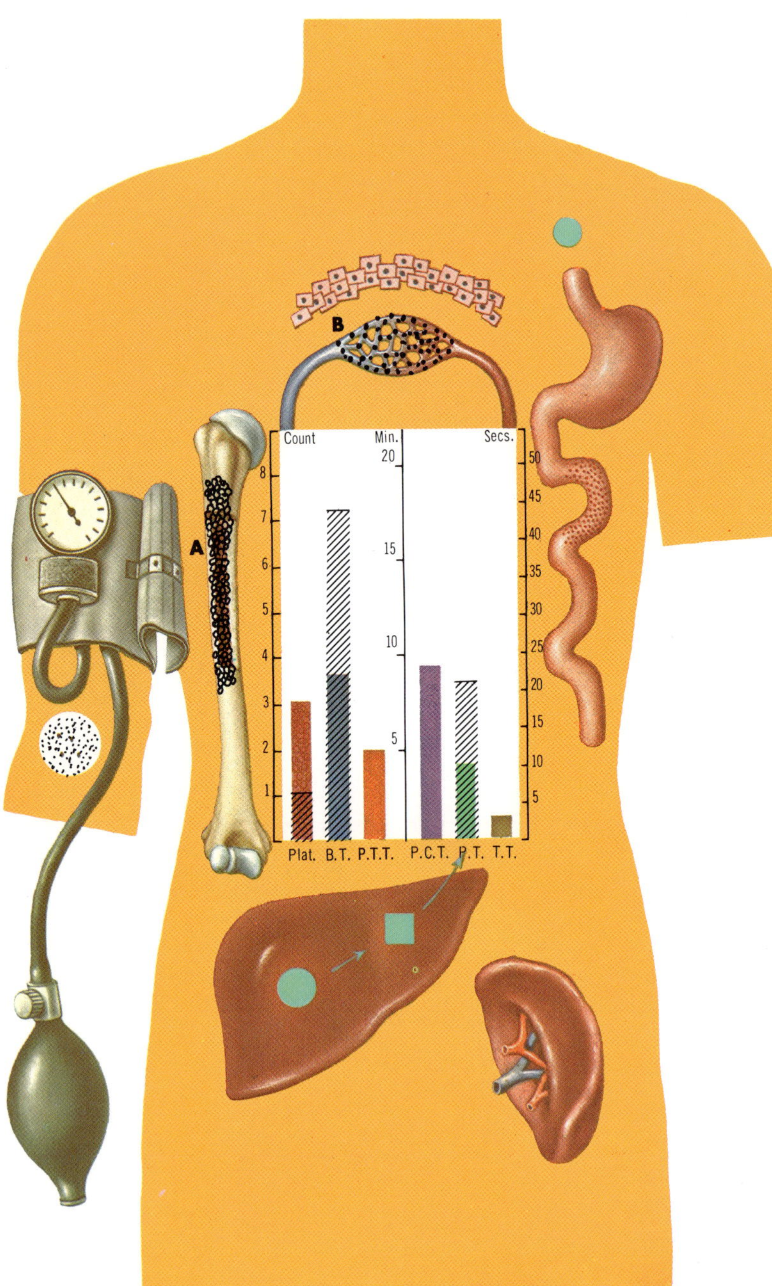

ACUTE LEUKEMIA

By infiltrating the bone marrow (A), leukemic cells reduce platelet production, and a *thrombocytopenia* results. Thus *bleeding time* and *capillary fragility* are *increased.* In addition, the vascular integrity is impaired by infiltration (B). Hypoprothrombinemia with a *prolonged prothrombin time* may also occur. Blood smears establish the diagnosis in most cases. Any neoplastic or other infiltrating disease of the bone marrow will produce a similar picture (p. 216).

Summary of Laboratory Findings:

Platelet count: Decreased
Bleeding time: Increased
Capillary fragility: Increased
Clotting time: Normal
Prothrombin consumption: Normal
Prothrombin time: Increased
Thrombin time: Normal

CIRRHOSIS OF THE LIVER

Since prothrombin, Factors VII, IX, and X are synthesized by the liver, these substances become deficient in any severe hepatocellular disorder (A). Thus the *prothrombin time* is prolonged, and the *partial thromboplastin time* is often *prolonged.* When Factors IX and X are sufficiently decreased in the blood, the *prothrombin consumption* test becomes *abnormal.* In addition, cirrhosis may lead to congestive splenomegaly (B) and consequent *thrombocytopenia.* If this is severe, *Bleeding time* is *prolonged.* Rarely is liver damage severe enough to cause diminished fibrinogen synthesis. There are also vascular and extravascular defects in this disorder. The diagnosis is confirmed by other liver function tests and a liver biopsy.

Summary of Laboratory Findings:

Platelet count: Normal or decreased
Bleeding time: Normal or increased
Capillary fragility: Normal or increased
Partial thromboplastin time: Increased
Prothrombin consumption: Normal or decreased
Prothrombin time: Increased
Thrombin time: Normal or increased

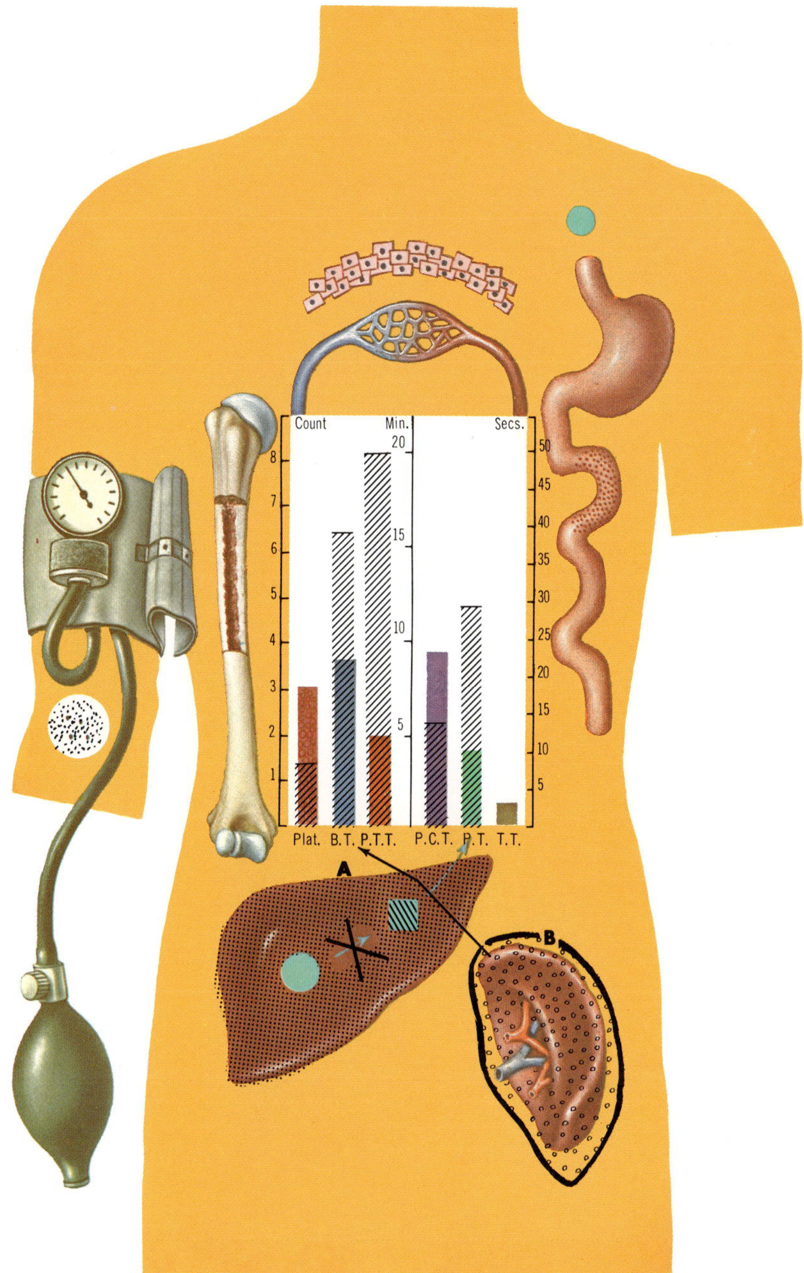

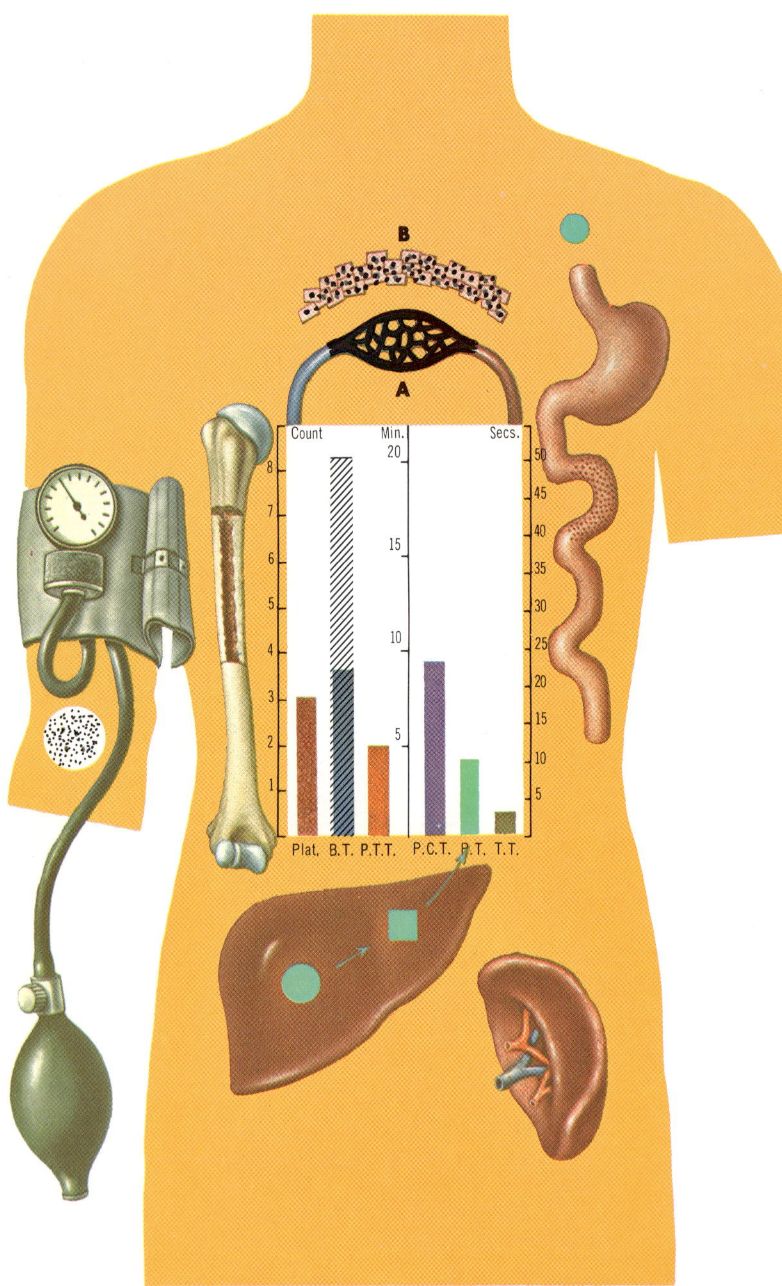

EHLERS-DANLOS SYNDROME

In this hereditary disorder the collagen tissue of the blood vessels (A) and the adjacent supporting tissue (B) is probably defective. Consequently, there are *increased capillary fragility* and a *prolonged bleeding time*. Other tests of hemostasis are generally normal.

Pseudoxanthoma elasticum is another disorder with a connective tissue abnormality, either elastic tissue or collagen. It produces a similar picture.

Summary of Laboratory Findings:

Platelet count: Normal
Bleeding time: Increased
Capillary fragility: Increased
Partial thromboplastin time: Normal
Prothrombin consumption: Normal
Prothrombin time: Normal
Thrombin time: Normal

POLYCYTHEMIA VERA

The increased proportion of red cells in the blood (A) results in a relative depletion of the plasma clotting factors and a deficient fibrillar network in the clot.* Fibrinogen and prothrombin are particularly decreased, and consequently there is an *increase* in the *thrombin* and *prothrombin times.* There is thrombocytosis, or occasionally thrombocytopenia, with their respective effects on bleeding time and capillary fragility. This diagnosis is supported by an increased blood volume and a normal arterial oxygen saturation.

Summary of Laboratory Findings:

Platelet count: Increased
Bleeding time: Usually normal
Capillary fragility: Usually normal
Partial thromboplastin time: Normal
Prothrombin consumption: Normal
Prothrombin time: Increased
Thrombin time: Increased

* Grollman, A.: The Functional Pathology of Disease. ed. 2, p. 581. New York, McGraw-Hill, 1963.

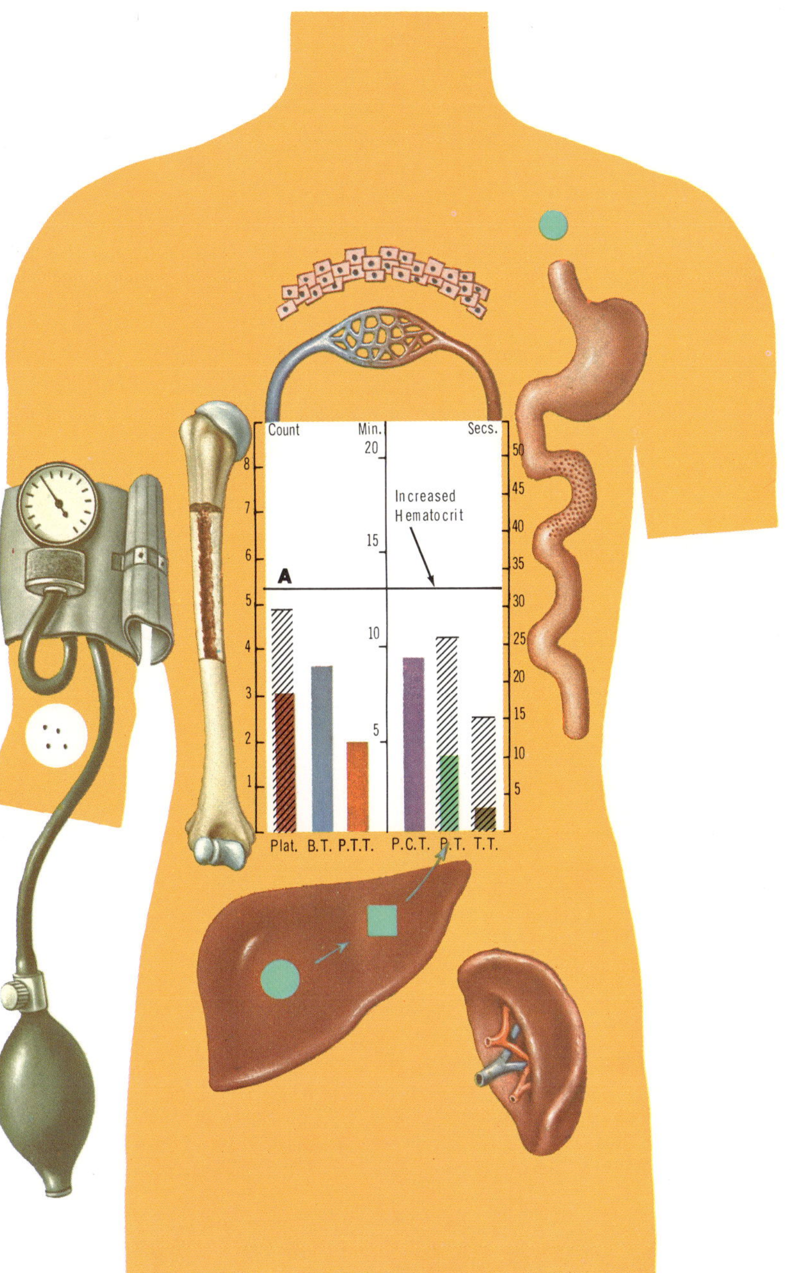

21 The Laboratory Diagnosis of Infectious Diseases

Basically, six classes of laboratory procedures are useful in the diagnosis of infectious diseases. Four of these, smears, cultures, animal inoculation, and tissue biopsy, may give direct evidence of the organism involved. The other two procedures, serologic tests and skin tests, give indirect evidence of the organism involved.

With the advent of the modern clinical laboratory, the physician's role in the performance of these tests has been largely assumed by the bacteriologist. Nevertheless, the physician retains a responsible role in the laboratory diagnosis of infectious diseases. It goes without saying that he must know what tests to order in each disease. These are listed in Table 21-1. Furthermore, he alone can properly interpret the bacteriologic findings.

Beyond these well-known responsibilities he must know how either to collect the specimen himself or to supervise others in its collection, and he must be able to perform certain tests in case a bacteriologist is not available. Finally, he needs a general understanding of the difficulties and pitfalls of bacteriologic diagnosis, so that he may effectively cooperate with the bacteriologist in the pursuit of a difficult diagnosis.

SMEARS AND CULTURES

Collection of the Specimen

Bacteriologic diagnosis begins with the proper collection of the specimen. This part of the work is too often delegated to untrained personnel, with the result that specimens frequently get lost or delayed in transit to the laboratory. Having reached the laboratory, they may be left to sit overnight without refrigeration before being plated.

In general, the collection of specimens should be as aseptic as possible. Specimens should be planted as soon as possible after collection. If this is not feasible, they may be refrigerated for a few hours. It should be noted, however, that some organisms (i.e., the meningococcus) will not be preserved by refrigeration.

Urine cultures may be refrigerated overnight at 4° to 6° C.

The practice of placing swabs directly into a broth medium before plating them is to be discouraged, as it may produce overgrowth of the pathogenic bacteria by contaminants.

The quantity of the specimen should be as large as possible. When only a small quantity is obtainable, swabs for collection should be moistened with sterile saline beforehand. This is particularly applicable in the collection of nasopharyngeal material.

All specimens should be collected as early in the course of the disease as possible and particularly before chemotherapy or antibiotics have been given. Specimens should be properly labeled, and information on clinical diagnosis, microorganisms suspected, and previous infections should be notated. The proper choice of culture media is based on a knowledge of the organism suspected.

Specimens for viral isolation should be collected within the first 5 days of illness. They must be frozen immediately on collection and shipped in dry ice to the viral laboratory.

Additional instructions for collection apply to the source of the specimen and the organism being sought. *Cultures of the nasopharynx* are best obtained by a 28-gauge Nichrome wire wrapped with cotton passed through a Pyrex tube inserted in the nose to prevent contamination from the anterior portion of the nasal passage. When the *sputum* is scanty, a better specimen may be obtained by passing a French catheter into the larynx to stimulate coughing. A saline aerosol may be used. Perhaps most effective of all is to inject 5 cc. of saline into the trachea via the crycothyroid membrane with a #22 gauge 1½ inch

Table 21-1. Laboratory Diagnosis of Infectious Diseases

Disease	Organism	Isolation of Organism: Source of Specimen	Isolation of Organism: Smear	Isolation of Organism: Culture	Animal Inoculation	Serologic Tests: Specific	Serologic Tests: Nonspecific	Skin Test	Biopsy
Bacteria									
Anthrax	*Bacillus anthracis*	Sore Blood Sputum	‡ (Wright's stain)	‡	‡	‡			
Bartonellosis (Oroya fever)	*Bartonella bacilliformis*	Blood Skin	‡	‡					‡
Boils, carbuncles, food poisoning, etc.	*Staphylococcus aureus*	Skin, stool Sputum Blood	‡	‡					
Brucellosis: see p. 280 Undulant fever									
Bubonic plague	*Pasteurella pestis*	Buboes Blood Sputum	‡	‡	‡	‡			
Chancre, soft (Chancroid)	*Haemophilus ducreyi*	Penis	‡	‡ *				‡	‡ Skin
Cholera	*Vibrio cholerae*	Stool	‡	‡					
Diphtheria	*Corynebacterium diphtheriae*	Pharynx	‡	‡ *				‡ Schick	
Dysentery	*Shigella dysenteriae*	Stool		‡ *		‡ †			
Glander's disease	*Actinobacillus mallei*	Sore in skin	‡	‡ *	‡	‡			
Gonorrhea	*Neisseria gonorrhoeae*	Vagina Urethra Blood Joint fluid CSF	‡	‡ *		‡			
Granuloma inguinale	*Donovania granulomatis*	Penis Groin	‡	‡ *					
Leprosy (Hansen's disease)	*Mycobacterium leprae*	Skin scrapings	‡		‡			‡ Histamine Lepromin	‡ Skin Nerve
Listeriosis	*Listeria monocytogenes*	Pharynx CSF Blood	‡	‡	‡	‡			
Meningococcal disease	*Neisseria meningitidis*	Pharynx CSF Blood	‡	‡					
Pharyngitis	*Streptococcus pyogenes*	Sputum Pharyngeal swab	‡	‡			ASO, CRP ‡	‡ Schultz-Charlton	
Pneumonia	*Haemophilus influenzae*	Pharynx CSF Joint effusion	‡	‡ *					

* Special media required. † Not practical or special personnel required. ‡ Valuable bacteriological procedures.

Table 21-1. Laboratory Diagnosis of Infectious Diseases *(Continued)*

		Isolation of Organism				Serologic Tests			
Disease	Organism	Source of Specimen	Smear	Culture	Animal Inoculation	Specific	Nonspecific	Skin Test	Biopsy
Pneumonia (*Cont.*)	*Klebsiella pneumoniae* *Staphylococcus aureus*	CSF Sputum Stool Blood	‡	‡					
Pneumonia (*Cont.*)	*Diplococcus pneumoniae*	Eye Ear Sputum, blood, CSF	‡	‡	‡				
Scarlet fever	(Group A hemolytic) *Streptococcus pyogenes*	Sputum Pharyngeal swab	‡	‡			ASO, CRP ‡	‡ Schultz-Charlton Dick test	
Subacute bacterial endocarditis	*Streptococcus viridans*	Blood Bone marrow	‡ (of petechiae)	‡					
Tetanus	*Clostridium tetani*	Wound	‡	‡	‡	(Isolation does not prove existence of infection.)			
Tuberculosis	*Mycobacterium tuberculosis*	Sputum Gastric washings Urine Tissue CSF	‡	‡ *	‡			‡	‡
Tularemia	*Pasteurella tularensis*	Skin Lymph node Pharynx		‡ *		‡		‡ Foshay	
Typhoid	*Salmonella typhosa*	Blood, first week Stool, after second week		‡		‡			
Undulant fever (Brucellosis)	*Brucella melitensis, Br. abortus, Br. suis*	Blood Bone marrow		‡ *		‡		‡	
Whooping cough	*Bordetella pertussis*	Trachea Bronchi Nasopharynx		‡ *		‡			
Spirochetes									
Pinta	*Treponema carateum*	Skin	‡			‡	‡		
	Spirillum minus	Skin (bite)	‡		‡		‡		
Rat-bite fever	*Streptobacillus moniliformis*	Blood Joint fluid		‡	‡	‡			
Relapsing fever	*Borrelia recurrentis*	Blood	‡	‡	‡	‡ †	‡		
Syphilis	*Treponema pallidum*	Skin	‡ Darkfield			‡ TPI, FTA-Ab	‡		
Weil's disease	*Leptospira icterohaemorrhagicae*	Urine Blood	‡ †	‡ *	‡	‡			‡ Muscle
Yaws	*Treponema pertenue*	Skin	‡			‡	‡		
Rickettsiae									
Q Fever	*Coxiella burnetii*		‡ (skin exudate)			‡	Weil-Felix (negative)		

* Special media required. † Not practical or special personnel required. ‡ Valuable bacteriological procedures.

Table 21-1. Laboratory Diagnosis of Infectious Diseases *(Continued)*

Disease	Organism	Isolation of Organism: Source of Specimen	Isolation of Organism: Smear	Isolation of Organism: Culture	Animal Inoculation	Serologic Tests: Specific	Serologic Tests: Nonspecific	Skin Test	Biopsy
Rocky Mountain spotted fever	*Rickettsia rickettsii*		‡ (skin exudate)	‡ (Blood)		‡	Weil-Felix		
Scrub typhus	*Rickettsia tsutsugamushi*		‡ (skin exudate)	‡ (Blood)		‡	Weil-Felix		
Typhus fever	*Rickettsia prowazekii*				‡ *	‡	Weil-Felix		
Viruses									
Cat-scratch fever	Not isolated							‡	‡ Lymph node
Colorado tick fever	Arbor virus	Blood or serum			‡	‡			
Common cold	Virus Bacteria Allergy	(No laboratory test available)							
Cytomegalic inclusion disease	Name unimportant	Urine Sputum		‡		‡			‡
Dengue	Arbor virus	Blood			‡	‡ †			
Eastern equine encephalitis	Arbor virus			‡		‡			
Eaton-agent pneumonia (Pap-1° atypical pneumonia)	*Mycoplasma pneumoniae*	Sputum		‡ *			‡ (Cold agglutinin, Strep. MG)		
Hepatitis	Type A Type B						HAA		
Herpangina	Coxsackie virus	Throat		‡ †		‡			
Influenza		Sputum Throat washings		‡ †		‡			
Infectious mononucleosis	Barr-Epstein virus					‡			
Japanese B encephalitis	Arbor virus					‡			
Lymphogranuloma venereum	Name unimportant				‡	‡	VDRL	‡ Frei	
Measles	Name unimportant	Throat Sputum Blood	‡	‡ †		‡			‡ Giant cells in nasal exudate
Mumps	Name unimportant	Saliva CSF		‡ †		‡ †		‡	
Poliomyelitis	Name unimportant	Stool		‡ †		‡			
Psittacosis (Parrot fever)	Name unimportant	Blood Sputum Lung tissue		‡ *		‡			‡
Rabies	Name unimportant	Saliva		‡ †	‡				
Rubella	Name unimportant			‡ (nasopharynx)		‡			

* Special media required. † Not practical or special personnel required. ‡ Valuable bacteriological procedures.

Table 21-1. Laboratory Diagnosis of Infectious Diseases *(Continued)*

Disease	Organism	Isolation of Organism: Source of Specimen	Smear	Culture	Animal Inoculation	Serologic Tests: Specific	Nonspecific	Skin Test	Biopsy
St. Louis encephalitis	Arbor virus					‡			
Smallpox	Name unimportant	Skin lesions	‡	‡ †		‡			
Trachoma	Name unimportant	Conjunctiva	‡ (Inclusion bodies)	‡ †		‡			
Varicella; Herpes zoster	Name unimportant					‡ †			‡ Giant cells (skin scrapings)
West Nile fever	Arbor virus	Blood			‡	‡			
Yellow fever	Arbor virus	Blood			‡	‡			‡ Liver
Fungi									
Actinomycosis	*Actinomyces israeli*	Skin Subcutaneous tissue Sputum	‡	‡ *					‡
Blastomycosis, North America	*Blastomyces dermatitidis*	Skin Sputum	‡	‡ *		‡		‡	
Candidiasis	*Candida albicans*	Mucous membrane Sputum	‡	‡ *					
Coccidioidomycosis	*Coccidioides immitis*	Sputum	‡	‡ * (Dangerous)	‡	‡		‡	‡
Histoplasmosis	*Histoplasma capsulatum*	Sputum Urine Blood Bone marrow	‡	‡ *	‡	‡		‡	‡
Mucormycosis	*Mucorales:* *Absidia,* *Rhizopus,* *Mucor*	Nose Pharynx Stool CSF		‡ *					‡
Nocardiosis	*Nocardia asteroides,* *N. brasiliensis*	Sputum Spinal fluid	‡	‡ *					‡
Sporotrichosis	*Sporotrichum schenckii*	Skin		‡ *					‡
Torulosis	*Cryptococcus neoformans*	Sputum Spinal fluid	‡ India ink	‡ *					
Parasites									
Amebiasis	*Entamoeba histolytica*	Stool	‡			‡			‡ Rectal
Ascariasis	*Ascaris lumbricoides*	Stool Sputum	‡						
Cestodiasis, intestinal	*Taenia saginata,* *Taenia solium,* *Diphyllobothrium latum*	Stool	‡ (Scotch tape)						
Chagas' disease	*Trypanosoma cruzi*	Blood Spinal fluid	‡		‡				

* Special media required. † Not practical or special personnel required. ‡ Valuable bacteriological procedures.

Table 21-1. Laboratory Diagnosis of Infectious Diseases *(Continued)*

Disease	Organism	Isolation of Organism: Source of Specimen	Smear	Culture	Animal Inoculation	Serologic Tests: Specific	Nonspecific	Skin Test	Biopsy
Cysticercosis	*Taenia solium* larvae								‡ Muscle Brain cyst
Echinococcosis	*Echinococcus granulosus*	Sputum Urine	‡			‡		‡ Casoni	‡ Liver Bone
Enterobiasis	*Enterobius vermicularis*	Stool	‡ (Scotch tape)						
Filariasis	*Wuchereria bancrofti*	Blood	‡			‡			‡ Lymph node
Hookworm disease	*Ancylostoma duodenale,* *Necator americanus*	Stool	‡						
Kala-azar	*Leishmania donovani*	Liver Bone marrow Blood	‡	‡	‡				‡ Lymph node Spleen
Malaria	*Plasmodium falciparum,* *P. malariae,* *P. vivax, P. ovale*	Blood Bone marrow	‡			‡	‡ (Wassermann)		
Onchocerciasis	*Onchocerca volvulus*								‡ Skin
Paragonimiasis	*Paragonimus westermani*	Sputum Stool	‡			‡		‡	
Scabies	*Sarcoptes scabiei*	Skin	‡						‡ Skin
Schistosomiasis, intestinal	*Schistosoma mansoni,* *S. japonicum*	Stool	‡			‡ †		‡ †	‡ Rectal Liver
Schistosomiasis, vesical	*Schistosoma haematobium*	Urine	‡			‡ †		‡ †	‡ Bladder
Strongyloidiasis	*Strongyloides stercoralis*	Stool Duodenal aspirate	‡						
Toxoplasmosis	*Toxoplasma gondii*				‡	‡	‡	‡	
Trichinosis	*Trichinella spiralis*					‡		‡	‡ Muscle
Trichomoniasis	*Trichomonas vaginalis*	Vagina Urethra	‡	‡ *					
Trichuriasis	*Trichuris trichiura*	Stool	‡						
Trypanosomiasis, African	*Trypanosoma rhodesiense,* *T. gambiense*	Blood Spinal fluid Lymph node	‡		‡	‡			
Visceral larva migrans	*Toxocara canis,* *T. cati*					‡		‡	‡ Liver

* Special media required. † Not practical or special personnel required. ‡ Valuable bacteriological procedures.

needle. This procedure will be followed by a prompt productive cough. *Gastric washings* for acid-fast bacilli must be neutralized and cultured soon after collection.

Stools should be delivered to the laboratory immediately after collection for the most accurate results. Certain coliform bacilli produce antibiotic substances that destroy enteric pathogens. Warm stools are also best for detecting ova and parasites. A cathartic (diarrheal) stool will sometimes give results when this fails. In enterobiasis and cestodiasis a plaster of Scotch tape placed on the anus in the morning is the best method of recovering the eggs.

Urine specimens are now collected in midstream after proper cleansing of the external genitalia. This practice is very adequate in males but does not always prevent contamination by diphtheroids, staphylococci, and other organisms from the vagina in females.* That is the reason that colony counts are so important on urine cultures in females. Suprapubic needle aspiration of the bladder may replace the use of the washed midstream specimen in females. A morning specimen of urine is preferable to a 24-hour specimen in isolating the tubercle bacillus. Special care must be exercised in washing the external genitalia before the collection of urine for tubercle bacilli, because non-tuberculous acid-fast bacilli are often present in the smegma.

Specimens of *blood* and of *pleural, peritoneal,* and *synovial fluids* must be obtained under especially aseptic conditions to prevent contamination by the flora of the skin. The skin over the site of puncture should be scrubbed with pHisoHex and swabbed with iodine before inserting the needle. The needle should be flamed after obtaining the specimen if it is to be used for injecting the material into the culture media.

Since *gonococci* are very sensitive to drying, urethral or synovial specimens should be plated at the bedside when these organisms are suspected. A special medium in a tube called Gonocult has recently been introduced by Smith, Kline, and French Laboratories for this purpose. Urethral and cervical smears should also be plated immediately. Women should have rectal smears via an anoscope as well if vaginal smears are negative. Delay in inoculation of sputum is also undesirable when *histoplasmosis* is being sought. A Chievitz and Meyer cough plate may be used to collect specimens for *pertussis.* When the patient cannot cooperate in coughing (e.g., infants), a cotton swab wrapped on the end of a flexible wire is passed into the nasopharynx by way of the nose and left there during several paroxysms of coughing. *Tubercle bacilli* may be best cultured from the pedicle that forms in the spinal fluid after standing.

* Clancy, C. F.: Bacteriological studies in office practice. Med. Clin. N. Am., *44*:1545, 1960.

Performance of Smears

The preparation and reading of most smears on hospitalized patients is rightly delegated to the bacteriologist. However, the clinician should be capable of performing smears for certain organisms in urgent situations when a bacteriologist is not available. This applies particularly to Gram stains of sputum, wounds, urine, spinal fluid, and urethral discharge. In addition, certain smear techniques are well within the capacity and needs of the office laboratory.

Every practitioner should be able to perform Gram's stain for bacteria, a Ziehl-Neelsen stain for tubercle bacilli, a potassium hydroxide or fresh wet preparation for fungi, and wet preparations of stools or vaginal discharge for ova or parasites. In certain geographical areas he will want to perform Wright's or Giemsa's stain of the blood for parasites (malaria, filariae, etc.).

The physician should be able to recognize in office practice and hospital emergencies any of the following list.

A List of Organisms and Their Morphologic Characteristics

Bacteria

Staphylococci: Gram's stain reveals clusters of densely stained gram-positive cocci, some within leukocytes or surrounded by them. They are usually single but may occur in pairs or chains.

Streptococci: Gram's stain reveals ovoid gram-positive cocci associated in chains.

Diplococcus pneumoniae: Gram's stain usually reveals gram-positive paired cocci. Each cell possesses a capsule in the virulent form. The adjacent ends are rounded, whereas the distal ends are pointed. They may be singular or in chains.

Neisseria gonorrhoeae: Gram's stain reveals gram-negative paired cocci in apposition like a pair of kidney beans. Many may exist intracellularly within leukocytes. They have no true capsule.

Neisseria meningitidis: Gram's stain reveals gram-negative paired cocci in apposition like a pair of kidney beans. They resemble gonococci in every way. Carbohydrate reactions are used to differentiate them.

Escherichia coli: Gram's stain reveals gram-negative, straight rods, usually singular but occasionally in chains.

Klebsiella: Gram's stain reveals ovoid gram-negative rods possessing a well-defined capsule. These are usually singular but may be paired.

Haemophilus influenzae: Gram's stain reveals small pleomorphic gram-negative rods which may be long and slender or so short that they look like cocci and must be differentiated from meningococci by culture.

Haemophilus ducreyi: Gram's stain reveals minute gram-negative bacilli 1 to 2 microns in length. They are in pairs, chains, or "fish-school" formation.

Calymmatobacterium granulomatis (organism of granuloma inguinale): Wright's stain reveals encapsulated coccobacillary or rodlike Donovan bodies within the mononuclear cells.

Tubercle bacilli: Ziehl-Neelsen stain reveals rod-shaped beaded cells that retain their red color after processing with acid alcohol.

Spirochaeta

Treponema pallidum: Darkfield examination reveals fine spiral motile organisms about 5 to 20 microns in length that appear light against a dark background.

Fungi

Candida albicans: Fresh preparation with saline or 10 per cent potassium hydroxide or Gram's stain reveals oval or budding yeastlike cells with a few pseudomycelia of varying thickness and length. They are gram-positive.

Cryptococcus neoformans: These appear similar to lymphocytes on a routine smear of spinal fluid. However, an India ink preparation delineates the large capsule of the yeast cells, because India ink outlines the capsular material.

Nocardia: A Gram stain from aerobic cultures reveals gram-positive branching filaments with or without clubs. Some filaments retain their red color after a Ziehl-Neelsen stain.

Actinomyces bovis: Gram's stain reveals the "sulfur granules" to consist of gram-positive, nonacid-fast, narrow branched filaments. The ends of the radial hyphae are often sheathed with a gelatinous mass (clubs).

Parasites

Enterobius vermicularis: A fresh preparation of anal scrapings or a preparation using the Scotch tape technique reveals eggs that have a thick shell, are flattened on one side, and contain a partially developed larva.

Leishmania donovani: Wright's stain reveals small round unicellular organisms with large rounded eccentric nuclei and a kinetoplast that looks like a minute dot or tiny oblique rod. The cytoplasm stains pale blue, whereas the nucleus stains red or violet. These organisms are found intracellularly in macrophages.

Entamoeba histolytica: These organisms may be found in the motile trophozoite stage or the encysted stage. The trophozoites are motile, rapidly moving organisms with hyaline pseudopodia. They are 15 to 30 microns in size and possess a finely granular cytoplasm with no food inclusions except red blood cells. Their nuclei are indistinct. The cysts are 6 to 15 microns in diameter, spherical, usually containing three to four nuclei. The cytoplasm is glassy clear. The nuclei are spherical and have a distinct rim and a central dot, the karyosome.

Malarial parasites: The appearance of the trophozoite, the signet ring forms of the developing schizont, and the number of merozoites of each species of the malarial parasites is quite characteristic. The young *trophozoite* in the red cell is a small blue-staining mass of cytoplasm with a *signet ring* stage, in which a vacuole or unstained central area develops, surrounded by a rim of blue cytoplasm with a chromatin dot at one side. In the *schizont stage* the cell has accumulated more cytoplasm and is divided into 2 to 16 chromatin masses. The red cell finally ruptures, liberating the individual *merozoites,* which penetrate new red cells and repeat the schizogony. The *gametocytes* of *Plasmodium vivax* and *P. malariae* are spherical and contain blue cytoplasm with a single chromatin mass. There are numerous pigment granules scattered throughout the cytoplasm. The gametocytes of *P. falciparum* are banana-shaped. For further differentiation of the various species of malarial parasites, standard texts on parasitology should be consulted.

Trichomonas vaginalis: A saline preparation of vaginal discharge reveals motile organisms shaped like a mouse's head and about 2-4 times bigger than a white cell with a whipping tail (flagella) at one end. The organisms may spin in a cylindrical fashion or twist like a fish while moving.

Performance of Cultures

Today the clinician in most localities can rely on an experienced bacteriologist to perform cultures on both hospital and office patients. However, it is relatively simple and inexpensive for the practitioner to culture common organisms in his office.* Staphylococci, streptococci, and coliform bacilli may be isolated in this way. However, some organisms will not grow on "universal" culture media such as blood agar and thioglycollate media. An erroneous negative result may then be obtained.

The bacteriologist has a wide variety of culture media at his disposal to suit the nutritional, moisture, and oxygen requirements of each organism, and he knows the requirements of each organism. He is experienced in reading cultures and smears. His knowledge of the many biochemical tests helps him further to differentiate similar organisms. Therefore, it is advisable to leave the culturing of microorganisms to him.

Yet he is severely handicapped if the physician does not provide him with clinical data. To select the appropriate culture media, he must know what organism is being sought. Knowing this is most important in dealing with those organisms that require special media or special handling for their isolation.

Organisms Requiring Special Media or Special Handling

Bacillus anthracis
Bordetella pertussis
Brucella organisms
Clostridia organisms
Corynebacterium diphtheriae
Fungi
Haemophilus ducreyi
Haemophilus influenzae
Mycobacterium tuberculosis
Neisseria gonorrhoeae
Neisseria meningitidis
Pasteurella tularensis
Sphirochetes
Streptobacillus moniliformis
Viruses

Special Comment. Some of the above deserve special mention. *Brucella* organisms are particularly difficult to isolate, and repeated blood cultures are necessary. *Corynebacterium diphtheriae* organisms are difficult to distinguish from diphtheroids and require either animal inoculation or careful microscopic and cultural study for several days. Serologic study of the toxic products is also helpful.

Most fungi may be grown on Sabouraud's French proof agar. However, it is dangerous to culture *Coccidioides,* as it may infect laboratory personnel. Animal inoculation is preferred here. *Histoplasma* organisms require immediate planting for their isolation.

Guinea pig inoculation is desirable in all cases of suspected tuberculosis not confirmed by smears. Spirochetes can rarely be isolated by culture, and animal inoculation is recommended. It should be noted that certain strains of group A hemolytic streptococci require anaerobic conditions for demonstration of beta hemolysis. The enteric bacteria require special media to distinguish the pathogens from the normal flora.

When the clinician cannot specify the organism sought, a knowledge of the source of the specimen is helpful in deciding what culture media to use. For example, all pus from wounds and sputum from cases of bronchiectasis or lung abscess should be cultured aerobically and anaerobically. This underscores the value of a knowledge of the clinical findings to the bacteriologist.

The physician is inclined to give up hope of isolating an organism once antibiotic therapy has been instituted. This attitude is not entirely justified. Thioglycollate medium neutralizes many antibiotics to some extent. Penicillinase may be added to reduce the inhibitory effects of penicillin on the organisms. Magnesium sulfate will antagonize tetracyclines. Semicarbazide antagonizes streptomycin. The bacteriologist will apply these techniques if he is notified that antibiotic therapy has been started and what antibiotics are being used.

Interpretation of Results

Only the clinician is in a position to interpret correctly the bacteriologic results, for he alone has full knowledge of the clinical findings and the course of the illness. Of most importance in assisting him in this task is a knowledge of the normal and pathogenic flora of each tissue or body fluid. These are listed in Table 21-2.

The reader will note that many organisms are found in certain fluids in both health and disease. When these organisms are reported, the clinician will need to know the quantity of the organisms present. For example, urine cultures of *Escherichia coli* are not definitely significant unless they contain more than 100,000 organisms

* Clancy, C. F.: *Ibid.*

Table 21-2. Microorganisms Found in Body Tissues and Fluid in Health and Disease*

Tissue or Specimen	Normal Flora	Pathogens
Nasopharynx	Alpha hemolytic streptococci *Neisseria catarrhalis* Coagulase-negative staphylococci Occasionally *Staphylococcus aureus* *Haemophilus haemolyticus* *Haemophilus influenzae* Diphtheroid bacilli Nonhemolytic streptococci *Candida albicans*	Beta hemolytic streptococci Group A, occasionally Groups B, C, and G *Corynebacterium diphtheriae* *Bordetella pertussis* Meningococcus *Staphylococcus aureus* (coagulase positive) *Haemophilus influenzae* in large numbers Pneumococci in large numbers *Candida albicans*
Sputum	Same as Nasopharynx	Pneumococcus *Klebsiella* species *Haemophilus influenzae* *Staphylococcus aureus* (coagulase positive) Hemolytic streptococci *Pasteurella pestis* *Pasteurella tularensis* *Mycobacterium tuberculosis* *Coccidioides immitis* *Histoplasma capsulatum* *Blastomyces dermatitidis* *Candida albicans* *Bordetella pertussis*
Stool	Enterococci (streptococci) *Escherichia coli* Clostridia Staphylococci *Proteus* species *Pseudomonas* Occasionally *Salmonella* in carriers *Candida albicans* yeast	*Salmonella* species (*typhosa*, etc.) *Shigella* species *Vibrio comma* *Myobacterium tuberculosis* *Escherichia coli*† (infants) Staphylococci *Clostridium botulinum* toxin *Proteus* (in large numbers) *Pseudomonas* (in large numbers) *Candida albicans* *Entamoeba histolytica* Other parasites
Urine		Coliform bacilli *Proteus* species *Pseudomonas aeruginosa* Enterococci Staphylococci, coagulase positive and coagulase negative
Urine (*Cont.*)		Beta hemolytic streptococci, usually Groups B and D Gonococcus *Mycobacterium tuberculosis* *Trichomonas vaginalis* *Klebsiella* frequently
Urethral discharge	Staphylococci, coagulase-negative Coliform bacilli Enterococci *Mycobacterium smegmatis*	*Neisseria gonorrhoeae* *Treponema pallidum* *Haemophilus ducreyi* *Mima polymorpha* *Trichomonas vaginalis*
Vaginal discharge	Döderlein's bacillus Coagulase-negative staphylococci Coliform bacilli Enterococci Nonpathogenic mycobacteria *Haemophilus vaginalis* Bacteroides Anaerobic streptococci	*Neisseria gonorrhoeae* *Haemophilus ducreyi* *Treponema pallidum* *Haemophilus vaginalis* *Listeria monocytogenes* *Trichomonas vaginalis* *Candida albicans* Enterococci
Skin	Diphtheroids Staphylococci, coagulase-negative Coliform bacilli Enterococci *Proteus* species *Clostridium* species	*Staphylococcus aureus* (coagulase positive) *Streptococcus pyogenes* Coliform bacilli *Proteus* species *Pseudomonas* species *Clostridium* species *Bacteroides* species Fungi (*sporotrichum, Actinomyces, Nocardia, Candida albicans, Trichophyton, Microsporum, Epidermophyton*)
Blood	None‡	*Staphylococcus pyogenes* *Streptococcus pyogenes* Coliform bacilli Pneumococci *Haemophilus influenzae* *Neisseria meningitidis* *Salmonella* species *Brucella* species *Pasteurella tularensis* *Leptospira* species Malaria Trypanosomes Filariae Bacteroides *Listeria monocytogenes* Rickettsiae

* Does not include viruses. † Pathogenic serotypes. ‡ But may be contaminated by normal skin flora.

(Continued on overleaf)

Table 21-2. Microorganisms Found in Body Tissues and Fluid in Health and Disease (*Continued*)

Tissue or Specimen	Normal Flora	Pathogens
Cerebrospinal fluid	None‡	Pneumococci *Neisseria meningitidis* *Haemophilus influenzae* (infants and children particularly) Staphylococci *Mycobacterium tuberculosis* Streptococci Coliform bacilli *Listeria monocytogenes* *Leptospira* species *Bacteroides* species *Cryptococcus* and other fungi
Pleural effusion	None‡	Same as Sputum
Peritoneal effusion	None‡	Pneumococci *Neisseria gonorrhoeae* Otherwise, same organisms as Stool
Conjunctiva	Same as Skin, plus *Corynebacterium xerose*	*Staphylococcus aureus* *Neisseria gonorrhoeae* Pneumococcus Alpha and beta hemolytic streptococci Koch-Weeks bacillus (*Haemophilus aegyptius*) *Pseudomonas* species *Moraxella lacunata*
Ear	Staphylococci, coagulase negative Diphtheroids and *Gaffkya tetragena*	*Pseudomonas aeruginosa* *Staphylococcus aureus* *Proteus* species Alpha and beta hemolytic streptococci Pneumococci Coliform bacilli Fungus (*Aspergillus*)

‡But may be contaminated by normal skin flora.

per milliliter. Therefore, a colony count should be ordered when these are reported. *Candida albicans* in large numbers in the stool is considered pathogenic in the presence of previous antibiotic therapy. Alteration of regional flora by antibiotic therapy may convert other normally harmless organisms into pathogens.

On the other hand, organisms generally considered pathogenic are not invariably so. At least 15 to 20 per cent of normal adults are carriers of *Staphylococcus aureus*. Five to 10 per cent are carriers of group A hemolytic streptococci. A few are carriers of *Salmonella typhosa* in their stools.

As noted in Table 21-2, specimens of blood and peritoneal, pleural, and spinal fluids do not normally contain "normal" flora. However, contaminants from the skin will be reported if sterile precautions have not been taken. Repeat cultures are indicated in such instances.

Positive blood culture results do not necessarily indicate septicemia. Many organisms produce transient bacteremia in their early stages of invasion of the host (pneumococci, *Salmonella*, etc.).

An infection may be due to two or more pathogens acting together. This is often true in lung abscesses.

Additional factors must be considered in the diagnosis of each particular infection:

1. All *hemolytic streptococci* may not cause pharyngitis. Group B organisms may come from a drink of milk.
2. All acid-fast bacilli are not *tuberculous*. Some of these are atypical mycobacteria that can produce illnesses similar to tuberculosis. Mycobacteria in urine specimens may be *Mycobacterium smegmatis* from the smegma.
3. Certain serologic types of *Escherichia coli* may be pathogenic in the stool, particularly in infants. The same is true of *Proteus* and *Pseudomonas*.
4. Toxin-producing organisms such as *Clostridia* are not pathogenic unless there is proof that they are producing toxins. This is true also of *Staphylococci* isolated in enteritis.
5. *Gonococci* are particularly difficult to isolate from synovial fluid or cervical discharge. Repeated cultures without detection do not exclude this diagnosis. Rectal cultures should also be done.
6. *Brucella* time and again escapes detection in blood cultures; therefore several cultures of blood and bone marrow must be taken.
7. Since bacteremia is relatively consistent in *subacute bacterial endocarditis*, at least one of 4 to 5 cultures taken in a 24- to 48-hour period will usually be positive.

8. In *typhoid fever, tularemia, plague,* and other illnesses, blood cultures are positive only in certain stages of the illness (during the first week, etc.).

9. Many laboratories fail to distinguish enterococci from group A hemolytic streptococci. Enterococci do not cause pharyngitis.

10. The presence of *tubercle bacilli* in stool cultures does not mean that they definitely come from the bowels. They may come from swallowed sputum.

11. Detection of organisms on a gram stain or unstained examination of uncentrifuged urine usually signifies the presence of at least 100,000 organisms per milliliter, and therefore infection may be implied. A colony count (see above) is more positive.

12. *Cryptococci* are easily mistaken for lymphocytes in the spinal fluid. An India ink preparation is useful in differentiating these two.

13. Harmless saprophytic *fungi* of the sputum and skin may be confused with pathogens on smears.

14. Aseptic meningitis is not invariably due to a virus. *Leptospira* cause a number of cases. Viruses most likely to be associated with this condition are group B Coxsackie, mumps, ECHO, lymphocytic choriomeningitis, polio virus, arbor virus, and herpes simplex.

15. The isolation of a virus does not establish it as a pathogen. *Coxsackie, herpes,* or *polio virus* may persist in the body for years without precipitating a disease state.

16. The same clinical syndrome may be produced by a variety of viruses.

Pursuit of the Diagnosis

When the first smears or cultures do not support the clinical impression, there is a strong tendency to drop the diagnosis. This is most regrettable. When the clinical findings strongly support the diagnosis, the clinician should not give up easily his pursuit of laboratory confirmation. There are further steps that he may take.

Obviously, he may order one of the other tests in Table 21-1. But, more important than this, he should be certain that he has gained all he can from the smears and cultures. The clinician should check details of the collection of the specimen, making sure that it was properly collected. He should consult the bacteriologist about what culture media were used. For example, anaerobic culturing may not have been done. Repeated cultures or animal inoculation are often necessary to isolate certain organisms. Utilizing centrifuged specimens of larger amounts of spinal fluid, urine, pleural and peritoneal fluids for cultures may yield positive results. A cathartic (diarrheal) stool may yield the suspected parasite. A bone marrow culture may pick up *Streptococcus viridans, Brucella,* and *Histoplasma* organisms when blood cultures are consistently negative. A thick blood smear may turn up the malarial parasite when thin ones fail.

Just as negative cultures may lead to unwarranted despair, positive cultures may lead to unwarranted security. For example, the isolation of *Clostridium botulinum* from the stool does not ascertain its role in a case of enteritis. The bacteriologist must be asked to find out whether it is toxin-producing. As heretofore mentioned all acid-fast bacilli are not tuberculous. The clinician might ask for a niacin test or an animal inoculation to ascertain whether the bacillus is a human strain. Gram-negative diplococci in vaginal discharge are not invariably gonococci. Carbohydrate reactions must be used to distinguish these from meningococci and from members of the tribe *Mimeae*.

Close cooperation between the clinician and the bacteriologist facilitates the diagnosis of many infectious diseases.

Sensitivity

Many physicians routinely order a sensitivity along with the culture at considerable expense to the patient. It may be wiser to rely on the knowledge of which antibiotics usually are effective against the organism isolated than the sensitivity report. This is because it is an in vitro test and the antibiotic will be working in vivo. For example, sulfa drugs frequently will be effective in vivo when sensitivity tests demonstrate resistance. If an antibiotic can not reach the area of infection in sufficient quantities, then the organism will be "resistant" regardless of sensitivity tests in vitro. Also, to be accurate the organism in question must be able to grow rapidly (within 24 hours) and be aerobic. It is likely that clinicians will continue to use sensitivity tests despite what has been said here.

ANIMAL INOCULATION

Animal inoculation is used in the isolation of many bacteria when other means of isolation fail. Guinea pig inoculation should be employed in all cases of suspected tuberculosis with negative smears. It has also proved to be a good virulence test in this disorder. *Pasteurella pestis* and *Pasteurella tularensis* are frequently isolated by this method. Animal inoculation is the procedure of choice in isolating many viruses, almost all spirochetes, and certain fungi (e.g., *Histoplasma*) and parasites (e.g., trypanosomes).

SEROLOGIC TESTS

These are only of diagnostic value late in the course of the infection. In short-term illnesses they are merely of epidemiologic significance. In patients with mild infections or in those who have received antibiotics prematurely, they may be the only means of diagnosis.

Collection of Specimens

In general, specimens of blood for serologic studies should be obtained immediately after admission and repeated in the convalescent phase of the illness (usually, 3 or 4 weeks after the onset of the illness). This applies to bacterial as well as viral infections, a point that is insufficiently emphasized. For example, when febrile agglutinins for typhoid, etc., are ordered, a repeat specimen should be drawn in 2 to 3 weeks to observe for an increase in the titer.

Blood should be drawn prior to skin testing, because skin tests may stimulate the production of antibodies. Specimens should be sent to the laboratory and examined before hemolysis. If specimens of plasma must be sent to a larger laboratory, they should be frozen immediately. As with culture requests, requests for serologic studies should contain clinical data, such as diagnosis, therapy, and previous infections or vaccinations.

Performance

Serologic tests are largely performed by the hospital or specialized clinical laboratory. Consequently, the technique of performing these tests will not be discussed here. There are four serologic tests in common use. These are the complement fixation test, the neutralization test, the hemagglutinin inhibition test, and the nonspecific agglutination test. Recently fluorescent antibody techniques have been developed and will simplify serologic methods considerably. Since each laboratory can usually give advice to the clinician about which serologic test is best for diagnosing each infection, these tests are not specifically noted in the table.

Interpretation

Certain facts must be kept in mind in the interpretation of serologic tests. A knowledge of the specificity of each test is essential. Cross reactions between various strains of bacteria, fungi, and viruses reduce the specificity of some of these tests. Serologic titers are also influenced by previous infections or vaccinations, as well as the anamnestic response. This is the reason that a single titer is of little value. The demonstration of a rising titer (an increase in the titer between the acute-phase serum and the convalescent-phase serum) is much more significant. Nevertheless, certain levels are considered to be very suspicious in themselves. What constitutes a significant titer varies from one laboratory to another, and therefore the clinician should consult the laboratory about the interpretation of these tests.

Nonspecific Tests

Nonspecific serologic tests are useful in the diagnosis of syphilis, rheumatic fever, rheumatoid arthritis, infectious mononucleosis, rickettsial diseases, and primary atypical pneumonia.

Syphilis. Various nonspecific tests (Wassermann, Kolmer, Mazzini flocculation, etc.) utilizing the antigen cardiolipin (alcohol soluble lipid from beef heart) are in common use. These lend strong support to the clinical diagnosis when positive, but are not 100 per cent diagnostic. Both false negatives and false positives do occur. If there is strong clinical evidence of syphilis in the face of a negative Wassermann, a *Treponema pallidum* immobilization test (TPI) should be ordered. Even these have been falsely negative, and the more sensitive fluorescent treponemal antibody test (FTA) is now gaining acceptance.

False positive Wassermann reactions have been observed in lupus erythematosus, infectious mononucleosis, smallpox, malaria, leprosy, measles, and all spirochetal diseases (rat-bite fever, Weil's disease, etc.). A TPI or FTA should be done on these cases also to differentiate them from true syphilis.

Rheumatic Fever. Since this disorder is definitely related to infections with group A hemolytic streptococci, the antistreptolysin O titer is almost always significantly elevated. It should be remembered, however, that streptococcal infections occur without rheumatic fever, and that the mere presence of an elevated ASO titer is not diagnostic of the latter disorder. Furthermore, the ASO titer may not be increased in the early stages of rheumatic fever. Repeat titers later in the course of the infection will frequently show a significant rise. Blood should be drawn for a repeat titer even when the initial titer is elevated, because a rising titer is more conclusive of a recent streptococcal infection. Although the ASO titer is not elevated in 10 to 15 per cent of patients with rheumatic fever, immunologic evidence of a recent streptococcal infection can be obtained in 100 per cent of these cases if tests for antibodies to other toxins of streptococci (streptokinase, etc.) are employed.

Rheumatoid Arthritis. Patients with this disorder have a factor in their sera capable of agglutinating latex particles or sheep red cells that have been sensitized with a special antisheep cell amboceptor. About 70 per cent of adult patients with rheumatoid arthritis possess this factor.

Infectious Mononucleosis. Patients with this disorder also have a factor in their sera that agglutinates sheep red cells. This factor is absorbed by beef red cells, but not by guinea pig kidney, which absorbs the factor found in normal serum and the sera of patients with serum sickness. This test is further discussed on page 253.

Rickettsial Diseases. Various rickettsiae have been found to agglutinate certain strains of *Proteus vulgaris* designated OX. This test is still routinely performed, but the more specific complement-fixation and precipitin tests have become available.

Primary Atypical Pneumonia. The organism responsible for this disorder has certain antigens in common with MG streptococci. Agglutinins for these organisms appear in one half of the cases and are fairly specific for this disease. In addition, cold hemagglutinins are found in high titers. However, these are also found in mumps, hemolytic anemias, and some respiratory and peripheral vascular diseases.

ANA Test. The antinuclear antibody test for *Lupus erythematosus* is positive in almost 100 per cent of cases of active *L. E.* However, all antigens (DNA, RNA, etc.) must be tested, and multiple techniques (immunofluorescence, radioimmunoassay, etc.) must be used.

Specific Tests

Reference to Table 21-1 shows that specific serologic tests are available for the diagnosis of *viral diseases,* such as poliomyelitis, lymphocytic choriomeningitis, psittacosis and mumps, *rickettsial diseases,* many *spirochetal diseases,* and *bacterial diseases,* such as typhoid, brucellosis, and gonorrhea. They are also of value in certain *parasitic infestations* (schistosomiasis, amoebiasis, toxoplasmosis, etc.).

The Communicable Disease Center of the United States Public Health Service in Atlanta, Georgia, may be consulted when a particular serologic test is not performed by the local laboratory. These tests will not be discussed in detail. However, some of them deserve special mention because of the problems in interpretation.

Brucellosis. The test is not reliable if a brucellergen skin test has been performed recently.

Gonorrhea. Although heralded as a useful adjunct in the diagnosis of gonorrheal arthritis, this serologic test is not too reliable. Many false positive and false negative results have been obtained.

Histoplasmosis. Because of the difficulty in culturing *Histoplasma,* this is a very important diagnostic test. Serial skin testing may increase the titer in positive reactors.

Typhoid Fever. Rising O titers usually indicate a recent infection. Elevated H titers are less significant, as they may indicate previous vaccination or infection.

SKIN TESTS

Skin tests are of value in the diagnosis of tuberculosis, brucellosis, tularemia, lymphogranuloma venereum, mumps, coccidioidomycosis, histoplasmosis, blastomycosis, trichinosis, echinococcosis, and toxoplasmosis (Table 21-1).

Performance

Skin tests should be performed by the clinician or experienced laboratory personnel. Too often the injection is made subcutaneously and therefore yields a false negative result. The manufacturer's directions should be followed. In general, 0.1 ml. is injected intradermally into the volar surface of the forearm. A control is employed whenever possible. The material must be fresh. The test is usually read 24 hours after the injection, but in some cases (e.g., the Dick Test, etc.) tests are read in 48 hours, and in others (e.g., tuberculin) they are read in 72 hours. Erythema or induration of more than 1 cm. in diameter is considered significant. A central area of necrosis is even more suspicious. A relatively quantitative test can be performed by utilizing serial dilutions of the test material.

These tests are definitely limited by the fact that once skin sensitivity is established, it often persists for life. Thus, they may indicate either past or present infection. Furthermore, this sensitivity may be lost in an overwhelming infection. Skin tests do not usually become positive until 3 to 4 weeks after the onset of the infection. Consequently, they are useless in short-term illness.

Interpretation

Certain additional points should be kept in mind in interpreting skin tests in the following disorders:

Blastomycosis. Cross immunity with histoplasmosis has been noted.

Brucellosis. This test is negative in 5 to 39 per cent of cases. It should be performed only *after* blood for serologic studies has been drawn, since the test may stimulate agglutinin and opsonin production. Its accuracy is affected by the prozone phenomena.

Coccidioidomycosis. Cross immunity with histoplasmosis and blastomycosis organisms occurs.

Histoplasmosis. Cross immunity with coccidioidomycosis and blastomycosis organisms occurs.

Leprosy. Patients with the lepromatous form of the disease do not usually react to the lepromin antigen. The transformation of a negative reactor to a positive reactor in the course of therapy is a good prognostic sign. Cross immunity with other mycobacteria (e.g., *Mycobacterium tuberculosis*) occurs. Thus a positive reaction is not diagnostic.

Lymphogranuloma Venereum. The Frei test may be positive in psittacosis infections.

Tularemia. The skin test becomes positive earlier in the disease than the serologic tests, making it of distinct value in diagnosis.

Tuberculosis. Up to 59 per cent of patients with suggestive radiologic findings of the disease may manifest negative reactions to the tuberculin skin tests. Patients with overwhelming miliary tuberculosis are occasionally insensitive, whereas patients with sarcoidosis, lymphoma, and hypogammaglobulinemia are frequently insensitive to the tuberculin skin test.

22 The Office Laboratory

Every primary physician—family physician, internist, or pediatrician—could benefit himself and his patients by performing certain laboratory procedures in his office. It is convenient to the patient, and many a diagnosis can be discovered when the motivation for diagnosis is at its peak (when the patient first presents the problem). To be used as an office procedure, a test should be simple, inexpensive, and commonly required. A certified laboratory technician can be hired if necessary, but a good nurse or other physician's assistant can be taught to do most of these procedures accurately. Possibly three exceptions to this are examining the blood smear, Gram's stain, and urine sediment. In Table 22-1 is a list of procedures that can easily be done in the office. The techniques of their performance will now be discussed.

HEMATOLOGY

Hemoglobin. The simplest method is by visual comparison with the Sahli hemoglobinometer. Blood (0.02 ml.) is drawn into a pipette and placed into a specially calibrated tube containing N/10 HCl at the 20 mark. Standing at room temperature for 10 minutes, the hemoglobin is converted to acid hematin. Then additional N/10 HCl is added to make the solution match the permanent standard of the comparator block in the hemoglobinometer. The percentage of hemoglobin is read from the calibration on the tube to which the solution was diluted. The normal is 13 to 17 gm. per 100 ml.

A more accurate method is to use a photoelectric colorimeter such as the Unimeter made by Biodynamics Laboratory. Tubes with premeasured amounts of potassium ferrocyanide and sodium cyanide can be used. The method is fast and easy for inexperienced personnel.

Hematocrit. A Clay-Adams microhematocrit, heparinized capillary tubes, and a sealing compound are necessary. Capillary or venous blood is drawn into 2 capillary tubes so they are 80-90% filled. The end opposite the one used for filling is sealed with the special compound. The tubes are then placed opposite each other in the centrifuge (the end with the sealing compound points out) and the centrifuge run for 5 minutes. Afterward the hematocrit values can be read from the gauge in the centrifuge. Normal values are 40-54% for men and 37-47% for women.

White Blood Cell Count. Draw capillary or venous blood to the 0.5 mark on a Thoma white cell pipette and add diluting fluid (2-3% aqueous solution of acetic acid and gentian violet) to the 11 mark. Agitate or shake the tube 2-3 minutes for good mixing. Discard the first 3-4 drops of fluid from the pipette. With the index finger over the upper end place the bottom tip of the pipette at the edge of the cover-slip of the hemocytometer (Neubauer or Fuch-Rosenthal) and allow sufficient (but not too much) fluid to escape. Fill the counting chamber by adjusting the pressure of the index finger at the upper end. The fluid is drawn into the chamber by capillary action. Place the hemocytometer under the microscope with a low-power objective (× 10) and count the number of cells in 4 large squares. The actual number of WBC's per cu. mm. is determined by the following formula:

$$\text{number of WBC's/cu. mm. of blood} = \frac{\text{number in 4 large squares} \times 10 \times 20}{4}$$

Normal values for adults vary between 5,000 and 10,000 cells per cu. mm.

Blood Smear. A drop of capillary or venous blood is placed 1-2

Table 22-1
OFFICE LABORATORY PROCEDURES

A. Hematology
   1. Hemoglobin
   2. Hematocrit
   3. WBC
   4. Blood smear
   5. Platelet count
   6. Clotting time
   7. Prothrombin time
   8. Rumpel-Leede test
   9. Sedimentation rate
B. Blood Chemistries
   1. Blood sugar
   2. Lipid profile
   3. Miscellaneous
C. Urinalysis
   1. Specific gravity
   2. Chemistry
   3. Cell count
   4. Fishberg concentration test
D. Stool
   1. Occult blood
   2. Ovum and parasites
   3. Scotch tape test
   4. Trypsin
E. Bacteriology
   1. Gram stain
   2. Saline preparation
   3. KOH preparation
   4. Cultures
      a. Nose and throat
      b. Urine
      c. Urethral
      d. Vaginal and cervical
F. Cytology—vaginal smear
G. Immunology
   1. Pregnosticon
   2. Monosticon
   3. Rheumosticon
H. Semen Analysis
I. Special Procedures
   1. Spinal tap
   2. Synovianalysis
   3. Gastric analysis
   4. Pulmonary function tests
   5. Venous pressure and circulation time
J. Skin Tests

cm. from the end of a glass slide. The edge of a second slide is placed at the center of the first slide at a 30 degree angle and drawn back to touch the drop of blood gently. As soon as the drop spreads along the entire edge of the second slide, the second slide is pushed forward along the first. The more rapid the movement, the thicker the smear. The bigger the angle, the thicker the smear. After some practice, smears can be made the desired thickness. The smear is air dried and placed film side up on a staining rack. Wright's stain (available already mixed) is then dripped onto the slide (to completely cover it) and the slide is allowed to stand 1 minute. Then distilled water (an equal amount) is dripped onto the slide carefully, so that the Wright's stain is not removed After 2-4 minutes the solution is washed off the slide with distilled water and the slide allowed to dry. Then the slide is placed under the microscope and observed with both low power and the high dry objective for the quality of the smear. A drop of immersion oil is placed on the slide and the oil immersion objective used. The character of the red cells is observed for size, shape, and content of hemoglobin. Atypical leucocytes are looked for. Two hundred white cells are counted and classified in a systematic manner so the percentage of neutrophils, lymphocytes, eosinophils, basophils, and monocytes can be determined.

Platelet Count. With the blood smear prepared above, the platelet count can be estimated as accurately as by performing one directly.

One platelet/oil immersion field = 10,000/cu. mm.

Clotting Time. Immediately after 5 cc. of whole venous blood is drawn into a clean, dry glass syringe, a stop watch is started. One ml. of blood is placed into each of 4 10 × 1 cm. dry glass test tubes at 37°C. After 3 minutes the tubes are tilted every 30 seconds. The clotting–time end point is determined by the average time it takes until the tubes can be inverted without the blood spilling out. The normal clotting time is 4 to 10 minutes.

Prothrombin Time. For this procedure it is wise to purchase a Fibrometer (Baltimore Biological Laboratories) with an automatic pipette. Thromboplastin reagent (0.2 ml.) with added calcium is placed in each of two cups and warmed at 37°C on the block for 5 minutes. Then 0.1 ml. of control plasma is pipetted into the first cup, the Fibrometer automatically drops 2 electrodes into the solution, and the timer is started. As soon as a firm clot is produced a spark jumps between the electrodes, stopping the timer. The control should be less than 15 seconds. The same procedure is repeated with 0.1 ml of the patient's plasma.

Rumpel-Leede Test. Using a sphygmomanometer the patient's blood pressure is determined, and then the cuff is inflated until the pressure is midway between the systolic and diastolic blood pressure. It is left there for 5 minutes. Then the number of petechiae are counted in a quarter-sized circle in the antecubital fossa. The normal is less than 10.

Sedimentation Rate. This is performed with Wintrobe hematocrit tubes graduated from 1 to 100 in 1 mm. divisions. Blood is drawn and placed in double oxalate test tubes. It is then transferred to the Wintrobe tube with a Wright pipette. The tube is filled to the 100 mm. mark and placed in an absolutely vertical position (either in a special rack or taped to the wall) for 1 hour. Normally the blood cells will settle up to 9 mm. in 1 hour. This must be adjusted according to the hematocrit, as the "normal" value for sedimentation rate will rise in relation to the degree of anemia.

BLOOD CHEMISTRIES

It is worth purchasing a photocolorimeter or blood chemistry system such as the Unimeter made by Biodynamics Laboratories if a physician's practice carries a large volume of diabetic patients. With the large automated laboratories available throughout the country, it is unnecessary and indeed more expensive to do other chemistries in the office. With the Unimeter, inexperienced personnel can perform several blood sugars fairly accurately in a short period of time. This saves the diabetic patient an extra visit to the office or outside laboratory, as he can have his blood sugar determined at the same time as his follow-up office visit if it is scheduled in the morning. Many physicians prefer testing their diabetic patients with a 2–hour postprandial blood sugar so the patient does not need to fast.

Some physicians test their diabetic patients with the Ames Dextrostix. A strip of paper impregnated with glucose oxidase and a color reagent is coated with a drop of blood and the color compared to a chart. Values between 40 and 130 mg./100 ml. have a deviation of ±20 to 40 mg. With more than 130 mg./100 ml., the test is less accurate. Thus the Dextrostix cannot be recommended.

Another simple "blood chemistry" that can be performed in the office is the *visual test* for classifying the types of *lipoproteinemia*. Five cc. of plasma is allowed to stand in the refrigerator overnight at 4°C. In type I a creamy layer develops with clear plasma beneath. In type II the plasma is uniformly clear with no creamy layer. In types III and IV the plasma is turbid throughout, usually with no creamy layer. In type V there is turbid plasma with a creamy layer on top. It is very important to distinguish the type of lipoproteinemia, since the treatment is different for each type.

URINALYSIS

Specific Gravity. Urine is placed in a special beaker with a microurinometer float and a reading for specific gravity can be measured. The urinometer can be checked for accuracy by testing with distilled water, which should measure 1.000. Normal urine specific gravity is 1.010 to 1.025. The specific gravity of small volumes of urine—even one drop— may be determined by a refractometer (purchased from American Optical Association).

All Other Chemistries. The pH, glucose, acetone, protein, bilirubin, and occult blood in urine can be easily checked by commercially available reagent strips (Combistix, Lab-stix, etc.). No special training is needed for this.

Microscopic Examination. Identifying red cells, white cells, casts, bacteria, and crystals in urine takes considerable experience, so this must be done by a trained laboratory technician or the doctor himself. Sternheimer-Malbin stain (Sedistain) has made identity of cells easier, but bacteria are very difficult to distinguish and must be looked for separately. The first step is to examine a drop of fresh unspun urine. If more than 2-3 WBC's or 2-3 motile bacteria are seen per h.p.f., a urinary tract infection is pretty certain. If the urine is negative on this examination, the urine is centrifuged for 5 minutes at 1500 to 2500 r.p.m. and the supernatant removed, preferably by special pipettes. The plug of material at the bottom is resuspended in what urine is left at the bottom of the tube. The Ames Microhematocrit has a special attachment to centrifuge urine which utilizes special tubes that eliminate the need for pipetting. The tube merely needs to be tipped over quickly and back again. The resuspended cells and debris are examined under the microscope and red cells, white cells, casts, etc. are easily seen. Urinary tract infection is likely if more than 10 WBC's per h.p.f. are seen in a clean–catch urine. White cell casts usually signify infection in the kidney (pyelonephritis). Glitter cells are larger than white cells and contain moving cytoplasm. They stain blue or not at all with Sedistain. They usually indicate pyelonephritis. Trichomonas organisms (page 285) can often be seen in the urine.

Fishberg Concentration Test. This is a simple but excellent screening test of renal function. It is useful in ruling out significant renal disease other than pyelonephritis before the BUN is elevated. The patient is instructed to omit all fluid after 6 PM the evening before the urine to be tested is collected. At 8 AM the next morning he empties his bladder, and specimens are collected at 9 AM., 10 AM., and 11 AM. The specific gravity of each urine is checked. To be considered normal, at least one urine has to have a specific gravity over 1.025.

STOOL

Occult Blood. Hematest tablets or Occultest pads are used. These tests are sensitive, and if positive they should be repeated after a meat–free diet for 3 days, or the test should be confirmed with the Guacacum reagent (hydrogen peroxide and guacacum resin).

Ovum and Parasites. A pea-sized portion of fresh stool is mixed well with 3 cc. of saline in a test tube, and a drop from the top layer of saline is examined microscopically for amebae and eggs of various parasites. This test takes experience but will be rewarding in isolated cases. Other laboratory texts should be consulted for a description of the ova and parasites. The Scotch tape test for pin worms is even more useful (see page 285).

Trypsin. Examining the stool for trypsin is useful in differentiating chronic pancreatitis from other causes of malabsorption and should be done on all patients with chronic diarrhea. A diluted portion of stool is placed on photographic film (x-ray or other), and if trypsin is present the gelatin coating the film will be digested away. Presence of trypsin is good evidence to rule out chronic pancreatitis, but proteolytic bacteria produce false positive results. The stool should be examined for fat also, but this can be more difficult unless a trained technician is available.

BACTERIOLOGY

Gram Stain. This is required in any primary physician's office, especially when a hospital is not near. A diagnosis of pneumococcal pneumonia can be made immediately from a Gram stain of the sputum, and a diagnosis of gonorrhea from immediate examination of the urethral or cervical discharge. A Gram–staining kit can be purchased. Then the following procedure may be used:

a. Place a small drop of mucus or sputum on a slide and smear with the wooden end of a sterile cotton applicator or sterile wire loop.
b. Fix the smear by gently warming over a Bunsen burner for a few seconds, being careful not to get the slide too hot.
c. Place the slide on a rack over the sink and cover with crystal violet for 1 minute.
d. Then wash off with Gram's iodine and leave additional iodine on for 1 minute.
e. Decolorize with alcohol for ½ to 1 minute until no more blue can be washed out.
f. Wash with tap water.
g. Counterstain with carbolfuchsin for 1 minute.
h. Rinse in water and dry.

Saline and KOH 10% Solutions are used to prepare slides of vaginal discharge to look for Trichomonas (in saline) and Monilias (in 10% KOH). See page 285 for description.

Cultures.

a. *Throat.* The back of the throat is swabbed with a sterile cotton applicator previously moistened in sterile saline, and then a blood agar plate is streaked. These plates can be purchased from Baltimore Biological Laboratories 10 at a time. After incubation at 35°C for 24-48 hours the β-hemolytic strept colonies grow with a clear zone of hemolysis around them. If bacitracin discs are placed on the blood agar further support to the diagnosis is indicated by the zone of inhibition of the growth of strept colonies around the discs.
b. *Urine cultures.* Excellent kits for culturing urine are available, such as UTI-tect (Abbott Laboratories) and Uricult (from Finland) produced by Bristol Pharmaceutical Co. These allow for colony counts and excellent differentiation of the organisms. Sensitivity tests can be made on blood agar or Endo after the organism is identified. Sterile urine should be placed in thioglycollate medium to confirm the growth on the media. There should be no difficulty in performing these tests accurately in the office.

c. *Urethral cultures.* To grow gonococci special medium called Gonocult (by Smith, Kline and French Laboratories) is now available and easy to use.

d. *Vaginal and cervical cultures.* In addition to Gonocult for females with a discharge a Monotube (also by Smith, Kline and French) can be purchased to grow *Candida albicans*.

CYTOLOGY

Vaginal smears have been a routine examination in most physicians' offices for years. Therefore they will not be discussed in detail here. Scrapings from the cervix and endocervix should be done, mucus from the posterior fornix should be aspirated and smeared on a slide, and all suspicious areas of the cervix should be biopsied unless an extensive biopsy procedure is necessary.

IMMUNOLOGICAL TESTS

Simple slide tests for infectious mononucleosis (Monosticon kit), rheumatoid arthritis (Rheumosticon kit), and pregnancy (Pregnosticon kit) can be purchased through Organon Laboratories. These are accurate and easy for a nurse or a laboratory technician to perform.

SEMEN ANALYSIS

This is a procedure that every family doctor should be able to perform, because at least 5% of married couples fail to conceive. Furthermore, a sperm count should be done monthly for 3 months after a vasectomy or until azoospermia is found. The semen must be collected in a sterile wide-mouth jar and examined within 1 hour of collection. Condoms are unsatisfactory for collection because they are powdered with a spermicidal material. A drop of semen is placed on a slide and covered with a cover glass sealed with petroleum jelly and examined for *motility* and *morphology*. In a normal sample at least 60% of the sperm are motile. Using a white–cell counting pipette, semen is drawn to the 0.5 mark, and a diluting fluid composed of 1% formalin and 3% trisodium citrate (the hospital pharmacist will mix this for you) is drawn to the 11 mark. The pipette is shaken until the fluid is homogenous. The contents of the stem are discarded, and then a Neubauer counting chamber is filled. The number of sperm in the two large ruled areas are counted, and the count is calculated by the following formula:

$$\text{sperm/ml.} = \frac{\text{N (number of sperm in 2 large squares)} \times 10}{2} \times 10 \times 1000$$

Normally 60 million sperm/ml. or more are found.

SPECIAL PROCEDURES

Spinal Tap. This can easily be performed in the office. Afterwards the patient can be transferred to the back seat of a car with a little assistance and taken home. If a number 22 spinal needle is used, the incidence of post-spinal headache can be reduced considerably. Baxter Laboratories have disposable kits with everything but sterile gloves and zephiran solution, which can be purchased separately. The pressure can be recorded. Accurate *cell counts* can be done on the fluid just as on blood (page 293); but if the fluid appears grossly clear, examination of a drop of fluid under the high–dry objective will suffice. If there are even a few cells, a count should be done. Protein can be measured by the commercially available reagent strips (Combistix, etc.). Fluid should be sent to a hospital or commercial laboratory for Wassermann and other procedures when indicated.

Synovianalysis. Joint fluid can be easily examined in the office. This procedure can be very rewarding when gout is suspected. Uric acid crystals may be hexagonal, prism–shaped, or like sheaves. Pseudogout crystals are rodlike. Regardless of the shape, the presence of crystals means further studies are in order.

Gastric Analysis. Bring the patient to the office after an overnight fast. A nurse or laboratory technician can be easily taught to pass a Levine tube. Two fasting specimens are aspirated, and 2 drops of Topfer's reagent are added to each. If the solution remains yellow, free HCl is absent. If it turns red, free HCl is present. If free HCl is absent, then Histalog 1.7 mg. per kg. is given subcutaneously, and further specimens of gastric juice are taken and checked as above. If there is no free acid after this procedure, then pernicious anemia is likely and a Schilling test (page 183) should be ordered. The presence of free acid virtually excludes pernicious anemia.

Pulmonary Function Tests. An accurate vital capacity, timed vital capacity, and maximum expiratory flow rate can be made with the Vitalor manufactured by the Scott-McKesson Company. The machine is inexpensive (less than two hundred dollars), and the directions are easy to follow. With this machine obstructive lung disease, both emphysema and bronchial asthma, may be diagnosed (prolonged timed vital capacity) and congestive heart failure suspected (reduced vital capacity). Chapter 9 should be consulted for further interpretation of these tests. Recently the Spirostat, manufactured by Marion Laboratories, Incorporated, in Kansas City, Missouri, has made the performance of these tests even simpler. In addition it can test a maximum breathing capacity. The machine is more expensive, however, than the Vitalor.

Venous Pressure and Circulation Time. When the diagnosis of congestive heart failure is suspected but not certain, this test should be performed. Baxter Laboratories of Deerfield, Illinois, puts out a disposable kit for this purpose. The arm–to–tongue circulation time can be done with 3 cc. of Decholin injected into the antecubital vein. The end point occurs when the patient gets a bitter taste on his tongue. An arm–to–tongue circulation time above 15 seconds should be repeated, but if consistent results are obtained this test is good evidence of congestive failure.

SKIN TESTS

Tuberculin tine and histoplasmin tine tests are commercially available and should be used in office practice. The technique is simple, and directions come with each kit.

MISCELLANEOUS

Vision testing can be done easily with the Titmus Vision Tester or an ordinary chart. Audiometry can be performed by a good technician using a Belltone audiometer. Nurses can also be taught to use the Shiotz tonometer.

In summary, the use of an office laboratory is convenient, less expensive than a hospital laboratory, and often less time consuming for both patient and doctor alike.

23 Following Diseases With Laboratory Tests

Laboratory tests are not used only in diagnosis. They are also essential in following the course of many diseases. In this section common disorders which require periodic laboratory tests for proper clinical management will be discussed.

Alcoholism. It is not enough to ask the alcoholic if he has been drinking. Liver function tests including SGOT, bilirubin, alkaline phosphatase, and B.S.P. should be done periodically, and frequently if cirrhosis is suspected. Blood–alcohol levels should be done when the patient appears inebriated clinically but denies drinking.

Angina Pectoris. Patients who have an anginal attack lasting more than 1 hour or one not relieved by nitroglycerin should have an ECG, SGOT, C.P.K., and L.D.H., and be hospitalized in the coronary–care unit for observation for at least 48 hours.

Aplastic Anemia. These patients require platelet and C.B.C.'s at least monthly and occasional bone marrows to evaluate their status. If symptomatic, more frequent evaluation or hospitalization is necessary.

Asthma. Yearly chest x-rays and pulmonary function tests are valuable in following these patients.

Bell's Palsy. Repeated electromyography may be valuable in following this condition.

Bronchopneumonia. If these patients are sick enough to be hospitalized, a chest x-ray, W.B.C. and differential, and 24-hour sputum analysis every other day should be done to be alert for complications such as atelectasis, lung abscess, and septicemia.

Carcinoma of the Cervix and Endometrium. After appropriate treatment, Papanicolaou smears should be done at least every 6 months, and every 3 months on the more advanced cases.

Carcinoma of the Colon. Repeat barium enema and/or sigmoidoscopy and a CEA at yearly intervals in those who are believed to be cured, but more frequently in those who may not be, or in patients with continued complications.

Carcinoma of the Lung. Sputums for Papanicolaou smears and a chest x-ray should be done every 3 months in cases where a cure is expected, but more frequently when there is no cure and radiation or chemotherapy is being used.

Carcinoma of the Pancreas. Most cases require no laboratory follow-up, but occasional liver function studies may evaluate severity of biliary obstruction or the development of liver metastasis and help the physician decide if a cholecystojejunostomy is worthwhile.

Carcinoma of the Stomach. A G.I. series and/or a gastroscopy may evaluate degree of obstruction and whether a gastrostomy or gastrojejunostomy is worthwhile to relieve obstruction.

Celiac Disease. Follow the d-xylose absorption and urine 5-HIAA every 2 weeks until normal results are obtained. Occasionally a mucosal biopsy is done in follow-up.

Cellulitis or Caruncles. If these are clearing slowly or causing systemic symptoms, blood cultures, W.B.C. and differential, and culture of the wound should be repeated frequently.

Cerebral Abscess. Repeated spinal fluid examinations at least every 3 days and brain scans at least weekly are helpful in follow-up.

Cerebral Embolism. If initial spinal fluid was bloody, a repeat tap to be sure it is clean should be done before discharge.

Cerebral Hemorrhage. (see Embolism).

Cholecystitis. If surgery is to be delayed until the inflammation is cooled down, daily W.B.C. and differentials, serum bilirubin, SGOT, alkaline phosphatase, and serum amylases should be done until all are normal on at least 2 successive occasions. To follow these cases without laboratory data is a mistake. Also, if a Levine tube is down, daily electrolytes and a BUN should be done.

Cholelithiasis. Patients with asymptomatic cholelithiasis who wish to delay surgery should have yearly cholecystograms and liver function tests to detect a nonfunctioning gall bladder or asymptomatic common duct stone.

Cirrhosis of the Liver. During the acute stage bilirubin, SGOT, albumin and globulin, C.B.C., alkaline phosphatase, and prothrombin time should be done at least every 2 days. A severe drop in albumin carries a bad prognosis. If there is hepatic coma, blood ammonia and electrolytes should be done daily. A thorough search for gastrointestinal bleeding is in order. If there is ascites, serum electrolytes, BUN, albumin, globulin, and other liver function tests may be needed monthly or more often.

Dehydration. Blood volume, BUN, and electrolytes should be done daily and maybe more frequently in diabetics and children.

Diabetes Mellitus. During *diabetic coma* or *acidosis* blood sugars, electrolytes, and plasma acetone are done at least every 2 hours. Blood pH, blood volume, and urinalysis should probably be done just as frequently, especially if there is an associated congestive heart failure, emphysema, or uremia.

The average *maturity onset diabetic* can be followed with blood sugars and urinalysis (for renal infection or glomerulosclerosis) at monthly intervals. If he is on no drugs this perhaps could be done every 2 or 3 months. *Juvenile diabetics* need monthly blood sugars and urinalysis at least, and must check their urine for sugar and acetone daily.

Emphysema. During intermittent positive pressure therapy for *CO_2 narcosis* frequent arterial blood gases and serum electrolytes and pH are a must. This may be necessary as often as every hour. The patient may go into respiratory alkalosis from too much IPPB, and this is just as dangerous as respiratory acidosis at times. During episodes of respiratory infection and right heart failure, pulmonary function tests, chest x-rays, and arterial blood gases should be done every 2-3 days to follow the course. In the outpatient department it may be wise to do pulmonary function tests at least yearly, and sometimes as often as every 3 months, while regulating therapy.

Epilepsy. An EEG every 2 years is commonly done in follow-up, but when adjusting medication it may be necessary monthly.

Erythroblastosis Fetalis. Serum bilirubin and CBC should be done 2-3 times a day on both diagnosed and suspicious cases of this disease so that one knows if exchange transfusion is necessary. A bilirubin above 20 mg./100 ml. in a mature infant and 15 mg./100 ml. in a premature infant or a hemoglobin below 13 gm./100 ml. is an indication for exchange transfusion.

Esophagitis. In asymptomatic cases an upper G.I. series and/or esophagoscopy should be done 3 months after the acute episode to evaluate therapy.

Glomerulonephritis. During the acute stage daily BUN's, creatinines, electrolytes, and urinalysis should be done to evaluate therapy. All patients should be on intake and output. Once diuresis has occurred (usually 7-14 days after onset) this may be reduced to every 2-3 days. After discharge biweekly or monthly evaluations of the BUN, urine, and even creatinine clearance should be done for at least 1 year. Although clinical recovery occurs in 90 per cent or more of these cases within 6 months, it is uncertain if complete recovery ever occurs. Clinical relapses may occur during the first year, especially during recurrent nonspecific respiratory infections.

Gonorrhea. Since there are so many resistant strains, women—and possibly men—who have a persistent light discharge should be recultured after treatment.

Gout. Serum uric acid should be done at monthly intervals in severe cases and at least every 6 months to a year in asymptomatic cases.

Hamman-Rich Syndrome. Chest x-ray, pulmonary function studies, and arterial blood gases should be performed at least every 3-4 months.

Heart Failure. During the acute stage—especially when treating with digitalis and diuretics—serum electrolytes, BUN, and ECG's should be done daily. All patients should be on intake and output. Central venous pressure should be monitored in very severe cases with associated renal disease and/or shock. Digitalis blood levels should be done when available. In outpatient follow-ups on asymptomatic cases a vital capacity and ECG might be helpful every 3-6 months. Chest x-rays should probably be done yearly.

Hemolytic Anemias. A monthly CBC and serum bilirubin should be done on all but the very mild cases. During a crisis these studies should be done as often as 2-3 times a day.

Hepatitis. Serum bilirubin, transaminase, and urine urobilinogen should be done every 2-4 days, and the patients should not be ambulated until the bilirubin is below 2 mg./100 ml. and the transaminase is less than twice normal.

Hodgkin's Disease. Chest x-ray and C.B.C. should be done every 3 months, and a lymphangiogram and scan of liver, spleen, or bone should be done whenever recurrence in these organs is suggested.

Hyperparathyroidism. Following surgery these patients need serum calcium and phosphorus as much as 3-4 times a day to detect tetany early.

Hypertension, Essential. Each time these patients visit the office they should have a urinalysis for protein and specific gravity (preferably a morning specimen), and an ECG should be done yearly to detect left ventricular hypertrophy and other cardiac complications.

Hyperthyroidism. Performing free thyroxines or T_4 by column every 2 weeks, and later monthly, is good sense for patients on antithyroid drugs or who have had radioactive iodine therapy. Some will have persistent elevations and require retreatment or surgery, and others may have low levels and require thyroid extract. Weekly WBC and differentials should be done on patients in the initial stage of treatment with antithyroid drugs. Later, monthly intervals are sufficient. After a thyroidectomy the above studies should be done daily. In addition serum calcium and phosphorus should be done 3-4 times a day for the first 2-3 days.

Hypothyroidism. Serum cholesterol, T_4 or TSH, and a photomotograph can be done monthly and later semiannually to keep the thyroxine in a therapeutic range.

Infectious Mononucleosis. The smear for atypical lymphocytes and serum transaminase should be repeated at monthly intervals to be sure they are normal before the patient resumes vigorous activity.

Iron-deficiency Anemia. Do a monthly CBC and blood smear until a good response is obtained. Initially a reticulocyte count can be done to evaluate immediate response to therapy.

Leukemia. Whether chronic or acute, these cases should be monitored with a CBC, differential, and platelet count at least monthly. In acute stages this is necessary daily until chemotherapy is definitely working. Bone marrows must be done frequently also.

Malabsorption Syndrome. (see Celiac Disease.)

Malaria. CBC and blood smears, both thick and thin, should be repeated daily until good therapeutic response is obtained.

Meniere's Disease. It is wise to do audiograms at 6–month intervals to evaluate therapy and prognosis.

Meningitis. In severe cases, especially with associated coma, spinal fluid examination should be done daily to evaluate therapy. If the patient is on intravenous therapy, daily electrolytes, BUN, and intake and output evaluation are needed.

Myasthenia Gravis. During a crisis a test-dose of Tensilon may have to be administered before each dose of prostigmine or other drugs.

Myocardial Infarction. Once diagnosis is established an ECG, SLDH, and SGOT may be ordered every 3-4 days to pick up an extension of the infarction or other complications (congestive heart failure, etc.). Other tests may be warranted if the clinical picture changes. After discharge from the hospital, it would be wise to have an electrocardiogram at every visit for 3-4 months and then every 6 months to a year. Prothrombin times should be done monthly, at least on all patients who are on anticoagulant therapy.

Nephritis. (see Glomerulonephritis or Pyelonephritis.)

Nephrotic Syndrome. In addition to the follow-up tests listed under Glomerulonephritis, these patients need frequent checks of their serum albumin and electrolytes to evaluate diuretic therapy.

Pancreatitis. Daily serum amylases, electrolytes, glucose, calcium, liver function tests, and BUN's would be valuable during the acute phase. In chronic pancreatitis an occasional serum amylase and lipase and screening for malabsorption may be beneficial.

Peptic Ulcer. It is wise to repeat the G.I. series and /or gastroscopy at 3 weeks, and again in 6 weeks, to be sure healing is taking place. During severe gastrointestinal bleeding a hemoglobin and hematocrit and BUN may have to be done every 2 hours. Electrolytes and blood volume may have to be done frequently, also.

Pernicious Anemia. Monthly CBC and blood smear are done during the initial stages of therapy, and later semiannually.

Phlebitis. (see Thrombophlebitis.)

Pneumoconiosis. Chest x-ray and pulmonary function tests should be done yearly. Arterial blood gas studies may also be needed at regular intervals.

Pneumothorax. Initially chest x-rays should be performed daily, and at least one or two times after discharge from the hospital and removal of the thoracotomy tube.

Polycythemia Vera. Monthly C.B.C. to evaluate need for phlebotomy or radioactive phosphorus.

Pregnancy. Follow with urinalysis at each visit. Some patients will require evaluation of blood count, Rh antibody titer, or blood sugars at each visit. During the first trimester a quantitative pregnosticon test is done if fetal death is suspected. If the pregnancy is complicated by toxemia, diabetes, or possible Rh incompatibility, frequent urinary estradiol levels should be done. A sudden drop from 12 to 6 is an indication for delivery.

Pulmonary Infarction. (see Myocardial Infarction)

Pyelonephritis. Urine cell counts and bacterial counts should be done every 3-4 days during the acute stage. A culture should be repeated after therapy is complete and again in 3 months. In chronic pyelonephritis urine cell counts and bacterial counts should be done every 2-3 months. A BUN and creatinine clearance may also be needed in follow-up.

Rheumatic Fever. A sedimentation rate at weekly intervals may be useful in following therapy. In obvious carditis ECG's may have to be done frequently.

Silicosis. (see Pneumoconiosis.)

Subacute Bacterial Endocarditis. These cases are best followed with WBC and differential and sedimentation rates every 2-3 days. With continuous intravenous therapy frequent serum electrolyte determinations and charting of intake and output should be done. Blood cultures are done weekly until negative, and 2-3 days after discontinuing therapy. In severe cases with unusual organisms blood cultures may be needed more frequently.

Subarachnoid Hemorrhage. The frequency of performing spinal taps in this condition is controversial because they may provoke more bleeding if done too frequently. If coma or delirium are felt to be due to increased intracranial pressure, they are, however, sometimes necessary. They should be done at least weekly to determine when the patient can go home or when arteriography might be safe. Of course, some do arteriography early in the course, so the latter may not be a consideration.

Syphilis. Once the ulcer is discovered and treated a serology should be done in 3 weeks, and if negative again in 6 weeks, 6 months, one year, and 2 years. If it is positive on any one of these occasions a spinal tap should be done before treatment. A quantitative Wassermann and FTA-ABS are done on the blood and spinal fluid. If positive, these are repeated 6 weeks and 6 months after retreatment. If spinal fluid Wassermann and/or FTA-ABS is positive with or without symptoms of syphilis of the nervous system, repeat spinal fluid FTA-ABS are done at least every 6 months for 4 years after treatment until FTA-ABS is found to be negative or no rising titer is seen. Even the FTA-ABS has a few false negatives and false positives.

Tapeworm Infections. Stool for ova and parasites should be done following treatment.

Thrombophlebitis. For those patients on Warfarin sodium, the prothrombin time should be done at least monthly.

Tuberculosis. On those patients who had positive smears and cultures on the sputum, these studies should be repeated weekly until negative on at least 2 occasions and this result correlates with improvement in the chest x-ray.

Ulcerative Colitis. A barium enema and sigmoidoscopy should be done at least every 2 years even on asymptomatic cases unless there is some other contraindication.

24 Multiphasic Screening of Asymptomatic Patients

In the past decade both the government and individual physicians have become increasingly concerned with preventive medicine, or keeping healthy people healthy. In this endeavor it is axiomatic to screen apparently healthy people for early disease utilizing laboratory and other diagnostic procedures. Physicians should be capable of performing these tests on outpatients as well as inpatients. It is wise to have them done at least every 2 years. Some tests should be performed every year on everyone over 40 years of age.

To qualify as a screening procedure, a test should meet the following criteria:

1. It should be simple to perform and inexpensive.
2. It should be an accurate procedure with very few false positives and false negatives.
3. It should not require a physician to perform it.
4. It should be as harmless and as painless as possible to the patient.
5. It should be a procedure to uncover a common or serious disease and hopefully one that is treatable.

The author has used the following battery of screening tests for his patients during the last 8 years.

Procedure for all patients:

1. SMA-12
2. Urinalysis and urine culture.
3. C.B.C.
4. Sedimentation rate
5. VDRL
6. Chest x-ray
7. Electrocardiogram and Master's two-step exercise test.
8. Pulmonary function tests
9. Tuberculin skin test
10. Tonometry
11. Audiometry
12. Vision test with eye chart
13. Sigmoidoscopy
14. Pap test (for women)

For *executives* an upper G.I. series, intravenous pyelogram, and cholecystogram are also done and repeated every 2 years.

A pediatric screen should include the following:

1. C.B.C.
2. Urinalysis, PKU, urine culture
3. Sedimentation rate
4. Throat culture
5. Vision test
6. Audiometry
7. Chest x-ray
8. Tuberculin tine test

In Negro children a sickle–cell prep should probably be done, and in children with a family history of diabetes a 2–hour postprandial blood sugar.

Obstetricians order certain tests routinely at the first prenatal visit. The following is one example of the prenatal battery:

1. Pap smear
2. Culture for gonococci
3. C.B.C.
4. Blood type
5. Two-hour postprandial blood sugar
6. Serology
7. Pregnancy test
8. Chest x-ray

CONCLUSION

The laboratory has earned a role in clinical medicine equal in importance to physical diagnosis. The value of the laboratory is underestimated by the experienced clinician who ignores laboratory terts and bases his diagnosis solely on the history and physical examination. It is overestimated by the neophyte physician who skips the history and physical examination and relegates the diagnosis to a "series of needle punctures." It is hoped that these attitudes will change.

Nevertheless, laboratory data must be interpreted with caution. It is wise to be skeptical of negative laboratory data in the face of strong clinical evidence to the contrary, and, conversely, to be skeptical of positive laboratory data in the absence of clinical findings. Repeated laboratory and physical examinations are of great value in these cases.

The laboratory must be utilized more in office practice. The continual development of simple laboratory procedures makes their use in the office both practical and enjoyable. The reward is greater because their help comes at a time when curiosity and incentive to reach the diagnosis are at their peak. Moreover, greater utilization of the office laboratory means that utilization of the hospital can be reduced at a time when Medicare is packing hospitals to capacity.

The laboratory must also be used more in hospital practice. The development of the Autoanalyzer has made it more practical to include a blood sugar, urea nitrogen, cholesterol, uric acid, and other tests as routine on all admissions.

This book has emphasized the stepwise process involved in the metabolism of each of the blood chemistries or elements. Interruption or change in each of these steps leads to a particular disease and a characteristic alteration in the blood chemistry or elements. As the metabolism is better elucidated, more and more tests will be developed to diagnose various disease states. The tests covered in this book are only the beginning.

Appendix I Normal Values

NOTE: The normal values will vary from one laboratory to another. The clinician should acquaint himself with the normal values of the laboratory that he uses.

Test	Normal value
Acetone, blood	0.3-2.0 mg./100 ml.
urine	Negative
Acidity, blood (pH)	7.35-7.45
gastric juice, free hydrochloric acid	25-50 degrees
urine (pH)	5.5-7.5
Acid phosphatase, serum	0.2-0.8 units per 100 ml. (Bodansky) 1-4 units per 100 ml. (King-Armstrong)
Albumin, serum	4.0-5.2 gm. per 100 ml.
urine	Negative
Aldosterone, 24-hour, urine	4-8 mcg. per 24 hours
Alkaline phosphatase, serum	1-4 units per 100 ml. (Bodansky) 8-14 units per 100 ml. (King-Armstrong)
Alpha amino nitrogen	64-199 mg./day
Ammonia, blood	0.7-2.0 mcg. per 100 ml.
urine	0.5-1.0 gm. per 24 hours
Amylase, serum	80-150 Somogyi units per 100 ml.
urine	2,200-3,000 Somogyi units per 24 hours
Bilirubin, serum, direct	0.1-0.2 mg. per 100 ml.
indirect	0.1-0.6 mg. per 100 ml.
urine	Negative
Bleeding time (Duke method)	1-5 minutes
Blood volume	Males: 69 ml. per kilogram of body weight Females: 64 ml. per kilogram of body weight
Breathing capacity, maximum	Adult males: 58-169 l. per minute, depending on age and size
Bromsulfalein excretion	Not more than 5 per cent of dye remaining at 45 minutes
Calcium, serum,	9-11 mg. per 100 ml. (4.5-5.5 mEq. per liter)
urine	100-150 mg. per 24 hours
Capillary fragility	less than 10 new petechiae in circle of 2.5 cm. diameter
Carbon dioxide, partial pressure of,	
arterial blood	40 mm. Hg
venous blood	46 mm. Hg
Carbon dioxide combining power	50-65 volumes per cent (21-28 mEq. per liter)
Carotene, serum	70-250 mcg. per 100 ml.
Catecholamines, urinary	20-40 gamma in 24 hours
Cephalin flocculation	2^+ or less in 48 hours
Chloride, cerebrospinal fluid	700-750 mg. per 100 ml. (120-130 mEq/l.)
serum	350-375 mg. per 100 ml. (100-106 mEq. per liter)
urine	119 mEq. per 24 hours
Cholesterol, total	150-250 mg. per 100 ml.
esters	68-76 per cent (of total cholesterol)
Clot retraction time	begins 30-120 minutes, complete in 24 hours
Coagulation time	5-12 minutes
Colloidal gold, spinal fluid	0000000000 to 1110000000
Complement, serum	101 to 189 mg./100 ml.
Copper, plasma	65-165 mcg. per 100 ml.
Creatine, blood	2-7 mg. per 100 ml.
urine	less than 100 mg. per 24 hours
Creatine phosphokinase (CPK)	0-4 units
Creatinine, serum	1-2 mg. per 100 ml.
urine	Adult males: 1.5-2.0 gm., per 24 hours Adult females: 0.8-1.5 gm. per 24 hours
D-xylose absorption test	6.5 ± 1.2 gm. in 5 hours
Electrolytes	*See specific electrolytes,* Sodium, etc.
Erythrocytes, blood	Males: 4.5-5.5 million cells per cubic millimeter Females: 4.2-5.2 million cells per cubic millimeter
cerebrospinal fluid	0
urine	less than 500,000 cells per 24 hours
Ethanol	0.3-0.4 per cent or above = marked intoxication
Fat, stool	7-27%
Follicle-stimulating hormone (FSH)	*See* Human pituitary gonadotropin
Fragility, capillary	*See* Capillary fragility
red cell	*See* Osmotic fragility

Test	Normal value
Globulin, total	2.0-3.9 gm. per 100 ml.
Glucose, blood	70-120 mg. per 100 ml. (fasting) (Folin-Wu)
cerebrospinal fluid	50-75 mg. per 100 ml.
urine	0.5-0.75 gm. per 24 hours
Glucose tolerance test, intravenous	Maximum rise: 180 mg. per 100 ml. Return to normal: 150 minutes
Hematocrit	Males: 40-54 per cent Females: 42 ± 5 per cent
Hemoglobin	Males: 14-17 gm. per 100 ml. Females: 12-15 gm. per 100 ml.
Human pituitary gonadotropin (HPG)	Males: 5-30 mouse units per 24 hours Females: 5-100 mouse units per 24 hours
5-Hydroxyindoleacetic acid (5-HIAA), urine	2-8 mg. per 24 hours
17-Hydroxysteroids, urine	5-15 mg. per 24 hours
Iodine, protein-bound	*See* Protein-bound iodine
Iron, serum	Adult males: 75-175 mcg. per 100 ml. Adult females: 60-150 mcg./100 ml.
Iron-binding capacity, serum	150-300 mcg. per 100 ml.
17-Ketosteroids, urine	Males: 8-20 mg. per 24 hours Females: 6-15 mg. per 24 hours
Lactic dehydrogenase, serum	50-400 units per 100 ml.
Leukocyte count	Adults: 5,000-10,000 cells per cubic millimeter
pleural and peritoneal fluids	up to 5,000 cells per cu. mm.
spinal fluid	less than 5 per cu. mm.
synovial fluid	50-200 per cu. mm., most being neutrophils
urine, 24-hour	1 to 2 million
Lipase, serum	0.2-1.5 Cherry-Crandall units/ml.
Magnesium, serum	1.5-2.5 mEq. per liter
Mean corpuscular hemoglobin (MCH)	27-32 micromicrograms
Mean corpuscular hemoglobin concentration (MCHC)	32-36 per cent
Mean corpuscular volume (MCV)	82-92 cubic microns
Nonprotein nitrogen, blood (NPN)	15-35 mg. per 100 ml.
Occult blood, stool	Negative
Osmotic fragility, red cells	0.45-0.39 per cent of NaCl (beginning of hemolysis)
Oxygen saturation, arterial blood	95 per cent or above
pH	7.35-7.45
Phosphate, inorganic, plasma	Adults: 3-4.5 mg. per cent Children: 4.5-6.5 mg. per cent
Phospholipids, serum	230-300 mg. per 100 ml.
Phosphorus, serum	Adults: 3-4.5 mg. per 100 ml. Children: 4-6.5 mg. per 100 ml.
Platelet count	140,000-340,000 per cubic millimeter
Porphobilinogen, urine	Negative
Potassium, serum	3.5-5.0 mEq. per liter
urine	25-100 mEq. per 24 hours
Protein-bound iodine (PBI)	4-8 mcg. per 100 ml.
Prothrombin consumption time	Over 80 per cent consumed in 1 hour
Prothrombin time	11-14 seconds, but depends on control
Radioactive iodine uptake	10-40 per cent
Reticulocyte count	Adults: 0.5-1.5 per cent Newborn: 2-4.8 per cent
Sedimentation rate of erythrocytes, Westergren	Males: 1-13 mm. per hour Females: 4-17 mm. per hour
Sodium, serum	135-147 mEq. per liter
urine	111 mEq. per 24 hours
Thrombocytes	*See* Platelets
Thymol turbidity	0-5 units
Transaminase (SGOT), serum	5-40 Karmen units per 100 ml.
Transaminase SGPT), serum	10-50 units per ml.
Transferrin, serum	*See* Iron-binding capacity, serum
Triglycerides, serum	0-150 mg. per 100 ml.
Urea nitrogen, blood (BUN)	8-25 mg. per 100 ml.
urine	20-35 gm. per 24 hours
Uric acid, serum	3-6 mg. per 100 ml.
Urobilinogen, stool	50-300 mg. per 24 hours
Urine	0-4 mg. per 24 hours
Vanillyl mandelic acid (VMA) urine	less than 10 mg. per 24 hours
Vital capacity	Males: 3-5 liters (average) Females: 2.5-4 liters (average)

Appendix II Laboratory Work-up of Symptoms*

Routine Orders

1. CBC
2. Urinalysis
3. Sedimentation rate
4. SMA-12
5. Wassermann
6. ECG (for patients over 40)
7. Chest x-ray and flat plate of abdomen
8. PPD, intermediate

Abdominal Pain

Routine Orders plus

A. Laboratory

1. Amylase
2. Lipase
3. 2-hour postprandial blood sugar
4. Transaminase series
5. LDH (lactic dehydrogenase) series
6. Urine culture and sensitivity
7. Save all urine and examine for stones
8. Vaginal culture (pelvic inflammatory disease)
9. Stool culture
10. Liver function studies
11. Uric acid
12. Calcium, phosphates, alkaline phosphatase (renal calculus)
13. Pregnancy test (ruptured ectopic pregnancy)
14. Blood lead level
15. Urine porphobilinogen
16. Wassermann
17. Stool for occult blood
18. Stool for ova and parasites
19. Gastric analysis
20. Spinal tap (spinal cord tumor)
21. Serum protein electrophoresis

B. X-ray

1. Flat plate, upright and lateral decubiti of abdomen
2. Cholecystogram or cholangiogram
3. Intravenous pyelogram
4. Upper G.I. series
5. Barium enema
6. Small bowel series
7. X-ray of lumbosacral spine
8. Myelogram
9. Aortography (dissecting aneurysm)
10. Liver scan

C. Special diagnostic procedures

1. Esophagoscopy
2. Gastroscopy
3. Sigmoidoscopy
4. Cystoscopy
5. Culdoscopy
6. Peritoneoscopy
7. ECG and Master's two-step test
8. 0.1 normal HCl drip (peptic esophagitis)
9. Catheterize for residual urine
10. Peritoneal tap
11. Lymph node biopsy (Hodgkin's disease)
12. Double enema (intestinal obstruction)
13. Exploratory laparotomy

* It is expected that the clinician has the necessary clinical judgment to know when each of these tests is indicated. Routine orders are selected.

Anemia

Routine Orders plus

A. Laboratory

1. Red cell count, indices
2. Reticulocyte count
3. Wright's stain of peripheral blood for cell morphology
4. Serum iron and iron-binding capacity
5. Gastric analysis
6. Stools for occult blood and chromium-tagged red cells
7. Stools for ova and parasites
8. Serum bilirubin
9. Urine and fecal urobilinogen
10. Blood cell fragility
11. Coombs' test
12. Radioactive chromium-tagged red cell survival
13. Ham's test
14. Sickle cell preparation
15. Platelet count
16. Repeated WBC and differential and smears for atypical cells
17. Blood lead level
18. Plasma hemoglobin, haptoglobin, and methemalbumin
19. Coagulation studies (see Purpura, this table)
20. Hemoglobin electrophoresis
21. Donath-Landsteiner test
22. PBI, T_4
23. Urine 17-ketosteroids and 17-hydroxysteroids
24. Serum protein electrophoresis
25. L.E. preparations
26. Blood smear for parasites
27. Blood cultures
28. Febrile agglutinins
29. Urine formiminoglutamic acid
30. Serum carotene, D-xylose absorption
31. Serum B_{12} assay

B. X-ray

1. Skull and long bones
2. Upper G.I. series
3. Barium enema

C. Special diagnostic procedures

1. Sigmoidoscopy
2. Esophagoscopy
3. Gastroscopy
4. Bone marrow aspiration or biopsy
5. Lymph node biopsy
6. Liver biopsy

Back Pain

A. Laboratory

1. CBC
2. Urine
3. Urine for Bence-Jones protein
4. Serum protein electrophoresis (multiple myeloma)
5. Calcium, phosphorus, alkaline phosphatase (metastatic carcinoma)
6. Sedimentation rate
7. Latex flocculation (rheumatoid spondylitis)
8. Serum amylase and lipase
9. Urine culture and sensitivity
10. Acid phosphatase
11. Spinal fluid examination and culture
12. Wassermann

B. X-ray

1. X-ray of thoracolumbar or lumbosacral spine
2. Chest x-ray
3. X-ray of long bones and skull
4. Myelogram
5. Barium enema
6. Intravenous pyelogram
7. Aortogram
8. Upper G.I. series
9. Gallbladder series

C. Special diagnostic procedures

1. ECG
2. Blood pressure in lower extremities (dissecting aneurysm)
3. Sigmoidoscopy
4. Cystoscopy
5. Culdoscopy
6. Nerve block
7. Procaine infiltration at site of pain
8. PPD, intermediate
9. Esophagoscopy

Convulsions

A. Laboratory
1. CBC
2. Na, K, Cl, CO_2
3. Calcium, phosphorus, alkaline phosphatase (hypoparathyroidism)
4. BUN
5. Blood lead level
6. Blood bromide level
7. Glucose tolerance test (islet cell adenoma)
8. 36-hour fast (islet cell adenoma)
9. Urine porphobilinogen
10. Warm stool for ova and parasites
11. Wassermann
12. Blood alcohol
13. Spinal fluid examination and culture

B. X-ray
1. Skull x-ray
2. Brain scan
3. Arteriography
4. Pneumoencephalography
5. Ventriculogram

C. Special diagnostic procedures
1. ECG
2. EEG (preferably sleep)
3. EEG with Megimide (idiopathic epilepsy)
4. Ophthalmodynamometry
5. Visual fields
6. Burr holes (subdural hematoma)
7. Echoencephalogram

Cough and Hemoptysis

Routine Orders plus

A. Laboratory
1. Sputum for routine smear and culture
2. Sputum or gastric washings for acid-fast bacilli
3. Sputum culture for fungi
4. Sputum analysis and 24-hour quantitation
5. Sputum for eosinophils
6. Sputum for Papanicolaou test
7. Nose and throat culture
8. Febrile agglutinins
9. Heterophil antibody titer
10. Histoplasma agglutinins
11. Acute and convalescent-phase sera for viral serologic studies
12. Cold agglutinins
13. MG streptococcus agglutinins
14. Sweat test

B. X-ray
1. Lateral and apical lordotic views of the chest
2. Tomograms
3. Bronchograms

C. Skin tests
1. PPD, intermediate
2. Coccidioidin
3. Blastomycin
4. Histoplasmin
5. Kveim test

D. Special diagnostic procedures
1. Bronchoscopy
2. Venous pressure and circulation time
3. Pulmonary function studies
4. Scalene node biopsy
5. Open lung biopsy
6. ECG
7. Allergic skin testing
8. Lung scan

Diarrhea

Routine Orders plus

A. Laboratory
1. Stools for routine culture
2. Stools for fungal culture
3. Stools for ova and parasites
4. Stools for occult blood
5. Stools for fat and trypsin
6. Serum carotene
7. D-xylose absorption test
8. Urine 5-HIAA (carcinoid tumor)

9. Sweat test (fibrocystic disease)
10. Gastric analysis (pernicious anemia and Zollinger-Ellison Syndrome)
11. PBI
12. Calcium, phosphorus, alkaline phosphatase (hyperparathyroidism)
13. Na, K, Cl, CO_2
14. Lactose tolerance test

B. X-ray
1. Flat plate of abdomen
2. Upper G.I. series
3. Small bowel series
4. Barium enema
5. Intravenous pyelogram

C. Special diagnostic studies
1. Sigmoidoscopy and colonoscopy
2. Response to nicotinic acid (pellagra)
3. Dietary elimination
4. Exploratory laparotomy

Dysphagia

Routine Orders plus

A. Laboratory
1. CBC, indices, Wright's stain of peripheral blood (Plummer-Vinson syndrome)
2. PBI, radioactive iodine uptake
3. Wassermann (aortic aneurysm)
4. Spinal fluid examination

B. X-ray
1. Upper G.I. series and esophagram
2. Chest x-ray
3. Aortogram
4. Tomography of mediastinum

C. Special diagnostic procedures
1. Tensilon test (myasthenia gravis)
2. Esophagoscopy
3. Gastroscopy
4. Attempt to pass Levin tube (esophageal atresia)
5. Mecholyl test (achalasia of esophagus)

Dyspnea

Routine Orders plus

A. Laboratory
1. Sputum culture and sensitivity
2. Sputum analysis (eosinophils, etc.)
3. PBI, T_4
4. CO_2-combining power
5. Arterial oxygen saturation
6. Test for methemoglobinemia
7. Urine for salicylates
8. Transaminase and LDH (lactic dehydrogenase)

B. X-ray
1. Chest x-ray
2. Bronchogram (foreign body)
3. Esophagram
4. Fluoroscopy

C. Special diagnostic procedures
1. Pulmonary function studies (emphysema, etc.)
2. Therapeutic trial of sublingual Isuprel (bronchial asthma)
3. Trial of Mercuhydrin (congestive heart failure)
4. Venous pressure and circulation time
5. ECG
6. PPD, intermediate
7. Bronchoscopy (foreign body)

Edema

A. Laboratory
1. CBC and urine
2. Sedimentation rate
3. Na, K, Cl, CO_2
4. Serum protein and albumin/globulin ratio
5. 24-hour urine protein and serum cholesterol
6. Addis count (nephritis)
7. Liver function tests (see Jaundice, this table)
8. Blood volume (congestive heart failure)
9. Stools for ova and parasites (*Taenia solium, etc.*)
10. PBI (myxedema)
11. Eosinophil count (trichinosis)
12. 24-hour urine 17-ketosteroids and 17-hydroxysteroids
13. Renal function tests

B. X-ray
1. Chest x-ray
2. Flat plate of abdomen (ovarian tumor)
3. X-ray of long bones (metastatic carcinoma)

C. Special diagnostic procedures
1. Venous pressure and circulation time
2. Muscle biopsy (trichinosis, etc.)
3. Lymph node biopsy (Hodgkin's disease)
4. Lymphangiogram
5. Liver scan

Epistaxis

Routine Orders plus

A. Laboratory
1. CBC
2. Prothrombin time
3. Partial thromboplastin time
4. Bleeding time
5. Platelet count
6. Rumpel-Leede test
7. Nasal smear for eosinophils (allergic rhinitis, asthma)
8. Liver function tests (cirrhosis)
9. ASO titer

B. X-ray
1. X-ray for paranasal sinuses

C. Special diagnostic procedures
1. Nasopharyngoscopy
2. Pulmonary function tests
3. Venous pressure and circulation time

Fatigue

A. Laboratory
1. Routine orders
2. Sedimentation rate
3. PPD, intermediate
4. Na, K, Cl, CO_2
5. 36-hour fast (hypoglycemia)
6. PBI, T_4, and RAI
7. 24-hour urine 17-ketosteroids and 17-hydroxysteroids
8. 24-hour urine aldosterone
9. Liver function tests (*see* Jaundice, this table)
10. Febrile agglutinins
11. Brucellin antibody titer
12. Heterophil antibody titer
13. L.E. preparations and ANA test
14. Calcium, phosphorus, alkaline phosphatase

B. X-ray
1. Skull and long bones (metastatic carcinoma)

C. Special diagnostic procedures
1. Response to vitamins and corrective diet
2. Exploratory laparotomy
3. Psychometric tests
4. Lymph node biopsy
5. Tensilon test

Fever of Unknown Origin

Routine Orders plus

A. Laboratory
1. Nose and throat culture
2. Routine sputum culture
3. Sputum for acid-fast bacilli smear and culture (or gastric washings)
4. Urine cultures
5. Blood cultures
6. Bone marrow smear and culture
7. Stool for ova and parasites
8. Blood smear for parasites and spirochetes
9. Febrile agglutinins
10. Heterophil antibody titer
11. ASO titer
12. Brucellin antibody titer
13. Cold agglutinins
14. Latex flocculation
15. L.E. preparations and ANA test
16. Serum protein electrophoresis
17. Acute and convalescent-phase sera for viral studies
18. Sickle cell preparation
19. Urine for porphobilinogen
20. Cerebrospinal fluid examination and culture
21. Liver function tests (*see* Jaundice, this table)
22. Urine for etiocholanolone

23. Fibrindex (Mediterranean fever)
24. Nitroblue tetrazolium (NBT) test (for chronic granulomas)

B. X-ray
1. Chest x-ray
2. Flat plate of abdomen
3. Upper G.I. series
4. Intravenous pyelogram (hypernephroma)
5. X-ray of long bones (metastatic carcinoma)
6. X-ray of teeth
7. X-ray of hands (sarcoidosis)

C. Special diagnostic procedures
1. PPD, intermediate
2. Histoplasmin skin test
3. Coccidioidin skin test
4. Blastomycin skin test
5. *Trichinella* skin test
6. Brucellergen skin test
7. Frei test
8. ECG (rheumatic fever)
9. Lymph node biopsy
10. Kveim test
11. Liver biopsy
12. Muscle biopsy
13. Exploratory laparotomy

Headache

Routine Orders plus

A. Laboratory
1. Wassermann
2. Spinal fluid examination and culture
3. Febrile agglutinins
4. CRP (C-reactive protein)
5. Nose and throat culture
6. 24-hour urine catecholamines

B. X-ray
1. Skull x-ray
2. X-ray of paranasal sinuses and mastoids
3. X-ray of teeth
4. X-ray of cervical spine
5. Angiography
6. Pneumoencephalography

C. Special diagnostic procedures
1. EEG
2. Histamine provocative test (migraine and histamine cephalgia)
3. Therapeutic trial of ergotamine
4. Visual fields (pituitary tumor)
5. Audiogram and caloric testing (acoustic neuroma)
6. Tonometry
7. Irrigation of sinuses
8. Brain scan
9. Allergic skin tests
10. Block of cervical nerves
11. Block of trigeminal nerve
12. Block of nerve roots of various teeth
13. Elimination diet

Hematemesis and Melena

Routine Orders plus

A. Laboratory
1. Stools for occult blood
2. Gastric analysis
3. Prothrombin time
4. Coagulation time and partial thromboplastin time
5. Platelet count
6. Bleeding time
7. BSP and other liver function test (*see* Jaundice, this table)

B. X-ray
1. Upper G.I. series and esophagram
2. Barium enema
3. Small intestinal series
4. Arteriography
5. Liver scan

C. Special diagnostic procedures
1. Sigmoidoscopy and colonoscopy
2. Esophagoscopy
3. Gastroscopy
4. Levin tube to see whether blood is coming from stomach
5. Fluorescein dye string test
6. Exploratory laparotomy and liver biopsy

Hematuria and Pyuria

Routine Orders plus

A. Laboratory

1. Repeated urinalysis
2. BUN
3. Uric acid
4. Calcium, phosphorus, alkaline phosphatase
5. Urine culture and sensitivity
6. Urine for acid-fast bacilli smear and culture
7. Serum complement
8. ASO titer
9. Addis count
10. 24-hour urine protein
11. Fishberg concentration test
12. Blood cultures
13. Blood smear for malarial parasites
14. Plasma hemoglobin and methemalbumin
15. Red cell fragility test, reticulocyte count, and serum bilirubin
16. Coombs' test
17. Prothrombin time (liver disease)
18. Coagulation time (hemophilia)
19. Bleeding time
20. Platelet count
21. L.E. preparations
22. Nose and throat culture (glomerulonephritis)
23. Urine myoglobin

B. X-ray

1. Flat plate of abdomen
2. Intravenous pyelogram
3. Retrograde pyelogram
4. X-rays of long bones (metastatic carcinoma)
5. Aortogram (embolism)
6. Renal scan

C. Special diagnostic procedures

1. Catheterize for residual urine
2. Cystoscopy
3. Three-glass test
4. Muscle biopsy (periarteritis nodosa)
5. PPD, intermediate
6. Renal biopsy
7. Exploration of kidney

Hypertension

Routine Orders plus

A. Laboratory

1. Blood electrolytes
2. Total eosinophil count
3. 12-hour Addis count
4. Fishberg concentration test
5. 24-hour urine protein
6. 24-hour urine potassium
7. 24-hour urine catecholamines
8. 24-hour urine aldosterone and plasma renin
9. 24-hour urine 17-ketosteroids and 17-hydroxysteroids
10. Urine culture
11. Morning urines for acid-fast bacilli smear and culture

B. X-ray

1. Intravenous pyelogram with 1-, 2-, 3-minute shots
2. Retrograde pyelogram
3. Renal scan
4. Renal angiography
5. Perirenal air insufflation

C. Special diagnostic studies

1. Direct recording of arterial pressure
2. Differential sodium excretion test
3. Histamine or Regitine test
4. Renal biopsy
5. Exploratory laparotomy
6. Angiotensin infusion test

Jaundice

Routine Orders plus

A. Laboratory

1. Transaminase
2. Thymol turbidity
3. Serum bilirubin
4. Urine bilirubin and urobilinogen
5. Stool for urobilinogen

6. Alkaline phosphatase
7. Total cholesterol and esters
8. Total protein and albumin/globulin ratio
9. Prothrombin time
10. Reticulocyte count and red cell fragility
11. Coombs' test
12. Blood ammonia level
13. BUN
14. Serum amylase and lipase
15. Stool for occult blood and parasites
16. Heterophil antibody titer
17. Eosinophil count (chlorpromazine sensitivity)
18. Febrile agglutinins
19. Brucellin antibody titer
20. Guinea pig inoculation of blood (Weil's disease)
21. Blood smear for parasites
22. Blood culture
23. HAA
24. CEA

B. X-ray

1. Flat plate of abdomen
2. Cholecystogram or cholangiogram after jaundice is subsiding
3. Upper G.I. series
4. Barium enema
5. Lymphangiogram

C. Special diagnostic procedures

1. Liver biopsy
2. Rectal biopsy
3. Sigmoidoscopy and colonoscopy
4. Gastroscopy
5. Lymph node biopsy
6. Occupational history
7. Duodenal analysis
8. Exploratory laparotomy
9. Peritoneoscopy

Joint Pain or Swelling

Routine Orders plus

A. Laboratory

1. Sedimentation rate
2. ASO titer
3. CRP (C-reactive protein)
4. Latex flocculation
5. Blood Blood cultures
6. Vaginal and/or urethral smears and cultures for gonococci
7. Sickle cell preparation
8. L.E. preparations and ANA
9. Blood uric acid
10. Febrile agglutinins
11. Heterophil antibody titer
12. Brucellin antibody titer
13. Eosinophil count (trichinosis, periarteritis)
14. Synovianalysis (for mucin clot, cell count, uric acid crystals, etc.)
15. Synovial fluid culture and sensitivity (for bacteria, fungi, and spirochetes)
16. Coagulation time (hemophilia)
17. Serum protein electrophoresis

B. X-ray

1. Chest x-ray
2. X-ray of joint involved
3. X-ray of additional joints
4. Lymphangiogram
5. Arthrogram

C. Special diagnostic procedures

1. Synovial biopsy
2. ECG (rheumatic fever)
3. Muscle biopsy (periarteritis nodosa)
4. Therapeutic trial with colchicine
5. Therapeutic trial with salicylates

Lymphadenopathy

A. Laboratory

1. CBC
2. Sedimentation rate
3. Nose and throat culture
4. Sputum for acid-fast bacilli smear and culture
5. Blood cultures
6. Heterophil antibody titer
7. Brucellin antibody titer
8. Febrile agglutinins

9. Wassermann
10. Bone marrow examination
11. Nitroblue tetrazolium (NBT) test (for chronic granulomas)

B. X-ray

1. Chest x-ray
2. X-ray of long bones (metastatic carcinoma)
3. X-ray of hands (sarcoidosis)
4. Lymphangiogram

C. Special diagnostic procedures

1. Lymph node biopsy
2. PPD, intermediate
3. Skin tests for fungi (histoplasmosis, etc.)
4. Brucellergen skin test
5. Kveim test

Neck Pain

A. Laboratory

1. CBC
2. Sedimentation rate
3. Calcium, phosphorus, alkaline phosphatase (metastatic carcinoma)
4. Serum protein electrophoresis (multiple myeloma)
5. Acid phosphatase
6. Bone marrow examination
7. Wassermann
8. Spinal fluid examination

B. X-ray

1. X-ray of cervical spine
2. Chest x-ray
3. Skull x-ray with special views of foramen magnum
4. X-ray of long bones
5. Myelogram

C. Special diagnostic procedures

1. PPD, intermediate
2. Nerve block
3. EMG

Purpura

A. Laboratory

1. CBC
2. Sedimentation rate
3. Coagulation time and partial thromboplastin time
4. Bleeding time
5. Prothrombin time
6. Platelet count
7. Rumpel-Leede test
8. Thromboplastin generation test
9. Bone marrow examination
10. L.E. preparations and ANA test
11. Blood cultures
12. Coombs' test
13. Heterophil antibody titer
14. Cold agglutinins

B. X-ray

1. Chest x-ray
2. Long bones
3. Flat plate of abdomen for size of spleen

C. Special diagnostic procedures

1. Response to corticosteroids
2. Skin biopsy (Ehlers-Danlos syndrome)
3. Muscle biopsy

Splenomegaly

A. Laboratory

1. CBC
2. Wright's stain of peripheral blood
3. Reticulocyte count
4. Platelet count and clot retraction
5. Radioactive chromium-tagged red cell survival
6. Serum bilirubin
7. Bone marrow examination
8. Blood cultures
9. Febrile agglutinins
10. Heterophil antibody titer
11. Brucellin agglutinins
12. Blood smear for parasites
13. Liver function studies (*see* Jaundice, this table)
14. Latex flocculation (Felty's disease)
14. Latex flocculation (Felty's disease)
15. L.E. preparations and ANA test
16. Serum protein electrophoresis

17. Hemoglobin electrophoresis

B. X-ray

1. Esophagram (esophageal varices)
2. X-ray of long bones (Gaucher's disease)
3. Flat plate of abdomen for spleen size

C. Special diagnostic procedures

1. Lymph node biopsy
2. Liver biopsy
3. Splenic aspirate
4. Splenoportogram and splenic pulp pressure
5. PPD, intermediate, and skin tests for various fungi (*see* Cough and Hemoptysis, this table)
6. Skin biopsy (hemochromatosis)
7. Muscle biopsy

Syncope and Coma

A. Laboratory

1. CBC
2. Urine
3. Sedimentation rate
4. FBS
5. BUN
6. Wassermann
7. Plasma acetone (diabetes mellitus)
8. Na, K, Cl, CO_2 (emphysema, diabetes mellitus, Addison's disease)
9. Blood bromide level
10. Blood lead level
11. Urine for barbiturates
12. Urine porphobilinogens
13. Blood alcohol
14. Serum pyruvic acid (beriberi)
15. Blood cultures (subacute bacterial endocarditis)
16. PBI and T_4 (hypothyroidism)
17. Blood ammonia level
18. Spinal fluid examination and culture
19. 48–hour fast

B. X-ray

1. Skull x-ray
2. Chest x-ray
3. Arteriography
4. Brain scan
5. Ventriculogram

C. Special diagnostic studies

1. ECG
2. EEG (with carotid compression in syncope)
3. Ophthalmodynamometry
4. Visual fields
5. Caloric testing
6. Audiogram
7. Blood pressure in recumbent and erect positions
8. Carotid sinus massage
9. Burr holes (subdural hematoma)
10. Echo encephalogram

Tachycardia

A. Laboratory

1. CBC
2. PBI, RAI, T_4
3. Blood cultures
4. FBS (hypoglycemia)
5. Febrile agglutinins
6. Sedimentation rate
7. ASO titer (rheumatic fever)
8. CRP (C-reactive protein)
9. 24-hour urine catecholamines
10. Na, K, Cl, CO_2
11. Blood volume
12. Arterial blood gases

C. Special diagnostic studies

1. ECG with carotid sinus massage
3. Temperature q. 4 hours
4. Sleeping pulse rate
5. Pulmonary function studies

Thoracic Pain

Routine Orders plus

A. Laboratory

1. Transaminase series
2. Lactic dehydrogenase series
3. CPK series

4. Serum amylase
5. Serum lipase
6. Wassermann (aortic aneurysm)
7. Spinal fluid examination
8. Serum bilirubin (cholecystitis)
9. L.E. preparations
10. Sickle cell preparation

B. X-ray

1. Chest x-ray, posteroanterior and laterals
2. Flat plate of abdomen
3. X-ray of cervical and thoracic spine
4. Upper G.I. series including esophagram
5. Cholecystogram
6. Fluoroscopy
7. Tomography
8. Myelography
9. Aortogram
10. Lung scan

C. Special diagnostic procedures

1. ECG
2. Master's two-step test
3. Bronchoscopy
4. Esophagoscopy
5. Gastroscopy
6. Therapeutic trial with nitroglycerin
7. Local procaine infiltration
8. Nerve block

Vertigo

A. Laboratory

1. CBC
2. FBS
3. BUN
4. Na, K, Cl, CO_2
5. Spinal fluid examination

B. X-ray

1. Chest
2. Skull x-ray
3. X-ray of mastoids and internal auditory foramen
4. X-ray of cervical spine
5. Brain scan
6. Pneumoencephalography
7. Arteriography

C. Special diagnostic procedures

1. ECG
2. EEG
3. Audiogram
4. Caloric tests
5. Ophthalmodynamometry
6. Carotid sinus massage
7. Blood pressure in recumbent and erect positions
8. Inflation of external auditory canal
9. Myringotomy

Vomiting

Routine Orders plus

A. Laboratory

1. FBS
2. Stools for occult blood
3. Stools for ova and parasites
4. Pregnancy test
5. Amylase
6. Lipase
7. Serum bilirubin (acute cholecystitis)
8. Transaminase and LDH (lactic dehydrogenase) (acute myocardial infarction)
9. Gastric analysis
10. Spinal fluid examination and culture
11. PBI
12. Calcium, phosphorus, alkaline phosphatase (hyperparathyroidism)
13. Na, K, Cl, CO_2
14. Liver function tests

B. X-ray

1. Chest x-ray
2. Flat plate of abdomen
3. Upper G.I. series and esophagram
4. Cholecystogram and/or I.V. cholangiogram
5. Intravenous pyelogram (renal calculus)

C. Special diagnostic procedures

1. Esophagoscopy

2. Gastroscopy
3. ECG
4. EEG (brain tumor, etc.)
5. Peritoneal tap
6. Culdoscopy
7. Histamine test (migraine)
8. Tonometry
9. Peritoneoscopy
10. Exploratory laparotomy

Weight Loss

Routine Orders plus

A. Laboratory

1. 2-hour postprandial blood sugar
2. Fractional urines
3. PBI, radioactive iodine uptake, and T_4
4. Calcium, phosphorus, alkaline phosphatase (hyperparathyroidism)
5. Electrolytes (Addison's disease)
6. Serum amylase and lipase
7. D-xylose uptake, radioactive triolein uptake (malabsorption syndrome)
8. Urine 5-HIAA
9. Stool for fat and trypsin
10. Stool for ova and parasites
11. Serum transaminase
12. Liver function tests (*see* Jaundice, this table)
13. Serum electrophoresis
14. Acid and alkaline phosphatase
15. Sputum for routine and acid-fast bacilli
16. Sputum for Papanicolaou test
17. Gastric analysis (carcinoma of the stomach, pernicious anemia)
18. Febrile agglutinins
19. Heterophil antibody titer
20. Brucellin antibody titer
21. Urine for Bence-Jones protein

B. X-ray

1. Chest x-ray
2. Long bone series (metastatic malignancy)
3. Upper G.I. series
4. Barium enema
5. Intravenous pyelogram
6. Lymphangiogram
7. Liver scan
8. Bone scan

C. Special diagnostic procedures

1. Sigmoidoscopy
2. Gastroscopy
3. PPD, intermediate, and other skin tests
4. Liver biopsy
5. Bone marrow aspiration
6. Lymph node biopsy
7. Exploratory laparotomy

Appendix III Laboratory Work-up of Diseases

Abortion, threatened: Urinary CGH and pregnanediol
Acoustic neuroma: skull x-ray, spinal tap, caloric test, audiogram
Acromegaly: skull x-ray, x-ray of hands, serum phosphorus, FBS, serum immunoassay of growth hormone, BMR, urine hydroxyproline
Actinomycosis: smear for sulfur granules, culture skin lesions
Addison's disease: urinary 17-hydroxycorticosteroids and 17-ketosteroids before and after ACTH, plasma cortisol, Robinson-Power-Kepler water test
Adrenogenital syndrome: urinary 17-ketosteroids and 17-hydroxycorticosteroids, ACTH test, dexamethasone suppression test, urine pregnanetriol, plasma cortisol
Agammaglobulinemia: serum electrophoresis and immunoelectrophoresis, blood type, lymph node biopsy
Agranulocytosis, idiopathic: CBC, platelet, bone marrow examination, spleen scan
Albright's syndrome: x-ray of long bones, bone biopsy
Alcaptonuria: urinary homogentisic acid, x-ray of spine
Alcoholism: liver function tests, blood alcohol, liver biopsy
Aldosteronism: serum electrolytes, 24-hour urine potassium, 24-hour urine aldosterone, plasma renin.
Alveolar proteinosis: LDH, sputum for PAS–positive material, PSP, lung biopsy.
Amebiasis: stool for ova and parasites, rectal biopsy
Amyloidosis (secondary and primary): Congo red test, rectal biopsy, liver biopsy, gingival biopsy
Angina pectoris: ECG, Master's test, nitroglycerin trial, coronary arteriography
Anthrax: smear and culture, skin biopsy
Aplastic anemia: bone marrow, lymph node biopsy, platelet count
Ascaris lumbricoides: cathartic stool for ova and parasites, eosinophil count
Asthma: sputum for eosinophils, pulmonary function tests, allergic skin testing
Atypical pneumonia (Eaton-agent pneumonia): cold agglutinins, MG streptococci agglutinins, chest x-ray, complement-fixation test
Ayerza's syndrome: pulmonary function tests, arterial oxygen saturation, cardiac catheterization

Bacillary dysentery: stool culture, febrile agglutinins
Balantidiasis: stool for trophozoites or cysts
Banti's syndrome: liver functions, bone marrow examination, spleen-liver ratio, epinephrine test
Barbiturate poisoning: blood or urine barbiturate level, EEG
Basilar artery insufficiency: brachial or vertebral arteriography
Bell's palsy: x-ray of skull and mastoids, clinical diagnosis, EMG
Beriberi: serum pyruvic acid, urine thiamine after load
Bilharziasis: stool or urine sediment for eggs
Biliary cirrhosis: liver function tests, cholesterol and phospholipids, liver biopsy
Blastomycosis: culture of pus from skin lesions (or other tissue), skin test
Boeck's sarcoid: Kveim test, x-ray of hands, scalene node biopsy, tuberculin test
Botulism: clinical diagnosis, culture of stool and food
Brain tumor: brain scan, arteriography, pneumoencephalography, EEG, skull x-ray, spinal tap
Brill-Symmer's disease: lymph node biopsy
Bromide poisoning: blood bromide level
Bronchiectasis: bronchogram, bronchoscopy, sputum culture, sweat test
Bronchitis: sputum culture, bronchoscopy, sputum analysis
Bronchopneumonia: sputum smear and culture, chest x-ray
Brucellosis: serologic tests, skin test, blood cultures

Bubonic plague: culture of bubo, blood or sputum; animal inoculation, serologic tests
Buerger's disease: biopsy of affected vessels

Carbon monoxide poisoning: carboxyhemoglobin determination
Carbon tetrachloride poisoning: liver function tests, infrared spectrometry, liver biopsy, blood carbon tetrachloride, renal function tests
Carcinoid syndrome: serum serotonin, urine 5-HIAA, exploratory laparotomy
Carcinoma of the cervix: Papanicolaou smears, cervical biopsy
Carcinoma of the colon: barium enema, sigmoidoscopy and biopsy, exploratory laparotomy, CEA
Carcinoma of the endometrium: Papanicolaou smear, D. and C.
Carcinoma of the esophagus: cytology of esophageal washings, esophagoscopy
Carcinoma of the lung: sputum for Papanicolaou test, bronchoscopy, open lung biopsy, scalene node biopsy
Carcinoma of the pancreas: duodenal drainage, liver function tests, liver biopsy, exploratory laparotomy, serum amylase, lipase, leucine aminopeptidase, pancreatic scan, CEA.
Carcinoma of the stomach: G.I. series, gastroscopy and biopsy, gastric cytology and analysis
Cat-scratch disease: skin test, lymph node biopsy
Celiac disease: D-xylose absorption, urine 5-HIAA, mucosal biopsy, small bowel series, radioactive triolein and olien uptake
Cellulitis: appraisal of clinical symptoms, smears and cultures of wound exudate
Cerebellar abscess: spinal fluid examination and culture, brain scan, pneumoencephalography, exploratory
Cerebellar ataxia: laboratory diagnosis by exclusion of other diseases
Cerebral abscess: spinal fluid examination and culture, arteriography, brain scan, pneumoencephalogram, exploratory
Cerebral aneurysm: skull x-ray, spinal tap, arteriography
Cerebral embolism: spinal tap, EEG, blood culture, arteriography
Cerebral hemorrhage: spinal tap, arteriography
Cerebral thrombosis: spinal tap, arteriography, spinal fluid GOT and LDH
Cervical spondylosis: spinal tap, x-ray of cervical spine, myelogram
Chagas' disease: blood smear and culture, smear or culture of CSF, bone marrow or tissue biopsy, animal inoculation, serologic tests
Chancroid: smear and culture of genital lesion, skin biopsy
Cholangioma: liver function tests, cholecystogram, liver biopsy, exploratory laparotomy
Cholangitis: liver function tests, liver biopsy, blood culture, WBC.
Cholecystitis: serum bilirubin, cholecystogram, BSP, alkaline phosphatase
Choledocholithiasis: liver function tests, I.V. cholangiogram, percutaneous cholangiogram
Cholelithiasis: cholecystogram, duodenal drainage for stones
Cholera: stool smear and culture
Choriocarcinoma: urine chorionic gonadotropin, D. and C.
Cirrhosis of the liver: liver function tests, liver biopsy, liver scan, BSP
Coarctation of the aorta: chest x-ray, clinical evaluation, aortograms rarely required
Congestive heart failure: ECG, chest x-ray, pulmonary function tests, blood volume
Coccidiomycosis: Culture, animal inoculation, skin tests, chest x-ray
Coronary insufficiency: ECG, Master's two-step, coronary arteriography, serum lipoproteins and lipid profile, GTT, uric acid
Costochrondritis (Tietze's syndrome): no abnormal findings
Craniopharyngioma: skull x-ray, PBI, urine 17-ketosteroids and 17-hydroxysteroids, FBS, urine HPG (human pituitary gonadotropin)
Cretinism: x-ray for bone age, PBI, T_4, RAI uptake
Crigler-Najjar syndrome: see Gilbert's disease
Cryoglobulinemia: serum protein electrophoresis and immunoelectrophoresis, SIA water test, cold agglutinins, R-A test
Cryptococcosis: spinal fluid examination, smear and culture, sputum or blood culture
Cushing's syndrome: plasma cortisol and urinary 17-ketosteroids and 17-hydroxysteroids before and after ACTH, dexamethasone suppression test
Cystic fibrosis of the pancreas: quantitative sweat test, saliva test, duodenal drainage, chest x-ray, stool for fat and trypsin
Cysticercosis: biopsy of subcutaneous cysticerci
Cystinosis: slit-lamp examination for crystals, liver biopsy
Cystinuria: serum and urine cystine and arginine
Cytomegalic inclusion disease: clinical diagnosis, urine for intraepithelial inclusion bodies

Dehydration: intake and output of fluid, blood volume, plasma sodium concentration, BUN, NPN
Dengue: viral isolation from blood or serum, serologic test
Dermatomyositis: muscle biopsy, electromyography, sedimentation

rate, serum transaminase, LDH and aldolase, Trichinella skin test, R-A test

Diabetes insipidus: Hickey-Hare test, intake and output before and after Pitressin, skull x-ray

Diabetes mellitus: FBS, 2-hour postprandial blood sugar, fractional urines, cortisone glucose tolerance test

Digitalis intoxication: ECG, observe effect of infusion of potassium on heart rate, atropine test, serum digitalis level.

DiGuglielmo's disease: bone marrow, peripheral blood study

Diphtheria: nose and throat culture on Loeffler's slant

Diphyllobothrium latum: stool for eggs of the worm, x-ray following a barium meal

Diplococcus pneumonia: blood culture, sputum smear and culture, throat culture

Dissecting aneurysm of the aorta: chest x-ray, aortography

Diverticulitis of colon: barium enema

Dracunculiasis: noting presence of worms in subcutaneous tissue

Dubin-Johnson syndrome: liver function tests, cholecystogram, liver biopsy

Ductus arteriosus, patent: fluoroscopy (hyperdynamic aortic pulse), cardiac catheterization, angiocardiography

Duodenal ulcer: see Peptic ulcer

Dwarfism: x-ray of bones; endocrine, renal, and gastrointestinal function tests

Echinococcosis: x-ray of long bones, Casoni intracutaneous test, serologic tests, liver biopsy of cyst wall, liver scan

Eclampsia: uric acid, renal function tests, renal biopsy, urinalysis

Ehlers-Danlos syndrome: skin biopsy, capillary fragility test, bleeding time

Emphysema: pulmonary function tests, arterial oxygen saturation, CO_2

Emphysema of the lung: chest x-ray (Bucky ray films), sputum culture, thoracocentesis and culture

Encephalitis: viral isolation from brain tissue and spinal fluid, serologic tests

Encephalomyelitis: viral isolation from brain tissue and spinal fluid, serologic tests

Endocardial fibroelastosis: ECG, chest x-ray

Epilepsy: FBS, 36-hour fast, calcium and phosphorus, skull x-ray, EEG, spinal tap, and contrast studies in adults, brain scan

Erythema multiforme: skin biopsy, patch test

Erythema nodosum: CBC, sedimentation rate, skin tests, chest x-ray

Erythroblastosis fetalis: bilirubin, CBC, agglutination of red cells by antiglobulin serum in human or bovine serum albumin, Coombs' test

Esophageal varices: barium swallow, esophagoscopy, injection of contrast material into spleen (splenovenography), liver function tests

Esophagitis: HCL drip, barium swallow, esophagoscopy

Extradural hematoma: spinal tap, skull x-ray, arteriography, burr holes

Fanconi syndrome: x-ray (pelvis, scapula, femur, humerus, ribs); urinary amino acid and glucose, calcium, potassium, phosphates, urates; serum alkaline phosphatase, uric acid

Filariasis: blood smears for microfilariae, *Dirofilaria* antigen intradermal test, complement-fixation test

Folic acid deficiency: gastric analysis, microbiologic assay of serum for folic acid activity, measurement of urinary excretion of formiminoglutamic acid, therapeutic trial, tests listed under malabsorption syndrome

Friedländer's pneumonia: sputum smears and culture, blood culture, lung puncture, x-ray

Friedreich's ataxia: clinical diagnosis

Galactosemia: blood and urinary galactose, galactose tolerance test, erythrocyte assay of the enzyme uridyl-diphosphogalactose transferase

Gallstones: cholecystogram, I.V. or percutaneous cholangiography, exploratory surgery

Gargoylism: urinary chondroitin sulfuric acid, x-ray of skull and long bones, biopsy

Gas gangrene: clinical diagnosis (organisms may be in wound exudate but not diagnostic)

Gastroenteritis: stool cultures, blood cultures

Gaucher's disease: bone marrow, x-ray of femur, acid and alkaline phosphatase

General paresis: spinal fluid examination, Wassermann test of blood and cerebrospinal fluid, TPI, FTA

Giardia lamblia: stool for cysts and trophozoites

Gigantism: skull x-ray, FBS, serum phosphorus, x-ray of long bones

Gilbert's disease: liver function tests, liver biopsy

Glanders: cultures of skin lesion, skin test, serologic tests, animal inoculation

Glanzmann's disease (see Thrombocytasthenia [thrombasthenia] this table): platelet count, clot retraction, prothrombin time, bleeding time, capillary fragility test

Glomerulonephritis: blood culture, L.E. cell preparation, muscle biopsy, IVP, cystoscopic examination with retrograde pyelography, renal biopsy, serial measurements of serum streptococcal antibodies, serum complement

Glossitis: culture of lesions, gastric analysis, gingival biopsy, therapeutic trial with vitamins or iron

Glycogen-storage disease: liver biopsy, glucose tolerance test, galactose tolerance test, epinephrine test

Goiter: BMR, PBI, RAI uptake and scan, serum cholesterol

Gonorrhea: urethral or vaginal smear and culture

Gout: serum or urinary uric acid, synovialysis for urate crystals, x-ray of bones

Granuloma inguinale: Wright's stain of scrapings from lesion

Graves' disease (see Hyperthyroidism, this table)

Guillain-Barré syndrome: spinal fluid examination

Gumma: serology, TPI

Haemophilus influenzae: nose, throat, and sputum culture or spinal fluid smear and culture

Hamman-Rich syndrome: chest x-ray, lung biopsy, pulmonary function tests

Hand-Schuller-Christian disease: x-ray of skull, bone biopsy, bone marrow examination

Hansen's disease: Wade's scraped incision procedure, x-ray hands and feet, biopsy of skin nerves

Hartnup disease: urinary amino acid, indican and indoleacetic acid

Hashimoto's thyroiditis: PBI, RAI, serum antibodies

Haverhill fever: agglutination titer, fluid aspiration from affected joint or abscess for *Streptobacillus moniliformis*

Hay fever: smears of nasal secretion for eosinophils, scratch and intracutaneous skin tests

Heart failure: vital capacity, venous pressure and circulation time, chest x-ray, ECG

Helminth infections: stool specimens, chest x-ray, serologic tests, skin tests, thymol turbidity, cephalin-cholesterol flocculation, urine urobilinogen

Hemangioblastoma: skull x-ray, spinal fluid examination, pneumoencephalogram

Hemochromatosis: serum iron and iron-binding capacity, liver or skin biopsy, glucose tolerance test, bone marrow biopsy

Hemoglobin C disease: blood smears for target cells, hemoglobin electrophoresis

Hemoglobinuria, paroxysmal cold: CBC, Coombs' test, Donath-Landsteiner test, VDRL, serum haptoglobins.

Hemoglobinuria, paroxysmal noctural: CBC, Ham test.

Hemolytic anemia: radioactive-chromium-tagged red cell survival, measurement of fecal urobilinogen excretion, Coombs' test, blood smears

Hemophilia: blood coagulation time, thromboplastin generation test

Hepatitis: liver function tests, liver biopsy, HAA

Hepatolenticular degeneration: urine amino acid and copper, serum ceruloplasmin, liver function tests, liver biopsy with histochemical staining of copper by rubeanic acid, slit-lamp examination of the cornea

Hepatoma: liver biopsy, liver function tests, exploratory laparotomy

Hernia, diaphragmatic: esophagram and G.I. series, esophagoscopy, exploratory laparotomy

Herniated disk: x-ray of cervical, thoracic, lumbar, and sacral spines, spinal tap, myelography, exploratory surgery

Herpangina: serologic tests, viral isolation

Herpes simplex: serologic tests, viral isolation

Herpes zoster: serologic tests (but clinical diagnosis usually sufficient)

Hiatal hernia: G.I. series, esophagoscopy, exploratory laparotomy, acid-perfusion of esophagus

Hirschsprung's disease: flat plate of abdomen, barium enema, rectal biopsy

Histamine cephalgia: test trial of histamine subcutaneously

Histoplasmosis: sputum culture, bone marrow smear and culture and animal inoculation, spinal tap, skin test, serologic tests, liver biopsy, chest x-ray

Hodgkin's disease: lymph node biopsy, bone marrow examination, lymphangiogram

Hookworm disease: stool for ova and parasites, eosinophil count

Huntington's chorea: clinical diagnosis

Hurler's syndrome: urinary acid mucopolysaccharides, tissue biopsy

Hyperaldosteronism: serum potassium, sodium, bicarbonate, pH, urine potassium, 24-hour urine aldosterone, plasma renin, exploratory surgery

Hypercholesterolemia, familial: lipoprotein electrophoresis, serum cholesterol, and triglycerides

Hyperlipemia, idiopathic: lipoprotein electrophoresis, serum cholesterol, and triglycerides

Hyperlipoproteinemias, familial: lipoprotein electrophoresis, serum cholesterol, and triglycerides
Hypernephroma: urinalysis, intravenous or retrograde pyelogram, renal angiogram, exploratory laparotomy
Hyperparathyroidism: serum calcium, phosphorus, alkaline phosphatase, phosphate reabsorption test, x-ray of mandible and long bones, urinary calcium, exploratory surgery
Hypersplenism: CBC, red cell survival, spleen-liver ratio, spleen scan, bone marrow, epinephrine test
Hypertension, essential: ECG, renal functions, renal biopsy, clinical observations, tests to exclude secondary hypertension (IVP, etc.)
Hyperthyroidism: PBI, RAI uptake, T_3 uptake, BMR, T_4 by isotope
Hypoparathyroidism: serum calcium, phosphorus, 24-hour urine calcium, alkaline phosphatase, skull x-ray
Hypopituitarism: PBI, 17-ketosteroids, 17-hydroxycorticosteroids, skull x-ray, visual fields, Hickey-Hare test, glucose tolerance test, urine HPG
Hypotension, idiopathic postural: clinical observations, response to Pitressin
Hypothyroidism: BMR, PBI, ECG, serum cholesterol, RAI uptake, T_4 by isotope, T_4 by column
Hypovitaminosis (see specific vitamin deficiency)

Ileitis (see Regional enteritis, this table)
Infarction, myocardial (see also Myocardial infarction, this table): ECG, vectorcardiography, serum enzymes (SGOT, SLDH, CPK)
Infectious mononucleosis: heterophil antibody titer, smear for atypical lymphocytes, liver function tests
Influenza: nasopharyngeal washings for viral isolation, complement-fixation test
Insulinoma (see Islet cell tumor, this table): blood sugar, glucose tolerance test, plasma insulin concentration, 36-hour fast, tolbutamide tolerance test, exploratory laparotomy
Intestinal obstruction: flat plate of abdomen, double enema, G.I. series with hypaque, exploratory laparotomy
Iron-deficiency anemia: serum iron and iron-binding capacity, CBC, bone marrow for hemosiderin content
Islet cell tumor: FBS, glucose tolerance test, 36-hour fast, tolbutamide tolerance test, exploratory laparotomy

Kala-azar: blood smear, bone marrow or splenic aspirate for parasites, serologic test
Klebsiella pneumoniae: sputum smear and culture, blood culture, chest x-ray, lung puncture for culture
Klinefelter's syndrome: sex chromatin pattern, testicular biopsy, urine HPG (human pituitary gonadotropin)
Kwashiorkor: serum albumin, CBC

Lactase deficiency: oral lactose tolerance test, mucosal biopsy
Laennec's cirrhosis: bromsulfalein, cephalin-flocculation test, serum protein albumin/globulin ratio, bilirubin, liver biopsy
Larva migrans, visceral: eosinophil count and serum globulin, skin testing, serologic tests, liver biopsy
Laryngitis: nose and throat culture and washings for viral studies
Lead intoxication: serum and urine lead content; urine for ALA, coproporphyrin, FEEP; test dose of EDTA, x-rays of long bones
Leishmaniasis: CBC, serum protein, cephalin-flocculation, thymol turbidity, blood and bone marrow smears for parasites, biopsy
Leprosy: Wade's scraped incision procedure, culture of lesion, biopsy of skin nerves, x-ray hands and feet, histamine test, lepromin test
Leptospirosis: animal inoculation, blood and urine culture, agglutinin titer, complement-fixation test, spinal tap, muscle biopsy
Letterer-Siwe disease: x-ray of bones, bone marrow aspirate or lymph node biopsy
Leukemia: hematologic examination of peripheral blood and bone marrow, total leukocyte count, BMR, uric acid, serum vitamin B_{12} concentration and iron-binding capacity
Lipoid pneumonia: chest x-ray, special sputum examination, surgical incision
Listeriosis: culture (blood or sputum) for microorganism, serum agglutinin titer, bone marrow biopsy
Liver abscess: liver aspiration and biopsy, blood culture, barium enema, stool culture for ova and parasites, exploratory laparotomy
Loeffler's syndrome: eosinophil count, sputum for eosinophils, stool for ova and parasites
Lung abscess: chest x-ray, tomography, sputum culture, bronchoscopy, thoracotomy, sputum cytology
Lupoid hepatitis: liver function tests and observe reversal on steroids, serum electrophoresis, serum haptoglobins, Coombs' test, LE smear
Lupus erythematosus: serologic tests, antinuclear antibody test, Coombs' test, clotting time, L.E. cell preparations; skin, tissue, muscle, lymph node, or kidney biopsy
Lymphangitis: CBC, sedimentation rate

Lymphoblastoma: lymph node biopsy, CBC, bone marrow examination

Lymphogranuloma inguinale: Lygranum test, serologic tests, tissue or node biopsy

Lymphogranuloma venereum: serum electrophoresis, Frei test, serologic tests, lymph node biopsy

Lymphoma (see Hodgkin's disease): lymph node biopsy; x-ray of chest, G.I. tract, G.I. system, bones; differential count, bone marrow; alkaline phosphatase, spinal tap

Lymphosarcoma: lymph node biopsy; x-ray of chest, G.I. tract, skeletal system; spinal tap; thoracocentesis; paracentesis; bone marrow

McArdle's syndrome: liver biopsy, FBS, enzyme assay of muscle phosphorylase

Macroglobulinemia: serum electrophoresis and ultracentrifugation, Sia water test

Malabsorption syndrome: mucosal biopsy; serum protein, carotene, calcium, cholesterol, potassium, magnesium; prothrombin time, D-xylose and glucose tolerance, stool for fat and trypsin, I^{131} triolein and I^{131} oleic acid, urinary 5-HIAA; small bowel series

Malaria: blood smear for parasites, bone marrow examination

Marfan's syndrome: x-ray long bones and ribs, slit-lamp examination of eyes, IVP, urinary hydroxyproline

Marie-Strumpell spondylitis: x-ray of lumbosacral spine, sedimentation rate, latex flocculation

Mastoiditis: nasopharyngeal culture, x-ray of mastoids, mastoidectomy

Measles: smear of nasal secretions for giant cells, serologic tests

Meckel's diverticulum: exploratory laparotomy

Mediastinitis: CBC, x-ray of chest, exploratory surgery

Medulloblastoma: skull x-ray, spinal tap, pneumoencephalogram

Megaloblastic anemia: (see Pernicious anemia, this table)

Meig's syndrome: thoracocentesis, culdoscopy, exploratory laparotomy

Melanoma: serum or urinary melanin, biopsy

Ménière's disease: skull x-ray with special views of each petrous pyramid and internal acoustic meatus, spinal tap, caloric tests, audiogram

Meningioma: x-ray of skull or spinal column, spinal tap, myelogram, pneumogram or arteriogram, craniotomy

Meningitis: spinal fluid examination, smear and culture; serum for viral serologic studies; blood cultures

Meningococcemia: blood cultures, spinal fluid examination, smear and culture, Gram stain of punctured petechiae

Menopause syndrome: urinary gonadotrophins, vaginal smear for estrogenic effects, therapeutic trial

Mental retardation: psychometric testing, skull x-ray, PKU test, urinary amino acids, PBI

Methemoglobinemia: erythrocyte methemoglobin, arterial oxygen saturation, blood diaphorase I

Migraine: histamine test, EEG, response to ergotamine

Mikulicz's disease: CBC, bone marrow, tuberculin test, biopsy of lesion

Milk-alkali syndrome: serum calcium, phosphorus, alkaline phosphatase, urinary calcium and phosphates

Milroy's disease: clinical diagnosis

Mitral stenosis: ECG, chest x-ray, cardiac catheterization, phonocardiogram

Mongolism: clinical diagnosis, psychometric tests, chromosome study, urinary beta-amino-isobutyric acid

Moniliasis: tissue smear or biopsy; culture

Mononucleosis, infectious: smear for atypical lymphocytes, heterophil agglutination test, liver function tests

Mucormycosis: nose and throat culture, biopsy

Mucoviscidosis (see Cystic fibrosis of pancreas): quantitative sweat test, duodenal assay of pancreatic enzymes and bicarbonate, chest x-ray

Multiple myeloma: serum protein electrophoresis, urine for Bence-Jones protein, bone marrow biopsy, serum calcium levels, skeletal survey

Multiple sclerosis: spinal fluid examination, clinical diagnosis

Mumps: skin test, serologic tests

Muscular dystrophy: serum CPK, SGOT, LDH, muscle biopsy

Myasthenia gravis: dynamometer test, maximum breathing capacity, test dose of neostigmine or Tensilon

Mycosis fungoides: skin biopsy

Myelitis: x-ray of spinal column, spinal tap, serologic tests, myelogram, exploratory laminectomy, gastric analysis

Myeloid metaplasia, agnogenic: red cell morphology, CBC, bone marrow examination, splenic aspirate, hepatic function tests, skeletal survey, leukocyte alkaline phosphatase, urine and serum erythropoietin

Myelophthisic anemia: CBC, bone marrow examination, skeletal survey, lymph node biopsy

Myocardial infarction: serial ECG, vectorcardiography, serial serum enzymes (SGOT, SLDH and, CPK)
Myocarditis: ECG, x-ray of chest, fluoroscopy
Myotonia atrophica: BMR, electromyography, urine creatinine, muscle biopsy

Nematodes: gastric analysis, muscle biopsy, eosinophil count, intradermal skin test; precipitin, complement-fixation, and flocculation techniques; ECG; Stoll's egg count in stool, stool cultures and smears; duodenal aspiration, G.I. series; rectal swab with Scotch tape
Nephritis: blood cultures, urine cultures, L.E. cell preparation, muscle biopsy, serum complement, ASO titer, urinalysis, renal function tests, renal biopsy
Nephrocalcinosis: urinary sediment, serum calcium, phosphorus and alkaline phosphatase, renal biopsy, x-ray of abdomen, IVP
Nephrolithiasis: urinary sediment, IVP, retrograde pyelogram, serum calcium, uric acid
Nephrotic syndrome: urinalysis, erythrocyte sedimentation rate, serum protein electrophoresis, total cholesterol concentration, BMR, PBI, renal function tests
Neurinoma, acoustic: spinal tap, skull x-ray with special views of internal auditory foramina, caloric tests, audiogram
Neuritis, peripheral (see also Neuropathy, this table): eosinophil count, L.E. cell preparation, neurologic examination, EMG
Neuroblastoma: urinary VMA, clinical observation, exploratory laparotomy
Neurofibromatosis: biopsy, x-ray of spinal column and long bones, spinal fluid examination, myelogram
Neuropathy: spinal tap, eosinophil count, FBS, urine porphobilinogen, muscle biopsy, blood lead level, hairs for arsenic content, urine for *N*-methylnicotinamide, EMG
Neurosyphilis: spinal tap, serologic tests (Wassermann, TPI, FTA)
Niacin deficiency (see Pellagra): urine *N*-methylnicotinamide
Niemann-Pick disease: demonstration of sphingomyelin in reticuloendothelial cells, bone marrow biopsy, tissue biopsy, x-ray of skull and long bones
Nocardiosis: sputum smear and culture
Nutritional neuropathy: serum pyruvic acid, blood pentose concentration, urine niacin or thiamine after loading dose

Ochronosis: urinalysis (Benedict's solution, isolation of homogentisic acid), x-ray of spine
Oppenheim's disease: electromyography, muscle biopsy
Optic atrophy: visual fields, spinal tap; x-ray of skull, orbits, and optic foramina
Osteitis deformans: serum calcium, phosphorus, alkaline phosphatase, skeletal survey
Osteoarthritis: x-ray of joints, synovianalysis
Osteogenic sarcoma: x-ray of bone, bone biopsy
Osteomalacia: serum calcium, phosphorus, alkaline phosphatase, x-ray of long bones, response to vitamin D and calcium
Osteomyelitis: blood culture, culture of bone biopsy material, x-ray of bones
Osteopetrosis: bone marrow examination, x-rays of bone
Osteoporosis: serum calcium, phosphorus, alkaline phosphatase, bone biopsy, x-ray of spine
Otitis media: nasopharyngeal or aural smear and culture, ASO titer, CBC, sedimentation rate

Paget's disease: skeletal survey, serum calcium, phosphorus, and alkaline and acid phosphatase
Pancreatitis, acute: blood glucose, serum calcium, glucose tolerance test, liver function test, serum amylase, and lipase, paracentesis, flat plate of abdomen
Pancreatitis, chronic: serum and urine amylase and lipase before and after secretin, glucose tolerance test, pancreatic juice volume, bicarbonate and enzyme concentration; G.I. series, cholecystogram, exploratory laparotomy, fecal fat, triolein I^{131} uptake
Panniculitis: bone marrow, skin and subcutaneous tissue biopsy
Paralysis agitans: clinical diagnosis
Pellagra: urinary *N*-methylnicotinamide
Pemphigus: skin biopsy, Tancz test
Peptic ulcer: gastric analysis, stool for occult blood, G.I. series, gastroscopy
Periarteritis nodosa: muscle, skin, and subcutaneous tissue biopsy; CBC, eosinophil count, urinary sediment
Pericarditis: ECG, pericardial tap, angiocardiography, echocardiography
Periodic paralysis, familial: serum potassium, ECG, response to sugar
Peritonitis: CBC, flat plate of abdomen, peritoneal tap, exploratory laparotomy
Pernicious anemia: CBC, blood smear, bone marrow, gastric analysis, Schilling test

Pertussis: CBC, nasopharyngeal smear and culture
Petite mal: EEG, skull x-ray, spinal tap, occasionally contrast studies
Peutz-Jeghers syndrome: small bowel series, exploratory laparotomy
Pharyngitis: CBC, ASO titer, sedimentation rate, C-reactive protein, pharyngeal culture
Phenylpyruvic oligophrenia: urinalysis for phenylpyruvic acid and phenylalanine, Guthrie test, serum phenylalanine
Pheochromocytoma: histamine provocative or Regitine blocking test, plasma and urine for epinephrine and norepinephrine, 24-hour urine test for VMA or catecholamines, IVP, presacral air insufflation, exploratory surgery, arteriography
Phlebitis (see Thrombophlebitis, this table): clinical diagnosis
Phlebotomus fever: serologic tests
Pickwickian syndrome: pulmonary function tests, CO_2 combining power, arterial oxygen saturation
Pinealoma: skull x-ray, spinal tap, pneumoencephalogram
Pinworm disease: Scotch tape swab of perianal region with microscopic examination for eggs
Pituitary adenoma: skull x-ray, PBI, serum TSH and cortisol, urinary 17-ketosteroids and 17-hydroxycorticosteroids, urine HPG (human pituitary gonadotropin)
Plague (see Bubonic plague, this table)
Platyhelminthes: stool for ova and parasites, serologic tests, eosinophil count, intradermal tests, liver function tests, urine sedimentation for eggs
Pleurisy: chest x-ray; pleural aspiration and culture; specific gravity, total protein, cell count differential, and cytologic examination of pleural fluid; pleural biopsy
Pleurodynia, epidemic: serologic tests, stool and throat cultures for Coxsackie B virus
Pneumococcal pneumonia: sputum smear and culture, blood culture, chest x-ray
Pneumoconiosis: chest x-ray, occupational history, sputum smear, lung biopsy, scalene node biopsy, pulmonary function tests, arterial O_2 and CO_2 content
Pneumonia (see Pneumococcal pneumonia, this table; also Cough and Hemoptysis, Table II)
Pneumothorax: chest x-ray, thoracocentesis, pulmonary function tests, PPD intermediate, sputum for AFB (acid-fat bacilli)
Poliomyelitis: viral isolation from stool, serologic tests
Polyarteritis: (see Periarteritis)
Polycystic ovary (see Stein-Leventhal syndrome, this table): culdoscopy, exploratory laparotomy
Polycythemia vera: CBC, platelet count, blood volume, BMR, serum uric acid, arterial oxygen saturation, pulmonary function tests
Polymyositis (see Dermatomyositis, this table)
Polyneuritis: spinal tap, heterophil antibody titer, urine for porphobilinogen, glucose tolerance test, muscle biopsy, electromyography, serum pyruvic acid, blood lead level, hairs for arsenic content
Porphyria: urine porphyrins and porphobilinogen
Portal cirrhosis (see Laennec's cirrhosis, this table)
Pott's disease: x-ray of spine, aspiration and culture of synovial fluid, synovial or bone biopsy, PPD, intermediate
Preeclampsia (see Eclampsia, this table)
Pregnancy: Friedman's test, Aschheim-Zondek, or serologic test for pregnancy
Prostatic carcinoma: serum acid phosphatase, x-ray of lumbosacral spine, biopsy of prostate
Protein–losing enteropathy: I^{131} polyvinylpyrrolidone test, serum protein electrophoresis
Pseudohypoparathyroidism: serum calcium, phosphorus, urine calcium, Ellsworth-Howard test, parathyroid tissue biopsy
Pseudotumor cerebri: skull x-ray, spinal tap, EEG, ventriculography
Psittacosis: chest x-ray, serologic tests, virus isolation
Pulmonary emphysema (see Emphysema, this table)
Pulmonary infarction: ECG, chest x-ray, serum bilirubin, and LDH (isozymes LD_2 and LD_3), thoracocentesis, lung scan, pulmonary angiography
Pulmonary hypertension, idiopathic: cardiac catheterization, pulmonary function tests, arterial oxygen saturation
Pyelonephritis: urine culture with colony counts, IVP, cystoscopy, renal biopsy
Pyloric stenosis: G.I. series and gastroscopy
Pyridoxine deficiency: serum iron concentration, urine concentration of xanthurenic acid, and trial of isoniazid, tryptophan tolerance test

Q Fever: serologic tests

Rabies: autopsy of infected animal, isolation of virus from saliva
Rat-bite fever: culture of lesion, aspiration and culture of regional lymph node, animal inoculation, serologic tests

Raynaud's disease: L.E. preparations, skin biopsy, muscle biopsy, serum protein electrophoresis, cold agglutinins, cryoglobulins
Regional enteritis: small bowel series, surgical exploration
Reiter's disease: clinical diagnosis, laboratory exclusion of other cause of joint pathology
Relapsing fever: peripheral blood for *Borrelia,* inoculation of rats and mice, serologic tests, total leukocytes, spinal tap
Renal tubular acidosis: serum electrolytes, calcium, phosphorus and alkaline phosphatase, urine calcium and phosphatase.
Reticuloendotheliosis: x-ray, erythrocyte count, tissue cholesterol content, biopsy skeletal lesion of bone marrow or lymph nodes
Reticulum cell sarcoma: alkaline phosphatase; lymph node biopsy; x-ray chest, G.I. tract, skeletal system; pyelogram, cytologic examination of pleural or ascitic fluid, spinal tap, bone marrow examination
Rheumatic fever: ASO titer, CRP, sedimentation rate, ECG, antihyaluronidase titer, antifibrinolysin titer
Rheumatoid arthritis: agglutination test using rheumatoid sera, x-ray of affected joints, serum iron, examination of synovial fluid; latex, sheep, erythrocyte, bentonite particle flocculation tests; C-reactive protein, electrophoretic tests, erythrocyte sedimentation rate
Riboflavin deficiency: clinical diagnosis, therapeutic trial
Rickets: x-ray of bones, serum calcium, phosphorus, alkaline phosphatase, urine calcium
Rickettsialpox: serologic tests
Rocky Mountain spotted fever: specific serologic tests, Weil-Felix test
Rubella: none
Rubeola (see Measles, this table)

Saddle embolus of aorta: oscillometry, aortography
Salicylate intoxication: serum electrolytes, urine and serum salicylates
Salmonellosis: stool culture, febrile agglutinins
Salpingitis: vaginal smear and culture, culdoscopy, exploratory surgery
Sarcoidosis (see Boeck's sarcoid, this table)
Scalenus anticus syndrome: x-ray of cervical spine, clinical observations
Scarlet fever: nose and throat culture, ASO titer, Schultz-Charlton reaction
Schilder's disease: skull x-ray, EEG, spinal tap, pneumoencephalogram, brain biopsy
Schistosomiasis: stool for ova or urine for ova, rectal biopsy, liver biopsy
Schönlein-Henoch purpura: urinalysis, platelet count, coagulation studies to exclude other causes of purpura
Schüller-Christian disease (see Hand-Schüller-Christian Disease, this table)
Scleroderma: skin biopsy, esophagram, work up for malabsorption
Scurvy: x-rays of bones, capillary fragility test, serum ascorbic acid, therapeutic trial
Seminoma: urine human pituitary gonadotropin, exploratory surgery
Septicemia: blood cultures
Sexual precocity: skull x-ray, urine 17-ketosteroids and 17-hydroxysteroids, exploratory surgery
Shigellosis: stool or rectal swab culture
Sickle cell anemia: CBC, Wright's stain of peripheral blood, serum bilirubin, sickle cell preparation, x-ray of skull and long bones, hemoglobin electrophoresis
Silicosis: chest x-ray, pulmonary function tests, lung biopsy
Silo-filler's disease: chest x-ray, clinical observations
Simmonds' disease (see Hypopituitarism, this table)
Sinusitis: x-ray of sinuses, nose and throat cultures, allergic skin testing, sinus irrigation
Sjögren's syndrome: Schirmer test for tear production, latex flocculation, thyroglobulin antibody titer, and other auto-immune antibody titers
Smallpox: smear of vesicular fluid for virus particles, viral isolation, serologic tests
Spherocytosis, hereditary: CBC, blood smear, reticulocyte count, serum haptoglobins and bilirubin
Spinal cord tumor: x-ray of spine, spinal tap, alkaline phosphatase, acid phosphatase, serum protein electrophoresis, myelogram
Sporotrichosis: culture of exudate from ulcer, serologic tests, skin tests
Sprue (see Celiac disease, this table)
Staphylococcal pneumonia: sputum smear and culture, blood culture, chest x-ray
Steatorrhea (see Celiac disease, this table)
Stein-Leventhal syndrome: culdoscopy, urine 17-ketosteroids, exploratory surgery
Stevens-Johnson syndrome: clinical diagnosis
Still's disease: latex flocculation, CRP, ASO titer, synovianalysis
Streptococcal pharyngitis: nose and throat culture, ASO titer

Strongyloidiasis: stool or duodenal aspirate for ova and parasites
Sturge-Weber syndrome: skull x-ray, clinical observation, EEG
Subacute bacterial endocarditis: blood cultures, urine cultures, bone marrow cultures, smear of petechiae
Subarachnoid hemorrhage: skull x-ray, spinal tap, arteriography
Subdiaphragmatic abscess: chest x-ray, fluoroscopy with phrenic nerve stimulation, needle aspiration, exploratory surgery
Subdural hematoma: skull x-ray, spinal tap, arteriography, burr holes
Subphrenic abscess (see Subdiaphragmatic abscess, this table)
Sulfhemoglobinemia: shaking of venous blood in test tube, spectroscopic examination of blood
Syphilis: blood and spinal fluid Wassermann, etc., TPI, FTA, darkfield microscopy
Syringomyelia: x-ray of spine, spinal tap, myelogram, exploratory surgery

Tabes dorsalis: blood Wassermann, etc., x-ray of spine, spinal fluid for colloidal gold and Wassermann or TPI
Takayasu disease: aortography, clinical observation, serum protein electrophoresis
Tapeworm infections: stool for ova and parasites
Tay-Sachs disease: cortical biopsy
Temporal arteritis: ophthalmodynamometry, biopsy of temporal artery
Tetanus: clinical diagnosis; positive culture does not establish diagnosis
Thalassemia, major: CBC, blood smear, reticulocyte count, serum bilirubin, serum haptoglobin, hemoglobin electrophoresis
Thromboangiitis obliterans (see Buerger's disease, this table)
Thrombocytasthenia (thrombasthenia): platelet count, bleeding time, clotting time, clot retraction
Thrombocytopenic purpura, idiopathic: platelet count, clot retraction, Rumpel-Leede test, bone marrow
Thrombophlebitis: clinical diagnosis
Thymoma: chest x-ray, tomography, barium swallow, exploratory thoracotomy
Thyroiditis, subacute: PBI, RAI uptake, sedimentation rate, antithyroid autoantibodies
Tonsillitis: nose and throat smear and culture, ASO titer, sedimentation rate
Torulosis (see Cryptococcosis, this table)
Toxemias of pregnancy (see Preeclampsia, this table)
Toxoplasmosis: Sabin-Feldman dye test for *Toxoplasma* antibodies, complement-fixation test, skin test
Trachoma: smear of conjunctival scrapings for inclusion bodies
Transfusion reaction: serum hemoglobin and haptoglobin, methemalbumin
Trichinosis: WBC and differential, muscle biopsy, *Trichinella* skin test, serologic tests
Trypanosomiasis: smears of blood, CSF, lymph node aspirate for parasites, animal inoculation
Tuberculosis: smear and culture of sputum or gastric washings, guinea pig inoculation, skin test, chest x-ray
Tuberosclerosis: skull x-ray, skin biopsy, cortical biopsy
Tularemia: culture of material from ulcer, lymph nodes, or nasopharynx; Foshay's skin test, serologic tests
Turner's syndrome: urine for human pituitary gonadotropin, buccal smear for chromatins, chromosomal studies
Typhoid fever: culture of blood, bone marrow, urine, or stool; febrile agglutinins (Widal reaction)
Typhus epidemic: serologic tests, Weil-Felix test
Typhus scrub: isolation from blood and Weil-Felix reaction, serologic tests

Ulcer (see Peptic ulcer, this table)
Ulcerative colitis: barium enema, sigmoidoscopy
Urethritis: urethral smear and culture, vaginal smear and culture, urine culture, cystoscopy
Urticaria: allergic skin testing, elimination diet

Varicella: serologic tests (although clinical diagnosis is usually sufficient)
Variola (see Smallpox, this table)
Visceral larva migrans: blood typing, serologic tests, biopsy
Vitamin A deficiency: serum vitamin A or carotene, dark-adaptation test, skin biopsy
Vitamin B deficiency (see Beriberi, this table)
Vitamin C deficiency (see Scurvy, this table)
Vitamin D deficiency: x-ray of skull, chest, and long bones; serum calcium, phosphorus and alkaline phosphatase, urine calcium
Vitamin K deficiency: prothrombin time, response to vitamin K
von Gierke's disease (see Glycogen-storage disease, this table)
von Willebrand's disease: bleeding time, coagulation time, thromboplastin-generation test

Waterhouse-Friderichsen syndrome: blood cultures, spinal fluid examination, nose and throat culture, urine 17-ketosteroids and 17-hydroxysteroids

Wegener's granulomatosis: x-ray of nose, sinuses, and chest; urinalysis, renal biopsy, lung biopsy.

Weil's disease: darkfield examination of blood for spirochetes, guinea pig inoculation, serologic tests, spinal fluid examination

Wernicke's encephalopathy: serum pyruvic acid, response to thiamine

Whipple's disease: small bowel series, lymph node biopsy, jejunal mucosa biopsy, malabsorption tests

Whooping cough: culture on Chievitz and Meyer cough plate, serologic tests

Wilson's disease: urine copper and amino acids, serum copper and ceruloplasmin, liver biopsy, slit-lamp examination of cornea, uric acid

Yaws: darkfield examination, serologic tests

Yellow fever: viral isolation, neutralization tests, other serologic tests, liver biopsy

Zollinger-Ellison syndrome: 12-hour quantitative and MAO gastric analysis, G.I. series, gastroscopy, exploratory laparotomy

Appendix IV Relatively Innocuous Nonspecific Tests of Organ Involvement

Adrenal cortex:
- Serum electrolytes
- Glucose tolerance test
- Plasma cortisol
- 24-hour urine 17-ketosteroids before and after ACTH
- 24-hour urine 17-hydroxysteroids before and after ACTH
- 24-hour urine aldosterone test
- Eosinophil count before and after ACTH
- Robinson-Power-Kepler water test
- Flat plate of abdomen

Heart:
- Chest x-ray with barium swallow
- ECG
- Venous pressure and circulation time
- Vital capacity
- Fluoroscopy
- Serum lactic dehydrogenase
- Serum transaminase
- Serum CPK
- Angiography
- Urine myoglobin

Kidney:
- BUN and creatinine
- Serum electrolytes, phosphorus, calcium
- Urinalysis
- Addis count
- Creatinine clearance
- Fishberg concentration test
- PSP dye test
- Intravenous pyelogram
- Cystoscopy

Large bowel:
- Stool for occult blood
- Barium enema
- Sigmoidoscopy
- Colonoscopy

Liver:
- BSP dye test
- Cardio-green dye test
- Serum bilirubin
- Thymol turbidity
- Serum transaminase (SGOT, SGPT)
- Alkaline phosphatase
- Serum protein and albumin/globulin ratio
- Prothrombin time
- Urine bile and urobilinogen
- Duodenal drainage
- Cholecystogram or I.V. cholangiogram
- Rose bengal I 131 uptake and scan
- Peritoneoscopy

Lung:
- Pulmonary function tests
- Chest x-ray
- Fluoroscopy
- Blood carbon dioxide
- Arterial oxygen saturation, CO_2
- Serum lactic dehydrogenase
- Bronchoscopy
- Bronchogram
- Lung scan

Muscle:
- Serum transaminase
- Serum lactic dehydrogenase
- Serum CPK
- 24-hour urine creatinine and creatine
- Electromyography

Nervous system:
- Spinal tap
- X-rays of the skull or spine
- Electroencephalography
- Visual fields
- Audiogram
- Caloric tests
- Brain scan
- Electromyography

Ovary:
- 24-hour urine gonadotropin and estrogen
- Vaginal smear for estrogen effects
- Temperature chart
- Cervical mucus

Pancreas:
1. Acinar cells
   - Serum amylase
   - Serum lipase
   - Duodenal drainage
   - Stool for fat and trypsin
   - Flat plate of abdomen
   - G.I. series
   - Radioactive triolein uptake
   - Pancreatic scan
2. Islet cells
   - Fasting blood sugar
   - Glucose tolerance test
   - Fractional urines
   - 36-hour fast

Parathyroid:
- Serum calcium
- Serum phosphorus
- Alkaline phosphatase
- 24-hour urine calcium
- Phosphate reabsorption tests (TRP)
- X-rays of skull and long bones

Pituitary:
- Plasma growth hormone radioimmunoassay
- See Adrenal cortex, Thyroid, Ovary, and Testicles, this table
- Skull x-ray
- Hickey-Hare test
- Pitressin test
- Plasma TSH

Reticuloendothelial system:
- CBC and smear of peripheral blood
- Platelet count
- Bone marrow aspiration or biopsy
- Serum bilirubin
- Flat plate of abdomen for spleen size
- X-rays of long bones
- Spleen and liver scan

Skeleton:
- Serum calcium
- Serum phosphorus
- Alkaline phosphatase
- X-rays of skull and long bones
- 24-hour urine calcium
- Bone scan

Small bowel:
- D-xylose absorption test
- Glucose tolerance test
- Serum carotene test
- Urine 5-HIAA
- Stool for fat content
- Radioactive triolein and olein uptake
- Small bowel series
- Mucosal biopsy
- Duodenoscopy

Stomach:
- Gastric analysis
- Upper G.I. series
- Gastroscopy

Testicles:
- Plasma testosterone
- 24-hour urine gonadotropin
- 24-hour urine 17-ketosteroids
- Semen analysis

Thyroid:
- BMR
- Serum cholesterol
- PBI or free thyroxine
- RAI uptake and scan
- T_3 uptake
- T_4 by column
- T_4 by isotope
- Free thyroxine index

Index

Abdominal compression, 191
Abdominal pain, 307–308
ABO incompatibility, 226, 230
Abruptio placentae, 268
Absorption, in metabolism. *See also* Reabsorption.
of blood electrolytes, 35, 41
disorders of, 41
of blood glucose, 58, 61, 62
of blood oxygen, 130–131, 132–133
blood oxygen content in, 138–140
of iron, 173
of lipids, 101–102, 106
of plasma proteins, 143, 146
of serum calcium, 21, 24–26
Acanthocytosis, lipids in, 114
Acetazolamide therapy, 31
Achilles reflex test, 80
Achlorhydria, 192, 234
Acid phosphatases. *See* Phosphatases.
Acidity, of body fluids, 37
Acidosis, 37
diabetic, 40, 56–57, 111
metabolic, 44, 46, 55
renal tubular, 31, 53, 54
respiratory, 47
Acids. *See also* Uric acid; specific acids.
Aciduria, 198
organic, 40
Acinar cells, 170
Acromegaly, blood glucose in, 70
hormones in, 83
protein catabolism in, 129
ACTH, 76, 79, 81, 84
stimulation test associated with, 80, 81, 93
Actinomyces bovis, 285
Actinomycosis, 282
Adrenal androgens, 77, 80
Adrenal cortex. *See also* Adrenal hormone disorders.
hormones of, 77
in diagnosis of hormone disorders, 80–81
in primary aldosteronism, 51
Adrenal cortical insufficiency, 49
Adrenal hormone disorders, Addison's disease, 90
adrenogenital syndrome, 93
Cushing's syndrome, 92
primary aldosteronism, 90
Adrenal medulla, catecholamines from, 171
Adrenocortical hormone, and glucose, 59
Adrenocorticotropin. *See* ACTH.
Adrenogenital syndrome, 93
Adrenoglomerulotropin, 79
Addison's disease, as hormonal disorder, 90
blood glucose in, 67
diagnosing, 80
leukocytes in, 247
protein catabolism in, 129
Agglutination, of donor cells, 226, 227, 229
of recipient red cells, 226, 228, 229
Agglutinins, 253
Agnogenic myeloid metaplasia, 256
Agranulocytosis, 254
Air, inspired, distribution of, 132–133
Air pump, in respiration, 130
Albinism, 175
Albumin, in autoanalyzer profiles, 202, 204, 206, 208
macroaggregated, 189
serum, plasma proteins and, 143, 144
disorders of, 145–149, 152–154
radioactive isotopes in, 183
Alcoholism, tests in management of, 299
Aldolase, 155, 160
Aldosterone, 49, 76, 77, 79–81, 90, 91
Aldosteronism, primary, 51, 91
Alkaline phosphatases. *See* Phosphatases.
Alkalosis, hydrogen ion in, 37
in pyloric obstruction, 43
metabolic, 51, 52
Alkaptonuria, 175
Allopurinol, 165
Alpha-1 antitrypsin deficiency, 151
Alveolar-capillary block, 47, 133
Alveolar-capillary membrane, 130, 131
overall area and character of, 133
thickening of, in blood oxygen disorders, 138
Alveoli, in pulmonary emphysema, 136
oxygen absorption in, 130–131
Amebiasis, 282
Ames Dextrostix, 295
Ames Microhematocrit, 295
Amino acids, 119
enzymes and, 155
impaired absorption of, 146
in urine, 198
plasma proteins and, 143, 144
β-aminoisobutyric aciduria, 198
ς-aminolevulinic acid, 175, 177
Ammonia, blood, 119
in cirrhosis of liver, 123
Ampulla of Vater, carcinoma of, 10, 18
Amylase, in peritoneal fluid, 199
serum, disorders of, 170–171
ANA test, 249, 291
Anaphylactoid purpura, 270
Androgens, 76
Anemia, acute lymphoblastic and chronic, lymphocytic, 231
aplastic, 299, 217,
cirrhosis of liver and, 232
Cooley's, 15
diagnosing, 212
nine tests for, 212
gastric, 212
hemolytic, 14, 174, 249
red cell survival time test for, 186
acquired, red cells in, 225
tests in management of, 300
hypochromic, of infancy, 213
in bleeding peptic ulcer, red cells in, 219
in Banti's syndrome, 233
in hypothyroidism, 234
in leukocyte disorders, 244, 246
iron-deficiency, 174, 213, 214, 221, 301
iron regulation in, 174
laboratory work-up of symptoms in, 308
myelophthisic, 216
normocytic, 231
in acute myeloblastic anemia, 231
normochromic, 247, 256
pernicious, 215
red cells in, 215
test for, 183
tests in management of, 301
sickle cell, 15, 223
simple chronic, 235
Angina pectoris, 299
Angiotensin, 79
Animal inoculation, 286, 289–290
tables on, 279–283
Ankylosing spondylitis, 137
Anoxemia, 130–131, 133
Anterior pituitary insufficiency, 69
Anthrax, 279
Anthrosilicosis, 138
Antibiotics, isolating organisms after use of, 286, 288
prolonged use of, 266
sensitivity report and, 289
Antibodies, auto-, in red cell disorders, 225
in blood type compatibilities, 226
in erythroblastosis fetalis, 230

Antibodies (*Cont.*)
iso-immune, 226
Anticoagulants, 259
Antidiuretic hormone, 36
in diabetes insipidus, 50
in tubular reabsorption, 182
in urine formation, 180
Antigen, carcinoembryonic (CEA), 202
Antihemophilic globulin, 264
Antinuclear antibody test, 249, 291
Antistreptolysin O titer, 290–291
Aplastic anemia, 299
Aplastic crisis, 223
Apoferritin, 173
Arachidonic acid, 101
Argininosuccinic aciduria, 198
Arsenic, in blood and urine, 177
Arterial blood oxygen saturation. *See* Oxygen saturation.
Arterioles, disorders of, 271
inflammation of walls of, 270
Arthritis, acute, crystals in synovial fluid in, 197
acute septic, bacteria in, 196
poor mucin in various types of, 193
rheumatoid, 291
Ascorbic acid, 210
Aspirin, and blood-salicylate levels, 178
Asthma, bronchial, 196, 197
test in management of, 299
Asthmatic bronchitis, 135
Audiometry, 298
Auer bodies, 240
Australian antigen, 159
Autoanalyzer, 200–209
Autoantibodies, 249

B_{12}, 183, 215
Bacilli, and white cells, 196
Bacillus subtilis, 175
Back pain, 308
Bacteria, list of, 284–285
Bacterial infections. *See also* Infectious diseases.
acute, 148, 195, 196, 251
chronic, 148, 196, 252
plasma proteins in acute and chronic, 148
white cells in, 196
Bacteriologic diagnosis, 278
Bacteriology, in office laboratory, 296–297
Bacteriologist, 284, 286, 289
Banti's syndrome, 233
Barbiturate intoxication, 142
Barbiturates, in blood and urine, 177
Barr-Epstein virus, 253
Bartonellosis, 279
Basal cells, in reduced estrogen secretion, 94, 96
Basophil, 236
Basophilic stippling, 225
Belltone audiometer, 298
Bell's palsy, 299
Bence-Jones proteins, 153, 197
Beryllium poisoning, 138
Bicarbonate, as blood electrolyte, 35, 37
in acute renal failure, 46
in aldosteronism, 51
in salicylate toxicity, 48
Bile, 190, 199
Bile duct(s), common, gallstones in, 20
obstruction of, 10, 14, 19
in obstructive jaundice 112, 267
Biliary calculi, 197
Biliary obstruction, extrahepatic, 161
in carcinoma, 18
in Laennec's cirrhosis, 17
Bilirubin, 13
in autoanalyzer profiles, 202
in cerebrospinal and peritoneal fluid, 199
indirect, 13, 15
in red cell disorders, 220, 222, 230
test, 212
serum, disorders of, 13–20
carcinoma of head of pancreas, 18
choledocholithiasis, 20
hepatitis, viral and chlorpromazine, 16, 19
hereditary spherocytosis, 15
Laennec's cirrhosis, 17
red cell disorders, 215, 223, 224, 226
normal metabolism of, 13–14
urine, and urobilinogen, in disorders of serum bilirubin, 15–20
Bilirubin, serum indirect, 15
Bilirubin concentration, serum, 13
Bilirubin diglucuronide, 13
Bilirubin stones, 15
Bilirubin tetrapyrrole, 13
Biochemical alterations in body fluids, 197–199. *See also* Blood chemistries; Body fluids.
Biopsy, tables on, 279–283
Blast cells, 231, 240
Blastomycosis, North American, 282
test for, 292
Bleeding, analysis of, 194–196
gastrointestinal, 194–195
test for, 183
massive, anemia from, 219
three lines of resistance to, 257–259
Bleeding diathesis, 246
Bleeding time, in hemostasis disorders, 262, 263, 269, 270, 272, 274–276
recording, 259
Blood in body fluids and feces, 193–194
microorganisms in, 287
occult, in stool, 296
specimens of, 284
in serologic tests, 290
Blood agar plate, 296
Blood calcium. *See* Calcium.
Blood cell study. *See also* Cells; Erythrocytes; Leucocytes; Red cells; White cells.
of body fluids, 195–196
Blood chemistries, 170–179
disorders in, amylase and lipase, 170–171
copper metabolism, 172
iron, serum, 173–174
melanin metabolism, 175
magnesium serum, 174–175
porphyrin metabolism, 175, 177
toxic substances in blood and urine, 177–178
urinary catecholamines, 171–172
urine 5-hydroxyindoleacetic acid (5-HIAA), 172–173
in office laboratory, 295
Blood electrolytes. *See* Electrolytes.
Blood loss, in cirrhosis of liver, 232
Blood oxygen. *See* Oxygen, blood.
Blood smear, for anemia, 212
in office laboratory, 293–294
Blood sugar. *See* Glucose; Hyperglycemia; Hypoglycemia; Sugar, blood.
Blood types, 226–229
Blood volume, 183
Bodansky units, 3, 7
Body fluids. *See also* Fluids; Water.
appearance, 193–194
biochemical alterations, 197–199
casts, 196
comparative analysis of, 190–199
crystals, 196–197
cytology, 199
examination for clotting, 193
kidney in regulation of, 36–37
lung in regulation of, 37
microorganisms in, 287–288
obtaining specimen, 190–191
specific gravity, 192–193
volume, 191–192
Body lipids. *See* Lipids.
Body tissues, microorganisms in, 287–288
Boeck's sarcoid, 24
Boils, 279
Bone(s), calcium and phosphate in, 21
in calcium disorders, 23
in chronic nephritis, 30
in hyperparathyroidism, 32
in hypoparathyroidism, 33
in rickets and osteomalacia, 9
metastatic carcinoma of, 29, 208, 209
Paget's disease of, 7
Bone marrow, erythrocytes and, 210, 211
disorders of, 212–218, 222—224, 233
hypercellular, 215
in hemostasis disorders, 274
in leukocyte disorders, 238, 240–245, 254, 256
lymphocytes and, 236
reading, 212
space-occupying lesions of, 216
Bone scanning, 189
Bone tumors, 5, 8
scanning in diagnosis of, 189
Brain, diagnosing lesions of, 188
Brain scanning, 188
Bromides, toxic levels of, 177
Bromsulphalein dye excretion, 14, 17
Bronchial adenomas, 173
Bronchitis, asthmatic, 135
Bronchopneumonia, tests in management of, 299
Bronchospasm, 135
Brucella organisms, 286, 288
Brucellosis, 279, 280
test for, 291, 292
BUN, in autoanalyzer profiles, 202, 204, 208
Burdick electrocardiograph machine, 80
Burkitt's lymphoma, 253

Calcium, autoanalyzer profiles and, 204, 206, 208
blood, in rickets and osteomalacia, 9
serum, disorders of, 21–34
approach to diagnosis of, 22
Boeck's sarcoid, 24
chronic nephritis, 30
Cushing's syndrome, 29
hyperparathyroidism, 32
hypoparathyroidism, 33
hypovitaminosis D, 25
malabsorption syndrome, 26
malnutrition, 23
metastatic carcinoma of bone, 29
nephrotic syndrome, 27
pseudopseudohypoparathyroidism, 34
renal tubular acidosis, 31
normal metabolism of, 21–22
urine, in serum calcium disorders, 23–26, 30–33
Calculi, 196, 197
Calymmatobacterium granulomatis, 285
Candida albicans, 285, 288, 297
Candidiasis, 282
Capillaries, abnormal, 269
disorders of, 270, 271
Capillary blood flow, pulmonary, 131, 133
Capillary fragility, in hemostasis disorders, 262, 263, 269, 270, 272, 274, 276
Carbohydrates, 40, 44
in blood glucose disorders, 60, 61, 74
in diabetes mellitus, 111
in triglyceride production, 102
Carbon dioxide
in blood, 131
blood electrolytes and, 37
in blood oxygen content disorders, 132, 135, 136, 142
impaired excretion of, in pulmonary emphysema, 47
partial pressure of, 132
in pulmonary emphysema, 47
in salicylate toxicity, 48
Carbon monoxide, toxic levels of, 177
Carbon tetrachloride, in blood and urine, 177
Carbonic acid, 37, 43
Carbonic anhydrase, 53
Carbuncles, 279, 299
Carcinoembryonic antigen, 202
Carcinoid tumors, malignant, 173
Carcinoma, cytologic examination for, 199
islet cell, 74
of bone, metastatic, 29
of cervix and endometrium, 299
of colon, 299
of liver, metastatic, 12, 204, 205
of lung, 299
of pancreas, 10, 18, 299
of stomach, 299
prostatic, metastatic, 6
Cardiac failure. *See* Heart failure.
Cardiolipin, 290
Cat-scratch fever, 281
Catecholamines, urinary, 171–172
Catheterization, 190
Celiac disease, 173, 299
See also Malabsorption syndrome.
Cell(s). *See also* Red cells; White cells.
band, 236, 241
damage to, producing, 249
immature, in leukemias, 240, 241
L.E., 249
mononuclear, 196
Cell counts, in spinal tap, 297
Cell study, of body fluids, 195–196
Cellulitis, tests in management of, 299
Central nervous system disorders, 188, 198
Cephalin-cholesterol flocculation, 144, 147
positive, 16, 17
Cerebral abscess, 299
Cerebral embolism, 299
Cerebral hemorrhage, of, 299
Cerebrosides, 101, 110
Cerebrospinal fluid. *See also* spinal fluid.
blood in, 195
cholesterol and bilirubin in, 199
clotting of, 193
microorganisms in, 288
specimen of, 190–191, 193
volume of, 191
white cells in, 196
Cerebro-vascular diseases, 199
Ceruloplasmin, in Wilson's disease, 172
Cervical cultures, 297
Cervical discharge, specimen of, 190
Cervix, carcinoma of, 299
Cestodiasis, intestinal, 282
Chagas' disease, 282
Chancre, soft, 279
Charcot-Leyden crystals, 197
Chemistry graph, serum-, 201
Chievitz and Meyer cough plant, 284
Chloride, as blood electrolyte, 35
in pulmonary emphysema, 47
spinal fluid, 199
Chlorpromazine hepatitis, 11, 19
Chlorothiazide diuretics, 53
Cholecystitis, tests in management of, 299
Choledocholithiasis, amylase and lipase in, 170–71
Cholelithiasis, tests in management of, 299
Cholera, 279
Cholestasis, extrahepatic, 20
intrahepatic, 11, 16, 19
Cholesterol, as body lipid, 101–103
excretion of, blocked, 18
in autoanalyzer profiles, 202, 206 ,208
in diet, 103
in esterified form, 101, 102, 113
normal serum total, 102
in serum lipids disorders, 105, 107–109, 112–116, 118
serum, in cirrhosis, 17
Chondrosarcomas, 8
Chorionic gonadotropin, 81, 97, 98
Chorionephithelioma, 98, 99
Chromosome, Philadelphia, 241
Chromium-tagged red cell excretion test, 194
Chromium-tagged red cell survival test, 222
Chylomicrons, 115
Cirrhosis,
of liver, advanced, 64
blood urea nitrogen in, 123
hemostasis in, 275
Laennec's, 17
autoanalyzer on, 202, 203
serum magnesium in, 174–175
red cells in, 232
portal, lipids in, 109
plasma proteins in, 147
postnecrotic and biliary, 147
tests in management of, 300
Circulation time, arm-to-tongue, 298
Clay-Adams, microhematocrit, 293
Clearance
creatinine, endogenous, 181
renal and standard urea, 181
Clostridia, 288
Clostridium botulinum, 289
Clot retraction, 259
defective, 262, 263
Clot retraction activity, 257
Clotting, of body fluids, 193
platelets in, 257
Clotting time, in hemostasis disorders, 267
of office laboratory, 294
Coagulation, bleeding due to disorders in 194, 195
disorders in, 258
disseminated intravascular, 260
stages in, 258–259
disorders in, 264–268
Coagulation factors, 257–259
disorders of, 264–269
Cobalt, radioactive, 183
Coccidiodomycosis, 282, 292
Coccidioides, 286
Colchicine therapy, 165
Colitis, ulcerative,
serum magnesium in, 174
tests in management of, 302
Collagen disorders, 167
Collagenous cement substance, 272
Collagenous diseases, 196
Colloidal gold test, 198
Colon, carcinoma of, 299
Colorimeter, 201, 293
Colorado tick fever, 281
Coma, tests for, 316
Common bile duct. *See* Bile duct.
Common cold, 281
Communicable Disease Center, 291
Competitive binding, 186
Concentration test, 182
Congestive heart failure. *See* Heart failure.
Conjunctiva, microorganisms in, 288
Connective tissue abnormality, 276
Convulsions, 309
Cooley's anemia, 15
Coombs' test, 222, 225, 230
Copper, plasma, 172
Copper metabolism, disorders of, 172–173
Coproporphyrin, 175, 177

Corticosteroids, in Cushing's syndrome, 92
Cortisol, 76, 77, 79, 80
excessive, 28
fatty acids and, 103
Corynebacterium diphtheria, 286
Costovertebral joints, 137
Cough, 309
Cough plate, Chievitz and Meyer, 284
Coulter Counter, 210
Cr_{51} quantitation of blood loss, 183
Creatine, 119, 121, 126
Creatine phosphokinase, disorders involving, 157, 160
normal metabolism, 155
Creatinine, 119
in autoanalyzer profiles, 124
in blood nonprotein nitrogen substances, 124, 126–129
Creatinine clearance, 181
Crossmatching, of blood, 226, 229
Cryptococcal organisms, 196
Cryptococci, 289
Cryptococcus neoformans, 285
Culture media, 286
Cultures and smears, 278–289
for bacteria, 296–297
performance of, 284–286
tables on, 279–283
Curschmann spirals, 196
Cushing's syndrome, 28, 68, 80, 248
Cutler-Power-Wilder test, 49
Cystic fibrosis, 197
Cysticercosis, 283
Cystinuria, 198

de Toni-Fanconi syndrome, 66
Dehydration, 39
Dehydroepiandrosterone, 76, 77
Dehydrogenases. *See* Lactic dehydrogenases.
Dengue, 281
Denver classification, 241
Deoxyribonucleic acid, 215
Dermatomyositis, 160
Destruction in metabolism, blood glucose, 58
of erythrocytes, 210, 222–226, 230
of leukocytes, 237, 249
of plasma proteins, 143
Detoxification, in metabolism of nonprotein nitrogen substances, 119
Dexamethasone suppression test, 93
Diabetes, blood chemistry for, 295
diagnosis of, 59
urine specific gravity in, 192–193
urine volume in various types of, 191
Diabetes insipidus, 50, 182
Diabetes mellitus, blood glucose in, 75
lipids in, 111
primary or symptomatic, 198
tests in management of, 300
Diabetic acidosis, 40, 56–57, 111
Diabetic glomerulosclerosis, 167
Diagnex Blue test, 192
Dialyzer, 200
Diaphoresis, 45
Diarrhea, 44, 191, 193, 296
laboratory work-up of symptoms, 309–310
Dicumarol therapy, 265
Digitalis toxicity, 177
Digoxin, 177
Diplococcus pneumoniae, 284
Diphtheria, 279
Disaccharides, 198
Diseases. *See also* Bacterial infections; Infectious diseases.
laboratory work-up of, 319–329
Disseminated intravascular coagulation, 260
Diuretics, 52, 53, 167
DNA, 215
Donath-Landsteiner test, 225
Dopamine, 171
Drugs. *See also* Antibiotics; Morphine.
as cause of hyperglycemia, 75
Dubin-Johnson syndrome, 13
Duffy factor, 226
Duodenal fluids, 199
crystals in, 197
mucoproteins in, 197
obtaining specimen of, 190
pH of, 192
volume of, 191
Duodenal ulcer, 171. *See also* Ulcer.
Duodenum, in intestinal obstruction, 171
Dysentery, 279
Dysmenorrhea, 405–406
Dysphagia, 310
Dyspnea, 310
Dysproteinemia, 149

Ear, microorganisms in, 288
Echinococcosis, 283
Eclampsia, acute, 204
Edema, 310–311
Ehlers-Danlos syndrome, 276
Ehrlich's reagent, 177
Elastic fibers, and casts, 196
Electrophoresis
hemoglobin, 223
lipoprotein, 103, 115–118
paper, 144
Electrolytes, blood, 35–57
disorders of, acute renal failure, 46
adrenal cortical insufficiency, 49
chlorothiazide diuretics, 53
chronic renal failure, 55
dehydration, 39
diabetes insipidus, 50
diabetic acidosis, 56–57
diarrhea, 44
diagnostic approach to, 37–38
malabsorption syndrome, 41
mercurial diuretics, 53
pathological diaphoresis, 45
primary aldosteronism, 51
pulmonary emphysema, 47
pyloric obstruction, 43
renal tubular acidosis, 53
salicylate toxicity, 48
starvation, 40
in normal metabolism, 35–37
Ellsworth-Howard test, 33
Embolism, pulmonary, 140, 189
Emphysema, pulmonary, 47, 136, 151
tests in management of, 300
Empyema, 198
Encephalitis, 281, 282
Endo, 296
Endocarditis, subacute bacterial, 280, 288
tests in management of, 302
Endocrine system, 76. *See also* Hormones.
and radioactive isotopes, 186
Endogenous creatinine clearance, 181
Endometrium, carcinoma of, 299
Entamoeba histolytica, 285
Enteritis, 289
Enterobiasis, 283
Enterobius vermicularis, 285
Enterococci, 289
Enzymes, disorders of, 155–69
Eosinopenia, 248
Eosinophil, 236
Eosinophilia, 238, 245, 247, 252, 255
Epilepsy, 300
Epinephrine, 171
fatty acids and, 103
glucose and, 59
Epistaxis, 311
Epsilon-amino-caproic acid, 259
"Erlenmeyer flask" deformity, 244
Erythroblastosis fetalis, 230, 300
Erythrocytes. *See also* red cells.
disorders of, 212–235
acquired hemolytic anemia, 225
acute myeloblastic leukemia, 231
approach to diagnosis of, 212
bleeding peptic ulcer, 219, 220
chronic congestive splenomegaly, 233
cirrhosis of liver, 232
erythroblastosis fetalis, 230
hemolytic transfusion reactions, 226–229
hereditary spherocytosis, 222
hypochromic anemia, 213
idiopathic aplastic anemia, 217
idiopathic steatorrhea, 214
in leukocyte disorders, 243
myelophthisic anemia, 216
pernicious anemia, 223
polycythemia vera, 218
sickle cell anemia, 223
simple chronic anemia, 235
thalassemia major, 224
in normal metabolism, 210–211
Erythropoiesis, 210
Erythropoietin, 173, 174, 211
Escherichia coli, 285, 286, 288
Esophagitis, 300
Esters, cholesterol, 101, 102
Estrogens, 76, 77, 79, 81, 96, 103
Ethyl alcohol, in blood and urine, 177
Excretion. *See also* secretion.
disorders of, 18–20
in normal metabolism and in disorders, blood electrolytes, 36–37, 46–48
blood glucose, 58, 66
blood oxygen, 131
blood oxygen content, 132, 135–137
hormones, 77
lipids, 103, 112
plasma proteins, 144, 154
phosphatases, 3, 10–11

Excretion (*Cont.*)
serum bilirubin, 13, 18–20
serum calcium, 21, 30, 31
transaminases, 161
uric acid, 163, 167–169
of leukocytes, 237
Expiration, 130
Extrahepatic cholestasis, 20
Extravascular resistance, to bleeding, 257
Exudates, specific gravity of, 193

Familial idiopathic dysproteinemia, 148
Fanconi syndrome, 31, 169
Farber test, 196
Fat(s). absorption of, 101–102
in body fluids, 197
in diet, 103
in malabsorption syndrome, 26
deposits of, 110
fecal, 102
stored, 102
Fatigue, 311
Fatty acids, 101–103
Feces. *See also* stools.
blood in, 194–195
fat in, 102
in absence of bilirubin, 14
in hereditary spherocytosis, 15
pus in, 196
specimen of, 190, 193
volume of, 191
Ferritin, 174
Fetus, in erythroblastosis fetalis, 230
Fever, of unknown origin, 311–312
Fibers, elastic or muscle, 196
Fibrinogen, 258–260, 268
Fibrinogenopenia, 268
Fibrinolysins, 260, 268
Fibrometer, 294–295
Filariasis, 283
Fishberg concentration test, 182, 296
Flora, normal, 287–288
Fluids. *See also* body fluids in water.
loss of, in pyloric obstruction, 43
of gastrointestinal tract, 35–36
Fluorescein string test, 194
Fluorescent treponemal antibody test, 290
Fluorine-16, 189
Folic acid, 210
deficiency of, 214
Folin-Wu method, 58
Follicle-stimulating hormone, 76, 77, 79, 81, 86, 100
Food poisoning, 279
Formiminoglutamic acid, 214
Fractionation, 144
Fungi, diseases caused by, 282
harmless, 289
list of, 285

Galactose, 63
Galactosemia, 63
Galactoside, 110
Gallstones, 20
Gametocytes, 285
Gamma globulins, 143, 144, 147–150. *See also* Globulins.
Gamma glutamyl transpeptidase, 16
Ganglioneuromas, 171–172
Ganglionic tissue, 171
Gastric analysis, in office laboratory, 297
overnight, 192–193
Gastric anemia, 212
Gastric juice, bloody, 194
in pyloric obstruction, 43
mucoproteins in, 199
obtaining specimen of, 190
appearance of, 193–194
pH of, 192
volume of, 191
Gastric secretions, 35, 36
Gastric ulcer, 122
Gastric washings, 284
Gastrointestinal bleeding,
analysis of, 194
lower, 195
tests for, 183
upper, 194–195
Gastrointestinal tract, isotopes in disorders of, 183
Gaucher's disease, 6, 110, 244
Geiger-Mueller tube, 186
General paresis, spinal fluid proteins in, 198
Giant-cell tumors, 8
Giemsa stain, 196
Gilbert's syndrome, 15
Glander's disease, 279
Glanzmann's disease, 263
Glitter cells, 195
Globin portion of hemoglobin, 13
Globulin(s). *See also* Gamma Globulin.
abnormal, 153
alpha-1, 151
antihemophilic, 264
plasma proteins and, 143, 144
in disorders of, 145–149, 152–154
Glomerular filtrate, 36, 37
Glomerular filtration, 180–181
Glomerular nephritis, 50
Glomerulitis, 196
Glomerulonephritis, acute, 182
casts and, 196
chronic, autoanalyzer profile on, 208
nonprotein nitrogen substances in, 128
uric acid in, 167
proteinuria in, 197
tests in management of, 300
white cells in urine in, 195
Glomerulosclerosis, 167
Glomerulus, 180, 196
Glucagon, 59
Glucocorticoids, in Cushing's syndrome,
lack of, 67
Glucose. *See also* Hyperglycemia; Hypoglycemia; Sugar, Blood.
blood, disorders of, 58–75
acromegaly, 70
Addison's disease, 67
advanced cirrhosis of liver, 64
chronic pancreatitis, 73
Cushing's syndrome, 68
diagnosis of, 59
galactosemia, 63
in diabetic acidosis, 56
idiopathic steatorrhea, 61
islet cell adenoma, 74
malnutrition, 60
pheochromocytoma, 72
renal glycosuria, 66
tachyalimentation hypoglycemia, 62
in normal metabolism, 58–59
in urine and spinal fluid, 198
Glucose-6-phosphatase, 65
Glucose tolerance test, 69, 61
Glutamic-oxalactic transaminase, 155
Glutamic-pyruvic transaminase, 155
Glycerol, in body lipids, 101, 102
Glycine, 175
Glycogen, liver, 58
Glycogen-storage disease, 65, 111
Glycogenalysis, 65
faster than glycolysis, 71
Glycosuria, 59, 68, 73, 198
renal, 66
Glycouronide conjugation system, 13
Gold test, colloidal, 198
Gonadotropins. *See also* Specific Gonadotropins.
chorionic, 81, 97, 98
secretion of, 76, 79
urinary, 81, 86, 94, 96, 99, 100
Gonococci, 284, 288
Gonocult, 284, 297
Gonadal dysfunction, 129
Gonorrhea, 279, 291, 300
Gout, 297
crystals in synovial fluid in, 197
tests in management of, 300
uric acid in, 165
Gram stain, 296
Granular motility cells, 195
Granules, cytoplasmic, 195
Granulocytes, 236
in leukocyte disorders, 254, 256
Granuloma inguinale, 279, 285
Growth hormone, 59, 70, 81, 103
Guaiac test, 194, 195
Guanidinoacetic acid, 119
Guillian-Barre's syndrome, 189
Guthrie test, 175

HAA, 159
Haemophilus ducreyi, 285
Haemophilus influenzae, 285
Hamman-Rich syndrome, 138, 300
Hand-Schüller-Christian disease, 110
Hansen's disease, 279
Hartnup disease, 198
Headache, 312
Heart failure, 158
congestive, blood electrolytes in, 42
blood oxyen content in, 141
blood urea and creatinine in, 124
chronic, mononuclear cells in, 196
test for, 298
tests in management of, 300
Heating bath, 201
Heboglobinemia, 225
Heinz bodies, 225
Hematemesis, 219, 312
Hematest, 195, 296
Hematocrit, 212
in erythrocyte disorders, 213, 215, 218, 220-224, 226, 230

Hematocrit (*Cont.*)
in office laboratory, 293
leukocytes and, 238
Hematology, in office laboratory, 293
Hematuria, 194, 313
Heme, 13
Hemochromatosis, 174
Hemocytometer, 293
Hemoglobin, 131
disintegration of, 13
in erythrocyte disorders, 213, 215, 218, 220–224, 226, 230
in office laboratory, 293
iron as, 174
leukocytes and, 238
Hemoglobin test, 212
Hemoglobin electrophoresis, 223
Hemoglobinometer, Sahli, 293
Hemolysis, severe, 15
Hemolytic anemias, 14, 174, 249
tests in management of, 300
Hemophilia, 264, 269
Hemopoietic disturbances, 6
Hemopoietic system, radioactive isotopes in diagnosis involving, 183, 186
Hemoproteins, 175, 177
Hemoptysis, 309
Hemorrhagic disease, 266
Hemosiderin, 174
Hemosiderosis, 174
Hemostasis, disorders of, 259–277
acute leukemia, 274
abruptio placentae, 268
anaphylactoid purpura, 270
cirrhosis of the liver, 275
diagnosis of, 259–261
Dicumarol therapy, 265
Ehlers-Danlos syndrome, 276
hemophilia A, 264
hemorrhagic disease, 266
heparin therapy and, 273
hereditary hemorrhagic thrombasthenia, 263
hereditary hemorrhagic telangiectasia, 271
idiopathic thrombocytopenic purpura, 262
obstructive jaundice, 267
polycythemia vera, 277
scurvy, 272
vascular hemophilia, 269
normal mechanisms of, 257–259
Henoch-Schönlein purpura, 270
Heparin, and lipids, 103
Heparin therapy, 273
Hepatic disease, 177
See also Hepatitis; Liver.
Hepatic dysfunction, constitutional, 15
Hepatic necrosis, 159
Hepatic parenchymal disease, 14
Hepatitis, chlorpromaxine, 11, 19
diagnosis of, 281
"serum", 159
tests in management of, 300
viral, 11, 16, 192, 159, 202
Hepatomas, primary, 12
Hepatomegaly, 3
Hereditary spherocytosis, 15
Herpangina, 281
Herpes zoster, 282
Heterophile agglutination test, 253
Hickey-Hare test, 50
Histalog, 190
Histamine, 190
Histamine-resistant achlorhydria, 215
Histoplasma organisms, 286
Histoplasmosis, 282, 284, 291, 292
Hodgkin's disease, 245, 300
Homogentisic acid oxidase, 175
Homovanillic acid, 172
Hookworm disease, 283
Hormones, disorders of, 76–100
adrenal, 90–93
diagnosis of, 79–82
ovarian, 94–96
pituitary, 83–86
thyroid, 87–89
functions of, 76
in chorionepithelioma, 98
in Klinefelter's syndrome, 100
in normal metabolism, 76–79
in pregnancy, 97
plasma proteins and, 144
seminoma and, 99
Human pituitary gonadotropin, 77
Hydatidiform mole, 98
Hydrogen ion, 37, 43
17-Hydroxycorticosteroids, 77, 80, 81
urinary, 84–86, 90, 92, 97
5-Hydroxyindoleacetic acid, disorders of, 172–73
Hypergammaglobulinemia, 152
Hyperglycemia, 59, 62, 73, 75
Hyperlipemia, familial, 103
Hyperlipoproteinemia, types I, II, III, and IV, 115–117
Hyperparathyroidism, 32
in serum calcium disorders, 22, 26, 30–32
primary, 9, 206
tests in management of, 300
Hypertension, consistent, catecholamines in, 171
essential, 300
tests for, 313
Hyperthyroidism, 71
as thyroid hormone disorder, 87
nonprotein nitrogen substances in, 129
radioactive isotopes in tests for, 186
tests in management of, 301
Hypogammaglobulinemia, 150
Hypoglycemia, cerebrospinal fluid sugar in, 198
in Laennec's cirrhosis, 17
tachyalimentation, 62
Hypogonadism, 86
Hypokalemia, 41
Hyponatremia, 41, 42
Hypoparathyroidism, 33, 34
serum magnesium in, 174
Hypoplasia, 223
Hypoproteinemia, 27
Hypoprothrombinemia, 274
Hypothalamus, and hormone regulation, 77, 79
Hypothyroidism, lipids in, 113
radioactive isotopes in tests for, 186
red cells in, 234
tests in management of, 301
Hypovitaminosis D, 25
Hypovolemic shock, 125
Hypoxanthine-guanine phosphoribosyl transferase, 165

I^{131} rose bengal, 188
Icterus praecox, 230
Idiopathic steatorrhea
blood glucose in, 61
folic acid deficiency in, 214
lipids in, 106
plasma proteins in, 146
Idiopathic thrombocytopenic purpura, platelets in, 262
Immunoelectrophoresis, 144, 153
Immunoglobulins, 153
Immunological tests, 297
Inclusion body, 249
Infarction, myocardial. *See* Myocardial infarction.
pulmonary, 162, 195
Infections, bacterial. *See* Bacterial infections.
hemolytic anemia as, 225
viral, acute, 250
white cells in, 195–196
Infectious diseases, laboratory diagnosis of, 278–292. *See also* Bacterial infections; Laboratory, diagnosis of infectious diseases in.
Infectious mononucleosis, 253, 281, 291
tests in management of, 301
Inflammation, white cells in, 195–196
Influenza, 281
Inhibin, 100
Inoculation, animal, 279–283, 286, 289–290
Inspired air, 132–133
Inspired gas, 131
Inspiration, 130
Insulin, glucose and, 58
in chronic pancreatitis, 73
in diabetic acidosis, 56
in diabetes mellitus, 75
in islet cell adenoma, 74
in synthesis of fatty acids, 103
Insulin radioimmunoassay, 59
Intestinal cells, and lipids, 101, 102
Intestinal obstruction, amylase and lipase in, 171
Intrahepatic cholestasis, 11, 16, 19
Intravascular resistance, to bleeding, 257–259
Intrinsic factor, 210
of Castle, 215
Inulin, 181
Iodide, 76–77
Iodine, 76–77. *See also* Protein bound iodine.
radioactive, 183, 186
Iron, absorption of, in hypothyroidism, 234
in red cell production, 210
loss of, in menorrhagia, 221
plasma, 174, 217
serum, disorders of, 174
in anemia, 212
in erythrocyte disorders, 213, 215, 235
normal metabolism of, 173–174

Iron-binding capacity, in red cell disorders, 235
Iron-deficiency anemia, 174, 213, 214, 221
  tests in management of, 301
Islet cell adenoma, 74
Islet cell destruction, 73
Islet cell hyperplasia and carcinoma, 74
Islet cells, in diabetes mellitus, 75
Isoagglutinins, 226
Isoenzymes, 155, 157
Isotopes, 183–189

Jaundice, chronic idiopathic, 13
  conjugated bilirubin and, 13
  due to hemolytic anemias, 14
  hepatocellular, 3
  obstructive, 3, 15, 112
    feces in, 14
    hemostasis in, 267
    lipids in, 112
  tests for, 313–314
Joints, pain or swelling of, 314
  synovial fluids of, 191–193

Kala-azar, 283
Kell factor, 226
Ketonemia, 44
Ketones, blood, in early starvation, 105
    in pyloric obstruction, 43
  in diabetic acidosis, 56, 111
17-Ketosteroids, 77, 80, 81
  urinary, in Addison's disease, 90
  in adrenogenital syndrome, 93
  in Cushing's syndrome, 91
  in polycystic ovaries, 95
  of hormonal disorders, 84–86
Kidneys. *See also* Renal.
  in control of body fluid, 36–37
  in diabetic acidosis, 56
  infections of, proteinuria in, 197
  in urine formation, 180
Kimmelsteil-Wilson's disease, 197
King-Armstrong units, 3
Klebsiella, 285
Klinefelter's syndrome, 100
Krebs cycle, 58
Kohlmer test, 290
Kulchitsky cells, 172, 173
Kyphoscoliosis, 137

Laboratory, diagnosis of infectious diseases in, 278–292. *See also* Bacterial Infections.
    animal inoculation, 289–290
    serologic tests, 290–291
    smears and cultures, 278–289
    tables on, 279–283, 287
  office, 293–298
  tests in, disorders requiring, 299–302
  use of, in office practice, 304
  work-up in, of diseases, 319–329
    of symptoms, 307–318
Lactase deficiency, 198
Lactic dehydrogenases, disorders of, 155, 157–62
Laennec's cirrhosis of the liver, 17, 174–175, 202, 203
Langhans cells, 97
Lead, toxic levels of, 177
Lead intoxication, 225
Lead poisoning, porphyrins in, 175, 177
Leishmania donovani, 285
Leprosy, 279, 292
Leptospira, 289
Lesch-Nyhan syndrome, 165
Leucine aminopeptidase, 155
Leukemia, acute, hemostasis in, 274
    leukocytes in, 240
  acute myeloblastic, 231
  aleukemic variety of, 231
  chronic lymphocytic, 242
  chronic myelogenous, 241, 256
  serum and uric acid in, 166
  tests in management of, 301
Leukocytes, 236–256. *See also* White Cells.
  disorders of, 238–256
    acute bacterial infectious, 251
    acute leukemia, 240
    acute viral infections, 250
    Addison's disease, 247
    agnogenic myeloid metaplasia, 256
    agranulocytosis, 254
    chronic bacterial infections, 252
    chronic lymphocytic leukemia, 242
    chronic myelogenous leukemia, 241
    Cushing's syndrome, 248
    diagnosis of, 238
    Gaucher's disease, 244
    infectious mononucleosis, 253
    lupus erythematosus, 249
    trichinosis, 255
    Waldenström's macroglobulinemia, 246
  metabolism of, 236–237
  multilobulated, 215
Leukocytosis,
  in leukocyte disorders, 251, 253
  in red cell disorders, 218, 219, 223, 224, 230, 231
Leukopenia, 214–216, 233, 244, 249, 250
Leukopoiesis, 236
Leydig cells, 100
Linoleic acid, 101
Linolenic acid, 101
Lipase, disorders of, 170–171
Lipids, serum,
  disorders of, 103–118
    acanthocytosis, 114
    approach to diagnosis of, 103–104
    diabetes mellitus, 111
    early starvation, 105
    hypothyroidism, 113
    idiopathic steatorrhea, 106
    malnutrition, 107
    nephrotic syndrome, 108
    obstructive jaundice, 112
    portal cirrhosis, 109
    type I hyperlipoproteinemias, 115–118
    with normal blood lipids, 110
    xanthoma disseminatum, 110
  in normal metabolism, 101–103
  nature of, 101–103
Lipoprotein electrophoresis, 103, 115–118
Lipoproteinemia, 144, 295
Lipoproteins, 102
  in lipid disorders, 107–109, 112, 114–118
Listeriosis, 279
Liver. *See also* Hepatic Disease; Hepatitis.
  cirrhosis of. *See* Cirrhosis.
  glucose and, 58
  hormones and, 77
  in serum bilirubin disorders, 13–14
  in viral hepatitis, 159
  metastatic carcinoma of, 12, 204, 205
Liver profile, 3
Liver scanning, 188
Lumbar punctures, 191
Lung(s), blood oxygen and, 131
  carcinoma of, 299
  in regulation of body fluids, 37
  in respiration, 132
  "malabsorption syndrome" of, 138
  scanning of, 189
  scleroderma of, 138
  total capacity of, 132
Lung capacity, total, 132
    in blood oxygen content disorders, 135–137, 141
Lupus erythematosus, 249, 291
Luteinizing hormone, 76, 77, 79, 81, 86
Lymph nodes, in Hodgkin's disease, 245
Lymph tissue, hypertrophied, 148
Lymphadenopathy, 314–315
Lymphoblast, 236, 240
Lymphocytes, 236, 237
  atypical, 253
  in leukocyte disorders, 242
Lymphocytosis
  atypical, 246
  in leukocyte disorders, 247, 252
Lymphogranuloma venereum, 281, 292
Lymphopenia, 248, 249
Lymphosarcoma, 245

Macrocytosis, 234
Macroglobulinemia, 153, 246
Magnesium, serum, disorders of, 174–175
  normal metabolism of, 174
Majocchi's disease, 270
Malabsorption syndrome, 26
  as serum calcium disorders, 26
  blood electrolytes in, 41
  of lung, 138
  radioactive isotopes in diagnosis of, 183
  severe, autoanalyzer profile on, 206, 207
Malaria, 225, 283, 301
Malarial parasites, 285
Malnutrition. *See also* Starvation.
  blood glucose in, 60
  lipids in, 107
  serum calcium in, 23
Maple sugar urine disease, 198
Marihuana, 177
Maximum acid output test, 192
Maximum breathing capacity, 132

Mazzini flocculation test, 290
Measles, 281
Media, culture, 286
Megaloblasts, 210
Melanin metabolism disorders, 175
Melanotic sarcoma, 175
Melena, 219, 312
Melituria, 66
Meniere's disease, 301
Meningitis, acute bacterial and viral, 196
  aseptic, 289
  bacterial, 198
    tuberculous and, 198
  cerebrospinal fluid in, 193
  tests in management of, 301
Meningococcal disease, 279
Menopausal syndrome, 96
Menorrhagia, chronic, 221
Menstrual bleeding, 221
Menstruation, 195
  iron and, 173, 174
Mercurial diuretics, 52
Merozoites, 285
Metabolic degradation, 171
Metabolism. *See also* storage, in metabolism.
  of amylase and lipase, 170
  of blood electrolytes, 35–37
  of blood glucose, 58
  of blood nonprotein nitrogen substances, 119–120
  of blood oxygen, 130–131
  of copper, 172
  of erythrocytes, 210–211
  of hormones, 76–79
  of iron, 173–174
  of leukocytes, 236–237
  of magnesium, serum, 174–175
  of melanin, 175
  of plasma proteins, 143–144
  of porphyrin, 175, 177
  of serum lipids, 101–103
  phosphatases in, 3
  serum bilirubin in, 13–14, 16–17
  of uric acid, 163
  spinal fluid proteins in, 198
  transaminases, 155–156
Metamyelocyte, 236
Metastases, osteoblastic, 5
Metastatic bone tumors, 5
Metastatic carcinoma of liver, 12
Metastatic liver disease, 3
Metastatic prostatic carcinoma, 6
Metyrapone test, 85
Microorganisms, in body tissues and fluid, in, 287–288
Microscopic examination of urine, 295–296
Mimeae, 289
Monoblast, 236
Monocytes, 236, 252
Mononucleosis, infectious, 253, 281, 291, 301
Monosticon kit, 297
Monotube, 297
Morphine, 161, 171
Mucin, 193
Mucormycosis, 282
Multiphasic screening of asymptomatic patients, 303–304
Multiple myeloma, 153, 204, 205, 243
Multiple sclerosis, 198
Mumps, 171, 281
Murphy-Pattee test, 80, 186
Muscle catabolism, 129
Muscle disease, 155, 160
Muscle fibers, and casts, 196
Muscular dystrophies, creatine and creatinine in, 126
  enzymes in, 155
Myasthenia gravis, tests in management of, 301
Mycobacterium smegmatis, 288
Mycobacterium tuberculosis, 292
Myeloblast, 236, 240
Myelocyte, 236, 241
Myeloid metaplasia, agnogenic, 256
Myelofibrosis, 216
Myeloma, multiple, 153, 204, 205, 243
Myelophthisis, 231
Myocardial infarction, creatine phosphokinases in, 156
  differentiated from cardiac failure, 158
  tests in management of, 301
  transaminases and dehydrogenases in, 156
Myoglobin, 174
Myxedema, 89
  autoanalyzer profile on, 206, 207
  radioactive I^{131} uptake in, 186

Nasopharynx, cultures of, 278
  microorganisms in, 287
Neck pain, 315
Neisseria gonorrhoeae, 284
Neisseria meningitidis, 284–285
Neoplasms. *See also* Tumors.
  of brain and spinal cord, 196
Nephritis, chronic, 30
    specific gravity of urine in, 192
    tubular reabsorption in, 182
  glycosuria in, 66
  toxic, 167
Nephrotic syndrome, autoanalyzer profile on, 208, 209
  casts in, 196
  ceruloplasmin in, 172
  plasma proteins in, 154
  serum calcium disorder, 27
  serum lipid disorder, 108
  tests in management of, 301
Nervous system, disorders of, 188
Neuroblastoma, and urinary catecholamines, 171–172
Neutrophilia, 248
Neutrophils, 195, 214, 236, 237, 250–252
Newborn, erythroblastosis fetalis and, 230, 300
  hemorrhagic disease of, 266
  intestinal obstruction of, 196
Nitrogen, urea, blood and urine, 121–124, 125, 127, 128
Nitrogen-emptying rate, 132
Nitrogenous substances, blood nonprotein disorders of, 121–129
    chronic glomerulonephritis, 128
    cirrhosis of the liver, 123
    congestive heart failure, 124
    gastric ulcer, bleeding, 122
    hyperthyroidism, 129
    hypovolemic shock, 125
    muscular dystrophies, 126
    obstructive uropathy, 127
    starvation, 121
  in normal metabolism, 119–120
Nocardia, 285
Nocardiosis, 282
Nodules, "hot" and "cold," in scanning, 186, 188, 189
Nonprotein nitrogenous substances. *See* Nitrogenous substances.
Norepinephrine, 171
Normal values, 305–306
Normoblasts, 210, 223, 225, 231
Nucleic acid, 163
  white cell, 166
Obstructive jaundice. *See* Jaundice.
Obstructive uropathy, 127
Occultest pads, 296
Office laboratory. *See* Laboratory.
Office practice, use of laboratory in, 304
Oleic acid, 101
Onchoceriasis, 283
Opiates, 171
Organs, relative innocuous nonspecific tests of, 330–332
Ornithine cycle, 119
Oroya fever, 279
Orthochromic normoblast, 210
Osmolality, urine, 192
Osmoreceptor-aldosterone system, 39
Osteitis deformans, 7
Osteoblastic activity, alkaline phosphatases and, 3, 5, 7, 9
  serum calcium and, 22
Osteoblastic metastases, 5
Osteoblasts, 208
Osteogenic sarcoma, 7, 8
Osteolytic lesions, 24
Osteomalacia, 9
Osteoporosis, 28
Ovarian hormones, disorders of, 81, 93–96
Ovaries, 81
  arrhenoblastomas of, 95
  polycystic, 93, 95
Ovum, in stool, 296
Oxygen, blood, normal metabolism of, 130–131
Oxygen content, of blood, disorders of, 130–142
    ankylosing spondylitis, 137
    asthmatic bronchitis, 135
    barbiturate intoxication, 142
    congestive heart failure, 141
    diagnosis of, 131–134
    pulmonary embolism, 140
    pulmonary emphysema, 136
    pulmonary hemangioma, 139
    sarcoidosis, 138
Oxygen saturation, in blood, 131–133
  oxygen disorders, 135, 136, 138–142
Oxygen test, single-breath, 132–133

Paget's disease, 7
Palmitoleic acid, 101
Pancreas, carcinoma of, 73, 170, 299
    of head of, 10, 18, 202

Pancreas (*Cont.*)
disease of, 26
Pancreatic juice, 190
Pancreatic scanning, 189
Pancreatitis, acute, 161, 170
chronic, 73, 146, 170, 183, 199, 296, 301
Pancytopenia, 217
Panhypopituitarism, 85
Papanicolaou smears, 199
Paper electrophoresis, 144
Paracentesis, 191
Paragonimiasis, 283
Parasites, in stool, 296
intracellular, 225
list of, 285–286
laboratory diagnosis of, 282–283
Parathyroid activity, in rickets and osteomalacia, 9
Parathyroid hormone, in serum calcium metabolism, 21–23
disorders of, 32
Parenchymal diseases, 128
Parotitis, infective, amylase level in, 171
Parrot fever, 281
Parthormone, radioimmunoassay of, 32
Pasteurella pestis, 289
Pasteurella tularensis, 289
PBI. *See* Protein-bound iodine.
Peptic ulcer. *See* Ulcer.
Peritoneal effusion, microorganisms in, 288
Peritoneal fluids, 195, 199
bilirubin and amylase in, 199
proteins in, 197
pus in, 196
specimen of, 190–191, 284
appearance of, 194
volume of, 191
Peritonitis, acute, 196
Pernicious anemia. *See* Anemia.
Pertussis, 284
pH, blood, 37
in salicylate toxicity, 48
of specimens, 192–193
Pharyngitis, 279
Phenistix, 175, 178
Pheochromocytoma, 72, 171
Phenosulfophthalein, in tubular secretion, 182
Phenothiazines, urine test for, 177–178
Phenylalanine hydroxylase, 175
Phenylketonuria, 175
amino acids in, 198
Phenylpyruvic acid, 175
Philadelphia chromosome, 241
Phlebitis. *See* Thrombophlebitis.
Phosphatases, serum alkaline, 3
in autoanalyzer profiles, 202, 204, 206, 208
in serum calcium disorders, 22–26, 29–32, 34
disorders of, 3–12
carcinoma of head of pancreas, 10
chlorpromazine hepatitis, 11
metastatic bone tumors, 5
metastatic carcinoma of liver, 12
metastatic prostatic carcinoma, 6
osteitis deformans, 7
osteogenic sarcoma, 8
rickets and osteomalacia, 9
in normal metabolism, 3
Phosphate(s), serum, in normal metabolism, 21
in serum calcium disorders, 23, 25, 26, 30–33
Phosphate reabsorption test, 32
Phosphatides, 101
Phosphocreatine, 119
Phospholipids, 101–103
in body lipid disorders, 105, 107, 108, 112, 113
Phosphorus, in autoanalyzer profiles, 206, 208
in chronic nephritis, 30
in normal metabolism, 21
Pinta, 280
Pitressin, 50
Pituitary, disease of posterior hormones of, 76, 77, 79
disorders of, 81, 83–86
acromegaly, 83
basophilic adenoma of pituitary, 84
feedback mechanism and, 77
panhypopituitarism, 85
pituitary hypogonadism, 86
Pituitary insufficiency, 69
Placenta, in abruptio placentae, 268
in hormone disorders, 81, 98
in pregnancy, 97
retained parts of, 195
Plasma, in urine formation, 180
Plasma cells, 236, 243
Plasma coagulation factors, 257, 258
Plasma proteins. *See* Proteins.
Plasmoblast, 236–237
Plasmocyte, 237
Plasmodium, 285
Platelet(s), description of, 258
in diagnosing anemia, 212
disorders of, 262–263
in hemostatis, 257–258
leukocytes and, 238, 241, 242, 256
in red cell disorders, 218, 219, 223, 230
Platelet count, in coagulation test, 259
in office laboratory, 294
Pleural effusion, microorganisms in, 288
Pleural fluids, blood in, 195
proteins in, 197
pus in, 196
specimens of, 190–191, 284
appearance of, 194
volume of, 191
Pneumonia(s), 279–280
Easton-agent, 281
primary atypical, 291
sputum in, 196
Pneumoconiosis, tests in management of, 301
Pneumothorax, tests in management of, 301
Poisons. *See* Toxic substances.
Poliomyelitis, 137, 281
Polycythemia, 248
Polycythemia vera, hemostasis in, 277
red cells in, 218
relative and secondary, 218
tests in management of, 301
Porphobilinogen, 175, 177
Porphyria erythropoietica, 177
Porphyria hepatica, acute intermittent type, 177
cutaneous type, 177
Porphyrin metabolism disorders, 175, 177
Portal cirrhosis, 109, 147
Portal hypertension, 233
Potassium, as blood electrolyte, 35
in aldosteronism, 51, 91
in diabetic acidosis, 56
Precornified cells, 96
Pregnancy, abnormal bleeding in, 195
hormones in, 97
iron in, 173
placenta in, 81
tests in management of, 301
toxemia of, 168
Pregnosticon kit, 297
Primaquine sensitivity, 225
Progesterone, 79, 81, 96
Proportioning pump, 200
Prostate, acid phosphatase and, 5, 6
metastatic carcinoma of, 6
Protamine sulfate test, 260, 268
Protein(s), in body fluids, 197
lipid-binding, 102
plasma, 143–154. *See also* Lipoprotein.
disorders of, bacterial infections, 148
hypogammaglobulinemia, 150
idiopathic steatorrhea, 146
multiple myeloma, 153
nephrotic syndrome, 108, 154
portal cirrhosis, 147
starvation, 145
viral hepatitis, 152
methods of study, 144
normal metabolism of, 143–144
serum, in nephrotic syndrome, 27
total, in autoanalyzer profiles, 202, 204, 206, 208
Protein-bound iodine, 77, 79–80
in hormone disorders, 85, 87–89
Protein catabolism, excessive, 129
Protein electrophoresis, 103
Protein moiety of hemoglobin, 13
Proteinuria, 197
Proteus, 288
Proteus vulgaris, 291
Prothrombin, 258–260
plasma, in carcinoma of head of pancreas, 18
Prothrombin consumption, in hemostasis disorders, 264, 273, 275
Prothrombin consumption test, 259
Prothrombin time, in hemostasis disorders, 266–268, 273–275, 277
in office laboratory, 294
test of, 259
Protoporphyrin, 13
Pseudogout, 297
Pseudohypoparathyroidism, 33, 34
Pseudomonas, 288
Pseudopseudohypoparathyroidism, 34
Pseudoxanthoma elasticum, 276
Psittacosis, 281
Pulmonary capillary blood flow, 131, 133

Pulmonary diffusing capacity, 133
Pulmonary embolism
blood oxygen content in, 140
bullae and, 189
Pulmonary emphysema, 47, 136, 151, 300
Pulmonary function tests, 297–298
Pulmonary hemangioma, 139
Pulmonary infarct, 162, 195
Purines, 163
Purpura,
anaphylactoid, 270
idiopathic thrombocytopenic, 262
tests for, 315
Pyelonephritis, proteins in, 198
tests in management of, 301
white cells casts in, 196
white cells in urine in, 195
Pyloric obstruction, blood electrolytes in, 43
Pyridoxine deficiency, 173
Pyuria, 195, 313

Q fever, 280
Queckenstedt test, 191
Quinidine, blood levels for, 178

Rabies, 281
Radioactive I^{131} uptake, 186
Radioactive iodine uptake test, 79, 87
Radioactive isotopes, 183–189
Radioactive PVP test, 197
Radioactive T_3 red cell uptake, 186
Radioactive triolein uptake, 183
Rat-bite fever, 280
Reabsorption, in urine formation, 180
tubular defective, 182
Reagent bottle, 200
Rectal bleeding, 195
Red blood cell fragility test, 222
Red cells. *See also* Erythrocytes.
hemolyzed, 222
in tests using radioactive isotopes, 183, 186
morphologic characteristics of, 210
nucleated, 230
Red cell excretion test, 194
Red cell indices, 212
Red cell survival time, 186
Regintine test, 171
Relapsing fever, 280
Renal. *See also* Kidneys.
Renal calculi, 196
Renal clearance, 181
Renal disease, 59
Renal failure, acute, 46
amylase and lipase in, 171
chronic, 55
Renal function tests, 180–182, 296
Renal glycosuria, 66
Renal plasma flow, 182
Renal tubular acidosis, 53, 54
Renal tubular disease, 182
Renal tubules. *See* Tubules, renal.
Residual volume, in blood oxygen disorders, 135
of air in lungs, 132, 136, 137
Respiration, 37
rate and depth of, 131
system of, four components of, 130
vital capacity in, 132
Respiratory system, radioisotopes in disorders of, 189
Reticulocyte, 210
Reticulocyte count, 212
in red cell disorders, 216, 220, 222–224, 231, 233
Reticulocytosis, in red cell disorders, 226, 230
Reticuloendothelioses, 6
Rh incompatibility, 226, 230
Rheumatic fever, serologic tests for, 290–291
tests in management of, 301–302
Rheumatoid arthritis, 291
Rheumosticon kit, 297
Rickets, 9
Rickettsiae, 280–281
Rickettsial diseases, 291
Robinson-Power-Kepler test, 49
Rocky Mountain spotted fever, 281
Rouleau formation, 243
Rubella, 281
Rumple-Leede test, 295

Salicylate toxicity, 48
Salicylates, 48, 178, 265
Salmonella typhosa, 288
Sarcoidosis, 47, 138
Scabies, 283
Scanning, bone, 189
brain, 188
liver, 188
pancreatic, 189
respiratory system, 189
scintillation, 186
Scarlet fever, 280
Schamberg's disease, 270
Schilling test, 183, 215
Schistosomiasis, vesical, 283
Schizont stage, 285
Scintillation scanning, 186
Scotch tape test for pin worms, 296
Screening tests, of asymptomatic patients, 303–304
Scrub typhus, 281
Scurvy, 272
Secretion. *See also* Excretion.
blood electrolyte, 35–36, 43–45
gastric, 35, 36
into urine, 180
tubular, 182
Sedimentation rate, 144, 295
Semen analysis, 81, 86, 297
Seminiferous tubules,
atrophy and hyalinization of, 100
neoplasm of, 99
Seminoma, 99
Sensitivity report, 289
Sensitivity tests, urine, 296
Serologic tests, 290–291
in diagnosis of infectious diseases, 279–283
Serotonin, 172, 173
Serum acid and alkaline phosphatases. *See* Phosphatases.
Serum bilirubin. *See* Bilirubin.
Serum bilirubin concentration, 13
Serum calcium. *See* Calcium
Serum-chemistry graph, 201
Serum glutamic pyruvic transaminase, 155
in autoanalyzer profiles, 202, 204, 206, 208
Serum indirect bilirubin, 15
Serum lipids. *See* Lipids.
Serum proteins. *See* Proteins.
Serum transaminase level, 152, 158
Serum-free thyroxine test, 80
Sex chromatin analysis, 100
Sex chromatin test, 94
Sex chromosomal abnormalities, 100
Shiotz tonometer, 298
Shorr trichrome technique, 81
Shunt, venous-to-arterial, 133, 140
Sickle cell anemia, 15, 223
Signet ring stage, 285
Silicosis, 47
Skin, microorganisms of, 287
Skin tests, 291–292, 298
tables on, 279–283
SMA 12/60 analyzer, 200–209
Smallpox, 281
Smear(s). blood, in office laboratory, 293–294
cultures and, in diagnosis, 278–289
tables on, 279–283
differential and peripheral, 238
Papanicolaou, 199
vaginal, 81, 297
Smogyi-Nelson method, 58
Sodium, as blood electrolyte, 35, 37
in aldosteronism, 51
in congestive heart failure, 42
Sodium bicarbonate, blood, 37, 56
Sodium chloride, in adrenal cortical insufficiency, 49
Sodium phytate, 33
Specimens, appearance of, 193–194
bleeding due to trauma in obtaining, 194
collection of, in infectious diseases, 278–284
obtaining, of body fluid, 190–191
for serologic tests, 290
Spherocytosis, hereditary, 15
Sphincter of Oddi, 170–171
Sphingomyelins, 101
Spinal cord tumor, 193
Spinal fluid, bilirubin in, 199
glucose and proteins in, 198
Spinal fluid pressure, 191
Spinal tap, 297
Spine, disorders of, 137
Spirochaeta, 285
Spirochetes, 280
Spirostat, 298
Spleen, enlarged, 222, 232, 233
Splenomegaly, chronic congestive, 233
tests in, 315–316
Spondylitis, ankylosing, 137
Sporotrichosis, 282
Sprue, 183
Sputum, bloody, 194
casts in, 196
crystals in, 197
microorganisms in, 287
pH of, 192
purulent, 195–196
specimen of, 199, 278, 284
appearance of, 193
obtaining, 190

Sputum (*Cont.*)
volume of, 191
Stages, in coagulation, 258–259, 264–268
Stains, 284, 285
Gram, 296
Staphylococci, 284, 288
Starvation. *See also* Malnutrition and related conditions
early, lipids in, 105
electrolytes in, 40
nonprotein nitrogen substances in, 121
plasma proteins in, 145
Steatorrhea. *See* Idiopathic steatorrhea.
Stein-Leventhal syndrome, 93, 95
Stercobilinogen, stool, 222, 223
Stercobilins, 14
Sternberg-Reed cells, 245
Sternheimer-Malbin stain, 195, 295, 296
Steroid hormone synthesis, 102
Steroids. *See* 17-Hydroxycorticosteroids; 17-Ketosteroids.
Stomach, carcinoma of, 299
Stones. *See also* calculi.
bilirubin, 15
in obstruction of common duct, 10
gallstones, 20
Stool(s). *See also* feces.
bacilli in, 289
"cathartic," 190
color of, 193
disaccharides in, 198
examination for trypsin in, 199
fat content of, 26
microorganisms in, 287
protein in, 197
radioactivity in, 194
specimens of, 190, 284
stercobilinogen in, 222, 223
tests on, 212, 296
Stool urobilinogen. *See* Urobilinogen.
Storage, in metabolism, and disorders of, blood electrolytes, 35
blood glucose, 58
hormones, 77
leukocytes, 237
lipids, 102, 110
nonprotein nitrogen substances, 126
plasma proteins, 143
red cells, 211
serum calcium, 21
uric acid, 163
Streptococcal infections, rheumatic fever and, 290–291
Streptococci, 284, 289
hemolytic, 288
Strongyloidiasis, 283
Strontium-85, radioactive, 189
Subacute bacterial endocarditis, 280, 288
tests in management of, 302
Subarachnoid block, 191
Subarachnoid hemorrhage, 193
tests in management of, 302
Succinate, 175
Sugar. *See also* Glucose.
blood, 69, 202
urine, 59
Sweat, electrolytes in, 36
Sweating, excessive, 45
Symptoms, laboratory work-up of, 307–318
Syncope, 316
Synovial fluids, bloody, 195
clotting of, 193
crystals in, 197
pus in, 196
specimens of, 190–191, 194, 284
volume of, 191–192
Synovianalysis, 297
Syphilis, 280, 290, 302

T_3 by radioimmunoassay, 80
T_3-uptake test, 79
T_4 by column test, 79, 80
T_4 isotope test, 186
Tabes dorsalis, 198
Tachyalimentation hypoglycemia, 62
Tachycardia, tests for, 316
Tapeworm infections, 302
Tay-Sachs disease, 110
Technetium-99m colloid, 188
Technetium-99m macroaggregated albumin, 189
Technetium-99m pertechnetate, 188
Technetium-99m polyphosphate, 189
Telangiectasia, hereditary hemorrhagic, 271
Testicles, embryonal tumors of, 99
hormone disorders and, 81
Testosterone, 76, 77, 79, 81, 86
Tests. *See also* Specific Tests.
autoanalyzer for, 200–209
for hemostasis disorders, 259
table on, 260
laboratory, disorders requiring, 299–302
laboratory work-up and,
of diseases, 319–329
of symptoms, 307–318
nonspecific, of organ involvement, 330–332
renal function, 180–182
serologic, 290–291
simple slide, immunological, 297
skin, 291–292
Tetanus, 280
Tetrapyrrole, bilirubin, 13
Thalassemia major, red cells in, 224
Therapeutic trials, 212
Thoracic pain, 316–317
Thorn test, 247
Throat cultures, 296
Thrombasthenia, hereditary hemorrhagic, 263
Thrombin, delayed formation of, 273
Thrombin time, in hemostasis disorders, 268, 273, 277
test of, 259–260
Thrombocytopenia, in hemostasis disorders, 272, 274, 275, 277
in leukocyte disorders, 240, 244, 246, 249
in red cell disorders, 214–216, 231, 233
platelets in, 262
Thrombocytosis, 277
Thrombophlebitis, tests in management of, 302
Thromboplastin, 258–260
Thromboplastin regeneration test, 264
Thromboplastin time, in hemostasis disorders, 265–268, 273, 275
partial, 264
Thromboplastin time test, partial, 259
Thrombopoietin, 258
Thymol turbidity, plasma proteins and, 144, 147
positive, 16, 17
Thyro-binding protein, 79, 80, 186
Thyroglobulin, 77
Thyroid, glucose and, 58
hormones of, 76–77
disorders of, 79–80, 87–89
radioactive isotopes in disorders of, 186
toxic adenomas of, 87
Thyroid-stimulating hormone, 76, 84, 87
test of, 81
Thyroiditis, 88, 89
Thyrotropin releasing hormone, 76
Thyroxine, 76–77, 79
by isotope test, 80
free, index, 80
in thyroid disorders, 87, 88
lipids and, 103
radioactive, 186
serum free, test, 80
Thyroxine-binding proteins, 77, 97
Thyroxine test, serum-free, 80
Tissues, body, microorganisms in, 287–288
collagen, 276
connective, abnormality of, 276
ganglionic, extra-adrenal, 171
hypertrophied, 148
Tissue integrity, and bleeding, 257
Titers, serologic, 290–291
Titmus vision tester, 298
Tolbutamide tolerance test, 74
Tonicity, of body fluids, 36
Torulosis, 282
Tourniquet test, of coagulation, 259
Toxemia of pregnancy, uric acid in, 168
Toxic substances, in blood and urine, 178–179
Toxicity, salicylate, 48
Toxin-producing organisms, 288
Toxoplasmosis, 283
Trachoma, 282
Transaminase level, serum, 152
Transaminases, 152
disorders of, 157–161
normal metabolism of, 155
Transcortin, 77
Transferrin, 173, 174
Transfusion reactions, between mother and child, 230
hemolytic, red cells in, 226–229
Transport system, in respiration, 130
Transudates, specific gravity of, 193
Traumatic tap, 193
Treponema pallidum, 285
Treponema pallidum immobilization test, 290
Trichinosis, 255, 283
Trichomonas vaginalis, 285–286
Trichomoniasis, 283

Trichuriasis, 283
Triglycerides, 101–103
in serum lipid disorders, 105, 108, 112–115, 117, 118
Triidothyronine, 77, 79, 80
radioactive (T_3), 186
Triolein uptake, radioactive, 183
Trophic hormones, 77, 79, 85
Trophozoite, 285
Tropical sprue, 146
Tryosine, 175
Trypanosomiasis, African, 283
Trypsin, in stool, 199, 296
Tubes, for obtaining specimens, 190, 293, 297
Tubules, renal, casts from, 196
in adrenal cortical insufficiency, 49
in diabetes insipidus, 50
in renal glycosuria, 66
in serum calcium disorders, 21–23, 32, 33
acidosis, 31
in urine formation, 180
Tubular acidosis, renal, 53, 54
Tubercle bacilli, 284, 285, 288, 289
Tuberculosis, diagnosis of, 280
miliary, 138
mononuclear cells in, 196
skin test for, 292
sputum specimen in, 190
tests in management of, 302
Tularemia, 280, 289, 292
Tumors, carcinoid malignant, 173
from adrenal medulla, 171
giant-cell, 8
metastatic bone, 5
scanning in diagnosis of, 186, 188
spinal cord, 193
Turner's syndrome, 94
Typhoid fever, 280, 289, 291
Typhus fever, 281
Typing, blood, 226
Tyramine, test using, 171
Tyrosinase, 175

Ulcer, duodenal, lipase and amylase in, 171
gastric, bleeding, urea nitrogen in, 122
peptic, bleeding, 219, 220
gastric analysis in, 192
tests in management of, 301
Ulcerative colitis, serum magnesium in, 174
Ultracentrifugation, 144
Undulant fever, 279, 280
Unimeter, 295
Universal culture media, 286
"Universal donor," 226, 229
Urea, as nonprotein nitrogenous substance, 119
in glomerular filtration, 181
in hypovolemic shock, 125
Urea clearance, standard, 181
Urea nitrogen. *See* Nitrogen, urea.
Urethral cultures, 297
Urethral discharge, microorganisms in, 287
Uric acid, autoanalyzer profile and, 204, 206, 208
blood and urine, 167–169
serum, 163–169
"Uric acid pool," 163, 165
Uricosuric agents, 169
Uricultu, 296
Uridyldiphosphogalactose transferase, absence of, 63
Urinalysis, in office laboratory, 295–296
Urinary catecholamines, 72, 171–172
Urinary gonadotropins, 24-hour, 81, 86, 94, 96, 99, 100
Urinary steroids. *See* 17-Hydroxycorticosteroids; 17-Ketosteroids.
Urine, amino acids in, 198
bilirubin in. *See* Bilirubin.
biochemical alterations in, some, 198
blood glucose disorders and, 63, 67–72
bloody, diagnosing, 194
calcium in. *See* Calcium.
casts in, 196
crystals in, 196
cultures, 296
electrolytes and, 36
formation of, 180
glucose in, 198
microorganisms in, 287
mycobacteria in, 288
organisms in, 289
pH of, 192
protein in, 197
specific gravity of, 180, 182, 192–193, 295
specimen of, 190, 193–194, 284
sugar in. *See* Sugar.
suprapubic aspiration of, 190
toxic substances in, 177–178
urobilinogen in, 14–16
See also Urobilinogens.
volume of, 191
white blood cells in, 195
Urobilinogens, 14
stool and urine, 15–20
Urogenital tree, obstruction of, 127
Uropathy, obstructive, 127
Uroporphyrin, 175, 177
UTI-tect, 296

Vaginal cultures, 297
Vaginal discharge, blood in, 195
microorganisms in, 287
pH of, 192
pus in, 196
specimen of, 190, 193
volume of, 191
Vaginal smear, 81, 297
Valsalva maneuver, 191
Vanillyl mandelic acid, 171, 172
Varicella, 282
Vascular diseases, proteinuria in, 197
Vascular resistance to bleeding, 257
disorders in, 269–272
Ventilatory function, 132
Venules, 271
Venous pressure, 191, 298
Vertigo, 317
Viral infections, acute, leukocytes in, 250
Viral isolation, specimens for, 278
Viruses, Barr-Epstein, 253
in diagnosis of infectious diseases, 289
table on, 281–282
Visceral larva migrans, 283
Vision testing, 298
Visual test, for lipoproteinemia, 295
Vital capacity, and timed vital capacity, 132
in blood oxygen content disorders, 135–138, 141, 142
Vitalor, 297–298
Vitamin(s), B_{12}, 183, 215
C, 272
D, 9, 21, 24, 25
K, 18, 259, 265–267
red cell production and, 210
Vomiting, 317–318
Vomitus, coffee-ground, 194
von Gierke's disease, 65, 111
von Willebrand's disease, 269

Waldenström's macroglobulinemia, 246
Wassermann test, 290
Water. *See also* Body Fluids; Fluids.
acute renal failure and, 46
body, in congestive heart failure, 42
in diabetic acidosis, 56
in diabetes insipidus, 50
in diarrhea, 44
intracellular, 35
in dehydration, 39
in malabsorption syndrome, 41
Water-insoluble compounds, rendering water-soluble, 13
Water-load test, for aldosterone secretion, 81
Weight loss, 318
Weil's disease, 280
West Nile fever, 282
Whipple's disease, 146
White Blood Cells(s). *See also* Leukocytes.
in body fluids, 195–196
in leukemia, 166
White blood cell count, 212
in infants and children, 239
in leukocyte disorders, 241, 242, 252, 254–256
in office laboratory, 293
in red cell disorders, 226
Whooping cough, 280
Wilson's disease, 169, 172
Worms, pin, Scotch tape test for, 296
Wright's stain, 196, 223, 231

Xanthoma disseminatum, 110
Xenon, radioactive, 189
d-xylose absorption test, 61

Yellow fever, 282

Zollinger-Ellison syndrome, 191, 192
Zwitterion effect, 144